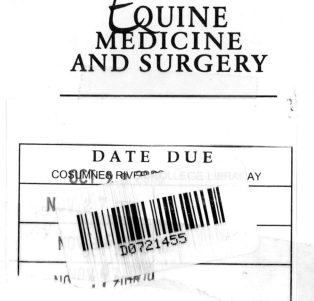

EQUINE
MEDICINE
AND SURGERY

MANUAL OF

EQUINE MEDICINE AND SURGERY

Prepared by
CHRISTINE KING, BVSc, MACVSc, MvetClinStud
Veterinary Editor

with
MARGARET E. McCANN, DVM, PhD
Merck and Company, Rahway, New Jersey

PATRICK T. COLAHAN, DVM, Dipl ACVS
College of Veterinary Medicine
University of Florida, Gainesville, Florida

ALFRED M. MERRITT, DVM, MS
College of Veterinary Medicine
University of Florida, Gainesville, Florida

JAMES N. MOORE, DVM, PhD, Dipl ACVS
College of Veterinary Medicine
University of Georgia, Athens, Georgia

IAN G. (JOE) MAYHEW, BVSc, PhD, FRCVS, Dipl ACVIM, ECVN
Royal (Dick) School of Veterinary Studies
University of Edinburgh, Easter Bush, Roslin, Midlothian, Scotland

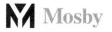 Mosby

St. Louis Baltimore Boston Carlsbad Chicago Minneapolis New York Philadelphia Portland
London Milan Sydney Tokyo Toronto

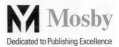

Dedicated to Publishing Excellence

Editor-in-Chief: John A. Schrefer
Executive Editor: Linda L. Duncan
Senior Developmental Editor: Teri Merchant
Project Manager: Mark Spann
Senior Production Editor: Beth Hayes
Design Manager: Gail Morey Hudson
Manufacturing Manager: Debbie LaRocca
Cover Design: Teresa Breckwoldt

Composition by Accu-color
Printing/binding by R.R. Donnelley & Sons Company

Mosby, Inc.
11830 Westline Industrial Drive
St. Louis, Missouri 64146

Library of Congress Cataloging in Publication Data

Manual of equine medicine and surgery / prepared by Christine King . . .[et al.].
    p. cm.
    Includes index.
    ISBN 0-8151-1741-8
        1. Horses–Diseases–Handbooks, manuals. etc.
        2. Horses–Surgery–Handbooks, manuals, etc.
        I. King, Christine. 1962–   .
SF951.M36 1999   98-35658
636.1'089–dc21   CIP

98 99 00 01 02 / 9 8 7 6 5 4 3 2 1

Contributors

Stephen B. Adams, DVM, MS, Dipl ACVS
Purdue University,
West Lafayette, Indiana

Dorothy M. Ainsworth, DVM, PhD, Dipl ACVIM
Cornell University, Ithaca, New York

Atwood C. Asbury, DVM, ACT
University of Florida,
Gainesville, Florida

Dr. Joerg A. Auer, Prof. Dr.Med.Vet., Dipl ACVS/ECVS
University of Zürich,
Zürich, Switzerland

A. N. Baird, DVM, MS, Dipl ACVS
University of Pennsylvania, Kennett
Square, Pennsylvania

Spencer M. Barber, DVM, Dipl ACVS
University of Saskatchewan
Saskatoon, Saskatchewan, Canada

Joy L. Barbet, DVM, Dipl ACVD
University of Florida,
Gainesville, Florida

Michelle Henry Barton, DVM, PhD
University of Georgia, Athens, Georgia

Gary M. Baxter, VMD, MS, Dipl ACVS
Colorado State University,
Fort Collins, Colorado

Ralph E. Beadle, DVM, PhD
Louisiana State University,
Baton Rouge, Louisiana

Jill Beech, VMD, Dipl ACVIM
University of Pennsylvania,
Kennett Square, Pennsylvania

William V. Bernard, DVM, Dipl ACVIM
Rood and Riddle Equine Hospital
Lexington, Kentucky

Clifford R. Berry, DVM, Dipl ACVR
University of Missouri,
Columbia, Missouri

Joseph J. Bertone, DVM, MS, Dipl ACVIM
Idaho Equine Hospital, Nampa, Idaho

Diane E. Bevier, DVM, Dipl ACVD
Heska Corporation,
Fort Collins, Colorado

John C. Bloom, DVM, PhD
Eli Lilly & Co., Indianapolis, Indiana

Lawrence R. Bramlage, DVM, MS, Dipl ACVS
Rood and Riddle Equine Hospital
Lexington, Kentucky

Corrie Brown, DVM, PhD, Dipl ACVP
University of Georgia, Athens, Georgia

Claus D. Buergelt, DVM, PhD, Dipl ACVP
University of Florida,
Gainesville, Florida

Martha Campbell-Thompson, DVM, PhD, Dipl ACVS
University of Florida,
Gainesville, Florida

John P. Caron, DVM, MVSc, Dipl ACVS
Michigan State University,
East Lansing, Michigan

G. Kent Carter, DVM, MS, Dipl ACVIM
Texas A&M University,
College Station, Texas

Noah D. Cohen, VMD, MPH, PhD, Dipl ACVIM
Texas A&M University,
College Station, Texas

Patrick T. Colahan, DVM, Dipl ACVS
College of Veterinary Medicine
University of Florida,
Gainesville, Florida

Chrysann Collatos, VMD, PhD, Dipl ACVIM
High Desert Veterinary Service,
Reno, Nevada

Frederick J. Derksen, DVM, PhD, Dipl ACVIM
Michigan State University,
Lansing, Michigan

Thomas J. Divers, DVM, Dipl ACVIM, ACVECC
Cornell University, Ithaca, New York

Howard Dobson, BVM&S, DVSc, Cert EO, Dipl ACVR
University of Guelph,
Guelph, Ontario, Canada

Sue J. Dyson, MA, VetMB, PhD, FRCVS
Animal Health Trust,
Newmarket, Suffolk, England

Susan Clark Eades, DVM, PhD, Dipl ACVIM
Louisiana State University,
Baton Rouge, Louisiana

J. Lane Easter, DVM
Texas A&M University,
College Station, Texas

Lucy M. Edens, DVM, MS, Dipl ACVIM
Encinitas, California

Ryland B. Edwards III, DVM, MS, Dipl ACVS
University of Wisconsin,
Madison, Wisconsin

Charles S. Farrow, DVM, Dr Med Vet, Dipl ACVR
University of Saskatchewan
Saskatoon, Saskatchewan, Canada

David T. Galligan, VMD, MBA
University of Pennsylvania, Kennett
Square, Pennsylvania

Sherril L. Green, DVM, PhD, Dipl ACVIM
Stanford University,
Stanford, California

Eleanor M. Green, DVM, Dipl ACVIM, ABVP
University of Florida,
Gainesville, Florida

Brent A. Hague, DVM, Dipl ACVS
Goldsby, Oklahoma

Caroline N. Hahn, DVM, MSc, MRCVS
University of Edinburgh
Easter Bush, Roslin, Midlothian,
United Kingdom

R. Reid Hanson, DVM, Dipl ACVS
Auburn University, Auburn, Alabama

Dan L. Hawkins, DVM, MS, Dipl ACVS
University of Florida,
Gainesville, Florida

William P. Hay, DVM, Dipl ACVS
University Of Georgia, Athens, Georgia

David R. Hodgson, BVSc(Hons), PhD, FACSM, FACBS, Dipl ACVIM
University of Sydney,
New South Wales, Australia

Clifford M. Honnas, DVM, Dipl ACVS
Texas A&M University,
College Station, Texas

Leo B. Jeffcott, MA, BVetMed, PhD, FRCVS, DVSc
University of Cambridge,
Cambridge, United Kingdom

Ian B. Johnstone, DVM, MSc, PhD
University of Guelph,
Guelph, Ontario, Canada

Carl A. Kirker-Head, MRCVS, Dipl ACVS
Tufts University,
North Grafton, Massachusetts

Thomas R. Klei, PhD
Louisiana State University,
Baton Rouge, Louisiana

Catherine W. Kohn, VMD
The Ohio State University,
Columbus, Ohio

Anne M. Koterba, DVM, PhD, Dipl ACVIM
University of Florida,
Gainesville, Florida

Ann E. Kraus-Hansen, DVM, Dipl ACVS
Pacific Equine Clinic,
Monroe, Washington

Thomas J. Lane, DVM
University of Florida,
Gainesville, Florida

Kenneth S. Latimer, DVM, PhD, Dipl ACVP
University of Georgia, Athens, Georgia

Douglas H. Leach , MSc, PhD
Lexington, Kentucky

Michelle M. LeBlanc, DVM, Dipl ACT
University of Florida,
Gainesville, Florida

Guy D. Lester, BVMS, PhD, Dipl ACVIM
University of Florida,
Gainesville, Florida

Dawn B. Logas, DVM
Veterinary Dermatology Center
Winter Park, Florida

Michael Q. Lowder, DVM, MS
University of Georgia, Athens, Georgia

D. Paul Lunn, BVSc, MS, PhD, MRCVS, Dipl ACVIM
University of Wisconsin,
Madison, Wisconsin

Robert J. MacKay, BVSc, PhD, Dipl ACVIM
University of Florida,
Gainesville, Florida

Edward A. Mahaffey, DVM, PhD, Dipl ACVP
University of Georgia, Athens, Georgia

Tim Mair, BVSc, PhD, MRCVS
Bell Equine Veterinary Clinic
Mereworth, Maidstone
Kent, England, United Kingdom

Richard A. Mansmann, DVM, PhD
Chapel Hill, North Carolina

Mark D. Markel, DVM, PhD, Dipl ACVS
University of Wisconsin,
Madison, Wisconsin

M.D. Marsden, BSc, PhD
Easter Bush Veterinary Centre
Roslin, Midlothian, Scotland

I.G. (Joe) Mayhew, BVSc, PhD, MRCVS, Dip ACVIM
Royal (Dick) School of
Veterinary Studies
University of Edinburgh, Easter Bush,
Roslin, Midlothian, Scotland

J. Trenton McClure, DVM, MS, Dipl ACVIM
University of Prince Edward Island
Charlottetown, Prince Edward
Island, Canada

Angus O. McKinnon, BVSc, Msc, Dipl ACT, ABPV
Goldburn Valley Equine Hospital
Shepperton, Victoria, Australia

Alfred M. Merritt, DVM, MS
University of Florida,
Gainesville, Florida

Elspeth Milne, BVM&S, PhD, MRCVS
Scottish Agricultural College
Veterinary Services
Dumfries, Scotland

Tony Douglas Mogg, BVSc(Hons), PhD, FACVSc, Dipl ACVIM, ACVCP
IVABS Massey University
Palmerston North, New Zealand

James N. Moore, DVM, PhD, Dipl ACVS
University of Georgia, Athens, Georgia

Rustin M. Moore, DVM, PhD, Dipl ACVS
Louisiana State University,
Baton Rouge, Louisiana

Debra Deem Morris, DVM, MS, Dipl ACVIM
North Jersey Animal Hospital,
Wayne, New Jersey

William A. Moyer, DVM
Texas A&M University,
College Station, Texas

P.O. Eric Mueller, DVM, PhD, Dipl ACVS
University of Georgia, Athens, Georgia

Gillian D. Muir, DVM, PhD
University of Saskatchewan
Saskatoon, Saskatchewan, Canada

Lisa Neuwirth, DVM, MS, Dipl ACVR
University of Georgia, Athens, Georgia

Alan J. Nixon, BVSc, MS, Dipl ACVS
Cornell University, Ithaca, New York

David Nunamaker, VMD, Dipl ACVS
University of Pennsylvania , Kennett
Square, Pennsylvania

Richard Panzer, DVM, MS
American Institute of Traditional
Chinese Veterinary Medicine
Seattle, Washington

Mary Rose Paradis, DVM, MS, Dipl ACVIM
Tufts University,
North Grafton, Massachusetts

Andrew H. Parks, VetMB, Dipl ACVS
University of Georgia, Athens, Georgia

Peter Pascoe, BVSc, DVA, Dipl ACVA, ECVA
University of California,
Davis, California

Lance E. Perryman, DVM, PhD, Dipl ACVP
North Carolina State University,
Raleigh, North Carolina

Peter Physick-Sheard, BVSc, Msc, MRCVS
University of Guelph,
Guelph, Ontario, Canada

Christopher C. Pollitt, BVSc, PhD
University of Queensland, Brisbane,
Queensland, Australia

Mimi Porter, MA, ATC
Equine Therapy, Inc,
Lexington, Kentucky

Gary D. Potter, PhD, PAS
Texas A&M University,
College Station, Texas

Patricia J. Provost, VMD, MS, Dipl ACVS
Tufts University,
North Grafton, Massachusetts

Norman W. Rantanen, DVM, MS, Dipl ACVR
Fallbrook, California

William C. Rebhun, DVM, Dip ACVIM, ACVO
Cornell University, Ithaca, New York

Virginia Reef , DVM, Dipl ACVIM
University of Pennsylvania,
Kennett Square, Pennsylvania

Johanna M. Reimer, VMD, Dipl ACVIM
Rood and Riddle Equine Hospital
Lexington, Kentucky

Dean W. Richardson, DVM, Dipl ACVS
University of Pennsylvania,
Kennett Square, Pennsylvania

N. Edward Robinson, BVet Med, PhD, MRCVS
Michigan State University,
East Lansing, Michigan

Reuben J. Rose, DVSc, PhD, Dipl Vet An, FRCVS, MACVSc
University of Sydney, New South
Wales, Australia

Michael W. Ross, DVM, Dipl ACVS
University of Pennsylvania, Kennett
Square, Pennsylvania

L. Chris Sanchez, DVM
University of Florida,
Gainesville, Florida

Catherine J. Savage, BVSc, MS, PhD, Dipl ACVIM
Colorado State University,
Fort Collins, Colorado

Michael C. Schramme, DrMedVet, CertEO, MRCVS, Dipl ECVS
University of London
Hertfordshire, England,
United Kingdom

James Schumacher, DVM, MS Dipl ACVS
Auburn University, Auburn, Alabama

Debra C. Sellon, DVM, PhD, Dipl ACVIM
Washington State University,
Pullman, Washington

Susan D. Semrad, VMD, PhD, Dipl ACVIM
University of Wisconsin,
Madison, Wisconsin

Roger K.W. Smith, MA, PhD, VetMB, CertEO, MRCVS
Royal Veterinary College
Hertfordshire, England,
United Kingdom

Janice E. Sojka, VMD, MS, Dipl ACVIM
Purdue University,
West Lafayette, Indiana

Louise L. Southwood, BVSc, BSc(Vet), MS
Colorado State University,
Fort Collins, Colorado

Theodore E. Specht, DVM, Dipl ACVS
Ocala, Florida

Edward L. Squires, PhD
Colorado State University,
Fort Collins, Colorado

John A. Stick, DVM, Dipl ACVS
Michigan State University,
East Lansing, Michigan

Kenneth E. Sullins, DVM, MS, Dipl ACVS
Virginia-Maryland Regional
College of Veterinary Medicine
Leesburg, Virginia

Farol N. Tomson, DVM, Dipl ACLAM
University of Florida,
Gainesville, Florida

Josie L. Traub-Dargatz, DVM, MS, Dipl
ACVIM
Colorado State University,
Fort Collins, Colorado

Cynthia M. Trim, BVSc, MRCVS, Dipl Vet
An, Dipl ACVA
University of Georgia, Athens, Georgia

Russell L. Tucker, DVM, Dipl ACVR
Washington State University,
Pullman, Washington

Eric P. Tulleners, DVM, Dipl ACVS
University of Pennsylvania,
Kennett Square, Pennsylvania

Tracy A. Turner, DVM, MS, Dipl ACVS
University of Minnesota,
St. Paul, Minnesota

Dickson D. Varner, DVM, MS, Dipl ACT
Texas A&M University,
College Station, Texas

Jeffrey P. Watkins, DVM, MS, Dipl ACVS
Texas A&M University,
College Station, Texas

Barbara J. Watrous, DVM, Dipl ACVR
Oregon State University,
Corvallis, Oregon

Peter M. Webbon, BVet Med, DVR, PhD,
MRCVS
The Jockey Club, London,
England, United Kingdom

Barbara B. Welsch, DVM, PhD, Dipl
ACVIM, ACVECC
University of Florida,
Gainesville, Florida

Robert D. Welch, DVM, Dipl ACVS
Scottish Rite Hospital, Dallas, Texas

Nathaniel A. White, DVM, MS, Dipl ACVS
Virginia-Maryland Regional
College of Veterinary Medicine
Leesburg, Virginia

R. David Whitley, DVM, MS, Dipl ACVO
Auburn University, Auburn, Alabama

Michael J. Wildenstein, AFA, CJF
Cornell University, Ithaca, New York

David G. Wilson, DVM, Dipl ACVS
University of Wisconsin,
Madison, Wisconsin

J. Dick Wright, MVSc, MVetClinStud,
FACVSc
University of Queensland,
Brisbane, Queensland, Australia

Ellen L. Ziemer, DVM, MS, PhD, Dipl
ACVIM, ACVP
Burlington, North Carolina

Preface

Manual of Equine Medicine and Surgery is designed as a handy, current reference for use by veterinarians, veterinary students, veterinary technicians, and other clinic staff. The goal of this manual is to provide readers with fast, helpful information on assessment, diagnosis, and treatment of the most common problems encountered in horses. In no way is it an exhaustive work; it is best used in conjunction with the fifth edition of *Equine Medicine and Surgery,* in which the reader will find more detailed discussions of relevant anatomy and physiology, pathophysiology, diagnostic testing, procedures, and underlying rationales for treatment options, as well as hundreds of supporting illustrations and extensive reference lists. Helpful page cross-references to the parent text have been provided throughout the manual to direct readers to more detailed information.

KEY FEATURES

◆ Focus on key information related to assessment, diagnosis, and treatment of common medical conditions in horses
◆ Organized by body system, with important sections on diagnostic approaches, critical care, neonatal care, and chemical restraint and anesthesia
◆ Convenient outline format

Manual of Equine Medicine and Surgery is your indispensable clinical quick reference!

Contents

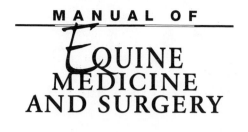

MANUAL OF

EQUINE
MEDICINE
AND SURGERY

1

Clinical Syndromes: Diagnostic Approaches to Common Presenting Complaints

The following are lists of conditions to consider when presented with a particular clinical problem, and diagnostic tools that may be helpful in establishing a diagnosis. Each item is discussed in the manual; consult the index. More complete discussions of the diagnostic approach to these problems are given in Chapter 1 of *Equine Medicine and Surgery*, edition V.

These lists are not intended to be comprehensive; rather, they are presented to remind the practitioner of the probable differential diagnoses or structures involved and the diagnostic approaches that are most likely to be useful in investigating the problem. As much as possible, the conditions are ranked, with the most likely conditions listed first. The practitioner should also consider physical examination findings and the horse's breed, activity, gender, and age, along with geographic location and other historical information, when deciding which conditions are most likely in a particular instance.

ABDOMINAL DISTENTION
Possible Causes
Adults
- pregnancy
- obesity

- poor-quality roughage diet ("hay belly")
- large intestinal obstruction (rapid distention)
- large colon displacement
- large or small colon impaction, foreign body, or fecolith
- large colon volvulus
- severe malnutrition or parasitism (relative distention)
- ileus
- peritonitis
- abdominal neoplasia (e.g., lymphosarcoma, mesothelioma)
- hemoperitoneum (see discussion of bleeding)

Foals
- meconium impaction
- small intestinal obstruction (e.g., intussusception, volvulus)
- ruptured bladder
- dietary intolerance
- enterocolitis
- colonic atresia or other congenital abnormality (e.g., myoenteric aganglionosis)
- gastric distention associated with an indwelling nasogastric tube

Diagnostic Approaches to Consider
- physical examination, including thorough abdominal auscultation ($\pm$ percussion)
- passage of a nasogastric tube and siphonage

- evaluation of the diet
- rectal palpation (adult horses); digital rectal examination in foals
- CBC and serum biochemistry panel
- abdominocentesis with fluid analysis and cytology (± culture)
  - peritoneal fluid electrolyte concentrations and peritoneal fluid:serum creatinine ratio in foals with suspected uroperitoneum
- ultrasonography
- radiography (foals)
- exploratory celiotomy

ABORTION
Possible Causes
- twinning
- placental insufficiency
- placentitis (bacterial or fungal)
- endotoxemia (e.g., colic, pleuropneumonia)
- equine herpesvirus 1 (EHV-1) infection
- equine viral arteritis (EVA)
- leptospirosis
- *Ehrlichia risticii* infection
- toxic plants and drugs
- hyperlipemia

Diagnostic Approaches to Consider
- physical examination of the mare
- thorough examination of the fetus and placenta (if available)
- necropsy of the fetus
- submission of placental and fetal tissue samples for histopathologic examination, culture, and virus isolation
- uterine swabbing and culture
- serologic evaluation for EHV-1, EVA, and leptospirosis

BACK PROBLEMS
Possible Causes
- the saddle and/or rider
- muscle spasms from lack of fitness or inability to perform the work demanded
- hind limb lameness (e.g., bone spavin)
- sacroiliac pain
- lumbar and lumbosacral arthrosis
- fractured dorsal spinous processes (especially at the withers)
- caudal cervical osteoarthropathy
- impinging or overriding dorsal spinous processes (may not cause back pain)
- exertional rhabdomyolysis

- pleuritis
- temperament or training problems (i.e., bad behavior manifested as back pain)

Diagnostic Approaches to Consider
- physical examination, including thorough palpation of the neck and back
- evaluation of saddle fit
- evaluation for hind limb lameness
- serum biochemistry panel, including measurement of CK and AST before and after exercise
- radiography
- nuclear scintigraphy (to distinguish soft tissue from skeletal problems)
- ultrasonography

BEHAVIORAL ABNORMALITIES
Possible Causes
- neonatal maladjustment syndrome (newborn foals)
- pain (mouth, neck, back, limbs)
- temperament or training problems
- vision deficit
- centrally acting drugs (e.g., intravascular procaine, tranquilizers)
- stereotypies ("vices")
- forebrain disease
  - viral encephalitis
  - leukoencephalomalacia
  - brain abscess
- epilepsy
- narcolepsy
- hepatoencephalopathy
- rabies

Diagnostic Approaches to Consider
- physical examination, including examination of the oral cavity
- evaluation for neck or back pain and lameness
- ophthalmologic examination
- neurologic examination
- CBC and serum biochemistry panel
- CSF collection for fluid analysis and cytology, ± culture or serology
- euthanasia and postmortem examination (especially in suspected rabies cases)

BLEEDING
Possible Causes
Generalized or any site
- wounds
- coagulopathy

- DIC
- drugs (e.g., heparin, warfarin-NSAID interaction)
- liver failure
- severe vasculitis

Head

- trauma to nasal mucosa or turbinates during nasogastric intubation
- mandibular fracture or other oral trauma
- external trauma to the facial bones (epistaxis) or cranium (bleeding from the ear)
- ethmoid hematoma
- guttural pouch mycosis
- granuloma or neoplasia of the nasal cavity
- exercise-induced pulmonary hemorrhage

Abdominal or pleural cavity (no external hemorrhage)

- ruptured uterine artery in periparturient mares
- ruptured spleen
- lacerated iliac artery from pelvic fracture
- ruptured aorta
- pulmonary laceration from rib fracture
- thoracic or abdominal neoplasia

Anus

- iatrogenic trauma (e.g., rectal tear during rectal palpation)
- colonic ulceration (e.g., NSAID toxicity, enterolith)
- coagulopathy

Vagina, penis, or prepuce

- parturition
- vaginal laceration during breeding
- varicose veins in the vaginal wall
- urolithiasis
- NSAID toxicity
- neoplasia
- cutaneous habronemiasis
- penile laceration during breeding or from trauma

Diagnostic Approaches to Consider

- Physical examination and, depending on the suspected site of origin:
- CBC, serum biochemistry panel, and coagulation profile
- endoscopy
- radiography
- ultrasonography
- abdominocentesis
- thoracocentesis
- urinalysis
- rectal examination

BLINDNESS

Possible Causes

- lesions of the cornea, anterior chamber, or lens (trauma, inflammation, cataract)
- retinal detachment
- optic nerve (cranial nerve II) trauma
- thalamic lesions
- forebrain lesions
  - cranial trauma
  - space-occupying lesion (e.g., abscess, tumor)
  - toxins (e.g., moldy corn)
- intracarotid injection
- hepatoencephalopathy
- neonatal maladjustment syndrome

Diagnostic Approaches to Consider

- physical examination
- ophthalmologic examination, with topical and perineural blockade as necessary
- fluorescein staining of the cornea
- neurologic examination, paying particular attention to cranial nerve function
- serum biochemistry panel, including serum ammonia and bile acid concentrations
- CSF collection and analysis

COLIC

Possible Causes

Mild-to-moderate abdominal pain in adults

- spasmodic colic
- colonic or cecal impaction
- simple large colon displacements
- sand colic
- enterolith
- ulceration of the gastric mucosa or right dorsal colon (e.g., NSAID toxicity)
- proximal enteritis (signs range from depression to severe abdominal pain)
- colitis
- peritonitis
- impending parturition
- grass sickness

Severe abdominal pain in adults

- strangulating obstruction of the small intestine
  - volvulus
  - incarceration (e.g., epiploic foramen, mesenteric rent, hernia)
  - strangulating lipoma (older horses; may also affect the small colon)

+ large colon volvulus
+ proximal enteritis (may simply cause depression and mild discomfort)
+ verminous arteritis and enteric thrombosis
+ dystocia
+ uterine torsion

Abdominal pain in foals and young horses
+ meconium impaction
+ gastroduodenal ulceration
+ enterocolitis
+ intussusception
+ small intestinal volvulus
+ ascarid impaction
+ ruptured bladder (causing stranguria)

Diagnostic Approaches to Consider
+ physical examination, including thorough abdominal auscultation
+ dental examination
+ evaluation of the diet
+ rectal examination (adult horses); digital rectal examination in foals
+ nasogastric intubation (to identify and relieve gastric distention)
+ CBC and serum biochemistry (especially PCV and total plasma protein)
+ abdominocentesis with fluid analysis and cytology
+ suspension of a fecal sample in water to check for accumulation of sand and coarse fibrous material
+ gastroscopy
+ radiography (foals and some adults)
+ ultrasonography
+ exploratory celiotomy

COLLAPSE
Possible Causes
+ drugs
  + anaphylaxis
  + intracarotid injection
+ shock (hemorrhagic or hypovolemic)
+ exhaustion, heat stroke
+ hyperkalemic periodic paralysis (HPP)
+ hypocalcemic tetany
+ head trauma
+ epilepsy
+ narcolepsy
+ syncope
+ botulism
+ congenital cardiovascular disorders (foals)
+ electric shock (ground currents)

+ lightning strike
+ cardiac tamponade
+ parturition

Diagnostic Approaches to Consider
+ physical examination
+ neurologic examination
+ CBC and serum biochemistry panel
+ genetic testing for HPP
+ radiography of the skull
+ assays of feed samples for *Clostridium botulinum* organisms or toxins
+ electrocardiography
+ echocardiography

COUGH
Possible Causes
+ viral respiratory infection (e.g., influenza, EHV-1 or EHV-4)
+ dust, other respiratory tract irritants
+ chronic obstructive pulmonary disease (COPD)
+ pharyngeal irritation
  + foreign body
  + abscess (e.g., strangles)
  + pharyngeal lymphoid hyperplasia (coughing during exercise or while eating)
+ laryngeal dysfunction (coughing during exercise or while eating or drinking)
  + excessive arytenoid abduction after prosthetic laryngoplasty
  + arytenoid chondritis
  + epiglottic entrapment
+ tracheal irritation
+ esophageal obstruction (choke)
+ lungworm (horses and ponies only; donkeys, mules, and asses are asymptomatic)
+ pneumonia, pleuropneumonia
+ *Rhodococcus equi* infection (foals)

Diagnostic Approaches to Consider
+ physical examination, including thoracic percussion and auscultation with a rebreathing bag
+ CBC and serum biochemistry panel
+ virus isolation on samples of upper airway secretions/exudate or mucosal swab
+ endoscopic examination of the upper airway and trachea (esophagoscopy for choke)
+ transtracheal aspiration with cytology and culture

- bronchoalveolar lavage with cytology
- ultrasonography of the pleural space
- thoracic radiography (especially in foals)
- thoracocentesis (in cases of suspected pleuropneumonia)

DEPRESSION
Possible Causes
- systemic illness, fever
  - viral respiratory disease (e.g. influenza, EHV-1 or EHV-4)
  - pleuropneumonia ("shipping fever")
- endotoxemia
- hypovolemia
  - severe dehydration (e.g., heat exhaustion, colitis)
  - severe, acute blood loss
- anemia (e.g., severe blood loss)
- severe pain (fractures, septic arthritis, meningitis)
- viral encephalitis (EEE, WEE, VEE)
- forebrain disease
- brainstem disease
- hepatoencephalopathy
Foals
- neonatal maladjustment syndrome
- septicemia
- neonatal isoerythrolysis

Diagnostic Approaches to Consider
- physical examination
- neurologic examination
- CBC and serum biochemistry panel, with attention to liver-specific enzymes
- virus isolation on samples of nasal discharge or mucosal swabs
- ultrasonography and/or radiography to detect intrathoracic disease
- abdominocentesis
- CSF collection (for suspected CNS disease)
  - fluid analysis and cytology
  - EEE and WEE titers (serum or CSF)
- blood culture (for foals with suspected septicemia)

EATING DIFFICULTIES
Possible Causes
- esophageal obstruction (choke)
- oral lesions, including dental problems
- mandibular or maxillary disease (e.g., fracture, masseter myositis)

- pharyngeal foreign body or mass (e.g., strangles abscess)
- botulism
- hyoid fracture
- cranial nerve lesions (V, VII, IX, X, XII)
  - guttural pouch disease
  - equine protozoal myeloencephalitis (EPM)
  - yellow star thistle toxicity
- botulism
- rabies
- lead toxicity
- tetanus
- grass sickness
Foals
- neonatal maladjustment syndrome
- guttural pouch tympany
- botulism
- white muscle disease
- cleft palate

Diagnostic Approaches to Consider
- physical examination
- thorough oral and dental examination (with sedation, speculum, and bright light) *and with due care if rabies is suspected*
- passage of nasogastric tube (with caution)
- neurologic examination, paying particular attention to cranial nerve function
- CBC and serum biochemistry panel
- endoscopic examination of the pharynx, guttural pouches, and esophagus
- radiography, focusing attention on the teeth and the pharynx
- CSF collection and analysis (if EPM or other CNS disease is suspected)

EYE PROBLEMS
Possible Causes
- conjunctivitis (dust, insects, infectious agents)
- nasolacrimal duct obstruction
- corneal ulcers
- corneal lacerations and foreign bodies
- recurrent uveitis
- corneal stromal abscess
- fungal keratitis
- ocular tumors, especially of the third eyelid
- chorioretinopathy
- lens opacity (cataract) or luxation

Diagnostic Approaches to Consider

+ physical examination
+ ophthalmologic examination, with topical and perineural blocks as necessary
+ fluorescein staining of the cornea
+ corneal scraping with cytology and culture (bacterial and fungal)

FECAL ABNORMALITIES
Possible Causes
Diarrhea in adults

+ dietary changes or stress (diarrhea generally is self-limiting)
+ parasitism (cyathostomiasis)
+ colitis
  • infectious (e.g., *Salmonella* spp., *Clostridium perfringens, Ehrlichia risticii* [Potomac horse fever])
  • sand ingestion
  • phenylbutazone toxicity (ulceration of the right dorsal colon)
  • blister beetle (cantharidin) toxicity
+ drugs, especially antibiotics (predispose to infectious colitis)
+ granulomatous bowel disease

Diarrhea in foals

+ "foal heat" (self-limiting diarrhea in foals 1 to 3 weeks of age)
+ intolerance to milk replacer diet
+ bacterial enterocolitis (typically enterobacteria such as *E. coli* and *Klebsiella* sp.)
+ viral enteritis (rotavirus, coronavirus)
+ parasitism (older foals and young horses)

Firm or dry feces

+ dehydration
+ poor-quality roughage diet
+ partial obstruction of the large or small colon
+ peritonitis
+ drugs that slow gut transit time (e.g., anticholinergics)
+ meconium impaction (newborn foals)
+ grass sickness

Diagnostic Approaches to Consider

+ physical examination
+ evaluation of diet and feedstuff
+ rectal examination (adults), digital rectal examination in foals
+ CBC and serum biochemistry panel
+ fecal examination for parasite ova/larvae and sand
+ assays on fecal samples for bacterial or viral antigens (e.g., PCR for *Salmonella* spp., on-site tests for rotavirus)

+ abdominocentesis with fluid analysis and cytology, ± culture
+ serology to determine *Ehrlichia risticii* antibody titers
+ culture of feces and rectal mucosal biopsy samples
+ blood culture (in young foals suspected of having bacterial enterocolitis)

FEVER
Possible Causes

+ respiratory system
  • viral respiratory diseases (e.g., influenza, EHV-1 or EHV-4)
  • pneumonia, pleuropneumonia ("shipping fever")
  • *Streptococcus equi* infection (strangles)
  • *Rhodococcus equi* infection in foals
+ endotoxemia resulting from gastrointestinal disease
+ proximal enteritis
+ colitis
+ equine viral arteritis (EVA)
+ peritonitis
+ abdominal abscess
+ septic tenosynovitis
+ cellulitis
+ viral encephalitis (EEE, WEE, and VEE)
+ neoplasia
+ neonatal infections, including pneumonia, enteritis, omphalitis, osteomyelitis, septic arthritis, meningitis, and septicemia
+ blister beetle toxicosis
+ hemolysis
+ heat stress
+ grass sickness

Diagnostic Approaches to Consider

+ physical examination
+ rectal palpation (if an intraabdominal process is suspected)
+ CBC and serum biochemistry panel
+ virus isolation on nasal discharge or mucosal swabs (for viral upper respiratory disease)
+ thoracic ultrasonography ± radiography
+ transtracheal aspiration and culture
+ thoracocentesis or abdominocentesis with fluid analysis, cytology, and culture
+ serum titers for viral diseases
+ blood culture in foals suspected of having septicemia

HAIR COAT ABNORMALITIES
Possible Causes
Alopecia
* harness rubs (e.g., girth galls, saddle sores, boot rubs)
* pruritus
  * insect hypersensitivity, especially to *Culicoides* spp.
  * external parasites (lice, mites, ticks)
  * pinworms (*Oxyuris equi;* pruritus and rubbing around the tail base)
  * cutaneous onchocerciasis (pruritus and rubbing mostly along the ventrum)
  * seasonal allergies
  * neurologic disorders (e.g., polyneuritis equi, self-mutilation syndrome, rabies)
  * hepatoencephalopathy
* ringworm (dermatophytosis)
* *Dermatophilus* sp. infection ("rain scald," "rain rot")
* sarcoids
* selenium toxicity (tail and mane)
Hirsutism
* pituitary adenoma (equine Cushing's disease)
* severe malnutrition and/or parasitism (failure to shed rather than true hirsutism)

Diagnostic Tests to Consider
* physical examination
* close inspection of the skin and hair coat for external parasites or their eggs
* visual inspection of plucked hairs with a Wood's lamp (for dermatophytosis)
* microscopic examination of plucked hairs
* acetate tape preparations (for *Oxyuris* eggs)
* impression smears of lesions or crusts
* skin scraping with cytology, ± culture
* skin biopsy
* intradermal skin testing
* pituitary-adrenal axis tests (e.g., dexa-methasone suppression, ACTH stimulation, insulin assays)

INFERTILITY IN MARES
Possible Causes
* poor management (nutrition, heat detection, timing of breeding)
* transitional estrus
* chronic endometritis with impaired uterine clearance ± fibrosis
* pneumovagina (resulting in persistent or recurrent bacterial endometritis)
* poor semen quality
* urine pooling
* cervical or uterine adhesions
* metritis, pyometra
* ovarian abnormalities

Diagnostic Approaches to Consider
* review of management procedures
* thorough physical examination
* rectal palpation of the ovaries, uterus, and cervix
* ultrasonography of the ovaries, uterus, and cervix
* visual inspection of the perineum and vulva
* visual (± manual) inspection of the vagina and external cervical os using a sterile speculum and light source
* endometrial swabbing with cytology and culture
* endometrial biopsy

INFERTILITY IN STALLIONS
Possible Causes
* abnormal sperm morphology or motility
* oligospermia (or azoospermia)
  * testicular atrophy or degeneration
  * epididymal lesions
* reduced sperm survival
  * hemospermia (penile, urethral, accessory gland, or testicular lesions)
  * urospermia
  * infection (e.g., orchitis, epididymitis, seminal vesiculitis)

Diagnostic Approaches to Consider
* physical examination, including palpation of external genitalia
* rectal examination
* semen collection and evaluation of volume, concentration, morphology, and motility
* semen culture
* ultrasonographic examination of the testicles and accessory glands

LAMENESS AND GAIT ABNORMALITIES
Possible Causes
Musculoskeletal conditions
* foot problems
  * abscess (subsolar or hoof wall ["gravel"])
  * sole bruise

- hoof wall defects
- navicular disease
- laminitis
- sprains (muscle, tendon, or ligament)
- synovitis, tenosynovitis
- tendonitis, suspensory desmitis
- arthritis (degenerative joint disease)
- osteochondrosis (OCD)
- bone problems
  - splints, dorsal metacarpal disease ("bucked shins")
  - sesamoiditis
  - physitis
  - fractures (chip fractures, incomplete fractures)
- exertional rhabdomyolysis
- septic arthritis (especially in young foals that are lame)
- angular or flexural limb deformities (foals and young horses)
- back pain

Neurologic conditions
- vertebral trauma
- equine protozoal myeloencephalitis (EPM)
- cervical vertebral malformation (cervical stenotic myelopathy)
- peripheral neuropathy (traumatic)
- EHV-1 myelitis

Diagnostic Approaches to Consider
- physical examination, including detailed examination of the feet, limbs, and back
- neurologic examination
- gait analysis and flexion tests
- diagnostic regional anesthesia (perineural or intrasynovial blocks)
- arthrocentesis with fluid analysis, cytology, and culture (for suspected septic arthritis)
- ultrasonography
- radiography
- nuclear scintigraphy
- serum CK and AST
- CSF collection and analysis

LUMPS AND BUMPS
Possible Causes
- hypersensitivity reaction (urticaria)
  - insect bites (e.g., mosquitoes, stable flies)
  - drugs
  - seasonal allergies
- nodular necrobiosis or eosinophilic granuloma

- fibropapilloma (mostly young horses)
- bruise or hematoma/seroma
- abscess
- tumors
  - sarcoid
  - melanoma
  - squamous cell carcinoma
- granulomatous diseases
  - excess granulation tissue ("proud flesh")
  - cutaneous habronemiasis
- normal structure (e.g., thyroid gland in the ventral throat latch area)

Diagnostic Approaches to Consider
- physical examination, including close inspection of the skin and hair coat
- ultrasonography
- fine-needle aspiration with cytologic evaluation ± culture (NOTE: *aspiration of a hematoma or seroma is not recommended*).
- excisional biopsy with impression smears and/or histopathologic examination

MALFORMATIONS AND CONGENITAL DEFECTS
Possible Causes
Cardiovascular and hemolymphatic systems
- cardiac defects (valvular and/or septal)
- major vessel anomalies
- combined immunodeficiency (CID)

Gastrointestinal system and skin
- intestinal stenosis or atresia
- lethal white foal syndrome or intestinal aganglionosis (overo-overo paint foals)
- albinism

Head and neck
- cleft palate
- parrot mouth
- wry nose
- occipitoatlantoaxial malformation (Arabians)

Trunk and limbs
- hernias
- digital flexor tendon contracture

Urogenital system
- gonadal dysgenesis
- intersex animals
- partial agenesis of the urinary tract

Diagnostic Approaches to Consider
- physical examination and the following as appropriate:

* immunologic assays
* radiography
* endoscopy
* ultrasonography
* karyotyping
* pedigree analysis
* DNA testing (CID, aganglionosis)

NASAL DISCHARGE
Possible Causes
Mucopurulent discharge
* viral upper respiratory disease (e.g., influenza, EHV-1 or EHV-4)
* sinusitis ± tooth root infection
* guttural pouch empyema
* guttural pouch mycosis
* severe pharyngeal lymphoid hyperplasia
* retropharyngeal lymph node abscessation (especially strangles)
* nasal polyp, granuloma, or tumor
* pneumonia or pleuropneumonia

Sanguineous or serosanguineous discharge
See discussion of bleeding.

Nasal discharge containing feed material
* esophageal obstruction (choke)
* dysphagia
* pharyngeal or laryngeal dysfunction
* botulism
* white muscle disease (especially foals)
* cleft palate (in foals, milk trickles from the nostrils after nursing)
* gastric distention and impending rupture
* rabies
* grass sickness

Diagnostic Approaches to Consider
* physical examination, including thorough oral examination, percussion of the paranasal sinuses, and thoracic auscultation with a rebreathing bag
* passage of a nasogastric tube for choke and impending gastric rupture
* endoscopic examination of the upper airway, guttural pouches, and trachea (esophagoscopy for choke)
* CBC and serum biochemistry
* radiography (head, neck, or thorax, depending on physical findings)
* bacterial culture (nasopharyngeal swab, guttural pouch exudate, sinuscentesis, transtracheal aspirate)

* virus isolation on nasal discharge or mucosal swab

NEONATAL DISORDERS
Possible Causes
* meconium impaction
* angular or flexural (laxity or contracture) limb deformities
* neonatal maladjustment syndrome ("dummy foal")
* failure of passive transfer of maternal antibodies, increasing susceptibility to infection
  * septicemia
  * bacterial enteritis (*Escherichia coli*, *Klebsiella* spp., *Actinobacillus* spp.)
  * bacterial pneumonia
  * septic arthritis ± osteomyelitis
  * meningitis
* prematurity/dysmaturity
* patent urachus, urachal/umbilical infection
* ruptured bladder
* neonatal isoerythrolysis
* congenital malformations (see discussion of malformations and congenital defects)

Diagnostic Approaches to Consider
* physical examination of the foal, including digital rectal examination
* examination of the placenta (if available) and the mare
* measurement of serum IgG
* CBC, serum biochemistry panel, and blood gases (arterial if pneumonia is suspected)
* radiography (thoracic, abdominal, cuboidal bones of carpus/tarsus)
* ultrasonography, especially of umbilical structures
* synoviocentesis with fluid analysis, cytology, and culture
* bacterial culture (blood, feces, transtracheal aspirate, umbilical discharge, CSF)
* abdominocentesis with measurement of creatinine and electrolytes in peritoneal fluid

PERFORMANCE PROBLEMS
Possible Causes
Musculoskeletal system
* lameness (may be subtle)
* back pain
* exercise-associated muscle disorders

Respiratory system
- viral respiratory disease or its sequelae
- environmental allergens, resulting in bronchoconstriction
- exercise-induced pulmonary hemorrhage (some cases)
- obstructive upper respiratory conditions
  - idiopathic laryngeal hemiplegia
  - dorsal displacement of the soft palate
  - epiglottic abnormalities and subepiglottic cysts
  - redundant alar folds
  - thickened nasal septum

Cardiovascular system
- structural abnormalities, such as mitral/tricuspid insufficiency and septal defects
- conduction disturbances
  - heart block
  - paroxysmal atrial fibrillation
  - ventricular premature contractions

Other
- anemia
- anhidrosis
- temperament and training problems
- lack of physical fitness and/or inherent athletic ability

Diagnostic Approaches to Consider
- physical examination
- lameness evaluation
- CBC and serum biochemistry panel (including CK and AST)
- endoscopy of the upper airway and trachea
- bronchoalveolar lavage
- electrocardiography
- Doppler echocardiography (if a murmur is detected)
- treadmill exercise test

RECUMBENCY OR INABILITY TO RISE
Possible Causes
- any of the causes of collapse listed above
- spinal cord trauma
- infectious, inflammatory, or neoplastic diseases involving the brain or spinal cord
  - EHV-1 myelitis
  - equine protozoal myeloencephalitis (EPM)

- rabies
- exertional rhabdomyolysis
- postanesthetic myopathy or neuropathy
- hypoglycemia (neonatal foals)
- long-bone fracture
- severe debilitation or terminal illness
- parturition

Diagnostic Approaches to Consider
- physical examination, including palpation of the limbs
- thorough neurologic examination
- CBC and serum biochemistry panel (including CK and AST)
- radiography
- CSF collection and analysis
  - EHV-1 titers
  - *Sarcocystis neurona* antibody and antigen assays
  - bacterial culture

RESPIRATORY NOISES AND DIFFICULTIES
Possible Causes
Respiratory noise during exercise
- idiopathic laryngeal hemiplegia
- dorsal displacement of the soft palate (may be intermittent)
- redundant alar folds ("false nostril" noise)
- epiglottic entrapment, subepiglottic cyst
- severe pharyngeal lymphoid hyperplasia
- arytenoid chondritis

Respiratory difficulty at rest
- chronic obstructive pulmonary disease (acute exacerbation)
- pneumonia
- pleuropneumonia
- pleural effusion
- strangles
- anaphylaxis with laryngeal edema
- bilateral nasal obstruction (traumatic, inflammatory, neoplastic)
- pharyngeal or laryngeal obstruction/dysfunction
- tracheal collapse, foreign body, or compression
- exercise-induced pulmonary hemorrhage (immediately after racing)
- thoracic trauma causing pneumothorax or hemothorax
- grass sickness (rhinitis sicca)
- hepatoencephalopathy

Diagnostic Approaches to Consider

* physical examination with thorough auscultation of the thorax using a rebreathing bag
* CBC and serum biochemistry
* endoscopy of the upper airway and trachea (endoscopy during treadmill exercise may be necessary to confirm some causes of respiratory noise)
* temporary abduction of the alar folds with a mattress suture (for redundant alar folds)
* transtracheal aspiration
* bronchoalveolar lavage
* ultrasonography of the pleural space
* radiography
* thoracocentesis
* thoracoscopy

SALIVATION (SIALISM, PTYALISM, HYPERSALIVATION)

Possible Causes

* oropharyngeal irritation or ulceration
  * caustic substances
  * irritant feeds (e.g., grass awns)
  * foreign bodies (e.g., wood, wire)
  * dental problems (more likely to cause "quidding")
* mandibular or maxillary fracture
* esophageal obstruction (choke)
* gastric ulcers in foals
* dysphagia
  * white muscle disease
  * botulism
  * stylohyoid fracture
  * guttural pouch disease
  * grass sickness
* rabies
* viral encephalitis (EEE or WEE)
* slaframine-contaminated forage (horses are otherwise healthy)

Diagnostic Approaches to Consider

* physical examination
* thorough oral examination, with sedation, speculum, and bright light
* examination of feedstuff
* neurologic examination, paying particular attention to the function of cranial nerves V, VII, IX, X, and XII
* CBC and serum biochemistry panel
* endoscopy of the upper airway, guttural pouches, and esophagus (+ gastroscopy in foals)
* radiography of the head

* CSF collection and analysis

SCRATCHING AND RUBBING

Possible Causes

* any of the causes of pruritus listed under *Hair Coat Abnormalities*
* healing wounds
* ringworm (dermatophytosis)
* drugs (toxic epidermal necrolysis)
* bacterial/fungal/seborrheic dermatoses
* trigeminal neuritis (rubbing of the muzzle)

Diagnostic Approaches to Consider

* physical examination, including close inspection of the skin and hair coat
* tools listed under *Hair Coat Abnormalities* (except for pituitary-adrenal axis tests)

STRAINING OR TENESMUS

Possible Causes

Adults

* passage of firm, dry feces (see *Fecal Abnormalities)*
* parturition
* rectal tear
* vaginitis, cystitis
* EHV-1 myelitis
* rabies
* cauda equina syndrome (sacral fracture or polyneuritis equi)
* colitis/proctitis
* peritonitis
* urethral obstruction
  * urolithiasis
  * inflammatory or neoplastic mass
* laminitis, colic, or exertional rhabdomyolysis ("sawhorse" stance can be mistaken for stranguria)

Foals

* meconium impaction
* ruptured bladder
* rectal damage or inflammation from administration of an enema
* enteritis or colitis

Diagnostic Approaches to Consider

* physical examination, including examination of accessible genitalia
* rectal examination (adults), digital rectal examination in foals (Note: *extreme care must be taken if rectal damage is the suspected cause of tenesmus)*
* CBC and serum biochemistry panel

- urinalysis
- abdominocentesis
- ultrasonography
- radiography
- endoscopic examination of the urethra and bladder
- CSF collection and analysis

SUDDEN (UNEXPECTED) DEATH
Possible Causes
- hemorrhage (see *Bleeding*)
- botulism
- anaphylaxis
- septic shock (e.g., ruptured stomach or intestine, peracute colitis)
- trauma to the head, resulting in basisphenoid fracture
- toxins (plants, chemicals, venom)
- lightning strike, electrocution
- malicious acts

Diagnostic Approaches to Consider
- thorough necropsy, beginning with close inspection of the carcass
- examination of the environment where the horse was found
- submission of blood, tissue samples, and gastric contents for toxicologic analysis
- submission of pasture or feed samples for toxicologic analysis

SWEATING ABNORMALITIES
Possible Causes
Abnormal increase or pattern
- stress, pain (e.g., severe colic)
- drugs (e.g., epinephrine, α_2-agonists [xylazine, detomidine, etc.])
- fever
- neurologic dysfunction
  - Horner's syndrome (sweating on face and neck)
  - other spinal cord or sympathetic peripheral nerve lesions
- pituitary adenoma (equine Cushing's disease)
- grass sickness

Abnormal decrease in sweating
- anhidrosis
- hypovolemia
- heat exhaustion

Diagnostic Approaches to Consider
- physical examination
- CBC and serum biochemistry panel
- neurologic examination

- tests of pituitary-adrenal axis function (see *Haircoat Abnormalities*)
- terbutaline skin test (for anhidrosis)

SWELLINGS
Possible Causes
Head, neck, trunk
- edema
  - cellulitis
  - vasculitis
  - hypoproteinemia
  - lymphatic obstruction
  - venous obstruction (e.g., swelling of the head with jugular thrombosis)
- hematoma/seroma (traumatic or resulting from coagulopathy)
- urticaria
- abscess
- tumor
- subcutaneous emphysema
Limbs
- as above for head, neck, and trunk
- joint or tendon sheath effusion
- tendonitis, desmitis
- hygroma
- exostosis

Diagnostic Approaches to Consider
- physical examination
- CBC and serum biochemistry panel
- ultrasonography
- fine-needle aspiration with cytologic examination ± culture (NOTE: *Aspiration is not recommended for hematomas or seromas*).
- radiography (plain ± contrast)
- biopsy

URINATION AND URINE ABNORMALITIES
Possible Causes
Production of grossly abnormal urine
- exertional rhabdomyolysis (gross myoglobinuria)
- prolonged exercise (e.g., endurance rides)
- intravascular hemolysis
  - drugs (e.g., penicillin)
  - immune-mediated hemolysis
  - red maple toxicity
- cystitis/pyelonephritis
- dehydration (horse may pass thick, dark-colored urine)
Abnormal urination
- polyuria

- estrus (normal behavior)
- polydipsia/polyuria (renal failure, pituitary adenoma, psychogenic water drinking or salt eating)
- iatrogenic overhydration or hyperglycemia
- drugs (e.g., frusemide, DMSO)
- ◆ oliguria or anuria
  - severe dehydration, shock
  - renal failure
  - neurologic conditions that inhibit normal voiding (e.g., EHV-1 myelitis, sacral fractures, cauda equina neuritis)
  - ◆ ruptured bladder (foals)
  - ◆ complete urethral obstruction with a calculus or mass
- ◆ urine dribbling or narrowed stream
  - partial urethral obstruction
  - urine pooling (broodmares)
  - patent urachus (foals)
  - ectopic ureter
  - retention with overflow (neurologic conditions that inhibit voiding)
- ◆ difficult or painful urination
  - urolithiasis
  - cystitis, urethritis
  - colic, laminitis, or exertional rhabdomyolysis-may be confused with stranguria

Diagnostic Approaches to Consider
- ◆ physical examination, including examination of external genitalia
- ◆ visual inspection of the vagina using a light source and speculum
- ◆ rectal palpation
- ◆ neurologic examination
- ◆ CBC and serum biochemistry
- ◆ urinalysis ± culture
- ◆ abdominocentesis (foals with suspected ruptured bladder)
- ◆ catheterization or endoscopy of the urethra and bladder
- ◆ ultrasonography
- ◆ measurement of water intake (± water deprivation test)

WEIGHT LOSS
Possible Causes
- ◆ malnutrition
- ◆ parasitism
- ◆ dental abnormalities
- ◆ inappetence/anorexia
  - fever

- systemic illness
- gastric ulceration
- ◆ diarrhea (see *Fecal Abnormalities*)
- ◆ maldigestion/malabsorption
- ◆ catabolism of chronic systemic illness
- ◆ motor neuron disease
- ◆ intraabdominal abscess
- ◆ protein sequestration or loss
  - pleuropneumonia or peritonitis
  - protein-losing enteropathy or nephropathy
- ◆ neoplasia
- ◆ liver disease
- ◆ grass sickness

Diagnostic Approaches to Consider
- ◆ physical examination
- ◆ dental examination
- ◆ rectal examination
- ◆ fecal flotation for parasite ova or larvae
- ◆ CBC, serum biochemistry panel, and urinalysis
- ◆ abdominocentesis
- ◆ thoracocentesis
- ◆ gastroscopy
- ◆ ultrasonography
- ◆ fecal culture
- ◆ carbohydrate absorption test (glucose or D-xylose)
- ◆ rectal mucosal biopsy

WOUNDS
Types of wounds
- ◆ abrasions—superficial skin damage
- ◆ contusions—subcutaneous tissue trauma with little or no skin damage
- ◆ incisions—wounds with sharp, clean edges, often amenable to primary closure
- ◆ lacerations—wounds with ragged edges, often with loss of tissue or devitalized tissue; contamination may be substantial
- ◆ punctures—deep, narrow wounds; contamination may be substantial, and primary closure is not advisable

Diagnostic Approaches to Consider
- ◆ physical examination
- ◆ arthrocentesis and lavage to determine if wound communicates with joint
- ◆ radiography ± sinography
- ◆ ultrasonography

2

Principles of Practice Management

Setting up, running, and marketing an equine practice are discussed in *Equine Medicine and Surgery V*, pages 51 through 75.

Insurance

(pages 65-67)

Thomas J. Lane

Malpractice and negligence are two of the most likely types of lawsuits that an equine practitioner may experience.

LEGAL DEFINITIONS

liability: the responsibility or obligation of an individual according to the law.

malpractice: professional misconduct or unreasonable lack of skill, which in practical terms means failure to exercise the degree of skill, learning, and care applied by the average prudent, reputable member of the profession. Malpractice pertains to inadequate or improper treatment, care, or handling of a client's animal.

negligence: the performance of an act that a person of ordinary prudence would not have done under similar circumstances or the failure to do what such a person would have done under the same or similar circumstances. The law of negligence pertains to personal injury to another individual, such as a client.

PROFESSIONAL LIABILITY INSURANCE

The owner of a veterinary practice should have professional liability insurance (this can be purchased from several sources, including the American Veterinary Medical Association).

- Ideally, the insurance policy should provide for defense against claims, pay the full amount to settle a claim, cover the entire cost of any defense, and take care of any court judgments up to the limits of the policy.
- Some companies insist on settling claims without the veterinarian's approval, but such an arrangement could affect the veterinarian's reputation and the future of his/her practice.
- Standard exclusions of professional liability policies include illegal acts, guarantee of results, and operation under the influence of alcohol or drugs.

EMPLOYED VETERINARIANS

Veterinarians employed by the practice usually are not parties to the owner's professional liability insurance policy, which only protects the owner from libelous acts of the employee. It is important that employed veterinarians have their own individual policies.

Extending Credit to Clients *(pages 70-72)*
Thomas J. Lane

The objective of a credit policy is to constrain the risk while maximizing the time and service component of the practice.

* Granting credit to clients may increase the workload or sales, but if the net result causes a disintegration of cash flow and requires the practice to borrow capital for operation, the total effect can be negative.
* A useful rule of thumb is to keep the accounts receivable at 10% or less of total gross income to date. Techniques include the following:
  * discounts on bills paid within a certain period
  * standardized periodic payments credited against current debt
  * incentive prepayment for future contracts

HOW MUCH CREDIT?

A veterinarian should extend credit on the basis of the client's ability to pay.

* The best guide is to evaluate the character, reputation, and abilities of the client and take into consideration the collateral circumstances.
* It is entirely appropriate for the veterinarian to request credit references and/or a financial statement in the course of a credit discussion.
* In large equine enterprises, in which billing and payment may require 90 days or more, credit references are necessary. In these instances, the fee structure may also reflect the extended use of the veterinarian's money by the client.

Each case is individual and significant in its own merit.

Compounded Drugs
(pages 72-74)
Joseph J. Bertone

Equine practitioners often find themselves faced with the dilemma of using formulations that are not approved for horses or approved formulations that are impractical to administer. In these situations, equine veterinarians often use compounded medications.

RESTRICTIONS

Ethical use of compounded medications is restricted by several stipulations, including the following:

* the development of a veterinarian-client-patient relationship
* prescription drug dispensing restrictions
* the need to improve animal well-being
* absence of an available product approved by the government regulatory agency in a suitable dosage form to treat the condition

Ensuring Safety and Efficacy

If practitioners choose to compound medications or to prescribe compounded medications, they accept the responsibility for formulation composition, effectiveness, and safety. Therefore the veterinarian should ask the following questions before choosing a firm to compound a prescribed formulation.

* *Does the firm compound medications for laypersons?* If so, extreme caution should be exercised; pharmaceutical guidelines specifically state that compounding of drugs should occur only by request of licensed medical professionals and by prescription only.
* *Is there a licensed pharmacist on the firm's staff?* Having a licensed pharmacist supervising the compounding process is essential for quality drug compounding, and in some states it is legally required. Licensed pharmacists have the legal and ethical responsibility to follow good compounding practices. Veterinarians should ask for the phar-

macist's name and state license number for verification.

• *If bulk product is used in the compounded formulation, is it produced using good manufacturing practices (GMP) at the source of origin?* Good manufacturing practices ensure that the product delivered to the compounding firm has the quality attributes identified by its label and a certificate of analysis. Quality compounding firms will not hesitate to provide certificates of analysis for the bulk drug they use.

NOTE: *Using bulk raw materials to compound drugs intended for use in animals (including horses) intended for human consumption is not appropriate, except in rare instances.*

• *What type of quality testing is performed?* If a compounded formulation is produced on a regular basis for a large group of animals, some form of test batch analysis should be expected. Even when GMP bulk drug of known strength and quality is used, loss of active ingredient or formulation errors may occur during compounding.

• *Are stability data available?* Because the nature of equine practice often taxes the stability of compounded products, it is worth determining if and under what conditions stability testing has been performed. Quality compounding firms collect data on controlled stability studies. The expiration date should be set at the time a given prescription will be entirely used.

Dramatic changes in drug bioavailability may occur with minor changes in compounding technique. Thus, approved drugs provide the highest assurance of quality, strength, purity, and stability, as well as the best opportunity for accurate dosing.

3

Patient Evaluation and Diagnosis

Patient Evaluation

(pages 76-95)

Reuben J. Rose and J. Dick Wright

The following are important steps in establishing an initial diagnosis:
* recording the presenting complaint and establishing the history relating to the problem
* undertaking a complete physical examination to localize the problem(s)
* establishing, in order of likelihood, a series of differential diagnoses
* undertaking any diagnostic tests that add further information to the clinical database, particularly those that rule out possible diagnoses

Specific emergencies, such as severe hemorrhage, shock, and colic, warrant immediate intervention. Complete evaluation can be undertaken once the horse's condition is stabilized.

SIGNALMENT

Knowledge of the horse's age, breed, gender, and use help in formulating a list of differential diagnoses and determining whether certain conditions are either more or less likely to be the cause of the presenting clinical signs.

Age
* *musculoskeletal diseases:* Septic arthritis involving multiple joints, osteochondrosis, and angular limb deformities are most common in

young horses. The incidence of degenerative joint disease increases with both age and degree of use.
* *respiratory diseases:* Infectious respiratory disease tends to be more severe in the neonatal and adolescent periods; in contrast, chronic obstructive pulmonary disease occurs principally in middle-age horses.
* *cardiac diseases:* Congestive heart failure occurs most commonly in older horses; congenital heart disease, although present from birth, may not manifest itself until the young horse begins training.
* *gastrointestinal diseases*
  * Consider gastric ulceration, pyloric stenosis, and ascarid impaction in foals with colic.
  * Small intestinal volvulus and intussusception occur more commonly in horses <3 years old.
  * Pedunculated lipomas, enterolithiasis, and incarceration of intestine in the epiploic foramen are common causes of small intestinal obstruction in horses >9 years of age.

Breed and Use
In combination with breed, the purpose for which the horse is used is of major importance in determining the likelihood of various abnormalities. Breed predilections exist for several conditions that cause gait abnormalities.

- Bucked shins are common in young Thoroughbreds and Quarter Horses in race training.
- Chip fractures of the carpal bones also are diagnosed more frequently in Thoroughbreds and Quarter Horses than in Standardbreds.
- Hind limb lameness and fractures of the distal phalanx (pedal bone) occur more commonly in Standardbreds than in Thoroughbreds or Quarter Horses.
- Navicular disease is common in Quarter Horses.
- Laminitis and upward fixation of the patella are more common in ponies than in other breeds.
- Cervical vertebral malformation (wobbler syndrome) is most common in Thoroughbreds and Warmbloods.
- Occipitoatlantoaxial malformation and cerebellar degeneration occur most often in Arabians.

Combined immunodeficiency, which often leads to adenovirus pneumonia, occurs primarily in Arabian foals. Laryngeal hemiplegia is more common in Thoroughbreds than in other breeds and generally is first noticed between 2 and 3 years of age.

Gender

Some conditions, such as inguinal hernias, occur only in colts and stallions.

Management and Geography

- Adolescent respiratory infections are more common on stud farms where there is overcrowding.
- *Rhodococcus equi* infections occur more commonly in certain geographic areas.

HISTORY

The *history of the current problem* begins with a discussion of the presenting clinical signs and an assessment as to whether the problem is static, regressing, or progressing.

The *general history* should commence with the history immediately before the onset of the problem and should include selective details from months to years previously, depending on the nature of the problem. Perti-

nent facts include the horse's appetite and history of weight gain or loss.

REFERRALS AND SECOND OPINIONS

For referrals to work effectively, it is essential that good communication be established between the referring and consulting veterinarians. Criticism of a colleague must never be made to a client or other third party.

Referral Process

- A colleague at a referral clinic or an expert in the horse's particular problem should be suggested to the client.
- A full written history should be supplied in a referral letter, as well as a clear description of the matters on which a second opinion or request for treatment are being sought.
- The referring veterinarian must fully inform the colleague on important clinical findings and any treatment initiated.
- With emergency cases, a telephone call or fax or e-mail message will suffice.
- Once a case is referred, the consulting veterinarian is solely responsible for the type of treatment selected; however, the referring veterinarian is entitled to a written report and appropriate telephone discussions about the progress, outcome, and future care of the case.

PHYSICAL RESTRAINT

Acceptable forms of physical restraint include:

- *holding the halter:* The person controlling the horse's head should stand on the same side as the operator.
- *lifting a limb:* If a forelimb is to be worked on, the opposite forelimb is lifted; if a hind limb requires attention, a forelimb on the same side is lifted.
- If an additional person is not available to hold the foot, a knee strap or leg rope can be used.
- *chain lead or rearing bit:* The chain end of a lead rope can be positioned either over the bridge of the horse's nose or under the upper lip.

Whether using a chain or a rearing bit, a single, sharp tug is applied only when restraint is needed.

* *Yankee war bridle:* A loop is made in a rope and placed around the back of the horse's ears and on the gum dorsal to the maxillary incisor teeth. A short, sharp tug on the free end is applied for restraint.
* *grasping a skin fold:* A fold of skin on the side of the neck is used.
* *twisting an ear:* The horse's ear is lightly grasped and twisted at the base.
* *twitch:* Either a rope or chain loop is applied to the upper lip; the person holding the twitch should stand at the horse's shoulder.
* *sidelines:* Single or double sidelines can be applied when stocks are not available.
* *tail restraint:* The horse's tail can be lifted up over its back for rectal or reproductive examination; stabilizing the tail is also a useful technique to use during anesthetic induction and recovery.
* *stocks:* When available, properly constructed stocks can be a very useful form of restraint.

Restraint of Foals

* The simplest way to restrain young foals (up to 2 months of age) for minor procedures is to have the handler gently twist the foal's ears (see above) while the foal's rear end is positioned in a corner of the stall.
* If restriction of movement is all that is required, the handler can place one arm around the foal's chest and hold the foal's tail up over its back with the other hand.

Handling Unbroken Horses

The Jeffery method of horse handling is invaluable when handling unbroken horses for veterinary treatment.

* A 6- to 7-m-long (20 to 25 feet) catching rope is used.
* With the horse in a restricted area, a large loop is formed in the catching rope and the rope is placed (not thrown) over the horse's head, using a long stick if necessary.
* A short, sharp "control pull" is made on the rope to turn the horse to face the handler, and then any tension in the rope is released.

* The handler then moves to a different spot and applies another "control pull."
* After four or five control pulls, the process of advance and retreat can begin, with the handler advancing toward the horse a little at a time and then retreating before the horse moves.
* After 15 to 20 minutes, most horses allow the handler to approach, stroke it, and perform any necessary tranquilization or treatment.

RECORD KEEPING

Accurate medical records are fundamentally important to a veterinary practitioner.

* They are legal documents, required to maintain accurate records.
* They provide an ongoing history of each animal.
* Record keeping also enables busy practitioners to keep track of services rendered so they may be fully compensated.

Details

A duplicate record system of all service calls is recommended.

* On completion of each call, the veterinarian should update the record, providing a copy to the client and keeping the original.
* The date, owner's name, and name and description of each horse are recorded.
* A brief description of the service or complaint, together with diagnosis, therapy, and treatment plan should be included.

PHYSICAL EXAMINATION

Initial examination comprises an overview of the horse, determining whether or not the horse is alert, depressed, or showing signs of pain and noting any asymmetry, swellings, or other irregularities. The horse should be viewed from the front, both sides, and the rear.

Examination of the Head and Neck

Regardless of the order in which the examination is conducted, the following areas should be thoroughly evaluated:

- *nares:* Check for symmetry, airflow, and the presence of abnormal odor or discharge.
- *mouth:* Measure capillary refill time (normally 1 to 2 seconds); inspect the incisors and molars for abnormalities, including sharp edges on the cheek teeth; estimate the horse's age.
- *maxillary and frontal sinuses:* Percussion may elicit evidence of pain or a dull sound that could indicate sinusitis.
- *eyes:* Examine for corneal scars, conjunctivitis, iridocyclitis, cataracts, and third eyelid lesions; evaluate the menace and pupillary light responses.
- *facial artery:* Evaluate the pulse rate and character as the artery passes ventral to the horizontal ramus of the mandible.
- *throat area:* Palpate the area between the rami of the mandibles and the region of Viborg's triangle to determine if the mandibular and retropharyngeal lymph nodes are enlarged.
- *larynx:* Palpate the dorsal aspect to detect asymmetry of the muscles.
- *cervical vertebrae:* Palpate the lateral processes and assess the range of lateral movement and neck flexion.
- *trachea:* Palpate the cervical trachea.
- *jugular veins:* Check both veins for patency and abnormal pulses.

Examination of the Thorax

Both sides of the thorax should be thoroughly examined.
- *respiration:* The normal respiratory rate of an adult horse at rest is 8 to 16 breaths/min, with little thoracic wall movement.
- *heart:* The normal resting heart rate of an adult horse is 28 to 36 beats/min. The heart should be ausculted for 1 minute over at least three sites, noting any disturbances of rhythm or the presence of murmurs.
- *trachea and lungs:* In most normal horses breathing quietly at rest, few sounds are heard on auscultation, except over the hilar area and trachea.
  - A rebreathing bag should be used if there is dyspnea, coughing, or any suspicion of abnormal sounds (crackles or wheezes). Al-

ternatively, the nares can be occluded for a short time, which causes the horse to take several deep breaths when the nares are released.
- The thorax should be percussed using a pleximeter (or dessert spoon) and rubber hammer or using the fingers (the tips of the first two fingers of one hand are used to strike the middle finger of the other hand, which is pressed firmly between adjacent ribs).

Examination of the respiratory system is discussed further in Chapter 9, Respiratory System, and cardiovascular examination is discussed in Chapter 8, Cardiovascular System.

Examination of the Abdomen

Examination of the abdomen should include the following:
- visual inspection for distention
- auscultation—the left and right sides should be ausculted over both the paralumbar fossae and ventral flank regions
  - At the right paralumbar fossa, ileocecal sounds (a brief "flushing" sound) are heard every 30 to 60 seconds.
  - It is important to determine whether gut sounds are normal, increased, decreased, or absent (see Chapter 10, Alimentary System).
- percussion and auscultation to detect pockets of gas (normal at cecal base)
- soft ballottement using a closed fist

Rectal Temperature

The normal range is 37° to 39° C (99° to 102° F) in adult horses and at the high end of this range in foals.

Examination of the Limbs

The limbs should be thoroughly and systematically examined in both weight-bearing and lifted positions, beginning with careful inspection for swellings and joint distention. Most problems occur in or below the carpus or hock. Many equine veterinarians begin the examination at the foot and work proximally. Examination of the forelimbs and hind limbs is discussed in Chapter 15, Musculoskeletal System.

Examination of the Back

The back should be checked for the following:

- scoliosis, lordosis, or kyphosis
- pain over the dorsal spinous processes of the thoracic and lumbar regions
- pain when firm pressure is applied over the tubers sacrale
  - Mild pressure at this site may cause horses with hind limb weakness or sacroiliac pain to crouch away from the examiner.
  - Stroking the thoracolumbar area and caudal sacral region with a blunt probe may provoke abnormal responses.
  - Stroking the thoracolumbar area normally causes extension of the thoracolumbar vertebral column.
  - Stroking the caudal sacral region causes the horse to flex its thoracolumbar vertebrae.
  - An abnormal response consists of the horse holding its back rigid, sinking very low, grunting, or showing some other pain response.
  - Some normal horses resent these manipulations and may crouch excessively.

Examination of the Genitalia

Unless the history indicates the possibility of a urogenital problem, detailed examination of the genitalia is not necessary. Basic examination includes the following:

- *stallions and geldings:* The preputial area should be examined for discharge that could indicate an infection, squamous cell carcinoma, or habronemiasis.
  - In colts and stallions, the testicles should be palpated to make sure the horse is not a cryptorchid.
- *fillies and mares:* The conformation of the perineum should be noted to determine the likelihood of ascending infection or pneumovagina.
  - If there is any discharge from the vulva or "scalding" around the hind limbs, a more detailed examination of the urogenital tract is indicated (see Chapter 13, Reproductive System: The Mare).

Rectal Examination

Rectal examination is not part of the routine examination procedure. However, it should be performed in the following instances:

- there is a history of weight loss
- a gastrointestinal, reproductive, or urinary system problem is suspected
- a sacral, pelvic, or lymphatic disorder is suspected

Restraint

The horse must be adequately restrained and, if necessary, tranquilized.

- Restraint is most safely achieved in stocks, although use of tail restraint with or without a sideline is quite effective.
- The following drugs may be used to relax the horse's rectum:
  - hyoscine and dipyrone (Buscopan compositum) 0.05 mL/kg IV
  - lidocaine enema (15 to 20 mL of 2% lidocaine with 30 mL of water or lubricant)
- copious amounts of water-soluble lubricant should be used

Normal findings

- The left lateral abdominal wall is palpated, and with further cranial exploration, the caudal pole of the spleen and the left kidney can be felt.
- The pelvic flexure of the large colon usually is palpable on the left side of the ventral caudal abdomen.
- The small colon (containing fecal balls) can be felt in the central abdomen.
- The cecum may be discernible, especially when distended with gas or impacted food.
  - The base can be felt toward the dorsal abdominal wall.
  - Most often the only reliable finding is the ventral taenia that is frequently felt running from the right dorsal to left ventral quadrants.
- Palpation of the cranial mesenteric artery is quite difficult in most large horses and impossible if there is abdominal pain.
- In stallions, the integrity of the internal inguinal rings (on the lateral parts of the ventral abdominal wall, just cranial to the pelvic canal) should be assessed.
- The pelvic organs can be evaluated (see Chapter 12, Reproductive System: The Stallion, and Chapter 16, Urinary System).

After completing a rectal examination, it is important to inspect the glove for blood, which could indicate a rectal tear or rupture.

Assessing the Gait

The extent of gait evaluation depends on whether there is a history of a musculoskeletal or neuromuscular problem. Minimum examination should include walking the horse toward and away from the investigator and in a circle to identify incoordination and trotting the horse on a firm surface to detect lameness.

Prepurchase Examination *(pages 95-103)*
Reuben J. Rose and J. Dick Wright

A complete examination should be performed in a methodic manner. Considerable care must be taken not only with the examination but also with recording the findings.

HORSE IDENTIFICATION

Adequate identification of the horse is very important, and should include the following:

♦ *height:* measured at the withers with a yardstick or estimated in hands (1 hand = 10 cm or 4 inches)
♦ *coat color:* (see *Equine Medicine and Surgery V,* page 96, for descriptions of the basic coat colors and variations)
♦ *gender:* the following classifications are used:
  • *colt:* uncastrated male ≤3 years of age
  • *stallion:* uncastrated male ≥4 years of age
  • *filly:* female ≤3 years of age
  • *mare:* female ≥4 years of age
♦ *age:* estimation made by inspection of the teeth is checked against the age supplied by the owner and that indicated by brands or tattoos

Natural Markings

An accurate description of markings is very important for identification. All markings and their extent and location should be precisely defined.

Head

Markings on the head are described as follows:

♦ *star:* a solid marking on the forehead; patches of white hairs should be described separately
♦ *stripe:* a solid white marking no wider than the flat surface of the nasal bones, running down the dorsal aspect of the face; may be continuous with (conjoined) or separated from (interrupted) a star
♦ *blaze:* a solid white marking covering the major portion of the forehead between the eyes, extending down the front of the face, usually to the muzzle, and involving the width of the nasal bones
♦ *snip:* an isolated white marking between or in the region of the nostrils

In addition, any white markings on the lip and muzzle must be accurately described and drawn on an appropriate diagram.

The limbs and trunk

The extent and location of white markings should be described, with special reference to variation in the height of the marking on various aspects of the limb. Other markings to be noted include:

♦ *whorls:* permanent irregular settings of coat hairs
  • Whorls may be simple (clockwise or counterclockwise) or feathered and single or in groups of two or three.
  • Description involves notation of location, type, and relationship to other structures and markings.
  • Whorls on the head should also be noted.
  • Whorls are of special importance in the identification of whole-colored animals (those with no other markings).
♦ *flesh marks:* patches where skin pigment is absent
♦ *ticking:* presence of isolated white hairs distributed throughout the coat
♦ *flecking:* small collections of white hairs distributed irregularly on any part of the body
♦ *spots:* small, circular collections of hair, differing from the general body color

- odd-colored hairs in the mane and tail

Congenital peculiarities

Congenital abnormalities and peculiarities should be noted, including the following:

- wall-eye
- Roman nose
- partly colored hoof
- undershot or overshot jaw
- muscle indentations (dimples)

Tattoos and Brands

All tattoos, brands, and other permanent acquired markings (including scars) require careful description and should be noted on the sketch of markings.

Tattoos

Thoroughbred horses in the United States and Canada are tattooed inside the upper lip. Thoroughbred horses bred in Europe or the United Kingdom are unlikely to carry brands or tattoos unless raced in the United States or Canada. Standardbreds also are tattooed inside the upper lip.

Freeze brands

In Australia and New Zealand, Thoroughbreds usually are branded on their right and left shoulders. In these countries, and in recent years in Canada, Standardbreds are identified by freeze branding on the right side of the neck. In the United States, Arabian horses also are identified by a freeze brand on the neck.

Electronic identification

Minute electronic microchips placed subcutaneously, usually in the neck, are becoming more widely used.

Sketch of Markings

A sketch of a horse, featuring all markings, should be part of the certification process.

- The position of whorls may be indicated by a circle, with an arrow showing direction of hairs.
- A few white hairs can be indicated by several lines, and flecking and ticking by small, light lines scattered over the area.
- Spots or markings on the body are best indicated by drawing the outline; white markings on the face and limbs should be further highlighted by light shading.

- Bordering around a marking should be noted by drawing a double outline.
- Flesh marks are best shown by drawing the outline with heavy shading.
- A small cross (X) can be used to denote the position of a scar.

EXAMINATION PROCEDURE

If possible, a statement should be obtained from the vendor (or agent) regarding the horse's history, including a schedule of medication. If an animal is to be examined for athletic serviceability, it is important to note the level of exercise in the months before inspection.

Initial Examination

The examination is best conducted in the horse's own environment, preferably in a stall. The horse's demeanor, general appearance, and condition are noted, and any vices such as crib biting, wind sucking, and weaving should be recorded. Note should also be made of the horse's temperament.

Clinical Examination

A careful and thorough physical examination, as described above, must be performed. It is also important to note any conformational abnormalities.

Observing the Gait

The horse is observed at the walk and trot and while turning and backing. It is important to look for ataxia, which generally can be accentuated by walking and turning the horse on an incline, particularly with its head elevated. Lunging the horse in circles can be used to accentuate a lameness. Flexion tests should be performed, with particular joints being held in flexion for 1 to 2 minutes, after which the horse is trotted.

Inspection with Exercise

If the horse cannot be exercised at the intensity required for the athletic event for which the horse is intended, it should be lunged for at least 10 minutes and the level of exercise noted on the certificate. In hot climates, the horse's ability to sweat after exercise should be recorded.

Evaluation after exercise
Immediately after exercise, the horse's thorax should be auscultated to detect abnormal respiratory sounds, cardiac arrhythmias, or heart murmurs. Low-grade systolic ejection murmurs often are identified in performance horses and are of no consequence.

Reevaluation after rest
The final phase of the examination involves observation of the horse while it is walked, trotted, turned, and backed after a 30-minute rest. Of particular interest is whether exercise followed by rest results in any stiffness or lameness.

Diagnostic Aids

Use of diagnostic aids such as radiography, endoscopy, ultrasonography, and electrocardiography should be discussed with the client and the advantages of such tests explained. Depending on the value of the horse and the particular use for which it is intended, some or all of these tests may be indicated. However, such specialized procedures should not be regarded as part of the routine prepurchase examination.

RECORDS AND CERTIFICATES

Certificates of examination must be dated and written or typed on letter-head stationery, and should include the following:
- name and address of the person requesting the certificate
- date and place of examination
- proper identification of the animal to which the certificate relates
  - A full description of the horse's breed, color, height, gender, distinguishing marks, and brands or tattoos should be recorded.
  - The horse should not be described by name without proof of identity.
- precise description of abnormalities detected on examination
- interpretation of the significance of these findings
  - Even though discretion should be used in expressing an opinion as to the potential loss of function associated with observed abnormalities, the client is entitled to some interpretation of the findings.

- Use of the term "in my opinion" as a qualifying statement has no legal value as a disclaimer.
- the examining veterinarian's signature and registered qualifications

Information gathered from a prepurchase examination must be supplied only to the person or agent who employed the veterinarian. Such information and should be passed to other parties only after permission has been obtained from the buyer.

Insurance Examination

(page 103)
Reuben J. Rose and J. Dick Wright

When an insurance examination is requested by the client, the veterinarian is required to report only the medical facts:
- Although the horse owner is paying for the examination and is thus the client, the information belongs to the insurance company.
- This can create a conflict of interest, especially when information about past treatment of the horse is required and may affect the animal's insurability.

Evidence of firing, blistering, neurectomy, or other surgery should be noted and its significance pointed out to the insurance company. Interpretation depends on whether insurance is sought for mortality or for loss of use.

EXAMINATION

The examination involves:
- positive identification
- a thorough and systematic inspection, similar to that for prepurchase examination
  - Foals usually cannot be exercised in a controlled manner, but should be observed running with the dam in a large yard or paddock.
  - Confirming passive transfer of maternal immunoglobulins and the absence of icterus in a serum sample at 24 hours of age is strongly recommended before passing a foal as suitable for insurance.

A copy of all the findings should be kept as part of the case record.

Investigation of Performance Problems

(pages 105-109)

Reuben J. Rose

Many horses experience loss of performance without clear indication in the history or clinical findings to identify the cause of the problem. In evaluating these horses a standardized, detailed investigation, concentrating on the cardiovascular, respiratory, and musculoskeletal systems, must be undertaken. The examination should not conclude when a singular problem has been identified.

HISTORY

In most cases the history is nonspecific and the presenting complaint is that the horse is failing to "run on" or is "fading" in the last 200 to 400 meters of a race, a sign caused by a great variety of clinical problems. Establishing the chronicity of the problem is helpful in making a diagnosis. Following are some other pertinent questions:

+ Has the reduction in performance been sudden or gradual?
+ Does the horse "blow" heavily after exercise?
+ Does the horse ever make a respiratory noise while galloping?
+ Is there any evidence of lameness?
+ Is there any history of ill health or change in the horse's appetite?

CLINICAL EXAMINATION

Reduced exercise capacity is a complex problem afflicting performance horses. Musculoskeletal conditions are common and are a probable cause of performance reduction in many horses. Other common abnormalities are heart murmurs and upper respiratory tract problems. Thus, although the general examination should be completed, the following key body systems should be given extra attention.

+ *respiratory* (see the earlier discussion of physical examination)
+ *cardiovascular*
  • Up to 80% of normal horses have localized murmurs that have no apparent effect on athletic performance; the majority are systolic and most are lower than grade III (out of V).
  • Doppler ultrasonography and assessment of cardiovascular function during treadmill exercise may be required to determine the functional effect of heart murmurs.
  • Vagally induced arrhythmias such as sinoatrial block and second-degree atrioventricular block do not appear to be associated with cardiac dysfunction.
  • Atrial fibrillation, ventricular tachycardia, ventricular premature contractions, and conditions giving rise to atrioventricular dissociation generally result in more obvious effects on performance.
  • If an arrhythmia is heard, an electrocardiogram should be performed.
+ *musculoskeletal*
  • The key high-mobility joints are the fetlock and carpus.
  • Back problems should not be overlooked in horses presented for poor performance.
  • Evaluation for ataxia is important in young horses (yearlings and 2-year-olds).
  • Conditions that commonly cause a reduction in exercise capacity include pedal osteitis, navicular disease, shin soreness, plantar fetlock chips, bone spavin, and rhabdomyolysis.
  • It is important to continue the examination even when a significant lameness is found, because it may not necessarily be the sole cause of reduced performance.

DIAGNOSTIC AIDS

Hematology and Plasma Biochemistry

Many apparent abnormalities evident on the hemogram and biochemistry profile are of no clinical significance. The hemogram is particularly subject to influence by excitement or apprehension and by the time of the day at which the sample is collected.

Upper Respiratory Tract Endoscopy

Endoscopy should always be performed in a horse with a history of reduced performance.

- Obstructive upper airway problems are common.
- Pharyngitis, purulent discharge from the guttural pouches, and purulent exudate in the trachea can represent underlying disease processes contributing to poor racing performance.
- If findings are of questionable significance, endoscopic examination during treadmill exercise is useful to evaluate possible effects on airflow

Bronchoalveolar Lavage

Bronchoalveolar lavage (BAL) is one of the most helpful diagnostic aids to detect subtle lower airway disease:

- In general, the presence of >15% neutrophils in BAL fluid suggests pulmonary lesions
- Hemosiderophages are a common finding in horses training at three-quarter pace or faster.
- Red-tinged BAL fluid indicates recent hemorrhage and may be taken to indicate the cause of the reduced performance.

Electrocardiography

An electrocardiogram (ECG) is part of the routine workup that should be used on all horses presented for poor racing performance.

Clinical Exercise Testing

Treadmill exercise testing assesses the key body systems involved in the oxygen transport chain under conditions of peak stress. It is a valuable means of interpreting the findings at rest, the significance of which is difficult to determine in some cases.

A range of abnormalities can be identified during exercise, including:

- higher heart rates during submaximal exercise in horses with heart murmurs
- lower PaO_2 and higher $PaCO_2$ at peak speeds in horses with low-grade idiopathic laryngeal hemiplegia

Low-grade lameness appears to have little effect on measurements made during exercise.

Traditional Chinese Veterinary Medical Diagnostics *(pages 109-119)*

Richard Panzer

Traditional Chinese veterinary medicine diagnostic techniques may be clinically useful to practitioners of Western equine medicine. The palpation techniques are probably most useful for directing the treatment of musculoskeletal problems, especially localization of musculoskeletal abnormalities in horses with no obvious signs of lameness.

Palpation may also support a presumptive diagnosis of internal disease (organ pathology). There are areas along the backs of horses that are "associated" with the heart, lungs, liver, digestive organs, and kidneys. Reactivity of these "association" acupoint areas is indicative of abnormalities in traditional Chinese veterinary medicine terms and may be suggestive of abnormalities in terms of Western medicine.

DIAGNOSTIC METHODS

The four diagnostic methods are:

- inspection
- inquisition
- auscultation and olfaction
- palpation for
  - temperature
  - skin (and hair coat) quality
  - muscle tone
  - pressure pain

Whenever an abnormality is identified, the acupoint is said to be "reactive."

The locations of the major acupoints are listed and illustrated in *Equine Medicine and Surgery V,* pages 111 through 118.

REFERRED ABNORMALITIES AT DISTAL ACUPOINTS

Reactivity may not necessarily indicate an abnormality in that area; it is common for musculoskeletal problems to manifest as referred reactivity.

- Reactivity can be found at the "master" acupoints of the limbs and at so-called opposite joints (the analogous joint on the diagonally opposite limb).

- The master acupoints are located in muscle grooves that overlie the main trunks of the brachial and pelvic nerves.
- When one of the master acupoints is reactive, abnormalities are to be suspected somewhere in that limb.
  - Opposite joint abnormalities can be useful in pinpointing the primary site of an abnormality.
    - For example, abnormalities of the right stifle can manifest as palpable abnormalities at the left elbow and vice versa.
    - This phenomenon may be explained by the fact that with many chronic musculoskeletal problems, long-term compensation may cause injury at multiple sites (limbs, neck, and back).

Necropsy *(pages 119-132)*
Claus D. Buergelt

A necropsy should be thorough and complete; gross examination alone often provides an incomplete diagnosis. Additional histopathologic, toxicologic, parasitologic, microbiologic, and virologic examinations may be needed to confirm the final diagnosis.

PRELIMINARY INFORMATION

Before necropsy, the history of the case should be reviewed, including:
- the animal's breed, gender, age, color, markings, tattoo, and use
- clinical signs
- precise medication history
  In all cases, written or telephone-witnessed permission should be obtained from the owner (or representative) and the insurance company before starting the necropsy. The dates and times that these contacts are made and the names of persons contacted should be recorded.

POSITIONING, EXAMINING, AND OPENING THE CARCASS
Initial Examination

After the body weight is obtained or estimated, the animal should be positioned in left lateral recumbency.

- In cases involving insurance or litigation a whole-body photograph should be made.
- All orifices, ocular sclerae, hooves (including coronary bands), and the condition of the hair coat are examined.
  - Dermal abrasions over bony structures (ocular arch, ileal wings, extremities) suggest antemortem pain or neurologic disturbances, with struggling or recumbency before death.
  - Careful examination of the jugular grooves, sides of the neck, and the skin over the gluteal musculature may reveal injection sites, which should be saved for toxicologic analyses if malicious intent or faulty injections are suspected.
- The tattoo or brand, if obtainable, is transcribed.
- The general color of the visible mucous membranes is recorded
  - Yellow mucosae suggest blood dyscrasia or liver failure.
  - White mucosae suggest blood loss or deficient bone marrow function.
  - Blue mucosae suggest insufficient oxygen supply or inadequate circulation.
  - Pinpoint red foci suggest septicemia, toxemia, thrombocytopenia, or vascular permeability disturbance.

Exposure of the Abdominal and Thoracic Contents

The necropsy proceeds with a ventral midline incision made through the abdominal skin.

- The incision is extended caudally toward the right coxofemoral joint, which is opened by incising the joint capsule and the ligament of the head of the femur; the right hind limb is reflected.
- The skin is removed over the abdomen and thorax.
- In male horses, a cut is made around the penis and sheath, reflecting both caudally over the ischial arch; the testes are removed from the scrotum.
- In female horses, the entire mammary gland is removed with the skin attached, and several sections

are cut through the mammary parenchyma and teats.

- The right forelimb is reflected by cutting into the subscapular tissues and muscles.
- The midline incision is extended along the neck toward the head.
- Exposed subcutaneous and muscular tissues are examined for nutritional and hydration status.
- The exposed superficial lymph nodes and, in young horses, the umbilicus are examined.

Opening the abdominal cavity

The abdominal cavity is opened by an incision through the abdominal wall, just caudal to the last rib.

- The adjacent viscera and abdominal fluid are inspected.
  - 100 to 200 mL of clear, straw-colored peritoneal fluid is normal.
  - If excessive fluid or exudate is present, a sample should be obtained aseptically for culture and cytology.
- The incision is extended through the abdominal midline and parallel to the transverse processes of the lumbar vertebrae.
- The abdominal viscera, in particular the intestinal tract, are checked for relative normal positions.
- Portions of the colon and cecum are partially removed to inspect the viscera in the left side of the abdomen. The sternal, diaphragmatic, and pelvic flexures are examined.

Opening the thoracic cavity

The diaphragm is punctured, and an in-rush of air indicates normal negative thoracic pressure.

- Using rib cutters or pruning shears, the entire right thoracic wall is opened.
- The thoracic cavity is visualized.
  - About 100 mL of straw-colored pleural fluid may be expected.
  - If indicated, fluid samples are collected for culture and cytology.
- In situ photographs of both the thoracic and abdominal cavities may be obtained for documentation purposes.

Evisceration and Examination of Abdominal and Pelvic Organs

The following order is recommended:

- The right adrenal gland, located medial and parallel to the right kidney, is gently removed.

- The cranial mesenteric arterial root can be inspected for patency and intimal smoothness in one of the following two ways:
  - The branches of the ileocecocolic artery are identified, lifted with one hand, and cut transversely. The dorsal portion is opened with scissors by cutting toward the aorta.
  - The abdominal aorta is opened and followed caudally toward the cranial mesenteric artery, which is opened from its origin by directing the scissors ventrally.
- The entire GI tract is removed by dissecting through its mesenteric attachment.
  - The small colon is cut near the pelvic inlet, and the esophagus is cut at the diaphragm.
  - The renosplenic ligament is severed, and the spleen is removed with the stomach.
- The liver is removed by cutting it from the diaphragmatic crura.
- The left adrenal gland and both kidneys are removed with the ureters attached (cut close to the urinary bladder).
- The mesenteric root and lymph nodes are severed from their dorsal attachment.
- The urinary bladder is opened in situ and the mucosal surfaces examined, unless a detailed examination is indicated.
  - The approximate volume of urine in the bladder is recorded, along with color and turbidity.
- The uterus and ovaries are removed by cutting caudal to the cervix.
- If it is necessary to examine the organs of the pelvic cavity more carefully (e.g., for a horse with a rectal tear), the bones of the pelvic cavity are cut with a handsaw.

Individual organs are examined, and the following are recorded: shape, dimensions, color, edges, consistency, nature of the cut surfaces, and, where appropriate, degree of symmetry, weight, and precise measurements (length, width, height).

Gastrointestinal tract, liver, and spleen

If the case history and internal gross examination suggest gastrointestinal disease, one should immediately proceed with a complete, thorough investigation of this system. Otherwise, dissection of the GI tract should be performed at the end of the necropsy, after other organs more susceptible to decomposition are examined.

Recommended order of examination:

- The spleen is detached from the stomach, and the stomach is opened along the greater curvature.
- The nature of the gastric contents and condition of the mucosa are recorded.
- The small intestinal tract is opened opposite to its mesenteric attachment, and the nature of the contents is recorded.
- The pancreas is removed from the base of the cecum, and its approximate dimensions, color, consistency, and degree of lobulation are noted.
- The colonic lymph nodes and vessels are examined before the cecum, ventral and dorsal colons, and the transverse and descending small colon are opened.
- The mesenteric lymph nodes are examined within the root of the mesentery.
- Multiple slices, 1 to 2 cm apart, are made through the liver and spleen.
  - The cut surfaces are examined for structural abnormalities.
  - The amount of blood exuding from the cut surfaces is judged and recorded.
  - The splenic lymph nodes are sliced and examined.

Kidneys and adrenal glands

- The kidneys are weighed and measured.
- Each kidney is cut sagittally from the outer cortex toward its pelvis delineation, and the color of the cortex and medulla are recorded. The shape of the renal pelvis, the extent to which it is dilated, and the appearance of its contents and mucosa are described.
- The renal capsule must be stripped to check for adhesions and to note the appearance of the outer cortex (which often reveals important but minute changes).
- Both adrenal glands are carefully sliced sagittally; the width and appearance of the cortex and medulla are recorded.

Reproductive tract

- The dimensions, consistency, and degree of bilateral symmetry of the ovaries or testes are described.
- Both ovaries are sliced, and the structures noted on cut section are recorded.
- The uterine body and horns are opened and the endometrial surface described.
- If present, any fetus and fetal membranes are removed and examined (see below).
- The spermatic cord and epididymis should be dissected from the testis before weighing and measuring each gonad.
  - A midsagittal incision is made into the testes, which causes the cut surface of a mature testis to bulge.
  - Each half should then be cut transversely into slices 0.5 to 1 cm wide, to reveal any small lesions, such as early tumors.
- The appearance of the male accessory organs, penis, and prepuce should be noted.

Removal and Examination of the Thoracic, Cervical, and Oral Organs

The entire pluck is removed *en bloc*.

- The tongue is removed by cutting through the periglossal tissues, parallel to the medial aspect of the mandibular ramus, and disarticulating the stylohyoid apparatus.
- The larynx, trachea, and esophagus are freed to the thoracic inlet.
- The cut is continued dorsal to the aorta, toward the diaphragm.
- The pericardial sac is dissected from its sternal attachment, and the entire pluck is lifted out.
- The parietal pleura is examined for moisture and transparency.
- If a thymus can be identified, its dimension and lobulation are recorded.
- The esophagus is opened along its entire length and removed from the trachea.
- Both thyroid glands are identified and examined, and midsagittal cuts are made to permit assessment of their degree of activity and to look for small tumors.

* The parathyroid glands are difficult to distinguish from small cervical lymph nodes.
  * A set of cranial parathyroid glands is located cranial and medial to the thyroid glands.
  * A set of caudal parathyroid glands usually is associated with the bicarotid trunk, ventral to the trachea, cranial to the thoracic inlet, and close to the first rib.
* The tonsils, pharynx, larynx, and epiglottis and dimensions of the retropharyngeal lymph nodes are described.
* The pericardial sac is opened to assess the volume and nature of the pericardial fluid. If indicated, a sample of the fluid is obtained for culture.
* The heart is removed from its vascular suspensions.
* The trachea is opened along its entire length, and the incision is extended into the bronchial tree.
* The tracheobronchial lymph nodes are assessed.
* The lungs are palpated and sectioned.
  * The color, degree of collapse, and presence of fluid exuding from cut surfaces are recorded.
  * Multiple transverse incisions are made through the lung parenchyma to search for small internal lesions.
  * The pulmonary arteries can be opened with scissors to search for thromboemboli.

Examination of the heart
Care should be taken not to destroy major cardiac structures.
* The left and right sides of the heart should first be identified; the pointed cardiac apex clearly identifies the left ventricle.
* The appearance of the epicardium and coronary grooves is recorded.
* The pulmonary arterial outflow tract is identified and incised.
  * This incision is extended caudally into the right ventricle and continued along the interventricular septum toward the right atrium.
* The left ventricle is opened, starting laterally and slightly above the apex.
  * The cut is directed toward the left atrium.

* The mitral valve leaflet is severed, and the ascending aorta is opened.
* The interior of the heart is rinsed with water, and the appearance of all internal structures is recorded.
  * The circumference of each valve ring and the ventricular wall thickness can be measured.
  * The degree of myocardial integrity and contraction can be determined by slicing tangentially into the myocardium.

Examination of the Locomotor System and Bone Marrow
Even if a detailed examination of joints, tendons, or muscles is not necessary, one should routinely open five sets of joints.
* The scapulohumeral, coxofemoral, femorotibial, tibiotarsal, and atlantooccipital joints usually are selected for routine examination.
* Additional joints are examined when the clinical history identifies their involvement in lameness; similarly, tendons and muscles are examined when necessary.
* The skin of the entire limb should be reflected before opening a joint.
* All major limb joints are opened from the medial side (ventral for the atlantooccipital joint).
  * Normally, a slight amount of viscous, straw-colored synovial fluid oozes from the opened joint.
  * Healthy articular cartilage has a smooth, light bluish-white surface.
* In cases of laminitis, the hooves can be sawed proximal to the coronary band and split into halves with a handsaw.
* A general statement should be made regarding the color and consistency of skeletal muscles.
* The bone marrow is exposed by scoring the cortices sagittally with a saw.
  * Bone marrow also can be obtained from cut ribs.
  * Bone marrow is best fixed in small, perforated plastic cassettes.

Examination of the Head and Brain
Before removing the head, a cerebrospinal fluid sample can be obtained from the atlantooccipital cistern if

CNS disease, especially equine proto-zoal myeloencephalitis, is suspected.

- Decapitation is performed at the at-lantooccipital joint.
- The guttural pouches are inspected.
  - The cranial cervical ganglion, lo-cated next to the carotid artery in the dorsocaudal aspect of the me-dial compartment, should be col-lected if grass sickness is suspected.
- The skin, soft tissues, and temporal muscles are removed from the skull.

Removal of the brain

- A handsaw is used to open the dorsal calvarium.
- A standard technique involves making a transverse cut through the frontal bones just caudal to the zygomatic arches (supraorbital pro-cesses) and two laterally angled then sagittal lines on the right and left sides of the calvarium, con-necting the frontal bone cut with the inner (medial) angle of both oc-cipital bone condyles.
  - The skull cap is loosened with a chisel, pried off, and carefully separated from the meninges.
  - The surface of the meninges is examined, and, if necessary, a sterile swab is taken for culture.
  - The brain is removed by tipping the skull and severing the vas-cular, meningeal, and cranial nerve attachments.
  - The basal surface of the meninges and brainstem may be swabbed for culture, if indicated.
  - The pituitary gland is lifted with forceps and severed from the basal fossa.
  - The optic chiasm is examined for symmetry.
- The brain is cut in transverse sec-tions.
  - The first cut separates the cere-brum into cranial and caudal halves.
  - The second cut separates the caudal half of the cerebrum into halves.
  - The third cut sections the cere-bellum and medulla oblongata transversely.
  - The brain sections are fixed *en bloc*, unless fresh tissue is needed for microbiologic, virologic, or toxicologic analyses.

- Other methods of brain removal:
  - A longitudinal handsaw cut can be made along the median plane of the head, and the halves (left and right) of the brain removed.
  - A transverse craniotomy can be made caudal to the last molar tooth, splitting the head into ros-tral and caudal parts.
  - Both of these alternatives are easier to perform after the mandible has been removed.
- The ocular globe is removed by grasping the skin around the eye with forceps and cutting deeply around the orbit, close to the bone, using scissors; the optic nerve is transected.

Examination of the Spinal Cord and Peripheral Nerves

An electric band saw facilitates access to the spinal cord without damaging it. The usual approach is through a dorsal laminectomy after removal of limbs, ribs, and surrounding muscle bulk from the vertebral column.

Removal of the spinal cord under field conditions

- One option is to split the vertebral column sagittally, just lateral to the spinal cord, using a meat cleaver.
  - This approach, however, may so damage the spinal cord as to pre-vent adequate histologic exami-nation.
- An alternative and preferable method is to divide the vertebral column into three or four major sections (cervical, thoracic, lumbar) with a handsaw.
  - Depending on the location of the lesion (see Chapter 11, Nervous System), one or all of these sec-tions is cut transversely through the arches and bodies of adjacent vertebrae, leaving the interverte-bral articulations intact.
  - The spinal cord segments are re-moved by cutting with scissors through the vertebral nerves in the epidural fat.
  - Each section of spinal cord is la-beled separately, and the dura is opened longitudinally to facilitate rapid penetration of the fixative.
- A third option is to saw the de-fleshed vertebral column into sec-

tions 15 to 30 cm (6 to 12 inches) in length, double bag the segments in formalin, and mail them to a laboratory equipped with a band saw.

Examination of "wobblers"

Cervical radiographs made before or after death can greatly assist in identifying the likely site(s) of spinal cord compression associated with cervical vertebral malformation, fractures, and vertebral osteomyelitis. In the case of "wobblers," the cervical vertebrae can be disarticulated.

- Disarticulation can be performed after the vertebrae are sectioned or with each vertebra intact.
  - With the latter technique, each spinal cord segment is removed before disarticulation.
  - The dorsal articular capsules are cut and the articular surfaces examined for symmetry and shape.
  - The exposed dorsal intervertebral space is examined for epidural fat, the presence of which indicates that spinal cord compression is unlikely to have occurred at that site.
  - The spinal cord segment is severed with a sharp cut and removed before disarticulation of the tight fibrous intervertebral disk.
- The atlantoaxial joint is disarticulated by cutting the strong ligaments of the dens using a ventral approach.
- The diameter of the vertebral canal is examined for narrowing at both ends of the disarticulated vertebra.
- Each vertebra and spinal cord segment is labeled separately for precise localization of the disease process.

Peripheral nerves

The peripheral nerves usually examined are the sciatic nerve (just caudal to the femur) and those of the brachial plexus (on the medial surface of the scapula).

EXAMINATION OF THE FETUS AND PLACENTAL TISSUES

Fetus

A complete necropsy should be performed on the fetus.

- The fetus is weighed, and its crown-to-rump length and umbilical cord length are measured.

- Blood is collected from the umbilical cord or fetal heart.
- The umbilical cord and either the ligated stomach or gastric contents should be submitted for virologic examination (or frozen at −70° C [−94° F] if virology is delayed).
- One adrenal gland can be frozen for virus isolation or fluorescent-antibody testing.
- Aqueous fluid can sometimes be used for immunologic and microbiologic testing.
- Fetal (and placental) tissues should be fixed in 10% buffered neutral formalin.

Placental Membranes

If complete placental membranes are available, they are weighed and thoroughly examined.

- The chorioallantois is stretched out in the shape of an **F**, and both surfaces are carefully inspected.
- The chorionic surface is examined for nonvillous or discolored areas.
- Placental samples for histologic examination should include sections of the chorioallantois from the uterine body and both horns and from the amnion and umbilicus.

ANCILLARY EXAMINATIONS AND TISSUE COLLECTION

Specimens for Bacteriology or Virology

Bacteriologic and virologic samples must be collected and handled in an aseptic manner, using an alcohol flame and sterile containers or swabs.

- The surfaces of organs to be cultured should be seared with a red-hot spatula.
- The seared surface is incised with a sterile scalpel blade and the specimen for culture is obtained with sterile scissors, swab, or needle (fluid aspiration).
- If immediate delivery is not feasible, samples should be shipped in sealed plastic bags surrounded by dry ice or freezer packs, using the fastest available transportation.
- Samples for virus isolation should be sealed in airtight bags and shipped cold, preferably on dry ice.

+ Serum should be refrigerated or frozen when sent for serologic analysis; whole blood should never be frozen.

Specimens for Parasitology

Direct fecal flotation and Baermann's method are recommended for detection of GI endoparasitic ova and lungworm larvae, respectively. If blood parasites are suspected, smears of blood and spleen should be prepared.

For helminth identification, parasites should be placed in physiologic saline (0.85% NaCl) and refrigerated for several hours to allow them to relax.

+ Trematodes and cestodes should then be fixed in AFA solution (85 mL of 85% ethanol, 10 mL of commercial formalin, 5 mL of glacial acetic acid).
+ Nematodes should be dipped in hot 70% ethanol and then transferred into glycerine-alcohol (90 mL of 10% ethanol, 10 mL of glycerine).

Specimens for Toxicology

Tissue collection for toxicologic analysis should be generous and encompass a variety of organs and body fluids. Duplicate samples should be collected. All material must be placed in clean, sealed glass containers, properly identified, and shipped frozen or on ice packs.

The following samples and quantities are recommended:

Urine: all available or 50 mL	Liver: 0.5 to 1.0 kg
Serum (clot removed): 10 mL	Kidney: 0.5 to 1.0 kg
Heart blood: 25 to 50 mL	Spleen: 0.5 to 1.0 kg
Body fat: 100 g	Heart: 0.5 to 1.0 kg
Stomach contents: 0.5 kg	Intestinal contents: 0.5 kg
Brain: ½ in formalin and ½ frozen	Lung: 0.5 to 1.0 kg
Intact eye with aqueous humor	

Other samples that should be considered include:

Feed: 2 kg
Water: 1 L
Bedding: 2 kg

Necropsy findings associated with various toxic compounds and the samples useful for diagnosis are listed in Tables 3-1 through 3-3.

Table 3-1
Toxic compounds, necropsy findings, and samples useful for diagnosis of some toxicoses of horses

Toxic compounds	Necropsy findings	Samples
Arsenic and arsenicals	Intense hyperemia of gastrointestinal tract, fluid hemorrhagic feces	Liver, kidney
Chlorinated hydrocarbons	Random petechiae	Blood, liver, fat, brain, stomach contents
Fluoroacetate	None	Stomach contents, liver, kidney
Nicotine	Nonspecific	Blood, liver, kidney, gut contents
Organophosphates and carbamates	Excessive fluid in lungs and gastrointestinal tract	Blood for cholinesterase, urine, brain, gut contents
Warfarin and other anticoagulants	Massive hemorrhage into a space or viscus	Liver, kidney, whole blood
Strychnine	Rapid onset of rigor mortis	Stomach contents, liver, kidney

Courtesy Dr. C. M. Brown.

Table 3-2
Animal toxins, necropsy findings, and samples useful for diagnosis of some toxicoses of horses

Animal toxins	Necropsy findings	Samples
Cantharidin (blister beetle)	Severe gastroenteritis with sloughing of mucosa, fluid gut contents, pale kidney, inflamed renal pelvis, bladder inflammation, myocardial degeneration	Foodstuffs (alfalfa hay), gut contents, urine
Snake and insect venom	Possible local swelling or evidence of acute anaphylaxis	None

Courtesy Dr. C. M. Brown.

Table 3-3
Plant toxins, necropsy findings, and samples useful for diagnosis of some toxicoses of horses

Plant toxins	Necropsy findings	Samples
Black nightshade *(Solanum nigrum)*	Nonspecific	Plants, gut contents to examine for poisonous plants
Blue-green algae	Nonspecific	Water sample
Castor bean *(Ricinus communis)*	Fluid gastrointestinal contents	Plants, gut contents to examine for poisonous plant
Chokecherry and other cyanogenic plants *(Prunus spp.)*	Bright red mucous membranes	Plants, gut contents to examine for poisonous plant
Oleander *(Nerium oleander)*	Nonspecific	Plants, gut contents to examine for poisonous plant
Red maple leaves *(Acer rubrum)*	Icterus; splenomegaly; swollen, black kidneys; brown urine; tubular nephrosis with hemoglobin casts	Plants
Poison hemlock *(Conium maculatum)*	Nonspecific	Plants, gut contents to examine for poisonous plant
Water hemlock, cowbane *(Cicuta* spp.)	Nonspecific	Plants, gut contents to examine for poisonous plant
Yew	Food often in mouth	Plants, gut contents to examine for poisonous plant
Pigweed *(Amaranthus retroflexus)* and other plants containing nitrate	Dark brownish blood and mucous membranes	Plants, gut contents to examine for poisonous plant

Courtesy Dr. C. M. Brown.

Specimens for Histopathology

Care should be taken to use an appropriate sample size (blocks of 1 × 1 × 0.5 cm) and fixative.

- 10% neutral buffered formalin (4% formaldehyde).
- Bouin's fixative (acetic/picric acid and formaldehyde).
- There should be at least 10 times as much fixative as tissue.

Sample Handling

- In the absence of gross lesions, any organ that may be associated with the clinical signs noted before death should be examined histopathologically.
- Bouin's fixative hardens tissue and is preferred for soft tissues, such as reproductive tract and bone marrow.

- Tissues are placed in Bouin's solution for 24 to 48 hours, then transferred to 10% formalin.
- Fixed tissues should be shipped in sealed plastic bags with cotton soaked in formalin; *tissues being submitted for histopathologic examination must not be frozen.*

RECORDING THE FINDINGS

All observations should be written down or tape-recorded, preferably before disposal of the carcass and organs.

- Gross necropsy findings should be descriptive in nature, incorporating all abnormal findings and including organ dimensions, shape, color, consistency, and nature of the cut surfaces.
- Terms understandable to the layman should be used and medical terms added in parentheses.
- Statements concerning the meaning of the findings should be reserved for the comment section of the report.
- All incidental findings or background pathologic lesions should be listed and their potential contribution to the disease process discussed; likewise, postmortem changes should be listed.

INSURANCE AND MEDICOLEGAL NECROPSY

A medicolegal necropsy must be conducted under the premise that the case may end up in court. The events of the necropsy should be substantiated through meticulous compilation of recorded physical findings, photographs, radiographs, preserved specimens, and laboratory results. The same procedure should be followed for insurance necropsies.

These types of necropsy require complete dissection and necessitate meticulous record keeping. The following four major considerations should be observed.

- The necropsy should be performed within 6 to 8 hours after death or euthanasia.
- The prosector should be qualified (preferably a veterinary pathologist).
- The events of the necropsy should be fully documented with written observations that include all normal findings.
- The report should be authenticated with the prosector's signature and the date the necropsy was performed, the time it was started and concluded, and the names of any witnesses.

Additional precautions
- Whole-body photographs and photographs of the animal's identifying marks should be obtained before starting the necropsy.
- Photographic documentation of major pathologic lesions should be procured in addition to written descriptions.
- Photographs of the immediate area where the animal was found dead also may be useful.
- A systematic dissection is imperative; all organ systems should be carefully examined.
- A thorough histologic tissue examination should be performed in the absence of gross lesions.
- Selected tissue samples and body fluids should be frozen for potential toxicologic or microbiologic analyses.

The report should list the results of all ancillary testing, photographs taken, and the nature of specimens retained. Specimens should be properly labeled, frozen, and stored in a safe environment for up to a year. Information relative to the case should not be released without the owner's signed permission.

4

Principles of Therapy

Intravenous Catheterization Techniques *(pages 136-146)*
Josie L. Traub-Dargatz

CATHETER SELECTION
Catheter Types
The three types of catheter most commonly used in horses, listed from most reactive to least reactive, are:
* polytetrafluoroethylene or Teflon
* polyurethane
* silicone rubber or Silastic

Teflon catheters are stiffer than the others and are therefore more prone to kinking and breaking (with the possible complication of a catheter embolus). However, they are easier to place, being threaded over a stylet. The other catheters are softer and most must be passed over a guide wire.

Selection Criteria
Catheter selection should be based on the following criteria:
* duration of anticipated catheter use
  * Teflon catheters should be replaced every 48 to 72 hours.
  * If IV treatment will likely be needed for >48 hours, a long-term polyurethane catheter should be considered (may be left in place for up to 3 weeks, with appropriate care)
* condition of the patient
  * Horses with clinical or laboratory evidence of hemostatic dysfunction or with diseases associated with hemostatic dysfunction (e.g., enterocolitis, intestinal strangulation/obstruction) should be catheterized with the least thrombogenic catheter available. However, horses with violently painful colic should be catheterized with a stylet type of (Teflon) catheter for immediate treatment.
  * A polyurethane catheter should be used in foals <1 month of age, for all except short-term IV treatments (e.g., plasma transfusion).
* vein to be used
  * The smallest-gauge catheter that will accommodate the treatment required and that can be readily placed in the selected vein should be used.
* ability to restrain the patient during catheter placement and the treatment period
  * Teflon catheters are easier to place, but they are also more likely to kink and break with excessive patient movement.
  * Placement of the softer catheters requires more time and better restraint (possibly even sedation); however, these catheters accommodate patient movement much better.
* expense of the catheter
  * Teflon catheters are the cheapest.
  * If catheterization is required for more than 48 to 72 hours, it is often more cost-effective to use a long-term polyurethane or silastic catheter.

- familiarity or experience of the person placing the catheter

CATHETER PLACEMENT AND MAINTENANCE

Techniques

Jugular vein

The jugular vein is the most commonly catheterized vein in horses.

- It is critical that both jugular veins be assessed for patency and overall health before placing a catheter in either vein.
  - If one jugular vein is already thrombosed or has clinical evidence of thrombophlebitis, use of the other jugular vein for catheterization or blood collection should be avoided.
  - The lateral thoracic vein in adults and the cephalic vein in neonatal foals are good alternatives (see below).
- All IV catheters should be placed aseptically, in a clean, dust-free environment.
- If the patient is very dehydrated or if a polyurethane catheter is used, it is advisable to make a stab skin incision with a no. 15 scalpel blade.
- The catheter and extension set should be flushed with sterile 0.9% saline containing heparin (10 IU/mL) and secured in place with either superglue or sutures.

Lateral thoracic vein

- The lateral thoracic vein runs along the ventrolateral thorax.
  - It is fairly large and lies partly embedded in cutaneous muscle.
  - It is readily visible and palpable in thin or athletic horses but can be difficult to locate in overweight horses.
- Some horses kick during placement of the catheter, so adequate restraint is necessary.
- Long-term polyurethane catheters are better tolerated and easier to place in this vein than are Teflon stylet catheters.
- The catheter is passed from caudal to cranial.

Cephalic vein

- The cephalic vein is recommended for catheterization in neonatal foals if the jugular vein cannot be used.
- Long-term polyurethane catheters are preferred.
- The foal is restrained in lateral recumbency, and the catheter is passed from distal to proximal.
- The catheter should be secured with sutures and a bandage.

Maintenance

All efforts should be made to maintain the catheter and administration system aseptically.

- The catheter system should be closed at all times, and all medications and fluids administered via the catheter should be sterile.
- All injection ports should be cleaned with 70% alcohol before injection, and male adapters (injection ports) should be changed daily.
- The catheter and vein should be assessed at least once daily (see below).
- The catheter and extension (if used) should be flushed with heparinized normal saline (10 IU heparin/mL) at least every 6 hours and before and after each treatment.

CATHETER-RELATED PROBLEMS

Catheter-related problems include:

- thrombosis, thrombophlebitis, or septic thrombophlebitis
  - Thrombophlebitis is the most common complication.
  - It causes pain, heat, swelling, and ropelike thickening within or around the vein.
  - Sepsis of the vein or surrounding tissues can also occur.
- septicemia
  - swelling of the part of the body drained by the affected vein
  - for example, head and neck if the jugular veins are involved)
- catheter failure requiring catheter replacement
- catheter failure resulting in local inflammation
- catheter failure resulting in a catheter embolus

Minimizing Complications

Guidelines to minimize complications from IV catheterization include:
* careful aseptic insertion and stabilization of catheters
* use of soft catheters in large veins
* use of topical antiseptic and sterile dressings over the catheter site
* daily inspection of catheter sites
  * Normally, the catheter can be palpated within the lumen of the vein, and this process does not cause the patient any discomfort.
  * Ultrasonography can be used to evaluate the vein if there is any question as to its status.
* removal of catheters at the first sign of phlebitis
* removal of catheters as soon as clinically prudent

Management of Catheter-Related Problems

* If thrombophlebitis occurs, the catheter should be promptly removed, and if sepsis is a risk, the catheter tip should be cultured.
* If the vein or surrounding tissue is painful or swollen, hot packs should be applied for 10 to 15 min q6h; topical treatment with DMSO is also indicated.
* If the patient has clinical signs of sepsis (e.g., fever, tachypnea, leukocytosis) or if there is local evidence of sepsis (e.g., purulent drainage from the catheter site or marked swelling and pain), broad-spectrum antimicrobials and possibly NSAIDs should be given.
* Any exudate should be submitted for bacterial culture.
* Perivascular tissue necrosis and abscess formation may necessitate surgical drainage.
* In some cases, septic thrombophlebitis will not resolve until the infected vein segment is surgically removed.
* If the horse is developing head edema as a result of jugular vein thrombosis, it should be fed from a feeder off the ground.
  Resolution of thrombophlebitis does not necessarily result in a return of patency of the vein; the vessel either recanalizes or collateral circulation becomes established.

Fluid and Electrolyte Therapy *(pages 146-152)*
Michelle Henry Barton and James N. Moore

BASIC FLUID THERAPY
Volume Needed

It is important to establish the goal of therapy: to replenish the horse's immediate needs or to simply meet its daily requirements. To determine how much fluid is needed, consider:
* maintenance fluid requirements
* estimates of fluid already lost (i.e., dehydration)
* estimates of continued losses above maintenance (e.g., diarrhea, gastric reflux)

Maintenance needs

Maintenance needs are influenced by diet, exercise, lactation, and ambient temperature.
* Adult horses typically require 40 to 60 mL/kg/d of water (may be as high as 100 mL/kg/d)
  * This is equivalent to 22 L/d for the average 450-kg (990 lb) horse.
* Basic fluid needs of equine neonates are 80 to 120 mL/kg/d.

Estimating existing losses

One method of estimating fluid needs and the effectiveness of fluid therapy is by serial measurement of body weight. When this is impractical, the horse's hydration status is estimated based on clinical signs associated with dehydration and on laboratory data.
* Table 4-1 lists guidelines for estimating the degree of dehydration from physical findings.
* In the absence of anemia, splenic contraction, and hypoproteinemia, the PCV and total protein increase by 5% to 10% and 1 g/dL, respectively, for each 2% to 3% increase in percent dehydration above 5%.
  To calculate the volume of fluid needed to correct dehydration use the following equation:

Liters of fluid needed = (Body weight in kilograms) × (% Dehydration)

Continued fluid losses must be taken into account and added to the volumes required for maintenance and for correction of dehydration.

Table 4-1
Estimation of water loss and dehydration based on clinical signs

Dehydration	% Water loss	Clinical signs
Mild	5-7	Depressed, dry mucous membranes, prolonged capillary refill time (2 seconds)
Moderate	8-10	Depressed, weak pulse; poor jugular distensibility; prolonged capillary refill time (2-4 seconds); decreased skin turgor, especially involving the eyelids; tachycardia
Severe	>10	Cold extremities, capillary refill time >5 seconds, recumbent, moribund, skin remains raised when pulled

Type of Fluid

For most conditions, isotonic polyionic fluid is the most appropriate and safest choice. If no electrolyte abnormalities are identified or suspected, the most commonly used fluid is acetated or lactated Ringer's solution.

Route of Administration

When selecting the route of administration, consider the following:
* volume of fluid to be administered
* type of fluid selected
* specific condition being treated
* availability of the route
* cost of fluids

Commonly used routes in horses include:
* *intravenous:* the most direct route; large volumes can be given rapidly, although the fluid must be sterile
* *subcutaneous:* rarely used because the volume that can be administered is limited
* *oral:* the horse must be (1) able to tolerate oral fluids *(do not use in a horse with gastric reflux),* (2) able to absorb the fluids, and (3) willing and able to either drink or receive the fluids via nasogastric tube
  * The volume intubated at one time is limited to 8 L q2-4h in adult horses.
  * The horse should be checked for excessive gastric fluid before fluid administration.
  * Oral fluids need not be isotonic; both hypertonic and hypotonic solutions are well tolerated, although excessively concentrated solutions may have an osmotic effect.

Rate of Intravenous Fluid Administration

The rate of administration depends on:
* the severity of the fluid loss (the disease being treated)
* the type of fluid needed
* the route of administration
* limitations dictated by correction of specific electrolyte abnormalities (see below)

Practical considerations
* When giving IV fluids by gravity flow, maximum rates of 10 to 20 mL/kg/h are achieved via a 16- or 14-gauge catheter.
* If this rate is insufficient to meet the horse's needs, fluid pumps or additional catheters may be used to increase the rate up to 40 to 80 mL/kg/h.
* Overzealous administration rates cause diuresis before adequate expansion of the extracellular fluid compartment and can result in pulmonary edema.

Monitoring Fluid Therapy

The most common method of evaluating the efficacy of and identifying problems associated with fluid therapy is by reassessing clinical signs and hydration status. Attention should be paid to:
* identification of continued fluid losses
* development of edema (subcutaneous and pulmonary edema)
* urine output
* measurement of temperature, pulse and respiratory rates, body weight and, where appropriate, central venous pressure

- serial measurements of PCV, total protein, creatinine, serum electrolytes, acid-base status, glucose, and calcium concentration
  - Serum total protein <4 g/dL accompanied by severe dehydration is best treated with concurrent administration of plasma.

COMMON ELECTROLYTE ABNORMALITIES

Sodium

Alterations in sodium concentration may lead to clinical signs (blindness, depression, seizures, ataxia) associated with cerebral edema or dehydration. These signs may develop at serum sodium concentrations <130 mEq/L or >150 mEq/L that persist for longer than 24 hours.

Hyponatremia

Hyponatremia is more common than hypernatremia.

- Colitis, renal failure, excessive sweating, and uroperitoneum are most often associated with hyponatremia and generally are accompanied by dehydration.
- The rate of development and degree of hyponatremia dictate the rate of sodium replacement.
  - If serum sodium is <120 mEq/L and signs of cerebral edema are evident, increase the sodium concentration to 125 mEq/L over 6 hours, using the following equation:

Na+ required (mEq) = (125 − patient's [Na+]) × 0.6 Body weight (kg)

  - Asymptomatic hyponatremia should be corrected slowly (increased by 12 mEq/L) over the first day.
- If the patient is volume depleted from GI or renal loss of sodium, isotonic saline or Ringer's solution (lactated or acetated) generally is appropriate for asymptomatic hyponatremia.
- Hyponatremia with a normal or increased ECF volume is uncommon in horses (may accompany excessive IV fluids or heart failure).
  - A diuretic (e.g., furosemide), along with sodium replacement and water restriction, may be needed.

Following are useful conversions:

- 1 g of NaCl = 17 mEq of Na+ and the same of Cl−
- 7.5 mL of salt in a syringe barrel = about 9 g of NaCl
- 9 g of salt in 1 L of water is isotonic

Hypernatremia

Hypernatremia (Na+ >160 mEq/L) is uncommon, but may occur iatrogenically or as a result of hypotonic water loss (e.g., colitis).

- Fluids deficient in Na+ must be given *slowly* to reduce the risk of cerebral edema.
  - To calculate the volume of water required to return Na+ to normal use the following equation:

Liters of water needed = [(Patient Na+/140) − 1] × 0.6 × Body weight (kg)

  - A value of 0.5 (instead of 0.6) may be more appropriate in volume-depleted patients.
- It is important to know if the hyponatremia is associated with a normal or decreased ECF volume, as occurs with diarrhea.
  - Dehydrated patients should receive 2.5% dextrose with 0.45% NaCl or 0.9% saline or Ringer's solution (lactated or acetated).
  - If the ECF volume is normal or increased (as can occur with renal failure), treatment also involves salt restriction and administration of diuretics.

Use of hypertonic saline

Creating hypernatremia may be transiently beneficial to horses in hypovolemic shock caused by acute hemorrhage or endotoxemia.

- Treatment with hypertonic saline (7% NaCl at 4 mL/kg) must be followed by administration of isotonic polyionic solutions.
- This therapy should not be used in patients with uncontrolled hemorrhage or those that have stabilized (with a lowered PCV) after acute blood loss.
- Hypertonic saline should be used judiciously in horses with preexisting sodium derangements.

Potassium

Hypokalemia

Hypokalemia commonly accompanies anorexia, acute GI diseases (especially colitis), excessive sweating, and renal disease.

+ Potassium should be supplemented when serum K^+ is <3 mEq/L, especially if the horse is anorectic.
+ It is also important to supplement potassium in acidotic horses when serum potassium is low or normal and an alkalinizing fluid is being administered.
+ KCl may be added to IV fluids (5 to 40 mEq K^+/L) and given at rate of 0.5 to 1 mEq/kg/h.
+ KCl may also be given orally at 5 to 40 g q6-12h.
  · Oral dosing with 10 g q6h is usually well tolerated.

Hyperkalemia

+ Hyperkalemia occurs in foals with uroperitoneum and in adult horses with periodic hyperkalemic paresis, renal failure, and, occasionally, acidosis.
+ Calcium gluconate may be given to offset the cardiotoxic effects of hyperkalemia.
+ Serum K^+ concentrations may be reduced by administering solutions of dextrose, $NaHCO_3$, or NaCl.

Chloride

Serum chloride tends to follow changes in serum sodium and is inversely related to the serum bicarbonate concentration.

+ The most common chloride derangement is hypochloremia caused by prolonged gastric reflux, excessive salivation or sweating, or intestinal loss associated with diarrhea.
+ Hypochloremic metabolic alkalosis is best treated with Ringer's solution or saline.

Acid-Base

Acid-base status is assessed by measuring blood gases, TCO_2, HCO_3^-, anion gap, and base deficit.

Anion gap

The anion gap is the calculated difference between measured cations and anions:

$$([Na^+] + [K^+]) - ([Cl^-] + [HCO_3^-])$$

+ It normally is 10 to 20 mEq/L.
+ The most common cause for increased anion gap is lactic acidosis

secondary to endotoxic or hypovolemic shock.

Metabolic acidosis

Metabolic acidosis is the most common acid-base derangement in horses. It occurs with lactic acidosis, hypovolemia, diarrhea, sepsis, endotoxemia, and renal failure.

The bicarbonate deficit in mEq is calculated as follows:

$$HCO_3^- \text{ deficit} = \text{Base deficit} \times ECF \times \text{Body weight (kg)}$$

The value for ECF is 0.3 in adults and 0.5 in neonates.

+ Mild metabolic acidosis can be treated with lactated or acetated Ringer's solution (both supply 27 mEq/L of bicarbonate).
+ If the base deficit is >10 to 15 mEq/L (serum $[HCO_3^-]$ <15 mEq/L), sodium bicarbonate should be administered.
  · Additional potassium should be administered if serum potassium is low or normal.
+ Paradoxical cerebral acidosis may occur if metabolic acidosis is corrected too rapidly.
  · Common practice is to replace half the deficit initially and the remainder over 24 hours
+ It is important to estimate continued losses and account for these with additional therapy.
  · In colitis cases, it may be necessary to supply 2 to 3 times the estimated deficit to account for continued loss.
+ Bicarbonate should not be added to fluids containing calcium (causes precipitation).
+ Bicarbonate can be replaced orally, but care should be taken to avoid administration of large amounts at a single time (may cause acute gastric distension and colic).
  · Up to 150 g of sodium bicarbonate can be given orally qh8 without ill effect.

Following are some useful conversions:

+ 1 g sodium bicarbonate = 12 mEq HCO_3^- and 12 mEq Na^+1 "mL" of baking soda in a syringe barrel = 1 g of sodium bicarbonate
+ isotonic bicarbonate = 1.3% = 13 g/L

Metabolic alkalosis

Metabolic alkalosis can occur in horses with heat stress or overexertion.

- Alkalosis decreases serum ionized calcium, so signs of hypocalcemia may be more apparent.
- Treatment involves identification and correction of the underlying problem.
- Fluid therapy involves administration of Ringer's solution, 5% dextrose, or normal saline.

Calcium

Hypocalcemia in horses may be caused by acute GI disease, exertion, lactation tetany, blister beetle toxicosis, alkalosis, and, less commonly, renal failure.

- Significant hypocalcemia causes clinical signs of ileus, tetany, or thumps (synchronous diaphragmatic flutter).
- Measurements of serum total calcium are influenced by albumin concentration and the acid-base status.
  - Protein-bound calcium decreases as the concentration of albumin decreases.
  - Serum ionized calcium increases with acidosis.
- The amount of calcium needed to treat an adult horse with hypocalcemia is 100 to 500 mL (or 0.25 to 1 mL/kg) of a 23% calcium gluconate solution IV.
  - If the horse's calcium status is unknown, it is best to dilute the calcium gluconate and monitor heart rate and rhythm during treatment.
- Calcium should not be added to solutions containing bicarbonate.

Glucose

Glucose is an important component of fluid therapy in neonates.

- It usually is administered as a 5% solution if serum glucose is <80 mg/dL.
  - 5% glucose can be safely given at 3 to 5 mL/kg/h.
- If severe hypoglycemia (<30 mg/dL) is encountered, a 10% dextrose solution (10 mL/kg for several minutes) may be used to rapidly raise serum glucose to 80 mg/dL.

- Continuous infusion of isotonic (5%) dextrose is more beneficial than intermittent boluses of hypertonic solutions and less irritating to the vein.
  - Blood or urine glucose should be monitored, and, if >250 or 500 mg/dL, respectively, the administration rate should be decreased.
- Supplementation may be required in adult horses with liver failure, lipemia, or fatty liver.
  - 5% dextrose is administered at 2 to 3 mL/kg/h (about 1 L/h).
  - Glucose may also be included in the treatment of hyperkalemia and to induce diuresis (solutions of 5% to 15%).

Blood and Blood Component Therapy

(pages 152-154)
Chrysann Collatos

WHOLE BLOOD TRANSFUSION
Indications and Precautions

Transfusion may be warranted:

- after accidental or surgical trauma resulting in acute, severe blood loss
- in the treatment of hemolytic processes such as red maple toxicity and neonatal isoerythrolysis
  Transfusion should be avoided unless absolutely necessary.
- Transfused erythrocytes suppress the host's bone marrow response to anemia.
- Transfused cells survive only 4 to 6 days.
- Adverse transfusion reactions are possible, and sensitization to heterologous donor RBC antigens is likely.
  If transfusion is not possible or advisable in a patient with clinical signs of whole blood loss, then volume expansion with isotonic or hypertonic fluid should be initiated.

Criteria for Transfusion
Clinical signs

Clinical signs of acute blood loss that may prompt transfusion include:

- increased heart and respiratory rates—transfusion may be warranted when the respiratory rate is >40

breaths/min and the heart rate is >80 beats/min
* generalized weakness
* mucous membrane pallor
* poor peripheral pulses

Laboratory data
* With external hemorrhage, both the PCV and plasma protein decrease.
  * These findings lag 12 to 24 hours behind acute hemorrhage.
* Horses with hemolytic anemia do not have volume depletion, and plasma protein is normal.
  * Icterus may be present, along with tachycardia, tachypnea, and weakness.
* In general, transfusion is indicated when the PCV drops below 12% (acute blood loss or hemolysis) or 8% (chronic blood loss).

Volume to Transfuse
Whole blood usually is transfused at a dose of 15 mL/kg.
* The average adult horse requires 6 to 8 L of transfused blood.
* The transfusion volume should not exceed 20% of blood volume (which is 8% of body weight).
* Volume overload may occur in smaller patients.
  * Foals with neonatal isoerythrolysis generally have a normal intravascular volume.
  * Packed RBCs (harvested following gravity sedimentation and resuspended in a small volume of isotonic saline) should be considered in these patients.
  * Bovine hemoglobin is an alternative.

Donor Selection
A suitable equine whole blood donor:
* weighs at least 450 kg (990 lb)
  * A 500-kg (1100 lb) horse with a PCV of 35% to 40% can safely give 8 L of blood every 30 days.
* has a normal PCV and plasma protein concentration
* has negative equine infectious anemia serology (Coggins' test)
* has never received a transfusion
* if female, should be a maiden mare
* should be Aa and Qa alloantigen negative

* should be negative for alloantibodies, particularly those directed against alloantigen Aa
  If no compatibility testing is possible and the donor blood type is unknown, a close relative to the recipient that meets the first five criteria is a good donor candidate.

Crossmatching
Ideally, compatibility testing should precede transfusion.
* Major cross match combines donor erythrocytes with recipient serum.
* Minor cross match combines donor serum with recipient erythrocytes.
* Incompatibility is indicated by agglutination.
* Hemolyzing antibodies are most likely to cause a severe transfusion reaction and may not be detected by routine agglutination cross match.

Blood Collection
Transfer systems specifically designed for large animal blood collection are commercially available. Alternatively, sterile 3-L IV fluid bags can be used. Acid-citrate-dextrose (ACD) or citrate-phosphate-dextrose (CPD) are recommended anticoagulants. Heparin (5 to 10 U/mL) and sodium citrate solutions can be used in an emergency.

ACD stock solution
ACD stock solution can be made with the following recipe:
  11 g dextrose (22 mL of 50% dextrose)
  9.9 g sodium citrate
  3.3 g citric acid
  Mix with distilled water to 300 mL.
  The solution is autoclaved and stored at room temperature. A 300-mL aliquot is added to a 3-L collection bag to provide a 1:9 ratio with blood. Whole blood in ACD can be stored refrigerated (4° C [39° F]) for up to 3 weeks.

Blood Administration
Blood is delivered at 0.1 mL/kg (slow drip) for 10 min while the patient is monitored for signs of adverse reaction, which may include:
* tachypnea, tachycardia
* trembling, restlessness
* urticaria
* sudden collapse

If no signs of adverse reaction are seen, the infusion rate is increased to 20 mL/kg/h and continued, with gentle and frequent mixing of blood, throughout administration.

Managing adverse reactions

If signs of adverse reaction occur:

* stop the transfusion
* administer flunixin meglumine 1.1 mg/kg IV
* wait 15 min; if signs abate, recommence transfusion at a slower rate in cases of severe reaction, consider:
* epinephrine (0.01 to 0.02 mL/kg at 1:1000, IM)
* high-volume IV polyionic fluids
* prednisolone sodium succinate 4.5 mg/kg IV

PLASMA TRANSFUSION

Indications for plasma transfusion include:

* neonatal failure of passive transfer
* severe hypoalbuminemia secondary to protein-losing enteropathy
* prevention of *R. equi* pneumonia in foals (hyperimmune plasma)
* treatment of acute endotoxemia (hyperimmune plasma)

Sources

Commercially prepared plasma is recommended for most practice settings. Plasma collection is also possible in a field setting.

* Whole blood is collected and hung for 2 hours.
* Plasma is then siphoned or decanted from the settled red cells.
* The plasma can be stored frozen at 0° C (32° F) for at least 1 year.

Administration

Infusion volume

* *foals:* 1 to 2 L of high-quality plasma usually is required to increase IgG to an acceptable range in foals with failure of passive transfer of antibodies.
* *adult horses:* At least 6 to 8 L of plasma is required to increase the total protein 5 to 10 g/L in horses with clinically significant hypoproteinemia.

Transfusion reaction

* Transfusion reaction is uncommon with plasma; however, recipients

may develop antibodies against foreign proteins in the plasma, increasing the likelihood of reaction with repeated transfusion.

* Sensitization to RBC alloantigens of the plasma donor is possible (unless the plasma was obtained by plasmapheresis).
  * In fillies or mares that received a plasma transfusion, cross matching with the intended stallion should be recommended before breeding.

ALTERNATIVE BLOOD PRODUCTS

Blood Components

Platelet-enriched plasma may be useful for treatment of immune-mediated thrombocytopenia. Fresh frozen plasma (separated and frozen within 6 hours) and cryoprecipitate (precipitate separated from fresh frozen plasma thawed at 4°C [39° F]) can be used as a source of clotting factors for animals with inherited or acquired (DIC) coagulation defects.

Growth Factors

Treatment of diseases characterized by leukopenia or neutropenia (e.g., ischemic GI lesions, neonatal septicemia) using granulocyte colony-stimulating factor has been investigated, with promising initial results.

Antiinflammatory Drug Therapy in Horses

(pages 155-163)

Rustin M. Moore

NONSTEROIDAL ANTIINFLAMMATORY DRUGS

Mechanism of Action

Nonsteroidal antiinflammatory drugs (NSAIDs) inhibit the production of prostaglandins and thromboxanes from arachidonic acid by inhibiting cyclooxygenase. Many of the actions attributed to NSAIDs are dose dependent; higher doses are necessary to reduce inflammation than are required to simply inhibit prostaglandin synthesis.

Therapeutic Uses

NSAIDs are indicated:

* in horses with inflammatory musculoskeletal conditions such as myositis, tendinitis, laminitis, osteoarthritis, septic arthritis, and surgically induced trauma
* for pretreatment of horses predisposed to developing endotoxemia or treatment of horses with suspected endotoxemia (to prevent endotoxic shock)
* for visceral analgesia in horses with acute abdominal pain
* for control of postoperative pain and prevention of excessive edema formation

Therapeutic differences among NSAIDs

There are differences in efficacy among the various NSAIDs, depending on the condition being treated.

* Phenylbutazone is more effective than flunixin meglumine in most horses with musculoskeletal disease.
  * It is more selective than flunixin meglumine in blocking the inhibitory effect of endotoxin on GI motility (at 2.2 mg/kg IV q12h).
* Flunixin meglumine is more effective than phenylbutazone in horses with colic or ocular pain.
  * It effectively inhibits the cardiovascular effects of endotoxin at low doses (0.25 mg/kg IV).
* Aspirin is most effective as an antithrombotic agent.
  * Platelet aggregation is inhibited for at least 7 days after a single oral dose of 20 mg/kg.
  * It may be useful for treatment or prophylaxis of thrombophlebitis, laminitis, intestinal ischemia, and nonstrangulating infarction.
  * Dipyrone is a potent antipyretic, but has only mild analgesic properties.

Toxicity

The two major toxic effects of NSAIDs are gastrointestinal ulceration and renal papillary necrosis. The toxic potential is greatest for phenylbutazone, less for flunixin, and least for ketoprofen and naproxen. Young animals are especially sensitive to the adverse effects of NSAIDs, and ponies are more susceptible than horses to the toxic effects of phenylbutazone.

Gastrointestinal ulceration

Administration of NSAIDs in excessive doses, for prolonged periods, or in the presence of dehydration or volume depletion can lead to ulceration of the gastric glandular or large colon mucosa.

* Ulceration is often accompanied by secondary anemia and hypoproteinemia (blood and plasma protein loss).
* Young horses are especially predisposed to gastric ulceration.
* Adult horses more commonly develop ulceration of the right dorsal colon, which results in abdominal pain, diarrhea, and protein-losing enteropathy.
  * Most reported cases have been in horses given phenylbutazone.

Renal toxicity

NSAID-induced papillary necrosis can occur with conditions that cause renal vasoconstriction, such as dehydration, volume depletion, and shock.

* Fluid volume should be normalized before (or during) NSAID therapy.
* Concurrent administration of aminoglycosides increases the risk of nephrotoxicity.

Other potential effects

* phlebitis/thrombophlebitis
  * Perivascular injection of phenylbutazone causes an intense phlebitis and necrosis.
  * Excessive doses of phenylbutazone can cause degeneration and dilation of the walls of small veins.
* suppression of cartilage repair—in general, NSAIDs have a suppressive effect on proteoglycan synthesis

Combination therapy

Because all NSAIDs have a similar mechanism of action, combination therapy can increase the potential for toxicity. Therefore it is important to adjust the dose of each NSAID administered in combination and to maintain hydration.

Pharmacokinetics

Following are some clinically useful facts:

* Orally administered NSAIDs bind to hay and other digesta, which can

Table 4-2
Recommended dosage regimens for antiinflammatory drugs in horses*

Drug	Route	Formulation	Dose	Duration
Acetylsalicylic acid (aspirin)	PO	Tablets, powder	25-35 mg/kg bid 5-50 mg/kg sid	
Dipyrone	IV, IM	Injectable	5-22 mg/kg 11.1 mg/kg qid	
Flunixin meglumine	IV, IM	Injectable	1.1 mg/kg sid-bid 0.25 mg/kg tid	≤5 days
	PO	Granules, paste	1.1 mg/kg sid-bid	
Ketoprofen	IV	Injectable	2.2 mg/kg sid	
Meclofenamic acid	PO	Granules	2.2 mg/kg sid then qod	5-7 days
Naproxen	PO	Granules	10 mg/kg bid then sid	≤14 days
Phenylbutazone	PO	Tablets, powder, paste	4.4 mg/kg bid 2.2 mg/kg bid 2.2 mg/kg sid	1 day 4 days 2 days
	IV	Injectable	2.2-4.4 mg/kg sid 4.2 mg/kg sid	≤5 days ≤4 days
Prednisolone sodium succinate	IV	Injectable	1-2 mg/kg	
Dexamethasone	IV, IM	Injectable	0.05-0.20 mg/kg	
Methylprednisolone acetate	IM	Injectable	2-4 mg/kg	Repeat as necessary
	IA	Injectable	20-240 mg/kg	
Triamcinolone acetonide	IV, IM	Injectable	0.05-0.20 mg/kg	
	IA	Injectable	6-18 mg/kg	
Dimethyl sulfoxide	IV	Injectable	0.1-1 g/kg of 10% solution	

Modified from Kallings P: *Vet Clin North Am Equine Pract* 9:523-541, 1993; Ferguson DC, Hoenig M. In Adams HR, ed: *Veterinary pharmacology and therapeutics,* Ames, Iowa, 1995, Iowa State University Press.
*Dosages are based on normal horses; may need to adjust dosages if horses are ill, dehydrated, or volume depleted or if administering NSAIDs in combination. Ponies and foals may require lower dosages.

delay the time to peak plasma concentration by 6 to 12 hours.
- NSAIDs administered to lactating mares are not excreted in milk in concentrations that yield measurable plasma levels in foals.
- Concurrent administration of other highly protein-bound drugs (e.g., chloramphenicol, thiobarbiturates) may cause displacement of the NSAID, which accentuates both its therapeutic and toxic effects.
- Neonates have a reduced ability to eliminate phenylbutazone, so the dosage must be adjusted accordingly.

The dose, interval, and route of administration for NSAIDs commonly used in horses are given in Table 4-2.

GLUCOCORTICOID THERAPY
Mechanisms of Action
Glucocorticoids exert their antiinflammatory effects by inhibiting membrane-bound phospholipase A_2, thereby inhibiting the release of arachidonic acid and production of inflammatory mediators including prostaglandins, thromboxanes, leukotrienes, and platelet activating factor.

Formulations
Parenteral formulations
- *rapid onset (<1 min) and short duration ($t_{1/2} = 1$ to 2 hours):* prednisolone sodium succinate, methylprednisolone sodium succinate

- *rapid onset (5 to 45 min) and intermediate duration ($t_{1/2}$ = 3 to 4 hours):* dexamethasone sodium phosphate or dexamethasone in propylene glycol
- *slow onset and long duration:* triamcinolone acetonide, methylprednisolone acetate, flumethasone

Oral formulations

- *rapid onset and short duration:* prednisone tablets
- *rapid onset and short-to-intermediate duration:* triamcinolone tablets or powder
- *slow onset and long duration:* dexamethasone tablets or powder

The dose, interval, and route of administration for corticosteroids commonly used in horses are given in Table 4-2.

Therapeutic Uses

Allergic disease

- *chronic obstructive pulmonary disease (COPD):* corticosteroids may be administered parenterally, orally, or via inhalation
  - Typically, initial therapy (e.g., dexamethasone) is given parenterally and maintenance therapy (e.g., prednisolone) is given per os.
- *allergic skin disease:* treatment often involves oral prednisone

Shock

Glucocorticoids can improve hemodynamic variables and increase survival in animals in endotoxic or hemorrhagic shock.

- Corticosteroids must be administered before or very early after the onset of shock to be beneficial.
- Short-term (<48 hours) use has relatively few side effects, and the potential benefits outweigh the risks.
- Typically, prednisolone sodium succinate or dexamethasone is administered IV.

Central nervous system disease

Corticosteroids often are administered to horses with traumatic or inflammatory CNS conditions.

- Injuries to the head or vertebral column and herpes myeloencephalopathy are the two most common types of CNS disease treated with corticosteroids.

- Chronic therapy with corticosteroids generally is contraindicated in horses with equine protozoal myeloencephalitis, although short-term administration can be beneficial in cases with rapidly deteriorating CNS signs.
  - Concurrent administration of appropriate antiprotozoal drugs is essential.
- Corticosteroids must be administered early in the course of disease to be beneficial.
- Dexamethasone (0.1 to 0.2 mg/kg IV or IM, q6-12h) is most commonly used.
  - The dosage is decreased to once daily after the first 24 hours and then gradually tapered over a few days.

Joint disease

Intraarticular injection of corticosteroids is effective in treating synovitis and arthritis.

- Aseptic technique is essential to prevent joint infection.
- Formulations approved for intraarticular use include triamcinolone acetonide, isoflupredone acetate, betamethasone acetate, methylprednisolone acetate, and flumethasone.

Adverse Effects of Intraarticular Corticosteroids

Detrimental effects of intraarticular corticosteroids include:

- decreased cartilage elasticity and glycosaminoglycan content, leading to progressive cartilage degeneration (thinning and fissuring)
- formation of calcium deposits on the surface of hyaline cartilage
- decreased synovial fluid viscosity and hyaluronic acid content

Clinically, the predominant adverse effects include:

- steroid arthropathy (see next section)
- postinjection flare—a nonseptic inflammatory response that causes joint heat, swelling, and pain
  - It can begin as early as a few hours after injection and may last for a few hours to several days.
- septic arthritis
- osseous metaplasia—can occur after inadvertent deposition of long-

acting corticosteroids in periarticular soft tissues
- Ossification may take several months to develop; mechanical interference can occur with large lesions.

Steroid arthropathy

Steroid arthropathy is characterized by:
- an increased rate of joint damage
  - Reduction of pain and inflammation allows continued strenuous exercise, thereby exacerbating degenerative joint disease.
- radiographic evidence of severe degenerative joint disease
- joint enlargement (capsular distention)
- osteophytic new bone growth
- decreased range of motion
- crepitation

This condition usually occurs in joints that already have appreciable cartilage damage and in those not rested sufficiently after injection. Corticosteroids administered at high doses or frequent intervals are more likely to cause this arthropathy.

Adverse Systemic Effects of Corticosteroids

Administration of corticosteroids in high doses or for extended periods can lead to adverse systemic effects, including:
- iatrogenic Cushing's syndrome
  - Adrenal insufficiency can occur on withdrawal of corticosteroids (prolonged use).
- immune suppression
- laminitis
  - Glucocorticoids sensitize vascular smooth muscle to the effects of catecholamines, thereby potentiating vasoconstriction.
  - Laminitis reportedly is more common with triamcinolone.

DIMETHYL SULFOXIDE

Mechanisms of Action and Pharmacologic Effects

Dimethyl sulfoxide (DMSO) is believed to exert its antiinflammatory action principally by scavenging hydroxyl radicals. Other pharmacologic effects include:
- immunomodulation—inhibition of leukocyte adhesion and migration, antibody production, and fibroblast proliferation
- modulation of enzyme activity
- vasodilatation (histamine-mediated)
- inhibition of platelet aggregation
- cryopreservation
- antimicrobial activity
- diuresis
- analgesia (exact mechanism unknown)

Pharmacokinetics

Plasma concentrations peak within 4 to 6 hours after *oral* administration of 1 g/kg; detectable plasma concentrations persist for up to 2 weeks. Following *topical* application, DMSO can be detected in all tissues within 20 min; the plasma concentration peaks in 2 hours.

Therapeutic Uses

Musculoskeletal injury

Traumatic or inflammatory musculoskeletal conditions often are treated with IV or topical DMSO. Exertional or anesthetic-associated rhabdomyolysis may also be treated with parenteral or topical DMSO.

CNS disease

- Traumatic injuries or inflammatory conditions involving the brain or spinal cord often are treated with IV DMSO.
- Peripheral nervous system (PNS) diseases, such as pressure-induced neuropathies, also are treated with DMSO.
- A common recommendation in horses with CNS or PNS disease is 1 g/kg IV, as a 10% solution in 5% dextrose or 0.9% saline.
  - This dose is given once or twice daily for the first 3 days, then three additional treatments are given either daily or on alternate days.

Other conditions

- *infected synovial structures:* DMSO occasionally is used for lavage.
- *laminitis:* DMSO often is administered IV or topically (over the coronary bands) to horses with acute laminitis.

Adverse Effects

DMSO has a wide margin of safety; however, toxicity can occur. Signs

associated with near-lethal IV doses
include:

* sedation
* diuresis
* intravascular hemolysis—dependent
  on the concentration and the rapidity of administration
* hematuria—may lead to nephropathy
  Ocular toxicity, typically involving
the lens, can occur with long-term
daily administration; it is more
common in young animals.

Antimicrobial Therapy in Horses *(pages 163-175)*

Rustin M. Moore

ANTIBIOTIC CLASSIFICATION
Inhibition of Cell Wall Synthesis

Penicillins and cephalosporins are the
two major categories of antibiotics
that interfere with bacterial cell wall
synthesis. Only bacteria that are undergoing active growth are affected by
such antibiotics.

Penicillins

Penicillins have a wide spectrum of
activity against numerous pathogenic
bacteria commonly isolated from
horses. Other than bacterial resistance
and occasional hypersensitivity, the
only limitation to their use is their
relatively poor systemic absorption
after oral administration.

Penicillin G:

* The *crystalline* salt of potassium or
  sodium is used when a rapid effect
  and high plasma concentration are
  desired.
  * IM injection results in slightly
    lower concentrations, but a
    longer duration of action, than
    IV administration.
* *Procaine* penicillin G is formulated
  only for IM administration and is
  absorbed relatively slowly.
  * Occasionally, horses have an ana-
    phylactic-like reaction to the pro-
    caine when injected in or near a
    blood vessel.
  * Some jurisdictions require with-
    drawal for 10 to 14 days before
    performance (showing or racing).
* *Benzathine* penicillin G provides
  slower absorption IM and results

in relatively low peak serum concentrations.
  * It generally is not useful in
    horses, but can be effective
    against very susceptible organ-
    isms or infections involving the
    urinary tract.

Semisynthetic penicillins:

* Semisynthetic penicillins include
  methicillin, oxacillin, nafcillin,
  cloxacillin, and dicloxacillin.
* They are penicillinase-resistant,
  so their primary indication is for
  treatment of infection caused
  by penicillinase-producing
  staphylococci.

Extended-spectrum penicillins:

* Extended-spectrum penicillins include ampicillin, amoxicillin, carbenicillin, ticarcillin, mezlocillin,
  azlocillin, and piperacillin.
* They have activity against some
  gram-negative bacteria but not
  against penicillinase-producing
  bacteria.
  * *Ampicillin* generally is less effec-
    tive than penicillin G against
    streptococci and clostridia.
  * Sodium ampicillin is the recom-
    mended formulation, and is
    given IV or IM.
  * Ampicillin has been associated
    with drug-induced diarrhea.
  * *Carbenicillin* and *ticarcillin* have an
    antibacterial spectrum similar to
    ampicillin.
  * Certain strains of *Pseudomonas
    aeruginosa, Proteus* spp., and *En-
    terobacter* spp. are susceptible;
    ticarcillin is more effective
    against *P. aeruginosa.*
  * These drugs often are used for
    intrauterine administration in
    mares.

Cephalosporins

Cephalosporins are semisynthetic
β-lactam drugs with similar structure
and mechanism of action to
penicillins.

* They are resistant to penicillinase
  but are susceptible to other
  β-lactamases.
* *First-generation* cephalosporins have
  a similar spectrum of activity.
  * Susceptible bacteria generally in-
    clude penicillinase-producing
    staphylococci, *Klebsiella* spp.,
    most streptococci other than ente-

rococci, and most obligate anaerobes (except *Bacteroides fragilis).*
- They include cephalothin,
cephapirin, cephradine, cefazolin, and cephaloridine.
- *Second-generation* cephalosporins
have a greater activity against Enterobacteriaceae and other gram-
negative bacilli, but they generally
are less effective against gram-positive bacteria, compared with first-
generation bacteria.
  - They include cefamandole and
cefoxitin.
- *Third-generation* cephalosporins
have greater affinity for gram-negative bacteria and are less effective
against gram-positive organisms
compared with first- and second-
generation cephalosporins.
  - They include cefotaxime, mox-
alactam, and ceftiofur.
- Cephalosporins are rapidly eliminated following IV injection; IM
administration provides a longer
duration of action.
- These drugs should be avoided in
horses with a history of allergic response to cephalosporins or severe, immediate hypersensitivity
to penicillins.
- Because cephalosporins will induce
production of β-lactamase by bacteria, *they should not be used in combination with penicillins.*
  Ceftiofur sodium:
- Ceftiofur sodium is the most commonly used cephalosporin in
horses.
- It is a β-lactamase–resistant antibiotic with potent antimicrobial activity against many gram-positive
and gram-negative bacterial
pathogens in horses.
- It is administered either IV or IM,
once or twice daily.
- Diarrhea has been reported when
ceftiofur is administered IV more
than twice daily.

Inhibition of Protein Synthesis

Antibiotics that inhibit protein synthesis can be divided into two main
categories: reversible inhibition or irreversible inhibition.

Chloramphenicol
- Chloramphenicol reversibly inhibits bacterial protein synthesis.

- It distributes into aqueous humor,
CNS, and pleural, peritoneal, and
synovial fluids, where it attains therapeutic intracellular concentrations.
- Chloramphenicol often is useful
for treating salmonellosis and
anaerobic infections.
- Bacterial resistance can develop.
- Chloramphenicol has been used
safely in horses, but can have toxic
(lethal) effects in humans.
  - It should not be administered to
horses intended for food.

Erythromycin
- Erythromycin is a macrolide antibiotic that reversibly inhibits bacterial protein synthesis.
- It distributes widely in the body,
including intracellular sites, and
tissue concentrations generally exceed serum concentrations.
- The major indication is treatment
of *R. equi* infection in foals, in
which case it usually is used in
combination with rifampin.
- Although the incidence is low, diarrhea is a potential side effect.
- Erythromycin should not be used in
combination with chloramphenicol.

Oxytetracycline
- Oxytetracycline is a bacteriostatic
antibiotic that reversibly inhibits
protein synthesis.
- Its spectrum of activity includes
many gram-positive and gram-negative bacteria and *Rickettsia, Mycoplasma,* and *Ehrlichia* organisms.
- Oxytetracycline distributes into
synovial and peritoneal fluids,
lung, bronchial fluid, and renal tissues and reaches high concentrations in equine urine.
- Bacterial resistance can develop.
- The main indication is treatment of
Potomac horse fever (*Ehrlichia risticii* infection).
- It also is commonly used to treat
respiratory infections in foals and
racehorses.
- In stressed animals, severe, potentially lethal diarrhea can develop
that may be associated with proliferation of pathogens such as
Clostridium perfringens type A and
Salmonella typhimurium.
- Renal tubular necrosis and hepatic
fatty degeneration have been reported.

- These effects are related to the dose and duration of treatment.
- The nephrotoxicity of tetracyclines is potentiated by endotoxin.

Aminoglycosides

- Aminoglycosides irreversibly inhibit bacterial protein synthesis.
- They include streptomycin, kanamycin, neomycin, gentamicin, amikacin, and tobramycin.
- Aminoglycosides must be administered parenterally to achieve systemic therapeutic concentrations.
  - Gentamicin does not attain appreciable intracellular concentrations.
- These drugs are most effective at an alkaline pH and in an aerobic environment
  - They may be inadequate in the presence of purulent material or necrotic tissue debris.
  - Anaerobic organisms are not susceptible because bacterial uptake of aminoglycosides is oxygen dependent.
  - Anaerobic conditions prevent the action of these drugs on bacteria that would otherwise be susceptible in an aerobic environment.
- Effective urine concentrations are attainable at doses that would be ineffective against systemic infections caused by the same organisms.
- Aminoglycosides are indicated in the initial treatment of life-threatening infections caused by gram-negative aerobic bacteria.
  - Gentamicin usually is the drug of choice, unless resistance is suspected or documented.
  - Amikacin is used when resistance to gentamicin occurs.
- The major toxic effects of aminoglycosides are nephrotoxicity, neuromuscular blockade (generally with concurrent use of anesthetic agents), and ototoxicity.
  - Nephrotoxicity is the major side effect and is related to the plasma drug concentration.
  - It can be potentiated by hypotension, loop diuretics, presence of other nephrotoxic agents, and age.
- Therapeutic drug monitoring should be used in patients with compromised renal function (see pp. 55-56).

Inhibition of Nucleic Acid Synthesis

Rifampin

- Rifampin is administered orally.
- It readily distributes to intracellular and extracellular sites, including CSF.
- Resistance to rifampin develops rapidly, so the drug must always be administered in combination with another antibiotic that is also effective against the offending organism.
- The principal use is for treatment of *R. equi* infection in foals, in combination with erythromycin.
- Clients should be informed that administration of rifampin may lead to an orange-red color to the urine, feces, saliva, sputum, tears, and sweat.

Metronidazole

- Metronidazole's antibacterial spectrum is limited to anaerobic and microaerophilic organisms.
- It is most useful in horses with infection caused by *B. fragilis.*
- Anorexia is a potential problem associated with oral metronidazole administration.

Fluoroquinolones

- Fluoroquinolones are bactericidal even when bacteria are in a stationary growth phase.
- These drugs readily penetrate phagocytic cells and have an appreciable postantibiotic effect.
- Fluoroquinolones have a relatively wide spectrum of activity with excellent activity against Enterobacteriaceae spp., *Pseudomonas* spp., and *Actinobacillus* spp.
  - They also have good activity against *Staphylococcus aureus* and *S. epidermidis*
  - They have variable activity against streptococci.
  - Anaerobic bacteria are considered resistant.
- Therapeutic concentrations are achieved in kidneys, liver, bile, prostate, female genital tract, skin, bone, body fluids, and CSF.
  - Urinary drug concentrations can be 100 to 300 times greater than serum concentrations.
- Enrofloxacin has good bioavailability following oral administra-

tion in horses, but ciprofloxacin does not.

- No plasmid resistance has been demonstrated, and the frequency of resistant mutants is low.
- Fluoroquinolones are antagonized by the actions of chloramphenicol and rifampin.
- The most significant adverse effect is articular cartilage damage in young animals.

Inhibition of Intermediary Metabolism

Sulfonamides and trimethoprim

- Sulfonamides and trimethoprim inhibit bacterial folate synthesis and metabolism.
- Trimethoprim and sulfadiazine readily enter synovial and peritoneal fluid following IV administration.
  - They also penetrate the blood-brain barrier when meningitis is present and achieve therapeutic concentrations in CSF.
- Trimethoprim and sulfonamides can be rendered inactive by cellular debris.

- Resistance is sufficiently common that susceptibility testing should be used to guide therapy.
- The major toxic effects of trimethoprim-sulfonamide combinations are leukopenia, anemia, and diarrhea.

CRITERIA FOR SELECTION OF ANTIBIOTICS

Criteria to be considered when selecting an antibiotic regimen in horses include:

- the presence or likelihood of an infectious process
- type of infectious process
- bacteria most likely to be isolated (see Table 4-3)
- age and immune status of the animal
- antibiotic characteristics
  - The bacteria must be susceptible to the drug's mechanism of action.
  - An appropriate concentration of drug must be achieved at the site of infection and maintained for a sufficient time to kill the organisms.

Table 4-3
Bacterial pathogens commonly isolated from horses with infectious processes affecting various body sites

Type of infection	Bacterial isolates
Pneumonia/ pleuropneumonia	E. coli, Actinobacillus spp., S. zooepidemicus, obligate anaerobes
Cellulitis	S. aureus, Clostridium spp.
Surgical wounds	β-Hemolytic streptococci, staphylococci, Enterobacteriaceae, Pseudomonas spp.
Traumatic wounds	Pseudomonas spp., streptococci
Iatrogenic septic arthritis	Coagulase-positive staphylococci
Traumatic septic arthritis	Hemolytic streptococci, staphylococci, Enterobacteriaceae, Pseudomonas spp.
Osteomyelitis	Hemolytic streptococci, staphylococci, Enterobacteriaceae, Pseudomonas spp.
Cystitis/pyelonephritis	Enterobacteriaceae, Corynebacterium renale
Uterine	β-Hemolytic streptococci, Enterobacteriaceae, Pseudomonas spp.
Peritonitis/abdominal abscess	β-Hemolytic streptococci, anaerobes, Enterobacteriaceae, R. equi
Enterocolitis	Salmonella spp., Clostridium spp.
Corneal	S. aureus, S. zooepidemicus, Pseudomonas spp.

- The microenvironment at the site of infection must be favorable for the antibiotic's action.
- cost of antibiotics
- ease of administration
- potential toxic effects

Table 4-4 lists antibiotics recommended for specific pathogens, and Table 4-5 lists drug dosages and regimens.

PROPHYLACTIC ANTIBIOTIC USE

Prophylactic antibiotics typically are administered perioperatively, although antibiotics are not always necessary in patients undergoing surgery.

Guidelines for Prophylactic Antibiotic Use

Preoperative antibiotics should only be used for procedures with a high rate of postoperative infection or in high-risk patients. They are indicated for:

- all clean-contaminated, contaminated, or dirty surgical wounds (i.e., when the GI, respiratory, or urogenital tract is entered, or when devitalized or exudative tissue is encountered)
- clean surgical wounds involving an implant or prosthesis
- any situation in which development of an infection is considered life-threatening

Table 4-4
Recommended antibiotics for specific pathogens isolated from horses with infectious disease processes

Bacteria	Initial antibiotic choice	Alternative choices
Actinobacillus spp.	Trimethoprim-sulfonamides	Chloramphenicol, cephalothin, gentamicin
Rhodococcus equi	Erythromycin	Erythromycin and rifampin, trimethoprim-sulfonamides, chloramphenicol
Escherichia coli	Gentamicin	Amikacin, extended-spectrum penicillins, cephalosporins, trimethoprim-sulfonamides
Klebsiella spp.	Amikacin	Trimethoprim-sulfonamides, gentamicin, extended-spectrum penicillins, cephalosporins
Enterobacter spp.	Gentamicin	Amikacin, chloramphenicol
Salmonella spp.	Trimethoprim-sulfonamides	Gentamicin, amikacin, chloramphenicol, ampicillin
Pseudomonas spp.	Gentamicin	Amikacin, ticarcillan, trimethoprim-sulfonamides, polymyxin B
Coagulase-positive staphylococci	Trimethoprim-sulfonamides	Methicillin, oxacillin, cephalosporin, aminoglycoside
Coagulase-negative staphylococci	Gentamicin	Amikacin, cephalosporin
Hemolytic streptococci	Penicillin G	Trimethoprim-sulfonamides, ampicillin, cephalosporins, chloramphenicol, erythromycin
Nonhemolytic streptococci	Chloramphenicol	Erythromycin, ampicillin
Anaerobes		
Bacteroides fragilis	Metronidazole	Chloramphenicol
Bacteroides spp.	Penicillin	Chloramphenicol, metronidazole
Clostridium spp.	Penicillin	Chloramphenicol, metronidazole
Fusobacterium necrophorum	Trimethoprim-sulfonamides	Cephalothin, metronidazole, ampicillin

Table 4-5
Recommended dosage regimens for antibiotics in horses

Drug	Dose (mg/kg)	Route	Frequency
Amikacin sulfate	6.6	IV, IM	q8h
	10	IV, IM	q12h
	21	IV, IM	q24h
Amoxicillin sodium	22	IM	q6-12h
Ampicillin sodium	25-100	IV	q6h
Ampicillin trihydrate	11-22	IM	q12h
Cephalexin	22-33	PO	q6h
Cephalothin/cefazolin	5	IV, IM	q6h
Cephapirin	20	IM	q8h
Ceftiofur sodium	2.2-10	IV, IM	q6-24h
Chloramphenicol	50	IV	q4-8h
	50	PO	q6-8h
Erythromycin estolate	25	PO	q8h
ethylsuccinate	25	PO	q8h
gluceptate	5	IV	q4-6h
lactobionate	2.5-3	IV	q6-8h
Gentamicin sulfate	2.2	IV, IM	q6h
	6.6	IV, IM	q24h
Kanamycin sulfate	5-10	IM	q8h
Metronidazole	15-25	PO, per rectum	q6-8h
Oxacillin sodium	16-50	IV, IM	q8-12h
	25	IM	q8-12h
Oxytetracycline	4.4-5	IV	q12h
	16.3	IV	q12h
Penicillin G K$^+$/Na$^+$	12,500-100,000 IU/kg	IV, IM	q4-6h
procaine	20,000-30,000 IU/kg	IM	q12h
Rifampin	5	PO	q12h
	5-10	PO	q12-24h
Tetracycline	5-7.5	IV	q12h
Ticarcillin	22-44	IM	q8h
	44	IV	q5h
Trimethoprim plus	15-30	PO	q12h
sulfamethoxazole			
or sulfadiazine			

- animals suffering from concurrent disease processes or receiving corticosteroids
- geriatric patients or those appreciably underweight or malnourished

Practical considerations

- Antibiotic prophylaxis is most effective when administered within 1 hour of bacterial inoculation and ineffective when administered 3 to 4 hours after bacteria inoculate the wound.
  - IV antibiotics should be given immediately before anesthetic induction (i.e., 30 min before surgery).
  - IM antibiotics should be given 1 to 2 hours before surgery.
- There is no apparent benefit in continuing antibiotic prophylaxis for more than 24 hours after surgery.
- If infection develops despite prophylactic antibiotics, the organism should be considered resistant or contamination of the surgical wound still exists.

Drug Selection

Systemic antibiotic therapy

The most commonly used antibiotics for systemic prophylaxis are penicillin with gentamicin, penicillin alone, trimethoprim-sulfonamides, and ceftiofur.

Topical antibiotic therapy

Topical antibiotics can be used prophylactically.

* Best results are achieved when the antibiotic is administered immediately after opening each tissue plane and when tissues are irrigated with the antibiotic throughout the surgical procedure, not just at closure.
* Antibiotics suitable for topical wound irrigation include penicillin, kanamycin, lincomycin, cephalothin, ampicillin, and a combination of neomycin, bacitracin, and polymyxin B.

ROUTES OF ADMINISTRATION

Parenteral vs. Enteral Administration

With few exceptions, antibiotics should be administered parenterally because of the unpredictable absorption of orally administered drugs in horses.

* IV administration results in high peak serum concentrations that decrease relatively rapidly.
* IM administration results in lower peak serum concentrations that persist for longer.
* In adults, oral administration is limited to trimethoprim-sulfonamides, metro-nidazole, erythromycin, rifampin, chloramphenicol, and enrofloxacin.
* Some antibiotics (e.g., metronidazole) can be administered rectally in horses that are anorexic or that have ileus with associated gastric reflux.

Local Antibiotic Administration

Topical administration

Topical antibiotics are useful for treatment of wound infections.

* The triple antibiotic combination of neomycin, bacitracin, and polymyxin B is useful for prophylaxis or treatment.
* Silver sulfadiazine is useful for treatment of wound infections caused by *Pseudomonas* spp.
* Addition of Tris-EDTA to an aminoglycoside such as gentamicin increases effectiveness against *Pseudomonas* spp.

Intrathecal administration

Intrasynovial administration of gentamicin (150 mg per joint) or amikacin (250 to 500 mg per joint) results in synovial fluid concentrations that remain above the MIC of most pathogenic bacteria for ≥ 24 hours.

Regional limb perfusion

Regional limb perfusion involves the delivery of antibiotic under pressure to a selected region of the limb via the venous system.

* It is an effective method of managing osteomyelitis and septic arthritis.
* The antibiotic can be delivered via an IV catheter placed in a superficial vein or through a catheter adapter placed in a 4.5-mm hole drilled in the bone.
* An elastic bandage is applied proximal to the site of infection.
* Perfusion usually is performed over 30 min at a maximum pressure of 450 psi.

Antibiotic-impregnated polymer

Antibiotic-impregnated polymethylmethacrylate (PMMA) has been used successfully for prophylaxis and treatment of musculoskeletal infections in horses:

* A combination of cefazolin and amikacin provides the best coverage against the most common bacteria isolated from horses with orthopedic infections.
* Antibiotics are added to the PMMA as it is being mixed, then round beads or cylindrical implants of PMAA are placed in the surgical wound.
* Although variable, there is sustained release of antibiotic from the implant into the surrounding tissue fluid.
* Antibiotic-impregnated PMMA can also be used for plate luting when repairing long-bone fractures.

SAFE USE OF AMINOGLYCOSIDES

Therapeutic Drug Monitoring

Conditions that alter ECF volume or drug distribution may affect the plasma concentrations of aminoglycosides. Examples include peritoneal or pleural effusion, colitis, dehydration, endotoxemia, and immaturity. Peak

serum concentrations of aminoglycosides are associated with the therapeutic effects, and trough levels are
associated with the toxic effects.
Guidelines for therapeutic monitoring
Following are guidelines:
* Samples should not be collected
  until after 2 to 3 days of treatment.
* Peak concentrations should be
  measured 30 min after IV and 1
  hour after IM administration
* Samples for measurement of
  trough concentrations are collected
  immediately before administration
  of the next dose.
* The recommended peak and
  trough serum concentrations for
  gentamicin are 10 to 15 µg/mL and
  ≤2 µg/mL, respectively.
* The recommended peak and trough
  values for amikacin are 25 to 35
  µg/mL and ≤4 µg/mL, respectively.
* A positive clinical response should
  be achieved if the maximal peak concentration is 8 to 10 times the MIC.

Once Daily Administration

Compared with bid or tid administration, single daily administration of
aminoglycosides may be superior in
regard to efficacy, duration of action,
safety, and convenience. High peak
and low trough concentrations are
characteristic of once daily aminoglycoside therapy.
* The recommended dosage for gentamicin is 6 to 8 mg/kg sid.
* Extrapolation for amikacin suggests
  a dose of 18 to 21 mg/kg sid.
* 2.2 mg/kg tid may be best for preoperative initiation of therapy because of the possible potentiation
  for neuromuscular blockade with
  anesthetic agents.

Principles of Nutrition

(pages 175-181)
David T. Galligan

FARM VISIT

An intensive inspection of the feeds
and feeding management, along with
examinations of the horses on a farm,
is essential to identify likely causes of
a problem and available options for
improvement.

Evaluation of Feeding Management

The uses of the horses must be clearly
defined and historical information on
diseases and performance problems
documented. General feeding management practices should be recorded.
A tour of the facilities better defines
any problem areas.
   Evaluation of feeding management
also involves:
* inspection of the feeds (cereal
  grains, supplements, hays, and pastures), storage facilities, and the
  feed-delivery system
* sampling and weighing feeds and
  calibrating scoops and flakes
* submitting feed samples to a forage
  laboratory for proximate analysis
* examination of individual horses

RATION FORMULATION

New rations are formulated on the
basis of the initial ration evaluation, results of feed analyses, and the feeding
system on the farm. The nutritional requirements listed in NRC publications
serve as a guide in formulation.
   Following are guidelines:
* Maintain a minimum roughage al-
  lowance of 1% body weight for all
  classes.
* Formulate grain mixes to balance
  the nutrients from forages available.
* Reformulate the diet with the
  fewest possible changes in feed staples and delivery system.
  * Generally, only the relative pro-
    portions of roughage to concen-
    trate require change.
* Make any changes in the ration
  over 7 to 10 days.
  * When changing the amount of
    grain fed per day, do not exceed
    0.2 kg increase or decrease per day.
* If the total amount of concentrate
  is >3.5 kg per feeding, encourage
  increased feeding frequency.

Parenteral Nutrition in Foals and Adult Horses

(pages 181-183)
Guy D. Lester

Newborn foals do not have significant energy stores and therefore do
not tolerate periods of caloric depri-

vation as well as adults. At least partial parenteral nutrition may be required in adult horses that cannot be fed enterally over a prolonged period.

PRACTICAL ASPECTS OF TOTAL PARENTERAL NUTRITION

Nutritional Requirements

The animal's nutritional requirements must be estimated before formulating the parenteral mixture.

- Neonatal foals require mixtures that provide 50 to 100 kcal/kg/d to maintain body weight and minimize protein catabolism.
- Maintenance requirements for adults depend on physiologic status.
  - Most healthy adult horses can maintain their body weight if supplied with 33 kcal/kg/d.
- Requirements in all animals are increased by sepsis or trauma.

Administration

Parenteral nutritional solutions are hypertonic and are therefore best administered into a large vein (e.g., the jugular vein).

- Silastic catheters are ideal, but polyurethane catheters are more cost-effective and easier to maintain.
- Teflon catheters are not recommended but can be used for up to <4 days.

Monitoring

It is critical to closely monitor all patients receiving parenteral nutrition. Complications include:

- hyperglycemia and glucosuria, which are more common in neonates
  - Young patients should receive glucose- or dextrose-containing solutions slowly if large amounts are being used (e.g., 12 to 15 g/kg/d).
- metabolic CO_2 production
- elevated BUN and blood ammonia
- lipemia
- sepsis
  - TPN formulations must be mixed under sterile conditions.
  - Unexplained, persistent fever should prompt investigation of the solution, fluid line, or catheter for possible contamination.

FORMULAS FOR FOALS

Calculations are based on amounts in g/kg/d of glucose (10 to 15), amino acids (2 to 3), and lipids (1 to 3). Following is a formulation that has been successfully used in newborn foals at the University of Florida Veterinary Medicine Teaching Hospital:

    1000 mL of 50% dextrose
    2000 mL of a 10% amino acid solution
    750 mL of a 20% lipid solution
    500 mL of 0.9% saline
    60 ml of KCl (2 mEq/mL)

This formulation provides 92 kcal/kg/d and is given by constant infusion at a rate of 180 mL/h. Micronutrients (e.g., "M.T.E.-6", containing chromium, selenium, iodine, manganese, copper, and zinc; 1.5mL/4 L bag of TPN) are added to the mixture if TPN is used for >3 days.

FORMULAS FOR ADULT HORSES

The following formulation is recommended for adult horses:

    4.5 L of 50% dextrose
    4 L of 10% amino acid solution
    2 L of 20% lipid solution

At 600 mL/h, this mixture provides 30 kcal/kg/d for a 450-kg (990 lb) horse. The final volume does not supply maintenance water requirements and must be supplemented with an electrolyte solution.

Equine Vaccination

(pages 183-191)

J. Trenton McClure and D. Paul Lunn

PRACTICAL CONSIDERATIONS

Vaccination Schedules

General recommendations for vaccination of foals and adult horses are given in Tables 4-6 and 4-7, respectively.

Primary vaccination regimens should be administered so that at least 2 to 3 weeks elapse between the final vaccination and potential exposure. Similarly, boosters should be administered at least 1 to 2 weeks before risk of exposure. It is important to remember that stress, illness, nutritional status, and concurrent medications

Table 4-6
Vaccination regimens for horses in the first year of life

Disease	Age for primary vaccination	Vaccination regimen	Comments
Tetanus	4 mo; if dam is not recently vaccinated, then after birth	Two doses 3-4 wk apart; booster at 1 yr of age	Vaccination in the face of maternal immunity appears to be effective
Equine encephalomyelitis	4-6 mo	Two doses 3-4 wk apart; booster at 1 yr of age	Vaccination of young foals, particularly in the face of maternal immunity (up to 3 mo) is frequently of limited efficacy. If born late in the year, protection may not be required until the following year and initial vaccination can be delayed
Equine influenza	6-12 mo	Three doses at 3-4 wk intervals; booster at 1 yr of age	Vaccination of young foals, particularly in the face of maternal immunity (up to 6 mo) is frequently of limited efficacy, and even beyond this age current vaccines may fail
Rhinopneumonitis	>6 mo	Three doses at 3-4 wk intervals; booster at 1 yr of age	Vaccination of young foals, particularly in the face of maternal immunity (up to 3-4 mo) is frequently of limited efficacy
Strangles	2-3 mo	Two to three doses 3-4 wk apart followed by boosters every 3 mo if at high risk	Principally a disease of young horses and particularly problematic on broodmare farms. Current vaccines of limited efficacy
Equine monocytic ehrlichiosis	4-6 mo	Two doses 3-4 wk apart; repeat vaccine every 3-6 mo until yearling	Limited efficacy and low prevalence in foals. May wait until following spring to vaccinate
Rabies	4-6 mo	Two doses 3-4 wk apart; booster at 1 yr of age	
Botulism	>6 mo	Three doses at 4-wk intervals	Typically used in pregnant mares to boost colostral immunity. Vaccination can be indicated in other ages. Only type B toxoid available, no commercial type C toxoid
Equine viral arteritis	6-9 mo for colts	Annual boosters	Only for colts with breeding potential. Vaccination with MLV in United States may require authorization of state authorities, and seroconversion may prevent future export
R. equi pneumonia	Administer hyperimmune plasma in first month of life	May administer twice in first month of life on endemic farm with very high risk of R. equi pneumonia	Expensive but effective on endemic farms

MLV, Modified live vaccine.
Shaded boxes denote importance of the use of this vaccine: ■ required, ▨ recommended, ☐ optional.

can affect immunologic responses to vaccination.

Vaccine Product Choices, Regimens, and Precautions

Equine encephalomyelitis

- In North America, vaccination with a bivalent product containing EEE and WEE viruses generally is adequate.
  - In states that border Mexico, it is sometimes necessary to use a trivalent vaccine that includes VEE.
- Protection after vaccination lasts <6 months in many horses.
  - In temperate regions where the vector season is short, annual spring vaccination generally is adequate.
  - In high-risk endemic regions, vaccination should be repeated every 2 to 4 months during the vector season.

Equine influenza

- A product containing a recent A/equine/2 isolate (late 1980s or the 1990s) should be used.
- Influenza vaccines can cause swelling and pain at the injection site (more likely with egg-culture products).

Rhinopneumonitis

- For prevention of abortion, a killed EHV-1 vaccine should be used during pregnancy.
  - Modified live virus vaccines should not be used in pregnant mares.
- Prevention of respiratory disease is best accomplished using a product containing both EHV-1 and EHV-4 antigens.
  - A bivalent vaccine is also recommended when vaccinating broodmares in their last month of pregnancy to boost colostral antibodies.
- The modified live virus vaccine against EHV-1 can cause transient fever and malaise.
- Vaccination does not appear to offer protection against the neurologic form of EHV-1 infection.

Strangles

- Current choices of *Streptococcus equi* vaccines are M-protein based or whole bacterin products.

- Strangles vaccines often cause injection site reactions; M-protein vaccines cause fewer reactions.
- There is a slight risk of purpura hemorrhagica after strangles vaccination or infection
  - Recently an intranasal avirulent live *S. equi* vaccine has been introduced and may improve protection.

Botulism

- The currently available equine vaccine is a *Clostridium botulinum* type B toxoid.
- *C. botulinum* type C is an important pathogen in some regions, but the type B toxoid is not cross protective.
  - A type C toxoid licensed for mink has been used in horses, but its safety and efficacy are unknown.

Controlling Internal Parasites *(pages 196-200)*
Thomas R. Klei

GENERAL GUIDELINES

Following are some guidelines for effective internal parasite control:

- Implement treatment schedules that maximize health while minimizing anthelmintic use.
- Use the proper dosage of anthelmintic based on accurate body weight assessment.
- Alternate classes of compounds annually to prolong the effectiveness of anthelmintics.
- Monitor deworming programs and drug efficacy on an annual basis using fecal egg counts.
- Use nonchemical control strategies when feasible.

ANTHELMINTICS
Avermictins and Milbemycins

The avermectins and milbemycins have the broadest range of activity and are effective against the adult stages and many migrating stages of nematodes.

Ivermectin

- Ivermectin has activity against adult and migrating larval nematodes and all stages of *Gastrophilus* spp. larvae.

Table 4-7
Vaccine regimens for horses over 1 year of age

Disease	Primary vaccination	Broodmare*
Tetanus	Two doses 3-4 wk apart	■ Annual, 2-4 wk before foaling
Equine encehaplomyelitis	Two doses 3-4 wk apart	■ Annual, 2-4 wk before foaling
Equine influenza	Two doses 3-4 wk apart	▨ Annual, 2-4 wk before foaling
Rhinopneumonitis	Two doses 3-4 wk apart	▨ EHV-1 killed: 3, 5, 7, 9 mo of pregnancy
Strangles	Two to three doses 3-4 wk apart	☐ Annual, 2-4 wk before foaling—only killed products licensed
Equine monocytic ehrlichiosis	Two doses 3-4 wk apart	☐ Annual, 2-4 wk before foaling
Rabies	Two doses 3-4 wk apart	☐ Not approved for pregnant mares
Equine viral arteritis (EVA)	One dose at least 3 wk before foaling in broodmare	☐ Annual, at least 2 wk before breeding. Required if stallion is a carrier
Botulism	Three doses 4 wk apart (last dose 2-4 wk before foaling in broodmare)	☐ Annual, 2-4 wk before foaling. Used in endemic areas
Rotavirus	Three doses 3-4 wk apart with last dose 2-4 wk before foaling	☐ Annual, 2-4 wk before foaling

MLV, Modified live vaccine.

*Broodmare vaccination recommendations are pertinent to maintenance of pregnancy and optimizing passive transfer of colostral immunity to the foal. Additional vaccinations may be required according to the pleasure or performance horse breed society recommendations.

Shaded boxes denote importance of the use of this vaccine: ■ required, ▨ recommended, ☐ optional

- It also reduces the prevalence of summer sores caused by larvae of *Draschia megastomum* or *Habronema* spp. organisms and dermatitis associated with *Onchocerca cervicalis* microfilariae.
- It is not effective against tapeworms, adults of *O. cervicalis*, or encysted cyathostome larvae.

Moxidectin
- Moxidectin has a range of activity similar to that of ivermectin.
- It also has activity against mucosal stages of developing cyathostome larvae.

- Resistance against reinfection with cyathostomes persists for at least 2 weeks.
- Fecal egg counts are suppressed for longer with moxidectin, so the recommended interval between treatments is 3 months (compared with 2 months for ivermectin).

Benzimidazoles
Benzimidazoles are highly effective against most nematodes living within the GI tract.
- Some benzimidazoles, including fenbendazole, are highly effective

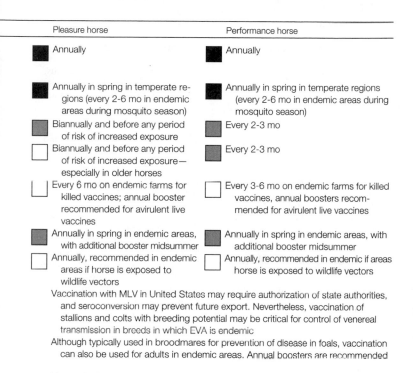

Pleasure horse	Performance horse
Annually	Annually
Annually in spring in temperate regions (every 2-6 mo in endemic areas during mosquito season)	Annually in spring in temperate regions (every 2-6 mo in endemic areas during mosquito season)
Biannually and before any period of risk of increased exposure	Every 2-3 mo
Biannually and before any period of risk of increased exposure—especially in older horses	Every 2-3 mo
Every 6 mo on endemic farms for killed vaccines; annual booster recommended for avirulent live vaccines	Every 3-6 mo on endemic farms for killed vaccines, annual boosters recommended for avirulent live vaccines
Annually in spring in endemic areas, with additional booster midsummer	Annually in spring in endemic areas, with additional booster midsummer
Annually, recommended in endemic areas if horse is exposed to wildlife vectors	Annually, recommended in endemic if areas horse is exposed to wildlife vectors

Vaccination with MLV in United States may require authorization of state authorities, and seroconversion may prevent future export. Nevertheless, vaccination of stallions and colts with breeding potential may be critical for control of venereal transmission in breeds in which EVA is endemic

Although typically used in broodmares for prevention of disease in foals, vaccination can also be used for adults in endemic areas. Annual boosters are recommended

Not applicable

against migrating large strongyles and encysted cyathostome larvae when used at higher-than-normal dosages for several days (e.g., fenbendazole at 10 mg/kg for 5 days).

- Resistance of cyathostomes to benzimidazoles is common.

Pyrimidines

These drugs include pyrantel pamoate and pyrantel tartrate.

- Daily dosing with pyrantel tartrate is prophylactic.

- Pyrantel salts are highly effective against the common tapeworm, *Anoplocephala perfoliata*, especially at twice the usual dosage.
- Resistance of cyathostomes has been reported, but is uncommon.

Other Anthelmintics

Mixtures that include benzimidazoles and organic phosphates or piperazine have a synergistic effect and may be useful as alternatives in controlling benzimidazole-resistant cyathostomes.

EVALUATING THE EFFECTIVENESS OF TREATMENT

Adult worm burdens of *Parascaris equorum* and *Strongyloides westeri* organisms, large strongyles, and cyathostomes can be estimated by fecal egg counts (in eggs per gram, or EPG).

- A drug's efficacy can be estimated by comparing EPGs of individual horses at the time of treatment and 10 to 14 days later.
  - The egg count should decrease by ≥90%; drug-resistant cyathostomes likely are present if the reduction is much less.
- Fecal flotation methods are not reliable for evaluating infections of *Anoplocephala* spp., spiruroid stomach worms, or *Oxyuris equi* organisms.

STRATEGIES FOR ANTHELMINTIC TREATMENT

Following are five basic anthelmintic strategies:

- *interval treatment:* These "fast rotation" programs use anthelmintics from different classes at predetermined periods during the year.
  - Drug selection allows for the annual elimination of seasonally susceptible parasites such as *A. perfoliata* and *Gastrophilus* spp. larvae.
- *annual rotation:* These "slow rotation" programs use the same anthelmintic at appropriate intervals throughout the year.
  - The class of anthelmintic is alternated each year.
- *no rotation:* This program involves the repeated use of a single, effective anthelmintic until it fails to reduce cyathostomes as indicated by fecal egg counts.
  - It presently is limited to periodic use of ivermectin or moxidectin, or daily administration of pyrantel tartrate in feed.
- *targeted treatments:* This program involves administration of anthelmintics only to horses with significant fecal egg counts (>100 to 200 EPG).
  - Implementation requires regular quantitative fecal examinations.
- *strategic treatment:* These programs are designed to eliminate luminal cyathostome burdens before the season of the year that is optimal for parasite development on pasture.
  - In northern temperate regions, treatments are administered in the spring, early summer, and fall.

DEWORMING YOUNG HORSES

The horse's immune system is important in the development of acquired resistance to *P. equorum* and *S. westeri* organisms; acquired resistance to strongyles is less well developed. Following are some practical considerations for designing parasite control programs in young horses:

- Initiation of vigorous control programs before the foal reaches 6 to 8 wks of age may impair the immune response and prolong parasite infection.
- Ideally, young horses should receive the minimal level of treatment sufficient to promote their optimal health.
- Nevertheless, foals and weanlings are very susceptible to *P. equorum.*
  - Efforts should be made to control these parasites before the foal reaches 10 weeks of age, the prepatent period of these worms.
  - Ivermectin and moxidectin are highly effective.

NONANTHELMINTIC METHODS OF CONTROL

Several methods have been described for reducing pasture contamination with infective larvae.

- rotating stock to clean pastures, particularly at times of the year when larval survival is expected to be minimal
- harrowing to scatter manure and reduce survival of strongyle larvae, particularly during dry seasons, can be detrimental to larval survival
  - However, foals raised on harrowed pastures can have greater parasite burdens than foals on other pastures.

- alternately grazing horses with ruminants
  - This method may expose horses to increased numbers of *Trichostrongylus axei.*
- biweekly mechanical removal of feces

Traditional Chinese Veterinary Medical Therapy *(pages 201-203)*

Richard Panzer

Traditional Chinese veterinary medicine is a useful complement or alternative to conventional Western equine medicine. Although the mechanisms of action of acupuncture and other traditional Chinese therapies are largely unexplained in terms of Western science, they can provide relief from numerous ailments, including:

- pain and spasm caused by arthritis
- sprain, strain, and trauma
- reversible traumatic paralysis
- laminitis
- colic
- diarrhea
- aggression and other behavioral problems during estrus
- anterior uveitis

Traditional Chinese veterinary medicine does not alter anatomy, so it is ineffective for management of cervical stenosis and other dysplasias. It also has limited efficacy against neoplasia and most infectious diseases, including equine protozoal myeloencephalitis.

5

Critical Care Medicine

Circulatory Shock

(pages 210-218)

Rustin M. Moore and James N. Moore

Circulatory shock is the inability of the cardiovascular system to provide adequate tissue perfusion, with resultant widespread cellular and organ dysfunction. Initially, this dysfunction is reversible; however, persistent hypoperfusion results in permanent cellular injury and necrosis.

The common causes of shock in horses are:

* endotoxemia—caused by GI ischemia or inflammation, metritis, pleuropneumonia, peritonitis, or other systemic infectious or inflammatory diseases
* dehydration—caused by diarrhea or extreme exercise
* sepsis
* hemorrhage

PATHOPHYSIOLOGIC CLASSIFICATION OF SHOCK

Shock can be classified according to the major hemodynamic abnormality:

* hypovolemic shock—pathologic loss of blood volume
  * Traumatic injuries and surgical trauma can result in loss of whole blood (see below).
  * Acute inflammatory conditions or severe burns can result in loss of plasma.
  * Fluid and electrolyte losses can occur subsequent to GI reflux, diarrhea, extreme sweating, and diuresis.

* maldistribution of blood volume— usually occurs subsequent to an inappropriate increase in venous capacitance (e.g., endotoxemia-associated venodilation) or secondary to obstruction of venous return (e.g., intestinal strangulation)
  * Blood volume loss may also occur as endotoxin or venous obstruction compromises vascular integrity, resulting in extravasation of blood or plasma into the tissues.
* maldistribution of blood flow—occurs from loss of circulatory control at the level of the arterioles
  * Dysfunction of circulatory control mechanisms results in some vascular beds being underperfused and others being overperfused; it may also involve arteriovenous shunting.
  * Sepsis often causes blood flow maldistribution; it may also lead to vascular obstruction, increased vascular permeability, and interstitial edema.

HEMORRHAGIC SHOCK

External hemorrhage is easily recognized, but hemorrhage into a body cavity (e.g., pleural or peritoneal cavity) may be more difficult to identify.

* Hypovolemic shock associated with hemorrhage is most often caused by spontaneous rupture of the middle uterine artery in mares or surgery involving the paranasal sinus, ethmoid, or nasal septum.
* Traumatic limb injuries can lacerate the dorsal metatarsal or digital arteries and the saphenous, cephalic, or digital veins.

• Traumatic injuries to the neck may damage the jugular veins or common carotid arteries.

Causes of Intraabdominal Hemorrhage

Sites or causes of intraabdominal hemorrhage include:

• *gastrointestinal:* cranial mesenteric artery aneurysm, GI ulcer, mesocolon avulsion during parturition, renosplenic or epiploic foramen entrapment, Meckel's diverticulum, small intestinal mesenteric vessel avulsion

• *urogenital:* umbilical artery, granulosa–theca cell tumor, urocystorrhexis, uteroovarian artery aneurysm or hematoma, ovarian or uterine neoplasia, follicular hematoma, urinary bladder or uterine rupture/tear, coital injuries to the vaginal wall, castration complications, mating injuries in stallions

• *musculoskeletal:* pelvic fracture, rib fractures

• *other:* coagulopathies, visceral neoplasia, traumatic splenic or hepatic rupture

Diagnostic Approach to Hemorrhagic Shock

Physical findings

Physical examination of horses with hemorrhagic shock usually reveals:

• lethargy and depression
• tachycardia and tachypnea
• blanched mucous membranes
• prolonged capillary refill time (>3 sec)
• weak peripheral pulse
• hypothermia
• systolic murmur (physiologic)

Reduced lung sounds ventrally or percussion of a fluid line provide supportive evidence of intrathoracic hemorrhage. On rectal examination, a hematoma can often be palpated in the uterus of mares with uterine artery rupture or in the pelvic area of horses with a pelvic fracture.

Laboratory data

• Initially, the PCV and total protein concentration are not decreased because equal proportion s of fluid and RBCs are lost.
  • Splenic contraction maintains the PCV in the normal range

for several hours after acute hemorrhage.
  • As intravascular volume is replaced with crystalloids and the fluid compartments redistribute, the PCV and total protein concentration both decrease.
  • Hypoproteinemia with a normal albumin:globulin ratio suggests acute blood loss or overhydration.
• Azotemia and hyperglycemia are common in horses with hemorrhagic shock.
• Thoracocentesis or abdominocentesis is indicated in horses suspected of having intrathoracic or intraabdominal hemorrhage.
  • Hemothorax or hemoperitoneum is confirmed by finding erythrophagocytosis, platelets, and a high PCV or erythrocyte count in the pleural or peritoneal fluid.
  • A PCV ≥5% and total protein concentration ≤3.5 g/dL are suggestive of hemothorax or hemoperitoneum.

Exploratory surgery

An exploratory celiotomy may be indicated in horses with intraabdominal hemorrhage. Uterine tears, mesenteric avulsions, or other sources of intraabdominal bleeding may be effectively treated surgically.

Treatment of Hemorrhagic Shock

The first goal of treatment is to identify the source and stop the bleeding. Depending on the location of the hemorrhaging vessel(s), digital pressure, a tight pressure bandage, temporary application of a hemostat, or ligation may be appropriate. Volume expansion and medical treatment also are necessary.

Fluid therapy

Volume replacement is an essential component of shock therapy.

• *isotonic fluids:* Isotonic, crystalloid solutions rapidly equilibrate with the interstitial fluid, so 3 to 4 times the volume of blood lost should be replaced with isotonic fluids.
  • If the volume lost cannot be determined, give 25 to 50 mL/kg IV rapidly.
  • Too rapid administration can lead to pulmonary or subcutaneous edema, hypoproteinemia, and anemia.

+ *hypertonic saline:* 4 to 6 mL/kg of 7% NaCl, given over 10 min can rapidly improve hemodynamic variables.
  • Experimentally, these beneficial effects last for 90 to 180 min.
  • *Administration of hypertonic saline must be immediately followed by administration of isotonic fluids.*
  • Use of hypertonic saline during uncontrolled hemorrhage is controversial; more severe hemorrhage may result from improved hemodynamics.
+ *colloids:* Colloidal solutions remain intravascular and draw fluid into the vascular space.
  • Colloids include plasma (fresh or frozen), hetastarch, pentastarch, and dextrans (40 or 70).
  • Plasma or other colloid is indicated when the total protein concentration is <3.5 g/dL.

• Colloidal solutions should be given with crystalloids.
• Transient, severe hemolysis, hemoglobinuria, and premature ventricular contractions may occur with dextran 70.

Blood replacement therapy
The need for a whole blood transfusion depends on the volume and rapidity with which blood is lost. A rapid reduction in PCV is less well tolerated than a more slow decline of the PCV of the same magnitude. Indications, precautions, and methods of blood replacement therapy are discussed in Chapter 4, Principles of Therapy.

Pharmacologic therapy
Dosages of drugs used to treat horses with hemorrhagic shock are given in Table 5-1.
+ *cardiovascular stimulants:* The drugs listed improve cardiac output; most

Table 5-1
Dose and route of administration of drugs used for treatment of hemorrhagic shock in horses

Drug	Dose	Route
CARDIOVASCULAR STIMULANTS		
Epinephrine	1-3 µg/kg	IV bolus
Isoproterenol	0.05-0.1 µg/kg/min	IV infusion
Dopamine	1-5 µg/kg/min	IV infusion
Dobutamine	1-5 µg/kg/min	IV infusion
Ephedrine	0.01-0.2 mg/kg	IV in 10-mg boluses
Phenylephrine	0.01 mg/kg	IV to effect
VASODILATOR DRUGS		
Acepromazine	0.02 mg/kg	IV
CORTICOSTEROIDS		
Prednisolone sodium succinate	1-2 mg/kg	IV bolus
Dexamethasone	2-4 mg/kg	IV bolus
NONSTEROIDAL ANTIINFLAMMATORY DRUGS		
Flunixin meglumine	1.1 mg/kg	IV bolus
Phenylbutazone	2.2-4.4 mg/kg	IV bolus
Ketoprofen	1 mg/kg	IV bolus
OPIATE ANTAGONISTS		
Naloxone	0.02 mg/kg	IV bolus
FLUID THERAPY		
Isotonic polyionic	3 times estimated blood loss or 25-50 mL/kg	IV rapid infusion
Hypertonic saline	4 mL/kg	IV over 10-15 min

of them also sensitize the myocardium to arrhythmias.
  • Some of these drugs improve
    blood flow to splanchnic and
    skeletal muscle beds, which,
    while improving tissue oxygena-
    tion in these tissues, can exacer-
    bate shock by reducing periph-
    eral vascular resistance and
    blood pressure.
• *vasodilators:* Acepromazine should
  be avoided in horses with severe
  blood loss or hypovolemia.
  • There is some evidence in other
    species that α-adrenergic blockers
    (including acepromazine) may be
    beneficial in restoring blood flow
    to vital organs during hypov-
    olemic or septic shock.
• *corticosteroids:* To be beneficial,
  corticosteroids must be administered before or very early after the
  onset of shock.
  • Potential adverse effects include
    laminitis, adrenal suppression,
    delayed healing, and immuno-
    suppression (see Chapter 4, Prin-
    ciples of Therapy).
  • Prednisolone sodium succinate is
    less likely to precipitate laminitis
    than is dexamethasone.
• *NSAIDs:* There have been no
  studies in horses to demonstrate a
  beneficial effect of NSAIDs during
  hemorrhagic shock.
  • Caution should be taken when
    administering these drugs to hy-
    povolemic or dehydrated horses.
• *naloxone:* Naloxone often is recommended for treatment of mares
  with hemorrhagic shock secondary
  to uterine artery rupture.
  • Extremely large doses are re-
    quired to inhibit the vasodilatory
    effects of β-endorphins in later
    stages of shock.

Antibiotics

Shock can disrupt the gastrointestinal
mucosal barrier, so broad-spectrum
antibiotics are recommended. Blood
volume should be expanded with
fluids before administering antibiotics, such as aminoglycosides, that
have nephrotoxic side effects.

Prognosis

The prognosis for horses with hemorrhagic shock depends on:

• the cause of hemorrhage
• the rapidity and magnitude of
  blood loss
  • Horses can tolerate an acute loss
    of up to 33% of their blood
    volume, or approximately 12 L
    in a 450-kg (990 lb) horse.
  • Larger acute losses rapidly result
    in death, unless aggressive treat-
    ment is instituted immediately.
• time elapsed between hemorrhage
  and onset of treatment
• institution of appropriate and aggressive treatment

ENDOTOXEMIA AND SEPTICEMIA

Clinical Manifestations of Endotoxemia

Endotoxins are structural components (lipopolysaccharides) of the
outer cell envelope of gram-negative
bacteria. They are released when bacteria die or replicate rapidly, and
may be absorbed into the systemic
circulation. Endotoxemia causes systemic hypotension, poor tissue perfusion, lactic acidosis, and a propensity toward thrombosis. The end
result is rapid onset of circulatory
shock.

Causes

Common causes of endotoxemia
include:
• colic
• colitis
• severe pneumonia or pleuropneu
  monia
• retained placenta
• peritonitis

Clinical findings

Typical findings include:
• alterations in mucous membrane
  color, with the presence of a "toxic
  line"
• prolonged capillary refill time
• increased heart and respiratory rates
• reduced borborygmi
• fever
• hemoconcentration
• neutropenia
• depression or abdominal pain

Intestinal abnormalities

• The conditions most commonly
  associated with endotoxemia are
  those involving severe intestinal
  displacements with obstruction of
  the blood supply and intestinal

lumen (e.g., volvulus, incarcerations).

- Endotoxemia also occurs when the intestinal wall is inflamed (e.g., colitis, proximal enteritis).
- The effects of endotoxin are not confined to the abnormal section of bowel.
  - The ability of the "normal" intestine to prevent the transmural movement of endotoxin also is impaired.
  - Consequently, the deleterious effects of endotoxin can persist for several days after surgical removal of the diseased bowel or, in the case of colitis or proximal enteritis, until the mucosal damage has resolved.

Clinical Manifestations of Septicemia

Septicemia develops when bacteria or their toxins enter the bloodstream. Many of the clinical manifestations of septicemia are the same as those of endotoxemia.

Causal organisms

Septicemia is most often encountered in neonatal foals with a nidus of bacterial infection. The most common organisms are gram-negative bacteria from the intestinal tract, most notably *Escherichia coli, Klebsiella, Enterobacter, Actinobacillus,* and *Pseudomonas* organisms. Septicemia also may be caused by gram-positive organisms, especially streptococcal species.

Therapy for Endotoxemia

When feasible, the single most important aspect of treating any endotoxemic patient is to eliminate the source of endotoxins. Other modes of therapy include:

- IV fluids to restore blood volume and prevent microvascular thrombosis
- pharmacologic agents that interfere with the synthesis or effects of specific inflammatory mediators
  - NSAIDs are the most commonly used drugs.
  - Reduced doses of flunixin meglumine (0.25 mg/kg IV q8h) often are recommended.
  - Ketoprofen (2.2 mg/kg IV q12h) appears to have similar beneficial effects.

Antibiotics

Antimicrobial drugs, most notably gentamicin, penicillin, and amikacin, often are administered to endotoxemic horses. They may not be indicated for adult horses that are not septicemic; however, many clinicians administer antibiotics to prevent secondary complications, such as septic phlebitis and dissemination of bacteria to other organs.

Hyperimmune plasma or serum

The efficacy of hyperimmune antiendotoxin plasma or serum is controversial. If this form of therapy is to be used, it should be initiated as early as possible in the disease.

Other treatments

Experimentally, a variety of other treatments show promise, including administration of monoclonal antibodies directed against equine tumor necrosis factor, pentoxifylline, α_2-adrenergic receptor antagonists, polymyxin B, and a combination of pentoxifylline and flunixin meglumine.

Disaster Medicine

(pages 226-237)
Farol N. Tomson
and Theodore E. Specht

RECOMMENDATIONS FOR RELIEF VETERINARIANS

- *Do not become a victim yourself.* Take care of yourself first and then begin relief efforts.
  - Bring maps, flashlights and batteries, a supply of water, nonperishable foods, proper clothing including gloves, and hard-soled shoes.
- *Use a well-equipped, dependable vehicle.* Ensure that the vehicle you use will not become disabled or stranded.
  - A high-clearance, four wheel drive vehicle with a trailer hitch and capacity to carry extra people and supplies is ideal.
  - Include a tire repair kit, extra fuel, and an emergency flashing red light for the roof.
- *Never go into a disaster area without direct communication with someone in charge via radio or cellular phone.*

◆ *Know and be prepared to use triage.*
◆ *Keep a well-equipped emergency kit containing:*
- *Antibiotics:* procaine G and potassium penicillin, trimethoprim-sulfa, gentamicin, metronidazole, oxytetracycline, and various ointments and creams
- *sedatives and anesthetics:* xylazine, butorphanol, acepromazine, ketamine, lidocaine, and mepivacaine
- *antiinflammatories:* phenylbutazone, flunixin meglumine, dexamethasone, prednisolone, and DMSO
- *fluids:* 0.9% saline, hypertonic saline, 5% dextrose, lactated Ringer's solution, and balanced electrolyte solutions
- *miscellaneous:* furosemide, tetanus toxoid and antitoxin, pentobarbital (for euthanasia), ivermectin, bandaging materials, catheters, and other equipment for IV administration
- Many of these items are in short supply during sustained relief efforts, so this list also serves as a guide of useful pharmaceutical supplies to be sent or donated to equine disaster relief.

More information on disaster medicine is given in *Equine Medicine and Surgery V* and in the AVMA's *Emergency Preparedness and Response Guide.*

6

Neonatal Evaluation and Management

Patient Evaluation

(pages 242-249)

L. Chris Sanchez

HISTORY

A complete history should include:
- specific questions relating to the mare before, during, and after parturition
  - for example, vaginal discharge during late gestation, early lactation, number of prior foalings, problems with prior foalings, and a description of the foaling process, if observed
  - examination findings indicative of dystocia, such as vaginal bruising or laceration
- placental examination findings
  - Placentitis (e.g., thickening, discoloration) may indicate that the foal is at risk for neonatal septicemia.
  - Meconium staining usually indicates in utero stress, placing the foal at risk for hypoxic ischemic encephalomyelopathy (see p. 74).
  - If the foal did not exit at the cervical star, premature placental separation may have occurred.
- gestation length (normal range in horses is 335 to 342 days)
- speed and ease of delivery, and extent of assistance (if any)
- color and texture of the colostrum
- specific questions relating to the newborn foal

- time to stand and suck
- Most normal foals stand within 1 hour, have a suck reflex within 30 minutes, and suck from the mare within 2 hours of birth.
- Any foal that fails to stand within 2 hours or fails to suck within 4 hours should be considered abnormal.
- strength of foal's suck reflex

PRESENTING SIGNS INDICATIVE OF SERIOUS DISEASE

Major warning signs include:
- signs of prematurity—domed forehead, silky hair coat, floppy ears or lips, joint laxity, small body size
- major alterations in mucous membrane appearance—injection, icterus, hyperemia, toxicity
synovial distention
- abdominal distention
- abdominal discomfort
- neurologic abnormalities—seizures, inability to stand, inability to suck

PHYSICAL RESTRAINT

Avoid direct pressure on the foal's thorax and abdomen, especially when lifting the foal.
- To lift the foal, grasp it in front of the shoulder and either behind the rump or just cranial to the stifles.
- When restraining foals in a standing position, apply pressure in front of the shoulder and either behind the rump or on the tail.

- Foals often are best restrained against a wall or backed into a corner of the stall.
- Normal foals may suddenly become limp or appear sleepy after prolonged or firm restraint.
  - Briefly reducing the amount of restraint usually encourages the foal to support its own weight.

PHYSICAL EXAMINATION

Routine physical examination of any neonate should include:

- rectal temperature
- pulse, heart rate and rhythm
- evaluation of respiratory rate and character
- thorough palpation of all joints
- careful auscultation of the trachea and thorax
- examination of oral, conjunctival, and vulvar (if applicable) mucous membranes
- auscultation of borborygmi
- ocular examination
- palpation and visual examination of the external umbilical stump
- visual examination of external genitalia
- assessment of mental status and ability to stand and ambulate

Cardiovascular System
Heart rate

The heart rate in newborn foals is 40 to 80 beats/min immediately after birth; it increases to approximately 120 beats/min after a few hours.

- For the first week of life, heart rates range from 80 to 100 beats/min.
- Heart rates consistently <60 or >160 beats/min indicate a current or impending problem.

Arrhythmias and murmurs

- Arrhythmias may be heard during the first 30 minutes of life, but the rhythm should quickly normalize.
- Murmurs are common in neonates.
  - Flow murmurs are easily heard over the aortic valve on the left side.
  - Less commonly, murmurs from a patent ductus arteriosus (PDA) can be heard up to 3 days of age, high on the left side.

- Murmurs that persist for longer than 3 to 4 days or arrhythmias that persist longer than 1 hour should be evaluated via echocardiography or electrocardiography, respectively.

Mucous membrane characteristics

- The mucous membranes should be pink and moist, with a capillary refill time of <1.5 seconds.
- Cyanosis indicates arterial oxygen tension (Pao_2) <40 mm Hg.
  - Causes include reversal of blood flow in a PDA as a result of pulmonary hypertension (subsequent to septicemia, dehydration, or hypoxemia), and congenital cardiac abnormalities (e.g., tetralogy of Fallot, truncus arteriosus, transposition of the great arteries, tricuspid atresia, and hypoplastic left heart syndrome).
  - Cyanotic foals should be placed on oxygen insufflation immediately.
- Icterus can be normal in neonates, but it may also be caused by serious problems such as neonatal isoerythrolysis, septicemia, and leptospirosis.
- Mild dehydration is indicated by dry mucous membranes.
  - Moderate-to-severe dehydration causes the mucous membranes to become dry and dark.
  - Additional signs of dehydration include poor skin turgor and, in severe dehydration, sunken eyes.

Pulmonary System
Physical findings

Careful auscultation of both lung fields is essential in neonates.

- Immediately after birth, fluid sounds and crackles can be heard (resulting from atelectasis).
  - In foals with pneumonia, findings on auscultation often do not correlate with the severity of pulmonary disease.
- Respiratory rate and effort often are more useful indicators of pulmonary disease.
  - Foals with significant pulmonary disease often breathe with flared nostrils, show marked abdominal movement with respiration,

and/or have persistently increased respiratory rates.

Arterial blood gas analysis

- The dorsal metatarsal artery (located on the lateral aspect of the hind limb, on the plantar edge of the third metatarsal bone) is the most often used site for arterial blood collection.
  - The sample is best taken with the foal in lateral recumbency, with the limb extended.
  - Other sampling sites include the brachial artery (on the medial aspect of the elbow joint) and the common carotid artery.
- A small-volume (1 to 3 mL) preheparinized syringe and a small-gauge (5/8-inch, 25 gauge) needle are preferred for collection; any air is purged from the syringe after blood collection.
- Pressure must be applied to the collection site to avoid hematoma formation.
- Samples not analyzed immediately may be placed on ice for up to 6 hours before analysis.
- Foals with a PaO_2 <60 mm Hg should receive supplemental oxygen via insufflation.
- Foals with a $PaCO_2$ >60 mm Hg should be closely monitored, because ventilatory support may be necessary.

Pneumonia

- Bacterial pneumonia is the most common neonatal respiratory disorder.
- Bacteria can be seeded hematogenously from another site (e.g., umbilicus, GI tract, bone) or directly via aspiration of infected amniotic fluids from mares with placentitis.
- Common isolates include *Escherichia coli, Klebsiella pneumoniae, Salmonella* spp., *Pasteurella* spp., *Actinobacillus* spp., *and Streptococcus zooepidemicus.*
- Transtracheal wash is the preferred method of sample collection, provided the foal is not in respiratory distress.
- Other culture sources include blood from the foal and, if placentitis is suspected, uterine or placental cultures from the mare.

- Herpesvirus (EHV-1) infection is the most important neonatal viral respiratory disease.
  - It is almost always fatal.
  - Other viral causes include EHV-4, equine influenza, and equine viral arteritis.

Aspiration of meconium

- Aspiration of meconium causes moderate-to-severe caudoventral pneumonia.
- While this is usually a sterile process, antibiotics are recommended to prevent secondary bacterial infection.
  - If aspiration of meconium occurs in the presence of placentitis, the pneumonia will likely have a bacterial component.
- When a large amount is aspirated, assisted ventilation may be required.

Alimentary System

Examination of the neonatal GI tract includes:

- auscultation of borborygmi
- passage of a nasogastric tube
  - Large quantities of reflux suggest obstructive small intestinal disease (e.g., volvulus, intussusception) or ileus.
- sampling and analysis of abdominal fluid
  - Peritoneal fluid from foals with strangulating lesions often has an increased total protein concentration (>2.5 g/dL) and elevated WBC count (>5000/μL).
  - Foals with nonstrangulating obstruction or enteritis usually have peritoneal fluid that either is normal or has a mild increase in total protein.
- digital rectal examination
- serial measurements of circumference—useful for detecting abdominal distention

Radiography and ultrasonography

- Radiographs of foals with small intestinal obstruction commonly show vertical U-shaped loops of gas-filled small intestine.
- Ultrasound of strangulating lesions may reveal one or more of the following:
  - moderate-to-marked bowel distention
  - nonmotile loops of small intestine

- increased free peritoneal fluid
◆ Ultrasound of an intussusception reveals a target, or bull's eye, appearance of the telescoped loops of bowel.

Meconium impaction
◆ Failure of meconium passage is one of the most common causes of colic in neonates.
  - Most foals should receive a prophylactic enema as part of the routine neonatal examination.
◆ Meconium impaction can usually be diagnosed by digital rectal palpation.
◆ If the impaction is over the pelvic brim, abdominal radiographs (± barium contrast) are useful.
◆ If no meconium is passed and the foal experiences progressively more pain, a congenital anomaly, such as atresia coli, is possible.
◆ Surgical intervention to relieve the impaction may be necessary

Gastroduodenal ulcer disease
◆ Gastroduodenal ulcers predominantly occur in weanlings (3 to 6 months of age).
◆ Classic signs of gastric ulcers in foals include rolling up into dorsal recumbency and teeth grinding; however, these signs are not pathognomonic.
◆ Prophylactic antiulcer therapy is recommended for hospitalized foals (see p. 80)
◆ Ulcers in the glandular mucosa are common in critically ill neonatal foals and with usage of NSAIDs.

Enteritis
◆ Foal diarrhea, or enteritis, is one of the most common causes of colic.
◆ Common causes include rotavirus infection, salmonellosis, foal heat diarrhea, and septicemia.
  - Other infectious causes include clostridia, cryptococcal organisms, and *E. coli*.
◆ Foals with enteritis display signs of varying degrees of pain.
◆ Signs may also be related to dehydration and electrolyte abnormalities (foals may develop severe hyponatremia, hypochloremia, and metabolic acidosis).

Urogenital System
Umbilical abnormalities
◆ Omphalophlebitis (infection of the umbilical vein) is a common problem in neonates and can serve as a source of ascending infection and septicemia.
◆ Presence of urine at the external umbilical opening likely indicates a patent urachus, which is commonly associated with infection of the umbilical remnants.
◆ Ultrasonography should be used to evaluate patent urachus, purulent discharge at the external opening, or enlargement of the external remnant.

Uroperitoneum
◆ Uroperitoneum is more common in colts than in fillies.
◆ It can be related to trauma during delivery or handling, but the cause often remains unknown.
◆ The bladder is the most frequent site of rupture, but leakage from the urachus, urethra, or ureters may also occur.
◆ Presenting complaints include colic, dysuria, and, in later stages, neurologic abnormalities caused by electrolyte alterations; abdominal distention may or may not be apparent.
◆ Severe electrolyte abnormalities often result, including severe metabolic acidosis, hyperkalemia, hyponatremia, and hypochloremia.
◆ Additional diagnostic procedures include ultrasonography, comparison of creatinine concentrations in the serum and abdominal fluid, and examination of peritoneal fluid for oxalate crystals.
  - Uroperitoneum is strongly suspected when abdominal fluid creatinine is twice that in serum.
◆ Surgery is necessary to correct the defect.
◆ The prognosis usually is good, provided the bladder wall is not severely damaged.

Neurologic System
Neurologic examination
Observation of the foal's behavior and movement in the stall with its dam provides useful information regarding its neurologic status. Neurologic examination is similar to that performed on adult horses, with the addition of spinal reflexes. The following specific differences between

adult and neonatal responses should be considered:

- Normal foals often have a choppy gait and a wide-based stance.
- Young foals normally have jerky, exaggerated head movements.
- The menace response usually is not present until several weeks of age, but foals should have a palpebral response and pupillary light reflex.
- Spinal reflexes may appear exaggerated compared with those of adults.
- Normal foals sleep a lot, but premature foals often are quieter and sleepier than normal.

Additional diagnostic procedures
Depending on the history and presenting signs, diagnostic procedures may include:

- skull and cervical vertebral radiographs
- cerebrospinal fluid analysis and possibly culture
- electrodiagnostics (electroencephalography, electromyography, and brainstem auditory evoked responses)
- advanced imaging techniques (MRI and CT)

Hypoxic ischemic encephalomyelopathy

- Also referred to as "dummy foal" and *neonatal maladjustment syndrome,* this is the most common neurologic problem in neonates.
- It likely occurs as a result of periparturient hypoxic damage to the brain or spinal cord.
- Affected foals can present with a wide variety of clinical signs; the most common are:
  - absence of a strong suck reflex
  - inability to rise
  - lack of affinity for the mare
- Onset of signs can vary from immediately after birth to 48 hours of age, depending on the severity of asphyxia and subsequent cerebral edema.
- Seizures may develop in severe cases (see below).
- Diagnosis is made by exclusion of other diseases and a history suggestive of ischemic insult.
  - Depending on the signalment, history, and signs, differential diagnoses may include electrolyte or metabolic abnormalities, trauma, bacterial or viral meningitis, botulism, tetanus, cerebellar abiotrophy, hydrocephalus, and atlantooccipital-axial malformation.
- If signs are mild to moderate and good supportive care is provided, the prognosis is good.

Seizures
A thorough history should be obtained for all foals experiencing seizures, including a detailed description of the seizures, if possible.

- Signs of tonic-clonic seizure activity can be subtle and include chewing, drooling, facial twitching or grimacing, champing, eye blinking or rapid eye movements, paddling, tachypnea, or abnormal breathing patterns.
- Generalized seizures must be treated immediately.
- Common anticonvulsant medications include:
  - diazepam: 5 to 10 mg (for a 45- to 50-kg foal [100-110 lb]) slowly IV; may be repeated
  - phenobarbital: loading dose: 10 to 20 mg/kg IV, diluted in 30 mL saline, given over 15 to 30 minutes; maintenance dose: 5 to 10 mg/kg IV or PO q8–12h
  - Phenytoin or general anesthesia may be used if the foal does not respond to diazepam or phenobarbital.
- The foal should be placed in a quiet, safe environment.
- Idiopathic epilepsy should be considered in Arabian foals; it is diagnosed by exclusion.

Musculoskeletal System
Key abnormalities to recognize in neonates include:

- angular limb deformities
- flexural deformities
- tendon, ligament, or joint laxity
- septic arthritis

Ophthalmic System
Neonates are susceptible to corneal trauma.

- All hospitalized neonates should have a daily ophthalmic examination, including fluorescein staining to evaluate corneal integrity.

- Foals with neurologic disease, especially seizures, often require prophylactic application of artificial tear ointment.
- Premature foals often have entropion, which leaves them at risk for corneal ulceration.
- Foals with corneal ulceration should be monitored closely for evidence of delayed healing.
  - Foals with indolent ulcers should undergo corneal scraping with culture to ensure appropriate antibiotic coverage.
  - Fungal keratitis is relatively common in warm, humid environments.

REFERRAL

Critically ill foals should be stabilized as much as possible before transport, specifically with regard to the following:

- maintenance of body temperature
- treatment of hypovolemia or hypoglycemia
- control of seizures
- evaluation of respiratory function

If the mare's udder is severely distended, she should be milked out. If the foal has not sucked and the mare has colostrum, the colostrum should be collected and either administered to the foal by stomach tube or sent with the foal to the referral hospital. If possible, the placenta should be sent with the newborn foal for examination, culture, and histopathology, if indicated.

ANCILLARY DIAGNOSTIC AIDS
Diagnostic Imaging
Radiography
- Radiographs provide a good indicator of the severity and progression of pulmonary disease in foals.
- Abdominal radiographs can help differentiate between large and small intestinal distention in foals exhibiting signs of colic.
  - Measurement of intestinal diameter can help differentiate between diseases requiring medical or surgical treatment.

Ultrasonography
- Thoracic ultrasound can be used to identify pleural irregularities, super-

ficial parenchymal abscesses and other abnormalities, pneumothorax, and cardiac abnormalities.
- Abdominal ultrasonography allows accurate evaluation of umbilical remnants, amount and character of free abdominal fluid, bladder integrity, intestinal wall thickness, small intestinal luminal diameter, and presence of intussusception and an estimate of intestinal motility.

Clinical Pathology

Several laboratory indices in foals vary from normal adult values:

- Normal PCV in the first few days of life is 28% to 46%, then 29% to 41% at 1 month, and 32% to 42% at 3 months.
- Total plasma protein concentration varies widely after birth.
  - It is not a good indicator of passive transfer of immunoglobulins.
- Differences in the biochemical profile often seen in normal foals include elevations in CK and bilirubin (for days), GGT, SDH, and AST (for weeks), and alkaline phosphatase (for weeks to months).
- Increased serum creatinine concentration immediately after birth may be normal, but they can often be attributed to renal or placental disease. Renal dysfunction or ruptured bladder should be considered if serum creatine does not decrease by 24 hours of age.

SEDATION AND ANESTHESIA
Special Considerations

During general anesthesia, changes in cardiac output, vasomotor tone, and pulmonary pressure can result in pulmonary hypertension and a return to fetal circulation (right-to-left shunting). Shunting is possible because the ductus arteriosus and foramen ovale, while functionally closed in normal neonates within 72 hours of birth, persist anatomically until 4 to 6 weeks of age.

Hypotension

Systemic hypotension during anesthesia in foals can be managed with dobutamine at 3 mg/kg/min IV.

Hypoxemia and hypercapnia

Neonatal foals are susceptible to hypoxemia, especially if any underlying respiratory disease is present.

- Supplemental oxygen should be provided and, if possible, arterial blood gases monitored during general anesthesia.
- Prematurity, hypothermia, hypoglycemia, electrolyte abnormalities, or other severe systemic illnesses may cause hypoventilation during anesthesia.
  - In such foals, a 2-L bellows with a respiratory rate of 12 to 18 breaths/min, a peak inspired pressure of 12 to 20 cm H_2O, and a tidal volume of 6 to 10 mL/kg are recommended.
  - If a higher level of ventilation is needed, increasing the rate rather than the peak inspired pressure avoids barotrauma.
- Intermittent positive-pressure ventilation usually is not necessary in healthy foals.

Hypothermia

Anesthetized foals are predisposed to hypothermia, especially during abdominal surgery.

- Careful monitoring of core body temperature is essential.
- Fluids used IV or for lavage should be warmed to body temperature and heating pads, heat lamps, and blankets used to keep the foal warm.

Hypovolemia

- Fluid loss, especially hemorrhage, is not well tolerated by neonates.
- Overzealous compensation for fluid losses leads to volume overload, so careful estimates of losses or dehydration should be made before replacement.

Sedation

Following are the drug dosages recommended for sedation in foals:

- *Diazepam* is commonly used, especially for sick foals.
  - A dose rate of 0.1 to 0.2 mg/kg slowly IV is recommended.
  - Doses up to 0.44 mg/kg can be used if needed.
  - Diazepam generally is safe in sick foals, but it offers poor analgesia.
- *Xylazine* can be safely administered at low doses (0.2 to 0.4 mg/kg IV or 0.6 mg/kg IM).

- Cardiopulmonary depression occurs with this drug, especially at higher doses.
- *Detomidine* can also be used in foals, at 10 μg/kg IV.
- *Drug combinations:* Acepromazine (0.03 mg/kg IV or IM) or butorphanol (0.01 to 0.04 mg/kg IV or IM) can be combined with xylazine (at the lowest end of the dosage range).

A common combination used to sedate the mare is acepromazine (0.02 mg/kg IV) and xylazine (0.2 to 0.3 mg/kg IV).

Anesthesia

Young or sick foals

Induction of anesthesia in young or sick foals is easily accomplished with either isoflurane or halothane:

- Isoflurane is preferred in critically ill foals.
- Induction can be accomplished using a face mask or a cuffed nasotracheal tube (quickest).
- After induction, a cuffed orotracheal tube is passed, and anesthesia is maintained with halothane or isoflurane.

Other foals

For older foals, foals in intense pain, or foals that are difficult to restrain, anesthesia may be induced with injectable agents.

- In young or sick foals xylazine (0.3 mg/kg IV) followed by ketamine (2.2 mg/kg IV) and diazepam (0.1 mg/kg IV) is preferred.
- In larger foals xylazine (0.2 to 0.5 mg/kg IV) followed by guaifenesin (60 to 100 mg/kg IV, to effect) then ketamine (2.2 mg/kg IV) or thiopental (4 to 6 mg/kg slowly IV) provides adequate induction.
- After induction, orotracheal intubation and maintenance of anesthesia are performed as for foals induced with inhalation agents.

Monitoring and recovery

- Anesthetized foals should be monitored similarly to adults, with special attention paid to cardiopulmonary function, body temperature, and blood glucose concentration.
- Foals should be watched carefully during recovery and assisted when attempting to rise.

◆ If possible, oxygen insufflation is continued until extubation.

Principles of Therapy

(pages 249-253)

L. Chris Sanchez

INTENSIVE CARE

Respiratory System

Maintaining nonambulatory foals in a sternal position as much as possible is essential to both the treatment of existing pulmonary disease and the prevention of problems during recovery. Following are some other recommendations:

◆ Thoracic coupâge helps break up thick lower airway secretions in foals with severe pneumonia, especially aspiration pneumonia.
◆ Oxygen insufflation is very important in foals with severe respiratory disease.
  • All cyanotic foals and those with a PaO_2 <60 mm Hg should be administered supplemental oxygen via nasal insufflation at a rate of 8 to 10 L/min.

Determining the need for assisted ventilation

The most common problems that cause respiratory failure and thus require ventilatory support are:

◆ *failure of central respiratory drive:* causes include hypoxic ischemic encephalomyelopathy and sepsis
◆ *ineffective ventilation resulting from weakness:* causes include prematurity, sepsis, and hypoxic ischemic encephalomyelopathy
◆ *primary lung disease:* aspiration pneumonia, bronchopneumonia, and interstitial disease

Criteria for placing foals on a ventilator vary. However, two general guidelines are:

◆ continued $PaCO_2$ >60 mm Hg *and/or*
◆ continued PaO_2 <60 mm Hg, despite oxygen insufflation

Fluid therapy

Maintenance Needs

◆ The daily fluid requirement for foals is 100 to 120 mL/kg, or 5 to 6 L for the average 45- to 50-kg (100 to 110 lb) foal.
◆ To meet its *caloric* needs, the average 45-kg foal consumes 9 to 11 L of mare's milk per day.

Replacing fluid and electrolyte losses

Calculating and replacing fluid and electrolyte losses in neonatal foals follow the same principles as those outlined for adult horses in Chapter 4, Principles of Therapy.

◆ An estimate of the degree of dehydration is made during the initial physical examination, using similar criteria as for adults, with the addition of urine specific gravity.
◆ A serum biochemical profile and venous or arterial blood gas analysis provide critical information about the foal's electrolyte, glucose, and acid-base status.

Choice of fluids

◆ Crystalloid solutions containing 5% glucose and supplemented with sodium bicarbonate, calcium, potassium, and magnesium as needed are appropriate in most foals.
  • Suitable fluids for replacement therapy include Plasmalyte 148 with 5% dextrose, Plasmalyte A, lactated Ringer's, and Multisol-R
  • Plasmalyte 56 with 5% dextrose is suitable for maintenance.
◆ Constant infusion provides the most physiologic method of fluid administration, but the daily requirement can be divided and given as boluses, especially in non–critical foals.
◆ Hypertonic saline (3 to 4 mL/kg) is occasionally indicated in cases of severe shock.
  • It is contraindicated in the presence of normonatremia or hypernatremia and should always be used with caution.
  • Hypertonic saline must be followed by isotonic crystalloids.
◆ Colloid solutions, such as whole blood, plasma, and synthetic colloids are indicated for severe blood loss, failure of passive transfer, and hypoproteinemia.

Fluid therapy for uroperitoneum

◆ Foals with uroperitoneum often have severe metabolic acidosis, hyperkalemia, hyponatremia, and hypochloremia.

- These foals can develop cardiac arrhythmias associated with hyperkalemia and should be initially treated with sodium chloride.
  - Addition of 5% to 10% dextrose increases intracellular movement of K^+, as does the addition of 5% sodium bicarbonate.

Fluid therapy for severe diarrhea

- Foals with severe diarrhea can develop severe metabolic acidosis, hypokalemia, hypochloremia, and hyponatremia.
- Addition of specific electrolytes to IV fluids should be guided by serum biochemical abnormalities; K^+ supplementation is almost always necessary.

Treating metabolic acidosis

- Mild acidosis often is better left untreated.
  - Overcorrection of bicarbonate deficits can cause paradoxical CSF acidosis.
- The bicarbonate need is estimated using the following formula:

$$\text{mEq deficit} = 0.4 \times \text{Body weight (kg)} \times \text{Base deficit (mEq/L)}$$

- Response to therapy and the need for further supplementation should be monitored by frequent venous blood gas evaluations.
- Severe diarrhea can cause ongoing bicarbonate losses that necessitate continued supplementation, but, in other cases, continued bicarbonate therapy usually is unnecessary.
- Sodium bicarbonate should be used with caution in hypocalcemic, hypokalemic, or hypernatremic foals.

Nutrition

Sick foals often are unable or unwilling to nurse with sufficient frequency to meet their caloric requirements; furthermore, these foals often have increased calorie needs. Provision of adequate nutrition is of critical importance to the outcome of sick or debilitated foals.

Meeting caloric requirements

- To meet their caloric requirements, normal foals consume 130 to 150 kcal/kg/day, or 21% to 25% of their body weight in mare's milk per day.

- Supplemental enteral feeding is preferred over parenteral feeding if the foal cannot nurse from the mare.
  - Bottle-feeding is an alternative for some foals; however, it carries an increased risk of aspiration pneumonia.
  - If the foal can tolerate large volumes of milk in its stomach but is too weak to drink on its own, an indwelling nasogastric tube can be used.
- When beginning an enteral feeding program for a sick foal, small amounts should be fed at first.
  - The volume fed is then gradually increased over 24 to 36 hours.
  - Smaller-volume, more frequent (e.g., hourly) feedings are preferred for sick foals.
  - If reflux is obtained before a feeding, signs of colic are noted, or the abdomen becomes distended, all feedings should be stopped.
- Commercial milk replacer or goat's milk can be substituted for mare's milk.
  - Cow's milk often causes diarrhea in foals.
- When a foal cannot tolerate enteral feeding, partial or total parenteral nutrition is necessary (see Chapter 4, Principles of Therapy).

ANTIBIOTIC THERAPY

Most antibiotic regimens used in neonates are adapted from those described for adult horses (see Chapter 4). In a farm setting, IV or IM routes are preferred. All available oral antibiotic formulations can cause diarrhea in foals, but some are frequently used with good success.

Antibiotic Selection

Obtaining samples for culture is always recommended.

- Blood, synovial fluid, and transtracheal wash cultures greatly influence antimicrobial selection.
- Common pathogens implicated in neonatal septicemia, pneumonia, and septic arthritis include *E. coli, Klebsiella pneumoniae, Salmonella* spp., *Pasteurella* spp., *Actinobacillus* spp., *and Streptococcus zooepidemicus.*

- Bactericidal antibiotics are best.
  - The most commonly used antibiotics in neonates are penicillins, cephalosporins, aminoglycosides, metronidazole, and trimethoprim-sulfonamides.

Specific infectious conditions
- ***neonatal septicemia or pneumonia:*** A combination of potassium penicillin (22,000 to 44,000 IU/kg IV q6h) and amikacin sulfate (20 mg/kg IV q24h) is recommended until culture results are known.
  - For foals with severe pneumonia, ceftazidime (25 mg/kg IV q8h) often is used.
- ***suspected anaerobic infections:*** *Bacteroides fragilis* or *Clostridium* spp. infections are treated with penicillin at the high end of the dose range of metronidazole (15 mg/kg qh8, or 7.5 mg/kg q6h after a loading dose of 15 mg/kg).

Adverse Effects

Renal function should be monitored when aminoglycosides are used for prolonged periods, in dehydrated foals, or if NSAIDs are used concurrently (see Chapter 4, Principles of Therapy). Serum creatinine concentration, urine output, and urine specific gravity can be used to detect developing renal problems. The use of fluoroquinolones in foals should be limited to cases in which the MIC suggests resistance to other agents.

IMMUNE THERAPY

Foals can develop complete (serum IgG <200 mg/dL) or partial (serum IgG of 200 to 800 mg/dL) failure of passive transfer (FPT). The most common reasons for FPT are:
- loss of colostrum (e.g., premature lactation)
- inadequate colostral IgG content
- inadequate colostral intake by the foal

In foals known to have consumed adequate amounts of good-quality colostrum, colostral malabsorption should be suspected. Septic foals require larger amounts of IgG than healthy foals to overcome altered IgG distribution and consumption.

Management of FPT

Before 12 hours of age

- If FPT is diagnosed before 12 hours age, oral IgG supplementation usually is effective.
- The best source is good-quality equine colostrum.
  - Colostral IgG content can be measured by RID (e.g., Gamma-Check C) or inferred by measuring specific gravity with a colostrometer.
  - Optimum IgG concentrations are consistent with an RID value of 3000 mg/dL or a specific gravity reading of 1.06.
- For a 40- to 50-kg (90 to 110 lb) foal, a total of 1 to 2 L of colostrum should be given via nasogastric tube or bottle hourly in 500-mL aliquots before the foal reaches 8 to 12 hours of age.
  - This volume should supply the necessary 1 g/kg body weight of IgG.
- If equine colostrum is unavailable, a commercial concentrated equine IgG product can be substituted, provided an adequate total amount of IgG is delivered.
- In all foals treated with oral IgG supplementation, serum IgG should be measured at or before 24 hours of age.

After 12 hours of age

- After 12 to 24 hours of age, foals with FPT should be treated IV with equine plasma, either fresh or from a commercial source.
  - In healthy foals, each liter of plasma increases the foal's IgG approximately 200 mg/dL.
- Plasma should be administered slowly for the first 15 minutes or 50 mL; subsequently, the rate can be increased to approximately 20 mL/kg/h.
- Foals should be monitored for tachycardia, tachypnea, weakness, and muscle fasciculations.
  - Crystalloid fluids and epinephrine (0.01 mg/kg IV, SC, or intratracheal) should be available in case of a transfusion reaction.

ANALGESICS

Indications for use of analgesics and antiinflammatory agents in foals include acute abdominal pain, severe pneumonia, trauma, severe neurologic disorders, and high fever.

Adverse Effects

Adverse effects are the same as those seen in adult horses (see Chapter 4, Principles of Therapy):

- Glandular ulceration is of specific concern in foals.
  - Prophylactic antiulcer therapy with ranitidine (6.6 mg/kg PO q8h or 2 mg/kg IV q6h) or cimetidine (18 to 20 mg/kg PO q8h) is indicated for foals needing repeated doses of NSAIDs.
  - A mucosal protectant such as sucralfate (20 mg/kg PO q6–8h) may also be used.
- Limiting or avoiding the use of NSAIDs in hypovolemic or dehydrated foals, especially in combination with potentially nephrotoxic antibiotics such as aminoglycosides and tetracyclines, decreases the risk of renal toxicity.

- Fluid therapy also reduces the risk in these foals.

Outcomes *(page 253)*
L. Chris Sanchez

Reported short-term survival rates for most neonatal ICUs currently range from 70% to 85%. Following are some specific prognoses:

- Hypoxic ischemic encephalomyelopathy and uncomplicated pneumonia carry a good prognosis for complete recovery.
- Neonatal septicemia, septic arthritis, and osteomyelitis carry a good prognosis for short-term survival, but a more guarded prognosis for future high-level athletic performance.
- Premature foals have the poorest prognosis of performing as top-level athletes.

7

Principles of Chemical Restraint, General Anesthesia, and Surgery

Chemical Restraint

(pages 256-258)

Cynthia M. Trim

XYLAZINE, DETOMIDINE, AND ROMIFIDINE

Xylazine, detomidine, and romifidine act by stimulation of α_2-adrenoreceptors. The behavioral effects and duration of action are dose related.

- Ataxia is a feature of moderate to profound sedation.
  - Xylazine and detomidine produce a greater degree of ataxia than does romifidine.
- Moderate to heavy sedation is sometimes accompanied by muscle twitches and head jerks.
  - Lightly touching the horse's hindquarters or legs may provoke an exaggerated muscle movement or kick, especially during sedation with detomidine.
  - Detomidine alone may not be useful for procedures involving the hind limbs.
- These agents produce less sedation in excited or nervous horses.
  - Detomidine produces more predictable sedation in an excited horse than does xylazine.
- The duration of sedation is longer with romifidine than with detomidine or xylazine.

- The IM dose rate for xylazine is twice the IV dose rate, and onset of action takes 20 minutes.
- Satisfactory sedation can be obtained by sublingual administration of detomidine (0.04 mg/kg, squirted under the tongue); sedation develops over 45 minutes.

Systemic Effects

Following are the major systemic effects of the α_2 agonists:

- ***cardiovascular system:*** Within 1 minute of IV injection, arterial blood pressure increases and is followed by bradycardia, often with second-degree atrioventricular heart block.
  - These effects are more pronounced with detomidine than with xylazine.
  - With time (15 minutes for xylazine, 40 minutes for detomidine), vasodilation develops and arterial pressure decreases.
- ***respiratory system:*** Respiratory rates may be low or within the normal range.
  - With xylazine, resistance to airflow through the upper airway increases, as does total pulmonary resistance and work of breathing.
  - PaO_2 is significantly decreased for 5 to 30 minutes after xylazine or romifidine and for longer after detomidine administration.

* *diuresis:* Diuresis occurs 30 minutes to 2 hours after xylazine or detomidine administration.
* *gastrointestinal motility:* Xylazine and detomidine decrease intestinal motility for several hours.
* *skin:* Sweating commonly occurs with these drugs, especially at the base of the ears, on the neck, and in the groin.
  * Detomidine sometimes causes piloerection on the shoulders and hindquarters.

Medetomidine

Medetomidine is an α_2-adrenoreceptor agonist licensed for sedation of dogs.

* It causes unacceptable ataxia in horses when used alone for sedation.
* However, it has potential use as premedication for emergency anesthesia with tiletamine-zolazepam at racetracks.

Antagonists

Tolazoline is a mixed α_1- and α_2-adrenoreceptor antagonist that reverses the effects of xylazine in horses.

* Onset of arousal is within 5 minutes of administration of tolazoline at 4 mg/kg IV.
* Reversal may not be complete if sedation is profound at the time of administration.
* Caution should be used when considering reversal of sedation in horses subjected to a painful procedure.
* Atipamezole is a specific antagonist of medetomidine in dogs, but will reverse the sedative and analgesic effects of detomidine in horses.

ACEPROMAZINE

Acepromazine is a commonly used phenothiazine tranquilizer that induces mild behavioral effects.

* It can provide adequate control of well-mannered horses for minor procedures and is a useful premedication for anesthesia with thiopental.
* Additional agents are needed for horses resenting restraint or for performance of a procedure.
* The combination of acepromazine with xylazine improves the degree of restraint over that produced by xylazine alone.

Systemic Effects

Following are the major systemic effects of acepromazine:

* *cardiovascular system:* Vasodilation may cause hypotension in geriatric or hypovolemic animals.
  * Decreases in cardiac output and arterial pressure are minimal in healthy horses.
* *paraphimosis:* Acepromazine is not recommended in breeding stallions because of the risk of causing paraphimosis.

OPIOIDS

Opioids generally are added to other drugs, such as acepromazine or an α_2-adrenoreceptor agonist, to produce neuroleptanalgesia (Table 7-1).

* Some opioids may cause CNS stimulation and excitement when given alone.
* Other opioids, including butorphanol, pentazocine, and meperidine, may be given alone without causing excitement.
  * However, these opioids cause little or no sedation.
* The combinations of butorphanol or morphine with xylazine, detomidine, or romifidine provide sufficient sedation for a wide variety of procedures.
  * High dose rates of xylazine (1.1 mg/kg IV), detomidine (0.04 mg/kg IV), or romifidine (0.1 mg/kg IV) with butorphanol (0.1 mg/kg IV) provide good analgesia and restraint; however, side effects are more prominent at these dose rates.
  * Lower dose rates reduce the intensity of undesirable effects and usually produce adequate restraint; local analgesia should be included where appropriate.
* The combination of an α_2-agonist and morphine produces profound sedation and analgesia and is particularly effective for procedures around the head and shoulders.
  * The intensity of sedation may lessen after 30 minutes; an additional small dose of α_2-agonist re-

Table 7-1
Suggested combinations of sedatives, tranquilizers, and opioids for restraint of the standing horse

Drug	Dose rate (mg/kg IV)	Concentration (mg/kg)	mL/500 kg
Acepromazine	0.04	20	1.0
Xylazine	0.6	100	3.0
Acepromazine	0.04	20	1.0
Meperidine	1.0	50	10
Detomidine	0.004	10	0.2
Xylazine	0.3-0.8	100	1.5-4.0
Xylazine	0.3-0.7	100	1.5-3.5
Butorphanol	0.02-0.03	10	1.0-1.5
Detomidine	0.005-0.02	10	0.25-1.0
Butorphanol	0.02-0.03	10	1.0-1.5
Acepromazine	0.04	20	1.0
Butorphanol	0.02-0.03	10	1.0-1.5
Xylazine	0.3-0.6	100	1.5-3.0
Xylazine	0.6-1.0	100	3.0-5.0
Morphine	0.2-0.7	15	10-20 (300 mg is maximum total dose)

stores neuroleptanalgesia (morphine provides analgesia for 15 to 60 minutes).

- This drug combination decreases intestinal motility for several hours.
- Administration of naloxone at 0.8 to 1.6 mg IV for a 450-kg (990 lb) horse can restore intestinal sounds within 5 minutes.

General Anesthesia

(pages 258-282)

Cynthia M. Trim

PREPARATION

Preparation for general anesthesia involves the following:

- consideration of pertinent facts in the history, such as an adverse response to previous anesthesia and recent administration of other drugs (e.g., organophosphate dewormers)
  - The horse's temperament may alter its reaction to sedatives, loss of consciousness, or recovery from anesthesia.
- examination of the horse
  - Evidence of cardiovascular or respiratory disease is important to note.
  - Hypovolemia, septicemia, endotoxemia, hyponatremia, and hypocalcemia increase the risk of hypotension during anesthesia.
  - The relative volume of distribution may be increased in lean horses and decreased in fat horses.
  - Laboratory tests for routine preanesthetic screening, such as CBC and measurement of total protein, fibrinogen, creatinine, and AST, are used by many clinics.
- consideration of the requirements or potentially adverse influences of the surgical or medical procedure
- preparation of the patient and equipment
  - Whenever possible, grain and fresh pasture should be withheld for 24 hours and hay for up to 12 hours before anesthesia; water is allowed.

- Foals may regurgitate and aspirate milk unless prevented from nursing by application of a muzzle for 30 to 60 minutes before induction.
- Older foals should be prevented from eating solid food for 3 to 4 hours before induction.
- Placement of an IV catheter is recommended if anesthesia is to be maintained for >30 minutes.
- consideration of potential drug interactions
  - IV administration of potassium and sodium penicillin cause significant cardiovascular depression and hypotension for up to 30 minutes. They should not be administered within 30 minutes of induction.
  - Potentiated sulfonamides have caused collapse and death when administered IV after sedation with detomidine or anesthesia with ketamine and halothane.

- Phenylbutazone displaces protein-bound thiopentone and halothane into their active unbound forms, so it should not be administered during anesthesia or recovery (although it can be administered preoperatively).

GENERAL ANESTHESIA WITH INTRAVENOUS AGENTS
Guaifenesin
Guaifenesin induces skeletal muscle relaxation.

- It is used to facilitate smooth induction of anesthesia with ketamine or thiopental.
  - It also allows the dose rate of ketamine or thiopental to be reduced, thereby minimizing cardiopulmonary depression.
- Either guaifenesin is administered immediately before ketamine or thiopental, or thiopental is added to the guaifenesin solution.

Table 7-2
Suggested anesthetic drug combinations for induction of anethesia

Premedication drugs	Dose rate (mg/kg IV)	Induction drug(s)	Dose rate (mg/kg IV)
Xylazine	1.1	Ketamine	2.2
Xylazine	1.1	Ketamine	2.2
Butorphanol	0.03		
Xylazine	1.1	Diazepam	0.05
Butorphanol	0.02	Ketamine	2.2
Detomidine	0.004	Diazepam	0.05
Xylazine	0.8	Ketamine	2.2
Xylazine	0.8-1.1	Guaifenesin	55
		Ketamine	1.7
Detomidine	0.02	Ketamine	2.2
Acepromazine	0.04	Guaifenesin	110
		Thiopental	4.4
Xylazine	0.6	Guaifenesin	80-100
		Thiopental	3.4-4.4
Detomidine	0.005-0.01	Guaifenesin	60-100
		Thiopental	3.4-4.4
Detomidine	0.02-0.04	Telazol	1.1-1.4

◆ A 5% (50 mg/mL) solution of guaifenesin should be used, because higher concentrations cause some degree of thrombophlebitis.

◆ There is a small decrease in blood pressure at recommended infusion rates; a large IV bolus dramatically decreases blood pressure.

Ketamine

Ketamine causes minimal cardiovascular depression.

◆ It allows the horse to recover rapidly from anesthesia, with less ataxia than after thiopental anesthesia.

◆ Its major drawback is that the depth and duration of anesthesia frequently are unpredictable.

Xylazine-ketamine

Several combinations of ketamine with sedatives, opioids, and muscle relaxing drugs are used (Table 7-2).

◆ Ketamine usually is given after administration of an α_2-adrenoceptor agonist.

• Xylazine (1.1 mg/kg IV) is followed in 3 to 5 minutes by ketamine (2.2 mg/kg IV)

• Anesthesia is induced in 50 to 60 seconds, but may be accompanied by increased muscle tone, muscle tremors, or jerks; the palpebral reflex is brisk, nystagmus usually is present, and swallowing may be elicited by passage of an endotracheal tube.

• Surgical anesthesia lasts 7 to 20 minutes (less in young animals, Thoroughbreds, and Arabians).

• Usually the horse stands within 30 min after administration of ketamine.

◆ Addition of butorphanol (0.02 to 0.03 mg/kg IV) to the xylazine ensures smooth induction.

◆ Muscle relaxation can be improved by administration of diazepam (0.05 mg/kg IV) immediately before injection of ketamine.

◆ Guaifenesin provides greater relaxation than diazepam and is a better choice for nervous or excited horses.

• The horse is sedated with xylazine and butorphanol, and anesthesia is induced with guaifenesin (45 to 55 mg/kg IV) followed by a bolus of ketamine (1.7 mg/kg IV).

Detomidine-ketamine

◆ Premedication with detomidine is similar to the procedure with xylazine, except that the interval between injections should be increased to 8 to 10 minutes.

◆ This combination is useful for induction before halothane or isoflurane anesthesia.

• Because of the disparity in duration of each drug's effects, anesthesia with detomidine-ketamine alone is not recommended.

◆ Recovery is associated with more ataxia than is seen with xylazine-ketamine.

Romifidine-ketamine

◆ Romifidine-ketamine induction is smooth and relaxed, and the duration of recumbency is slightly longer than with xylazine-ketamine.

◆ Recovery is quiet, with most horses standing on their first attempt.

Mules and donkeys

◆ Unsatisfactory anesthesia with xylazine-ketamine has been observed in mules and donkeys, possibly resulting from decreased effectiveness of xylazine.

• Anesthesia in donkeys is unpredictable and related to the degree of preanesthetic anxiety or stress.

◆ Addition of butorphanol (0.03 mg/kg IV) as a premedication improves the quality and duration of ketamine anesthesia and the quality of recovery.

Cardiopulmonary effects of ketamine

◆ Immediately after induction with ketamine, in a horse sedated with xylazine or detomidine, the heart rate is 26 to 40 beats/min and the respiratory rate is 10 to 20 breaths/min.

• Addition of butorphanol for premedication may result in a lower respiratory rate.

◆ Arterial pressure should remain relatively high (mean arterial pressure >80 mm Hg).

◆ The degree of peripheral vasoconstriction may make palpation of a peripheral pulse difficult.

Prolongation of anesthesia with ketamine

Ketamine anesthesia can be prolonged with additional doses of xylazine and ketamine by either intermittent injections or continuous infusion.

- Intermittent injections: Bolus injections of xylazine (0.37 mg/kg IV) and ketamine (0.73 mg/kg IV) are given at 12-minute intervals or when the plane of anesthesia becomes light (increased amplitude of nystagmus, sighing, ear movement).
- Continuous infusion: 1300 mg ketamine and 650 mg xylazine can be added to 1 L of 5% guaifenesin and infused at a rate of 2 mL/kg/h (GKX anesthesia).
  - Infusion should be started immediately after induction.
  - The horse will regain consciousness about 10 minutes after the infusion is discontinued and should stand 30 minutes (20 to 50 minutes) later.
  - In healthy horses, heart rates should remain between 26 and 40 beats/min and mean arterial pressure >80 mm Hg during GKX infusion.
- An alternative combination for continuous infusion is 500 mg xylazine and 1000 mg ketamine in 1 L of 5% guaifenesin and infusion at 2.75 mL/kg/h IV.
  - This combination delivers more guaifenesin, allowing greater control in excited horses.
  - Disadvantages are greater ataxia during recovery and less anesthesia time per bottle of guaifenesin.
  Xylazine-ketamine boluses or GKX may not ensure immobility in excited horses or provide sufficient analgesia during painful procedures or for major surgery.
- Inclusion of an opioid for premedication or use of local anesthetic agents may be needed for adequate analgesia.
- Additional opioids may have to be given during a long procedure; that is, it may be necessary to give an additional dose of butorphanol or morphine at 45 minutes of anesthesia.

Tiletamine-Zolazepam

Tiletamine-zolazepam is licensed for use in cats and dogs.
- In horses it is used at dose rates of 1.1 to 1.65 mg/kg, after premedication with xylazine (1.1 mg/kg) or detomidine (0.02 to 0.04 mg/kg).

- Xylazine-tiletamine-zolazepam produces smooth induction and a mean recumbency time of 25 to 30 minutes.
  - Recovery usually involves multiple attempts to stand.
  - This combination can be used to provide a smooth transition to halothane anesthesia; the initial vaporizer setting should be low to prevent anesthetic overdose.
- Detomidine (0.04 mg/kg) followed by tiletamine-zolazepam (1.4 mg/kg) produces considerably longer anesthesia and a smooth, quiet recovery.
- All combinations that include tiletamine-zolazepam decrease PaO_2.
  - Supplemental oxygen is recommended.

Thiopental

Thiopental is a barbiturate that predictably induces anesthesia in horses.
- Significant disadvantages are cardiovascular and respiratory depression and ataxia during recovery.
- Undesirable effects are lessened when thiopental is administered with guaifenesin, which allows the dose rate of thiopental to be halved.
- Heavy sedation is not essential before administration of guaifenesin and thiopental; acepromazine can be adequate for sedation.
- Dose rates for these drugs are inversely related to the degree of prior sedation and are up to 4.4 mg/kg for thiopental and up to 110 mg/kg for guaifenesin, IV.
- When guaifenesin and thiopental are given separately, the transition from standing to recumbency is accomplished rapidly and with minimal ataxia.
  - The calculated dose of guaifenesin is halved, with the first half (approximately 55 mg/kg) being infused before the IV injection of thiopental (3.5 to 4.4 mg/kg).
  - Part or all of the remaining guaifenesin is infused after the horse is recumbent.
  - Duration of anesthesia is 15 minutes, and the horse should be standing by 50 minutes.
- An alternative is to add 2 g of thiopental to 1 L of 5% (50 g) guaifenesin.

- The mixture is infused IV to the sedated horse at a dose rate of up to 2.2 mL/kg.
- The horse should be unable to stand after infusion of about 50% of the calculated dose.
- Heavy preanesthetic sedation decreases the total amount required for recumbency.

Monitoring thiopental anesthesia

- After anesthesia is induced, a palpebral reflex should be present but weak, and nystagmus and swallowing should be absent.
- Heart rates usually are 40 to 55 beats/min, and mean arterial pressure is 70 to 100 mm Hg.
- Rapid administration of thiopental may cause transient apnea.
- Ventilation is decreased, although respiratory rates should be within the normal range.

Prolongation of thiopental anesthesia

- Incremental doses of guaifenesin and thiopental (boluses of $1/10$ to $1/5$ of the initial dose), given as the depth of anesthesia lightens, can be used to prolong anesthesia.
- Multiple doses of thiopental are cumulative, resulting in an unacceptable degree of ataxia during recovery.
- Total thiopental dose should be limited to no more than twice the induction dose.

Propofol

Propofol is an IV anesthetic agent used in dogs and cats.

- It has a rapid onset of action, accompanied by good muscle relaxation; cardiovascular and respiratory effects are similar to those of thiopental.
- Recovery is rapid, even when multiple injections or infusions have been administered.
- Disadvantages in horses include the large volume needed and the variable quality of induction (limb paddling is common during the first 2 minutes of recumbency).
  - Average time to standing is 25 to 52 minutes after either a propofol bolus (2 mg/kg) or guaifenesin (100 mg/kg) with propofol (0.5 mg/kg).
- Horses are quiet and coordinated during recovery.
- Mean arterial pressure remains >115 mm Hg for all combinations

with propofol, but ventilation is depressed.
- Xylazine, detomidine, and ketamine can be used with propofol.

Oxygen Supplementation

Insufflation of oxygen is a wise precaution in emergencies and during prolonged anesthesia with injectable agents.

- A flow rate of at least 15 L/min is needed to increase arterial oxygenation in a 500-kg (1100 lb) horse.
- A demand valve can be used to provide artificial ventilation in an emergency.

GENERAL ANESTHESIA WITH INHALATION AGENTS

Advantages of inhalation anesthesia are:

- ability to produce a constant plane of anesthesia for long surgical procedures
- relatively rapid recovery
- facilitation of respiratory support by artificial ventilation and administration of oxygen

A disadvantage is significant cardiovascular depression, often requiring specific treatment, and this is linked with decreased muscle perfusion and development of postanesthetic myopathy.

Halothane and Isoflurane

Both halothane and isoflurane decrease cardiac output and arterial blood pressure and depress ventilation in a dose-dependent fashion.

- Cardiac output is decreased less with isoflurane than with halothane.
- Overall, there is little difference in the quality of recovery between halothane and isoflurane, although horses appear to be less alert and are ataxic for longer with halothane.

Sevoflurane

Sevoflurane decreases ventilation and cardiovascular function similar to other inhalation agents, but it results in a more rapid recovery than does halothane or isoflurane.

- Recovery is quiet and smooth, with little or no ataxia.
- Sevoflurane is degraded in soda lime to a compound that produces

renal toxicity in rats; until its toxicity in horses is determined, it is recommended that closed circuits be avoided.

Nitrous Oxide

Addition of nitrous oxide to halothane anesthesia increases analgesia and reduces the requirement for halothane.

- A significant disadvantage is that nitrous oxide accumulates in the intestinal lumen and causes abdominal distention.
  - Elimination of nitrous oxide from the intestine is slow.
- The lowest flow rates that should be used in a 500-kg (1100 lb) horse to ensure an inspired oxygen concentration >40% are 4 L/min O_2 and 4 L/min nitrous oxide.

Transition to Inhalation Anesthesia

The flow rate of oxygen should be high (6 to 8 L/min) for the first 10 to 15 minutes.

- The high flow rate rapidly increases the concentration of anesthetic in the reservoir bag, thereby ensuring a smooth transition from injectable drugs to inhalant.
- After about 15 minutes, the O_2 flow rate can be reduced to 3 to 4 L/min.
- The initial vaporizer setting depends on the drugs used for premedication and induction and on the physical status of the patient.
  - An initial vaporizer setting of 3.5% for halothane or isoflurane often is sufficient for a healthy horse premedicated with xylazine ± butorphanol and anesthetized with ketamine or guaifenesin and thiopental.
  - Detomidine and tiletamine-zolazepam greatly decrease the anesthetic requirement, so a vaporizer setting of 1.5% may be adequate for the first 30 minutes.

INHALATION ANESTHESIA IN FOALS

Isoflurane is the inhalation agent of choice for foals. Anesthesia can be induced with injectable agents or with isoflurane or halothane administered by face mask or nasotracheal tube.

- Inhalation induction in young or sick foals is facilitated by premedica-

tion with diazepam (0.05 mg/kg IV) and an opioid, such as pentazocine (0.3 to 0.5 mg/kg IV), with or without xylazine (0.15 mg/kg IV).
- When inducing anesthesia using a facemask, the mask is applied with the foal standing, and the foal breathes oxygen for 2 to 3 minutes before increasing the vaporizer setting in 0.5% increments every four breaths, up to 4%.
- Whether a mask or nasotracheal tube is used, an endotracheal tube should be placed after induction. Anesthesia in neonatal foals is discussed in Chapter 6.

POSITIONING DURING ANESTHESIA

Proper positioning of the limbs is of major importance in minimizing the incidence of myopathy.

- When the horse is in lateral recumbency, the lower forelimb should be pulled forward and the upper forelimb elevated to a horizontal position; excessive traction on the upper limb must be avoided.
- The hind limbs should be positioned perpendicular to the vertebral column, with the upper limb elevated to the horizontal position.
- When access to the medial surface of the lower hind limb is required, the upper hind limb should be flexed cranially and pulled close to the flank using a rope; the hind limb should never be pulled behind the horse for any length of time.

MONITORING INHALATION ANESTHESIA

Monitoring Depth of Anesthesia

For most horses, an adequate depth of anesthesia is indicated by a weak palpebral reflex. Other indicators are briefly described below:

- *eyeball position:* The eye is central, laterodorsal, or lateroventral during light anesthesia, rolled medioventrally during moderate anesthesia, and central during deep anesthesia.
- *nystagmus:* The presence of nystagmus during guaifenesin-thiopental or inhalation anesthesia indicates an excessively light plane of anesthesia.

- Small oscillations of varying amplitude can occur during deep inhalation anesthesia.
- ✦ *pupil:* Dilation of the pupil occurs during deep halothane or isoflurane anesthesia.

  Induction of anesthesia with ketamine often is associated with nystagmus and a brisk palpebral reflex, despite an adequate depth of anesthesia.

Cardiovascular Monitoring

Heart rates frequently remain constant at acceptable values throughout anesthesia, despite changes in depth of anesthesia or arterial pressure. Measurement of mean arterial pressure is of enormous value in early identification of cardiovascular depression and prevention of serious complications.

- ✦ Blood pressure can be noninvasively measured by placing a cuff around the tail and measuring pressure in the coccygeal artery with either an oscillometric technique (DINAMAP) or Doppler ultrasound.
  - Occasionally, a high blood pressure measurement is obtained using these techniques, when the horse's pressure is actually low.
- ✦ Arterial blood pressure may be measured directly by inserting a catheter in a peripheral artery (facial, transverse facial, great metatarsal) and using an aneroid manometer or more sophisticated equipment.
- ✦ Mean pressures of <70 mm Hg for more than 15 minutes are correlated with an increased incidence of postanesthetic complications.
- ✦ Mean pressures of <63 mm Hg are indicative of potentially life-threatening hypotension.
- ✦ Mucous membrane color and capillary refill time should also be assessed.
  - Pale mucous membranes and a capillary refill time >1.5 second indicate low cardiac output.

Respiratory System

An estimate of the adequacy of ventilation can be made by observing thoracic and reservoir bag excursions to determine the respiratory rate and depth.

- ✦ In most cases, a respiratory rate of <6 breaths/min indicates unacceptable hypoventilation.

- ◆ A recurring pattern of grouped breaths of descending volume or ascending then descending volume frequently is seen during xylazine-ketamine anesthesia.
- ◆ Coupled breaths often are observed during inhalation anesthesia.
- ◆ These patterns usually are associated with increased $PaCO_2$.

Methods of respiratory monitoring

- ◆ *capnography:* measures the concentration of CO_2 in expired air
- ◆ *measurement of arterial blood PCO_2 and PO_2:* most accurate method of determining adequacy of ventilation and oxygenation
- ◆ *pulse oximetry:* measures hemoglobin oxygen saturation noninvasively
  - It is a useful way to detect arterial hypoxemia in anesthetized horses.
  - The best site to attach the clip sensor is the tongue.

Temperature

Monitoring rectal temperature should be routine, because hypothermia can develop in horses anesthetized in air-conditioned surgery rooms.

- ◆ A rectal temperature of <35.6° C (96° F) is associated with increased ataxia during recovery.
- ◆ Hyperthermia rarely develops in anesthetized horses, but there are published reports of malignant hyperthermia occurring in horses (see p. 91).
  - Early recognition is essential if the animal is to survive.

TREATMENT OF COMPLICATIONS

Inadequate Depth of Anesthesia

Changing the halothane or isoflurane setting may take 5 minutes or more to make an impact on the depth of anesthesia. Consequently, it usually is advisable to temporarily increase the depth of anesthesia with an IV agent.

- ◆ Thiopental is the fastest-acting agent; the "top up" dose is 0.03 to 0.05 mg/kg.
- ◆ Within the first 10 minutes of induction with ketamine, supplemental doses of xylazine (50 mg) and ketamine (100 mg) work well in adult horses.
  - Later during anesthesia, xylazine (0.1 mg/kg) alone usually is suffi-

cient to cause muscle relaxation; larger doses have a significant adverse effect on cardiovascular function.

- Administration of an opioid may be appropriate during inhalation anesthesia, especially when effects of premedicant drugs are wearing off.
  - One choice is butorphanol (0.02 mg/kg IV) given at 40- to 60-minute intervals.

Hypotension

A horse is considered hypotensive when mean arterial pressure is ≤65 mm Hg.

- A mean pressure of 60 to 65 mm Hg is not immediately life-threatening, especially when it is short-lived and peripheral perfusion is good (pink mucous membranes and rapid CRT).
- However, a mean pressure of <70 mm Hg that persists for >15 minutes during inhalation anesthesia is associated with an increased risk for postanesthetic myopathy.

Treatment of hypotension

Treatment of hypotension should be directed at the cause.

- *anesthetic-induced vasodilation:* Rapid IV infusion of balanced electrolyte solution, such as lactated Ringer's solution (10 mL/kg) is appropriate,

especially in horses that were excited or anxious before anesthesia.
- Administration of lactated Ringer's solution (20 mL/kg IV) *before* induction is even more effective at preventing hypotension during anesthesia.
- *deep plane of anesthesia:* Hypotension is appropriately treated by decreasing anesthetic administration.
- *hypovolemia:* Hypertonic (7.5%) saline solution (4 mL/kg IV) administered before induction may prevent hypotension during anesthesia in horses with colic.
  - Balanced electrolyte solution (30 to 40 mL/kg IV) must subsequently be administered.

Cardiovascular stimulants

The cardiovascular stimulants most commonly used to treat hypotension are dopamine, dobutamine, and ephedrine (Table 7-3).

- *dopamine:* At low doses (2.5 µg/kg/min), arterial pressure may be unchanged or even decreased for the first 10 minutes of infusion.
  - Dopamine has a cumulative effect over 30 minutes, so the infusion rate can often be decreased after 20 minutes.
  - High dose rates (7 to 10 µg/kg/min) result in vasoconstriction, which is of value in

Table 7-3
Drugs to improve cardiovascular function during anesthesia

Drug/Product availability	Dose rates	Administration
Dobutamine 250 mg/20 mL	1-5 µg/kg/min (e.g., 500-kg horse: 2 µg/kg/min, 200 µg/mL; 10 drops/mL IV set = [(500 × 2) ÷ 200] × 10 = 50 drops/min	Add 4 mL to 500 mL saline to produce 100 µg/mL for foals, or add 8 mL or 20 mL to produce 200 µg/mL or 500 µg/mL for adults and give as continuous IV infusion
Dopamine 200 mg/5 mL	1-5 µg/kg/min to treat hypotension; 6-7 µg/kg/min to treat advanced atrioventricular heart block; up to 10 µg/kg/min to treat cardiac arrest	Add 1.25 mL to 500 mL saline to produce 100 µg/mL for foals, or add 5 mL to produce 400 µg/mL for adults and give as continuous IV infusion
Ephedrine 50 mg/mL	0.06 mg/kg IV; give half dose, add remainder in 5-10 min if response is inadequate	Give as an IV bolus, onset up to 10 min; duration 30-40 min

treatment of life-threatening hypotension, such as may occur with advanced atrioventricular heart block.

- Infusion of dopamine at 10 µg/kg/min in horses with less severe cardiovascular depression can result in tachycardia and life-threatening arrhythmias.

♦ *dobutamine:* Dobutamine causes significant increases in cardiac output and mean arterial pressure within a few minutes of beginning the infusion.

- It induces atrioventricular heart block and bradycardia in nearly 30% of patients; arrhythmias may be treated by decreasing the infusion rate and either adding an infusion of dopamine or administering an anticholinergic agent.
- Some horses with sepsis or endotoxemia are less responsive to dopamine and dobutamine.

♦ *ephedrine:* Arterial pressure usually begins to increase within 5 to 7 minutes, and the increase is sustained for 15 to 35 minutes.

- Tachycardia is less likely to occur if ephedrine is administered in incremental doses.
- The best response occurs in patients with moderately low blood pressure and pink mucous membranes.
- Ephedrine has little or no effect on blood pressure in some patients.

Hypoventilation

If the depth of anesthesia cannot be changed to reduce respiratory depression, artificial ventilation (assisted or controlled) is the appropriate treatment. An average rate of 10 (6 to 12) breaths/min and an inspiratory time of 1.5 to 2 seconds is recommended.

Malignant Hyperthermia

Malignant hyperthermia is characterized by a massive increase in metabolic rate within muscle, which initiates metabolic acidosis, hypercarbia, hyperkalemia, and hyperthermia; either hypertension or hypotension may develop. Some horses are unable to rise after anesthesia, and only a few survive. In predisposed individuals, the syndrome may be triggered by a variety of factors, including administration of halothane, isoflurane, and succinylcholine.

Warning signs

Malignant hyperthermia should be suspected during anesthesia in the following situations.

- The horse develops an irregular breathing pattern, tachycardia, and arrhythmias.
- The anesthetic circuit feels warm to touch.
- The CO_2 absorbent changes color earlier than usual.
- Rectal temperature is elevated.

Treatment of malignant hyperthermia

Treatment must be started early to be successful.

- Inhalation anesthesia should be discontinued and anesthesia maintained with IV agents as needed until the surgical procedure can be terminated abruptly.
- The CO_2 absorbent should be changed and the oxygen flow rate increased.
- The infusion rate of lactated Ringer's solution should be increased.
- Cold water hosing and ice packs should be used to lower the horse's temperature.
- Hyperkalemia should be treated.
- Sodium bicarbonate should be administered IV at a rate of 3 mEq/kg over 20 minutes.
- Dantrolene sodium is the specific treatment for malignant hyperthermia.
  - It is given either IV at 1 to 2 mg/kg or PO (via nasogastric tube) at 4 to 6 mg/kg.
  - Treatment of late complications must include diuresis to limit tubular necrosis; other supportive therapy should be given as necessary.

Hyperkalemic periodic paralysis

Hyperthermia, hypercarbia, and hyperkalemia during isoflurane anesthesia have been reported in horses with hyperkalemic periodic paralysis. However, unlike malignant hyperthermia, arterial blood pressure remains stable and body temperature rapidly decreases in response to external cooling.

RECOVERY FROM ANESTHESIA
Airway Management
Vigilance should not end when the horse is placed in the recovery room. Along with close observation and frequent monitoring, oxygen insufflation should be provided at 15 L/min.

Nasal edema
Nasal edema, causing partial or complete obstruction to breathing after removal of the endotracheal tube, can be managed in several ways.
- The endotracheal tube can be left in place during recovery and removed after the horse is standing (by which time the edema usually is resolved).
- The endotracheal tube can be removed and a smaller nasotracheal tube inserted until the horse is standing.
- The nasal passages can be sprayed with phenylephrine.

Laryngospasm
Laryngospasm is rare; it occurs most frequently as the horse struggles into a sternal or standing position. Following are some management suggestions:
- An endotracheal tube can be passed either nasally or orally, although some force may be needed.
- A tracheotomy is necessary in some cases.
- After the spasm is relieved, the horse should remain under close observation, because laryngospasm sometimes recurs several hours later.
- Laryngospasm may induce pulmonary edema, which becomes apparent after the horse stands (high respiratory rate and fluid flowing from the nostrils when the horse lowers its head).
  - Administration of furosemide and insufflation with oxygen are indicated.

Sedation and Analgesia
Sedation for smooth recovery
Some sedation is advisable after halothane or isoflurane anesthesia.
- When accepromazine has been used for premedication or when anesthesia time is short, no additional drugs may be needed for recovery.
- When xylazine has been used for premedication or when surgery time is >2 hours, an additional small dose of xylazine (0.1 mg/kg after halothane and 0.2 mg/kg after

isoflurane) may be useful when given 5 minutes after the vaporizer is turned off.
- In horses that were nervous or excited before anesthesia, administration of butorphanol (0.02 mg/kg) 10 minutes before the end of surgery and a small dose of xylazine after anesthesia ceases can promote a smooth recovery.

Postoperative pain relief
- Phenylbutazone, if used, should be administered *before* induction.
- Flunixin meglumine given during or after anesthesia is quite effective for pain relief after ocular surgery.
- Meperidine (0.7 to 1.0 mg/kg IM 20 minutes before the end of anesthesia) is an effective analgesic after orthopedic procedures, but its effects may not last longer than an hour.
- Butorphanol (0.02 mg/kg) also can be given for postoperative pain, but its duration of action is only about 1 hour; increasing the dose rate causes an unacceptable increase in ataxia.
- Alternative methods of analgesia include intraarticular administration of morphine or bupivacaine after joint surgery and topical application of bupivacaine or peripheral nerve blocks for other types of orthopedic surgery.

Assistance to Stand
Assistance, in the form of ropes tied to the tail and a halter, should be provided for horses that are:
- non–weight-bearing on one limb
- hypothermic
- hypovolemic from blood loss
- old
- endotoxemic
- recovering from anesthesia that lasted >3 hours or that were maintained in dorsal recumbency with hind limbs in a frog-leg position

Inability to Stand
The average time from turning off the halothane or isoflurane vaporizer to standing is 50 to 55 minutes, with the average horse making no movement for the first 45 minutes.
- Some horses are standing by 25 minutes, and some remain recumbent or sternal for 90 minutes.

- A 90-minute delay to standing is not a problem, provided the horse is quiet and breathing well; horses that make multiple unsuccessful attempts to stand are of concern.

There are many possible causes of a horse's inability to stand after anesthesia, ranging in severity from drug-induced muscle weakness to fracture or luxation (see Box 7-1 in *Equine Medicine and Surgery V*).

Management of postanesthetic myopathy

Treatment should be directed toward avoiding further injury by minimizing movement and preventing renal failure by inducing diuresis.

- Initially, acepromazine may be used for tranquilization; violent horses may require xylazine or other drugs
- Infusion of lactated Ringer's solution should be started early to minimize the risk of renal failure from myoglobinuria; fluid therapy may be necessary for 2 to 3 days.
- Flunixin meglumine and an opioid are indicated for muscle pain.
- DMSO (20 to 50 mg/kg IV in 1 L of fluid) may prevent reperfusion injury.
- Rectal temperature should be checked frequently and hyperthermia treated with cold hosing and ice packs.
- Dantrolene (1 to 2 mg/kg IV or 4 to 6 mg/kg PO) may be beneficial.
- If the horse is recumbent, it should be turned every few hours and the bladder catheterized to drain urine.

Laminitis is a potential sequela to postanesthetic myopathy.

PATIENTS WITH SPECIFIC PROBLEMS

Colic

Abdominal distention is just one factor that complicates anesthesia in horses with colic (see Box 7-2 in *Equine Medicine and Surgery V*). Hypotension is common, particularly when hypovolemia, endotoxemia, metabolic acidosis, hypocalcemia, or hypokalemia are present. Following are some practical suggestions:

- Pretreatment with lactated Ringer's solution (20 to 40 mL/kg), hyper-

tonic 7.5% saline (4 mL/kg), and, when indicated, calcium gluconate or sodium bicarbonate improves cardiovascular function during anesthesia.

- Dose rates of anesthetic drugs must be kept as low as possible.
- One effective combination is xylazine (0.5 to 1.1 mg/kg) and butorphanol (0.02 mg/kg) for premedication and diazepam (0.05 mg/kg) and ketamine (1.1 to 2.2 mg/kg) for induction; guaifenesin may be included for induction, and isoflurane used for maintenance

Foals

Foals <3 months of age respond differently to anesthesia and surgery than do adult horses.

Healthy foals

Following are some precautions for anesthesia in young foals:

- Anesthetic requirements are less in very young foals.
- Acepromazine premedication may prolong recovery.
- Xylazine (0.15 to 0.3 mg/kg IV) with diazepam (0.05 mg/kg IV) and either pentazocine (0.3 to 0.5 mg/kg IV) or butorphanol (0.02 mg/kg IV) may be used for premedication before induction with isoflurane or ketamine.
  - Xylazine should probably be avoided in foals <2 weeks of age, except for very small doses (0.15 to 0.2 mg/kg IV).
- Thiopental anesthesia should not be used in foals <1 month old, and ketamine is preferable to thiopental in foals <3 months old.
- In foals, cardiac output is largely governed by heart rate, so bradycardia and small decreases in plasma volume can produce significant changes in cardiovascular function.
  - Hypotension is a common problem during anesthesia in foals.
  - Blood pressure should be monitored using a DINAMAP cuff around the tail or metatarsus or directly with a catheter in the facial or metatarsal artery.
  - A bolus of lactated Ringer's solution (10 to 20 mL/kg IV) may expand blood volume sufficiently to increase blood pressure.

- Dopamine or dobutamine (5 µg/kg/min) or ephedrine (0.03 to 0.06 mg/kg IV) can be used to stimulate cardiovascular function.
- Blood glucose concentrations <100 mg/dL should be avoided by infusion of 5% dextrose in water (2 mL/kg/h, up to 5 mL/kg/h) with lactated Ringer's solution (8 to 10 mL/kg/h).
- Hypothermia can be prevented by using a hot water circulating heating pad and by keeping the oxygen flow rate at <20 mL/kg during inhalation anesthesia.

Ruptured urinary bladder

- Affected foals have CNS depression, a distended abdomen, hypovolemia, hyperkalemia, hypernatremia, hypochloremia, and azotemia.
- Their requirement for anesthetic drugs is minimal.
- They are at high risk for hypoventilation, hypotension, and cardiac arrhythmias, leading to cardiac arrest; rapid decompression of a distended abdomen may precipitate acute hypotension.
- Correction of existing abnormalities before anesthesia decreases the incidence of complications.
- Accumulation of urine in the abdomen continues, so haste is vital.
- Monitoring the ECG and blood pressure allows early treatment of potentially life-threatening cardiovascular changes.
- Advanced atrioventricular heart block may develop and can be successfully reversed by infusion of dopamine (6 to 7 µg/kg/min).

Sepsis

- Foals with an infected umbilicus, septic joint, or intestinal accident usually have severely decreased requirements for anesthetic drugs.
  - Oral endotracheal intubation can often be accomplished after only heavy sedation.
- Hypotension can develop unexpectedly during anesthesia.
- Hypoglycemia is common and should be treated with infusion of 5% dextrose in water.

Ophthalmic Procedures

Changes in eye position and reflexes are important in the assessment of anesthetic depth, so it can be difficult to maintain a smooth plane of anesthesia during ocular surgery.

- Anesthesia must be deeper for ophthalmic procedures, to prevent eye movement.
  - A stable plane of anesthesia should be achieved before the eye is draped, using a vaporizer setting that usually provides moderate-to-deep anesthesia.
  - Arterial blood pressure should be monitored for development of hypotension.
- Acepromazine or xylazine with guaifenesin-thiopental or a xylazine-ketamine combination is recommended for induction.
- Horses with corneal ulcers or lacerations requiring emergency surgery may have been recently fed and may develop bloat intraoperatively and colic postoperatively.
  - Oxygen administration during recovery is essential in these horses.
- Protection of the eye during recovery is advisable.

Neuromuscular block

Extraocular muscle paralysis can be achieved by administration of atracurium or vecuronium.

- Atracurium (0.1 to 0.15 mg/kg IV) provides 30 to 60 minutes of paralysis.
  - Supplemental doses of 0.02 to 0.06 mg/kg provide an additional 15 to 20 minutes of paralysis.
- Controlled ventilation is essential because the respiratory muscles are paralyzed.
- Edrophonium should be given at the end of surgery to reverse the blockade.
  - 0.5 mg/kg is given slowly IV over 1 minute while the ECG is monitored for heart rate changes.
  - Supplements of half this dose may be administered, if necessary, to a total of 1 mg/kg.

Principles of Surgery

(pages 282-291)

P.O. Eric Mueller and William P. Hay

Characteristics of commonly used suture materials are summarized in

Tables 7-9 and 7-10 in *Equine Medicine and Surgery V.* Below are some practical details on disinfectants and sterilization procedures.

SKIN PREPARATION
Disinfection
Following is a summary of the properties of the three most commonly used disinfectants:

- *povidone iodine:* fast-acting, broad-spectrum bactericidal agent with activity against many fungi, viruses, and protozoa
  - It is a poor sporicide and has minimal residual activity.
  - Its bactericidal activity is markedly reduced by organic materials.
  - Iodine can cause skin irritation and instrument corrosion.
- *chlorhexidine:* possesses rapid and persistent broad-spectrum bactericidal effects (up to 6 hours, even in the presence of organic material) while causing minimal tissue irritation
  - It has activity against many fungi, but is less effective against some species of *Pseudomonas* and has limited activity against viruses and spores.
- *isopropyl alcohol (70%):* rapidly bactericidal, but has limited activity against fungi and viruses and no sporicidal activity
  - It is inactivated by organic matter.
  - Alcohol most often is alternated with povidone iodine or chlorhexidine for surgical skin preparation.

Preparation of the Foot
Aseptic surgical procedures of the hoof require special preparation before surgery.
- The superficial layer of hoof wall, sole, and frog should be removed with a disinfected rasp and knife.
- The hoof is then wrapped in povidone iodine-soaked gauze for 12 hours.

STERILIZATION PROCEDURES
Thermal Sterilization
Instruments and drapes are almost always sterilized with moist heat (steam).

- Instruments should be clean, oil free, and loosely arranged with their box-locks open.
- Packaging wrappers must be permeable to steam and impermeable to microorganisms.
- An exposure time of 13 minutes at 121° C (250° F) is required for routine sterilization of instruments.
  - Linen packs require 30 minutes at 121° C.
  - Emergency (flash) sterilization is best performed in a prevacuum autoclave, with an exposure time of 3 minutes at 131° C (268° F).

Chemical Sterilization
The two most common forms of chemical sterilization are cold sterilization with glutaraldehyde and gas sterilization with ethylene oxide.

Glutaraldehyde
- Instruments must be thoroughly cleaned and dried before sterilization.
- The manufacturer's recommendations concerning solution concentration and shelf life should be strictly followed to ensure adequate antimicrobial activity.
- For *sterilization,* instruments must be immersed in 2% glutaraldehyde at room temperature (20° to 25° C [68° to 77° F]) for 10 hours.
- For intermediate-to-high-level *disinfection* (bactericidal, virucidal, and fungicidal activity, with minimal sporicidal activity), immersion times of 10 to 20 minutes are used.
  - This is sufficient for most arthroscopic, endoscopic, and laparoscopic instruments.
- Glutaraldehyde is extremely irritating to tissues, and repeated exposure may lead to the development of hypersensitivity reactions.
  - Gloves should be worn and instruments and equipment thoroughly rinsed with sterile saline.
  - Adequate ventilation must be available to exhaust glutaraldehyde vapor.

8

Cardiovascular System

Examination of the Cardiovascular System

(pages 296-314)

Peter W. Physick-Sheard

A detailed examination of the cardiovascular system is indicated.

• whenever the history or clinical signs suggest possible cardiovascular disease
• when abnormalities (e.g., murmur, pulse deficit) are detected on physical examination
• when the heart rate is higher or lower than other clinical findings suggest it should be
• during the course of severe systemic illness
• in cases of syncope or unsteadiness during exercise, suboptimal performance, or limited exercise tolerance

HISTORY

Detailed cardiovascular examination should start with a review of the history, including:

• analysis of exercise and training regimens and performance history
• consideration of previous clinical problems and general management
  • Nutritional history and changes of environment, trainer, or use should be considered.
• specific history of the presenting clinical problem(s), especially the clinical signs and circumstances of occurrence
• medications the horse has been receiving

INSPECTION AND PALPATION
General Observation

Details to note on visual inspection include:

• the horse's age, breed, gender, and apparent degree of fitness
• evidence of respiratory disease, such as increased inspiratory or expiratory effort, shallow respiration, or asymmetry of the respiratory pattern
• presence and distribution of any peripheral edema
  • Edema may indicate venous obstruction, pericarditis, or right heart failure, although cardiovascular disease is an uncommon cause of edema in horses.
  • Edema of the head may be seen with iatrogenic jugular thrombosis or heart-base masses.
  • Forelimb edema can also occur with thoracic masses.
• evidence of pulmonary edema
  • Cardiovascular causes include primary left heart failure (uncommon), acute severe left AV valvular regurgitation (e.g., ruptured chordae), and severe arrhythmias
• assessment of the horse's hydration status

Jugular Distention and Pulse

A jugular pulse may indicate abnormal cardiac activity, although more common causes are transmission of pressure from the underlying carotid artery and changes in intrathoracic pressure with ventilation. However, when a jugular pulse is observed, venous distention is the primary abnormality, not the pulsation.

Causes of jugular distention

Persistent jugular distention may result from:

- obstruction to venous return (e.g., intrathoracic mass, right AV stenosis and regurgitation, pericardial effusion)
- elevation of central venous pressure (e.g., right heart failure, iatrogenic volume overload)

Intermittent jugular distention (filling that varies from beat to beat) can be caused by:

- arrhythmias (e.g., second-degree AV block, AV dissociation, periods of severe bradycardia or tachycardia)
- respiratory disease (cor pulmonale)

Examination of the jugular veins

Following is the recommended protocol for examining the jugular veins:

- Examine the veins with the horse's head in a normal position, and check the extent and symmetry of fluid movement.
- Palpate both veins to detect and quantify scarring or obstruction.
- Obstruct each vein toward the top of the neck and empty the vein by sweeping the blood toward the heart; watch for refilling at the thoracic inlet while still obstructing flow.
  - Any tendency to fill proximally is abnormal.
- Compare jugular filling with the condition of other veins in the body.
  - Dependent veins, such as the cephalic and saphenous veins, are always distended.

Arterial Pulses

The following arteries may be palpated during routine physical examination:

- external maxillary (crosses the ventral border of the mandible)
- facial (runs along the rostral border of the masseter muscle)
- transverse facial (caudal to the lateral canthus of the eye)
- carotid (ventral neck)
- radial (medially, on the upper forelimb)
- medial palmar metacarpal (caudomedial aspect of the carpus)
- lateral and medial palmar/plantar digital (palmar/plantar aspect of the fetlock and pastern)
- coccygeal (underside of the tail)
- greater metatarsal (lateral aspect of proximal metatarsus)
- saphenous (beneath the leading edge of the saphenous vein)

Pulse rate

Following are normal heart rates for particular groups of horses:

- **adult horses:** Normal resting heart rate ranges from 28 to 40 beats/min.
  - Rates as low as 20 beats/min may be seen in mature, fit performance horses.
  - In ponies, the resting rate may be as high as 45 beats/min
- **foals:** A heart rate of around 70 beats/min often is observed within the first 5 minutes after birth, which rises to around 130 beats/min (range, 60 to 200 beats/min) as the foal attempts to rise.
  - By 48 hours after birth, the average heart rate is around 96 beats/min.
  - Usually, the heart rate falls to adult levels by 4 to 5 months of age.
- **pregnant mares:** The heart rate rises during pregnancy to around 60 beats/min in the last month and 80 beats/min as parturition approaches.

NOTE: *In any animal, a pulse rate that is inconsistent with the overall clinical picture may indicate the presence of a serious arrhythmia; not all arrhythmias cause an irregular cardiac rhythm.*

Pulse rhythm

Abnormalities of cardiac rhythm may be detected during palpation of the pulse, but it is always worth combining palpation of the pulse with auscultation of the heart. Arrhythmias may cause pulse deficits, in which ventricular contraction is not accompanied by a palpable pulse wave.

Pulse character

Pulse character consists of two components: width and contour. The pulse character in a normal, fit horse is long, surging, and full, and the contour consists of a rapid, strong rise to a peak, followed initially by a rapid fall, a hesitation (dicrotic notch), then a slower fall to diastolic pressure. Easily detectable pulse abnormalities are uncommon and may be found in cases of shock, aortic valve regurgitation ("wide" pulse pressure), and arterial obstruction (see p. 127).

Mucous Membranes

Capillary refill time

Capillary refill time is a crude test of peripheral perfusion. It is measured by gently pressing the mucous membrane, usually the gum, and noting how rapidly the color returns to the blanched area. Capillary refill time in a normal animal is <2 seconds.

Membrane color

In severely anemic animals the membranes are pale, and measurement of capillary refill time can be difficult. If poor cardiac output is contributing to the pale membranes, temperature of the periphery, pulse strength, and heart rate are more reliable indicators of cardiovascular dysfunction. Injected or dark purple mucous membranes typically occur during endotoxic shock. Uncomplicated cardiovascular insufficiency causes pale, not cyanotic, membranes; the only exception to this is congenital cardiac disease involving right-to-left shunts, which may cause cyanotic membranes.

Cardiac Impulse (Apex Beat)

The cardiac impulse can often be seen, and should be palpable, on the left side of the thorax.

- On the average horse, it is found 5 to 10 cm (2 to 4 inches) above, and slightly behind, the point of the elbow, at the fifth or sixth intercostal space.
- Abnormal location of the impulse usually involves caudal displacement of the heart.
  - Causes include cranial thoracic masses (e.g., lymphoma, pulmonary abscess) and cardiac enlargement.
- Seeing or feeling a cardiac impulse on the right side is a significant finding; it may indicate right ventricular hypertrophy or displacement of the heart caudally or to the right.
- Unilateral pleural effusion or pulmonary abscessation may both displace and reduce the intensity of the impulse on the affected side.
- Absence of a cardiac impulse may occur with marked increase in lung size (e.g., chronic airway disease) and with pleural effusion/pleuritis or pericardial effusion.
  - The cardiac impulse may also be difficult to feel in overweight horses.

Palpable thrills

A thrill is a vibration that is felt when palpating the cardiac impulse; it represents an intense, low-frequency component of a murmur (grade III/VI or greater). The thrill usually is most obvious over the point of maximum intensity (PMI) of the murmur, which is not necessarily directly over the cardiac impulse. Thrills are always clinically significant.

Palpation in neonatal foals

Simultaneous palpation of the cardiac impulse on both sides of the chest is easily achieved in neonates. In the case of ventricular shunts, the shunt flow may be detected moving from one side of the thorax to the other and is often associated with a palpable thrill.

Area of Cardiac Dullness

The area of cardiac dullness is the region behind the left elbow that is dull on percussion because the heart lies directly beneath the thoracic wall with no intervening lung.

- Normally, the caudal limit is the sixth intercostal space, and the dorsal limit is a horizontal line 8 to 10 cm (3 to 4 inches) above the point of the elbow.
- Enlargement of the area is seen with cardiomegaly and with caudal displacement of the heart.
  - Pulmonary consolidation or abscessation behind the heart confounds interpretation.
  - Observations cannot be made if there is pleural effusion.
- On the right side, there should be no area of dullness; its presence indicates pathology.

AUSCULTATION
General Considerations and Approach

A systematic approach ensures a thorough examination.

* Measure the heart rate.
* Assess the intensity and character of sounds, comparing the area over which heart sounds are clearly heard with the location of the cardiac impulse and area of cardiac dullness.
* Evaluate any murmurs.

It is important to auscultate both sides of the thorax; many cardiac abnormalities (e.g., right AV valvular regurgitation and simple ventricular septal defects) may be evident on only one side.

Heart sound amplitude and character

Muffled heart sounds have a remote, soft quality lacking in sounds that are merely quiet. Muffling implies cardiac displacement or the presence of some intervening medium such as fluid (e.g., pericardial or pleural effusion) or air. In shock and in heart failure, heart sounds may take on a hollow, complex character.

Normal Heart Sounds

Four heart sounds are commonly heard in each cardiac cycle in normal horses.

* The first sound in the cardiac cycle is the atrial contraction sound (ACS, or S_4). It is a short, quiet, low-frequency sound, best heard over the ventricles on either side of the chest. As the P-R interval shortens, the ACS merges with S_1.
* The so-called first heart sound (S_1) is generated by the events of ventricular contraction. The sound is of relatively long duration and low frequency, and over the left AV valve region is the most intense heart sound. It is palpated as the cardiac impulse.
* The second heart sound (S_2) is generated at the end of ventricular systole. It is most easily detected above the semilunar valves, at the heart base. It is a short, intense sound, but not as strong as S_1.
* The third heart sound (S_3), or ventricular filling sound, occurs early

in diastole, and is closely associated with S_2. It is of low frequency, soft, and can be heard on either side of the chest; occasionally, it is prolonged and high-pitched. S_3 is particularly prominent in fit, athletic horses.

Heart Sounds in Disease
Changes in intensity and quality

With atrial dysfunction, S_1 and S_2 may be modified in intensity and quality.

* After a dropped beat, there is a tendency for S_1 to be quiet and S_2 loud.
  * With a premature contraction, S_1 tends to be loud and S_2 sometimes inaudible.

A prominent S_3 may be heard during cardiac acceleration and deceleration; this is normal. However, a prominent S_3 during rest in the absence of obvious excitement, especially in an untrained animal, may be an indication of reduced ventricular compliance (e.g., cardiac hypertrophy or failure). In such cases, a loud S_3 usually is accompanied by other signs of cardiac dilation, such as tachycardia, jugular filling, or valvular regurgitation.

Splitting of heart sounds

Splitting of heart sounds is easily misinterpreted.

* Splitting of S_1 is unusual; such a sound usually consists of an ACS followed closely by S_1.
  * Intraventricular conduction abnormalities are a possible cause of split S_1.
* Splitting of S_2 can be heard in many normal horses, but an easily detected splitting may indicate ventricular asynchrony.
* Splitting of S_3 often is incorrectly diagnosed; S_3 closely follows S_2, but careful auscultation usually reveals that the sounds are separate.
* A split S_2 is most obvious at the heart base; S_2-S_3 is most obvious over the ventricles.

SPECIAL EXAMINATION OF THE RESPIRATORY SYSTEM

Examination of the respiratory system is discussed in Chapter 9,

Respiratory System. With reference to the cardiovascular examination, chronic small airway disease may result in a decreased area of auscultation and cardiac dullness. It may also lead to increased load on the right heart, which can cause splitting of S_2 and prominence of the cardiac impulse and heart sounds on the right side. Severely hypoxemic patients may exhibit cardiac arrhythmias, especially if they are toxemic.

EXAMINATION OF FOALS IN THE FIRST MONTH

When examining young foals, special attention should be paid to the foal's position, heart rate, cardiopulmonary interactions, mucous membranes, and exact age.

Evaluation
Murmurs
Following are some considerations when interpreting murmurs in young foals:
- "Postural" murmurs are especially problematic in foals; whenever possible, foals should be ausculted while they are standing.
- Benign, "physiologic" murmurs are common, with most foals having some systolic sounds in the first week of life.
- Many foals have a continuous murmur at the left heart base from shortly after birth to 3 weeks of age.
  - These sounds usually are of no clinical significance but are not always easily differentiated from congenital abnormalities by auscultation alone.
- Careful auscultation and simultaneous palpation of the cardiac impulse on both sides of the chest reveal most ventricular-level shunts and structural abnormalities of the outflow tracts.
  - In such cases, systolic murmurs often are accompanied by a palpable thrill.
- Arterial blood gas analysis should be performed on all cyanotic foals, whether or not a murmur is detected.

Persistent fetal circulation
Persistent fetal circulation can be induced by a variety of problems, including:
- congenital circulatory anomalies
- dystocia/prolonged delivery
- respiratory disease (e.g., pneumonia, respiratory distress syndrome) and associated anoxia
- meconium aspiration
- systemic disturbances (e.g., anoxia, severe acid-base and electrolyte disturbance)
- combinations of these conditions

Affected foals have a right-to-left shunt across the foramen ovale, and some have a patent ductus arteriosus. The possibility of secondary circulatory disturbance should be kept in mind when evaluating any seriously ill foal.

Effects of septicemia
Neonatal septicemia can induce quite intense physiologic (benign) murmurs and cause arrhythmias. Other cardiovascular complications of septicemia include:
- arterial thrombosis, particularly in older foals with *Salmonella septicemia*
  - Physical examination in septicemic foals should include palpation of all peripheral pulses and examination of regional skin temperature.
- pericarditis, endocarditis, and/or myocarditis with associated arrhythmias

Oxygen Therapy
Foals with congenital heart disease associated with right-to-left shunting and those with significant respiratory impairment show reduced exercise tolerance. Oxygen therapy has some diagnostic value in such foals, allowing the relative contributions of respiratory and cardiovascular disease to be evaluated.
- Assuming effective O_2 delivery and a normal respiratory system, hypoxia induced by right-to-left shunting shows little or no response to O_2 therapy.
- If there is respiratory disease, O_2 therapy should raise the PaO_2 significantly.

• When both problems are present, the outcome of O_2 therapy depends on the relative contributions to the hypoxia.

Ancillary Diagnostic Aids *(pages 314-337)*
Peter W. Physick-Sheard,
Howard Dobson, Virginia B. Reef,
and Peter J. Pascoe,

ELECTROCARDIOGRAPHY
Y or Base-Apex Lead
A Y, or base-apex, tracing is adequate in most circumstances; it is simple to obtain and usually provides large, easily identifiable complexes. In difficult cases other leads should be used. For rhythm monitoring using the base-apex lead, the black (positive) lead is attached over the xiphoid and the white (negative) lead at the caudodorsal right neck just in front of the scapula; the green, or ground, cable (the right leg cable on most machines) is attached at the base of the neck. The dial is turned to Lead I. Tracings should be analyzed in the following three stages:
• measure the heart rate
• evaluate the rhythm
• examine individual complexes

Interpretation
Following is a brief summary of ECG waveforms:
• The P wave, which is positive in the base-apex lead and usually bifid (notched), represents depolarization of the right atrium and interatrial septum.
  • An early negative component to the P wave may be seen in normal horses.
  • Wandering pacemaker, in which P wave conformation changes, is common in horses.
  • Increased magnitude of the second peak (P^2) could occur with left atrial enlargement, and widening of the P wave may be seen with right AV regurgitation.
• the QRS complex represents ventricular depolarization.

• Variation in vagal tone is the primary factor influencing the length of the P-R interval.
• The shape of QRS changes if the impulse originates in myocardium outside the conduction system or if there is obstruction in part of the conduction system.
• The T wave indicates ventricular repolarization.
  • In resting, relaxed horses, the T wave most often is biphasic (negative then positive in the base-apex lead), and the S-T segment is slightly elevated above the isoelectric line.

T wave changes
T wave changes in horses must not be overinterpreted; the waveform is extremely labile.
• Changes occur spontaneously in resting horses, sometimes in response to environmental stimuli or training and sometimes for no apparent reason.
• With excitement, electrolyte disturbances, increased myocardial workload (e.g., exercise), arrhythmias, and general anesthesia, the negative component becomes progressively smaller and the positive component larger; the entire T wave may be positive.
• Persistence of a T wave that appears inconsistent with the overall clinical picture warrants further investigation.

BLOOD GAS ANALYSIS
Arterial and venous oxygen tensions (PaO_2 and PvO_2) can be very useful in determining the functional significance of various congenital and acquired cardiac abnormalities.
• If the PvO_2 is <45 mm Hg, increased peripheral extraction is occurring.
  • Causes include significantly increased metabolic rate (which should be clinically evident), reduced PaO_2, and depressed cardiac output.
• With congenital defects involving shunting of blood from right to left, a fall in both PaO_2 and PvO_2

occurs, the extent depending on the severity of the shunt.

- In heart failure, PaO_2 is normal unless severe respiratory compromise (e.g., pulmonary edema or fibrosis) results.

RADIOGRAPHY

The Heart and Great Vessels

Radiographic examination of the heart and great vessels is possible in practice, although comprehensive evaluation generally is limited to neonatal foals.

- In foals, lateral projections of the cardiac silhouette can be made using rare-earth screens and high-speed film, with settings of 70 to 80 kVp and 10 to 15 mAs.
  - The foal should be positioned in lateral recumbency, with its forelimbs extended.
  - Motion artefact can be reduced by making the exposure at the end of expiration.
- In adult horses, lateral projections of the heart and great vessels can be obtained using a grid, a 200-cm film-focal spot distance, and a 20-cm air gap.
  - Suitable settings are in the order of 120 kVp and 20 mAs.
- Alteration in the size or shape of the cardiac silhouette may indicate cardiac disease.
- Assessment of the other thoracic structures is essential, particularly the great vessels and pulmonary parenchyma.
  - Pulmonary overcirculation with hypolucency and undercirculation with hyperlucency are manifestations of congenital and acquired cardiac diseases.
  - In left heart failure, pulmonary venous congestion progresses to pulmonary edema.

Peripheral Vessels

Peripheral angiography can be performed in practice, sometimes in the standing horse.

- Indications include investigation of guttural pouch mycosis and selected CNS diseases and identification of the site, extent, and development of collateral circulation in various vasoocclusive conditions (e.g., trauma, frostbite, thromboembolism).
- Typically, 20 to 50 mL of contrast material (250 to 300 mg/mL of iodine) are rapidly injected into the vessel under investigation.
- Fluoroscopy maximizes the usefulness of the study; if only a single radiograph can be made, it should be exposed at the end of injection.

NUCLEAR MEDICINE

Nuclear angiocardiography involves rapid IV injection of a radioactive tracer and evaluation of sequential images showing passage of the bolus through the right heart, lung, left heart, and great vessels. Several indices of cardiac function can be derived from this study. Valvular dysfunction or myocardial failure results in enlargement of one or more chambers or prolonged transit time. Cardiac shunts allow simultaneous visualization of both ventricles.

ECHOCARDIOGRAPHY

Echocardiography is a widely used noninvasive technique for evaluation of cardiac size and function in horses. The appearance of the valves and chambers are described using M-mode and two-dimensional real-time techniques, and flow profiles can be made using Doppler echocardiography. Often the most valuable information is the insight gained into actual and probable hemodynamic consequences of murmurs. Techniques are described in *Equine Medicine and Surgery V.*

MEASUREMENT OF ARTERIAL BLOOD PRESSURE

Blood pressure can be subjectively assessed by digital palpation of superficial arteries. However, the systolic-diastolic gap (which determines palpable pulse strength) may be reduced at high mean pressures and may be widened at lower pressures, giving an incorrect impression of pulse strength. Blood pressure is more accurately determined by one of the following two methods:

- *direct (invasive) measurement:* arterial puncture and insertion of a catheter connected to a suitable measuring device
- *indirect (noninvasive) measurement:* Doppler ultrasound or oscillometry (e.g., Dinamap 8300, Vet/BP)
  - Normal coccygeal blood pressure, measured by Doppler ultrasound, in resting adult horses ranges from 79/49 to 145/106.
  - Thoroughbreds tend to have pressures around 10 mm Hg higher than Standardbreds, which in turn have pressures about 7 mm Hg higher than other horses.

Techniques are described in *Equine Medicine and Surgery V.*

TWENTY-FOUR-HOUR RHYTHM MONITORING

Cardiac arrhythmias in horses may be frequent, intermittent, or persistent. Many horses have rhythm disturbances that are transient or intermittent; 24-hour continuous ECG (Holter) monitoring is indicated in these animals. Other indications include:

- evaluation of horses with a history of syncope or poor performance, in which no other abnormalities have been found
- evaluation of horses with known or suspected paroxysmal atrial fibrillation
- baseline assessment of the frequency of ventricular premature depolarizations
- assessing response to therapy
- ECG monitoring during exercise when radiotelemetry is not available

The equipment and technique are described in *Equine Medicine and Surgery V.*

Interpretation

Occasional premature depolarizations can occur in normal horses and probably are clinically insignificant. Supraventricular and ventricular premature depolarizations occurring less than once an hour are considered to be within normal limits; a more frequent occurrence should be considered investigated further.

EXERCISE

During clinical evaluation, exercise is used under two circumstances.

- when an abnormality, such as a murmur or arrhythmia, is found at rest
  - NOTE: *If there are obvious clinical signs of circulatory insufficiency at rest (e.g., tachycardia, venous distention), exercise is contraindicated.*
- to uncover any exercise-associated abnormalities during prepurchase examination or evaluation of horses considered to be performing suboptimally

The heart should be ausculted as soon as possible after the horse comes to a halt and auscultation continued until the heart rate decelerates into the range of 60 to 80 beats/min. Both sides of the chest should be ausculted.

Interpretation of Findings
Heart rate recovery

Recovery rate has been used as an indicator of fitness. But heart rate recovery is affected by several variables, including oxygen debt, heat load, hydration status, and acid-base balance. Prolonged recovery following moderately intense exercise can be the effect of respiratory disease, hyperthermia, pain, and significant metabolic disturbances, as well as cardiovascular disease.

Cardiac Sounds

Exercise to evaluate abnormal heart sounds usually requires that the heart rate be elevated only to 80 to 120 beats/min, which can be achieved by trotting and moderate cantering on a lunge line.

- Extra sounds, especially at midrange heart rates, are of questionable significance.
  - A gallop rhythm (exaggerated S_3 and/or S_4) is common during cardiac deceleration.
- A change in character of a murmur with exercise may be as important as its persistence.

Cardiac rhythm

Exercise using radiotelemetry or a Holter monitor can be used to evaluate the significance of occasional ectopic beats noted at rest or during excitement-induced tachycardia, along with dropped beats. The objective is to determine whether the arrhythmia becomes worse with exercise or disappears, and whether it could be limiting performance or presenting a physical danger:

- Syncope is always a possibility when exercising a horse to evaluate an arrhythmia.
  - If the problem is a bradyarrhythmia, such as severe second-degree AV block, exercise carries little risk, as long as the arrhythmia disappears with light exercise.
  - With ventricular tachyarrhythmias, exercise should never be attempted.
- Arrhythmias usually do not persist throughout all heart rates, except for atrial fibrillation.
  - Some arrhythmias disappear with exercise; others are present only at particular heart rates.
- Premature ventricular and supraventricular contractions occur most frequently at midrange heart rates (60 to 120 beats/min).
- Irregular cardiac rhythms sometimes occur during cardiac deceleration in normal horses.

Peripheral vascular response to exercise

Exercise can be used to assess regional blood flow by examining gait, skin temperature, distribution of sweating, venous drainage, and peripheral pulses. Delayed (>10 to 15 seconds) or asymmetric filling of regional veins is abnormal and suggests either reduced local arterial supply or distal venous obstruction. All limb pulses may seem less obvious immediately after exercise, but should return to normal within 30 to 60 seconds.

Upper respiratory tract

Premature depolarizations may occur with airway collapse, so the upper airway should be evaluated during treadmill exercise in horses with ventricular ectopic activity at exercise. Horses that are homozygous for hyperkalemic periodic paralysis experience dynamic pharyngeal collapse and have decreased PaO_2 values during peak exercise and an increased incidence of ventricular arrhythmias compared with heterozygous horses.

Abnormalities of Sound, Rate, and Rhythm

(pages 337-368)
Peter W. Physick-Sheard

MURMURS
Describing Murmurs
Intensity

The intensity (loudness) of a murmur generally is graded from I to VI.

- *Grade I:* the softest audible murmur, heard only after careful auscultation and limited to a small area of the thorax
- *Grade II:* a faint murmur, but clearly audible after a few seconds' auscultation
- *Grade III:* a localized murmur that is immediately audible when auscultation begins
- *Grade IV:* a loud murmur that is widespread but not associated with a thrill
- *Grade V:* a loud, widespread murmur accompanied by a palpable thrill
- *Grade VI:* a loud, widespread murmur, accompanied by a thrill, and still audible when the stethoscope is slightly lifted off the chest wall

Frequency

Murmurs of low frequency or pitch, especially if they are of low intensity (quiet), may be difficult to detect, but frequently are of clinical significance. Higher-frequency sounds, especially those with a musical quality, are easier to hear but often have limited importance.

Character

The quality, or character, of a murmur is described by such terms as noisy, soft and blowing, harsh, musical, and rumbling. For example, AV valve insufficiency can create a soft, blowing sound, whereas ventricular-level shunts cause a harsh, noisy murmur.

Timing

The timing of a murmur is described in terms of its relationship to events of the cardiac cycle, as indicated by the normal heart sounds:

* *systolic murmur:* begins with or after S_1 and ends before or with S_2
* *early systolic murmur:* begins with S_1 and ends about or before the middle of systole
* *late systolic murmur:* begins about the middle of systole and ends at or just before S_2
* *midsystolic murmur:* clearly begins after S_1 and clearly ends before S_2
  * These are also referred to as *ejection murmurs.*
  * The classical example is outflow tract (aortic or pulmonic) stenosis.
* *holosystolic murmur:* occupies all of systole, but does not interfere with either S_1 or S_2
  * Examples are AV valvular regurgitation, flail valve, ruptured chordae tendineae.
  * Holosystolic murmurs heard primarily on the left side usually are of clinical significance, whereas those heard primarily on the right tend to be of variable significance.
* *pansystolic murmur:* occupies all of systole but obliterates S_1 and S_2
  * Examples are ventricular septal defect and the systolic component of patent ductus arteriosus.
  * Pansystolic murmurs always indicate pathology.
* *diastolic murmur:* begins with or after S_2 and ends with or before S_1 of the next cycle
  * Aortic valve regurgitation causes a holodiastolic murmur.
  * Aortic aneurysms and aortic ring ruptures that dissect into a heart chamber can cause a pandiastolic murmur.
* *early diastolic murmur:* heard with or just after S_2
  * Examples are regurgitation at the semilunar valve and AV stenosis.
* *middiastolic murmur:* clearly begins after S_2 and finishes before S_1 of the next cycle
* *late diastolic murmur:* presystolic murmur; confined to the period immediately before S_1

* *continuous (machinery) murmurs:* heard throughout the cardiac cycle
  * The most common cause is persistent ductus arteriosus; the diastolic component often is of low grade and may not be obvious.

Location

There is no consistent association between the location of a murmur and an etiologic diagnosis, although some disorders tend to have a fairly characteristic distribution of sound.

* Murmurs generated in the outflow tracts tend to follow the tract dorsally, whereas their higher frequency components tend to radiate downward, toward the apex of the chamber of origin.
* Murmurs generated at the AV valves are heard best over the valve of origin.
  * An intense murmur of left AV valvular regurgitation is loudest on the left side, at the fourth to seventh intercostal space, at a level 2 to 4 cm (0.75 to 1.50 inch) below the shoulder joint.
  * Murmurs of right AV valvular origin tend to be loudest on the right side, although they can often be detected low down and well forward on the left.
* Murmurs associated with shunts tend to have wide distribution, but the direction of the shunt can often be inferred from the point of maximal intensity of the murmur.

Shape

A crescendo murmur progressively increases in intensity, and a decrescendo murmur starts out relatively loud and becomes progressively quieter. A crescendo-decrescendo murmur becomes loud then quiet; outflow tract stenosis often causes this type of sound, which is also referred to as an *ejection murmur.* Murmurs of fairly constant intensity are referred to as *band-shaped.*

Interference

The extent to which a murmur interferes with normal heart sounds has diagnostic value.

* The murmur of aortic stenosis starts shortly after S_1 and finishes just before S_2; there is no interference.
* The murmur of a ventricular-level shunt starts with S_1, often over-

rides S_2, and sometimes obliterates both sounds.

Determining Functional Significance

Horses are prone to benign flow sounds and to quite intense sounds during systemic stresses, such as colic and anemia. Murmurs should therefore be interpreted with caution and evaluated critically and individually. The following three general principles that apply when interpreting murmurs in horses:

- The presence of a murmur does not necessarily indicate significant cardiac disease, and the absence of a murmur does not mean all is well.
- Murmurs rarely provide information about the condition of the myocardium.
- Murmurs do not necessarily affect the horse's ability to perform.

If the murmur is similar following exercise to what was heard at rest, there likely are hemodynamic consequences associated with exercise. Detection of a murmur in a performance animal, particularly when present at exercise, requires echocardiographic examination.

"Benign" flow sounds

Early systolic, crescendo-decrescendo murmurs heard only at the heart base, and that are grade II or lower in intensity, are referred to as *innocent murmurs*.

- Reported occurrence in clinically normal horses is 49.5% on the left and 8.4% on the right.
- The sounds may be exaggerated during excitement or exercise.
- A similar murmur has been detected in foals and usually subsides by 3 to 10 months of age.

An early diastolic sound referred to as the "2-year-old squeak" is heard in about 10% of young horses. It comes and goes from beat to beat and disappears with maturity.

Adventitial sounds

Not all "murmurs" are of cardiac origin. Pericarditis, pleuritis, and pneumonia can all produce sounds synchronous with cardiac activity that may be mistaken for murmurs. Careful auscultation usually allows differentiation from true murmurs. Adventitial sounds characteristically are variable in character, duration from cycle to cycle, and precise relationship to normal heart sounds.

Management of Horses with Murmurs

Management is influenced by the underlying problem and generally is directed at career planning and campaign management.

- Obvious murmurs in young animals usually indicate congenital heart disease and should always be interpreted as being of probable clinical significance.
  - Murmurs associated with complex congenital heart disease always have a poor prognosis.
- Murmurs heard in old horses most likely indicate acquired valvular disease, usually with compensatory changes, such as eccentric hypertrophy of one or more chambers.
- Significance and progression in most other cases vary with the specific problem.
- Substantial progression within the animal's working life is most likely to occur in horses that perform maximally through a long career (e.g., eventers).

Ideally, the horse should be reevaluated every 6 to 12 months.

ABNORMALITIES OF HEART RATE

Tachycardia

Elevation in resting heart rate reflects increased demand for cardiac output (e.g., homeostatic disturbance, systemic illness), reduced ability of the heart to meet resting demands, increased sympathetic tone (e.g., pain, excitement), or arrhythmia:

- In most cases, the reason for the elevation is evident from the history and physical examination, with the degree of tachycardia reflecting the degree of systemic disturbance.
- Elevation of rate purely as a reflection of cardiovascular insufficiency is uncommon, but it is always serious, because it indicates decompensation and carries a poor prognosis.

- An ECG should be taken to confirm that a severe tachycardia is sinus in origin.
  - The sinus rate seldom exceeds 120 beats/min in sick horses, but the ventricular rate can reach 160 beats/min in a tachyarrhythmia.

Bradycardia

Bradycardia is uncommon. Causes include:

- aerobic fitness in mature horses (relative bradycardia of 24 to 28 beats/min)
- third-degree heart block (see p. 108)
- hypoglycemia in foals
- hyperkalemia
- increased intracranial pressure
- vagal stimulation (e.g., surgical manipulation of the vagosympathetic trunk, accidental deep perijugular injection of irritants)

An ECG should always be taken in bradycardic horses.

ATRIAL ARRHYTHMIAS

Table 8-1 lists arrhythmias according to their effect on heart rate and rhythm.

Sinus Arrhythmia

Sinus arrhythmia may be:

- A vagally mediated fluctuation in rhythm associated with respiration (respiratory sinus arrhythmia); this is rarely obvious in normal horses.
- An exercise-associated fluctuation in rhythm; this is normal, especially during cardiac deceleration in fit performance horses.
- A fluctuation in R-R interval with second-degree partial AV block (see p. 108)

When sinus arrhythmia is obvious (e.g., in horses with severe chronic respiratory disease), it is important to rule out extracardiac causes before assuming the presence of heart disease.

Sinoatrial Block and Sinus Arrest

Sinoatrial block

Sinoatrial block (SAB) is characterized by a normal rhythm with periodic dropped beats in which there is no auscultable sound and no electrical activity on ECG.

- Usually, only one beat is dropped; occasionally, two or three consecutive cycles are missed.

Table 8-1
Arrhythmias classified according to rate and rhythm

Disturbance of rhythm	Heart Rate		
	Low	Normal	Elevated
None	Sinus bradycardia, total heart block	Sinus rhythm, preexcitation, wandering pacemaker, bundle branch block	Atrial tachycardia, ventricular tachycardi (AV dissociation)
Regular	Second-degree partial AV block, sinoatrial block	Second-degree partial AV block, sinoatrial block	Exercise-associated sinus arrhythmia
Occasional	Sinus bradycardia with escape beats, sinoatrial block with escape beats	Atrial premature beats, ventricular premature beats, sinoatrial block with escape beats	Premature atrial contractions, premature ventricular contractions, ventricular tachyarrhythmias
Absolute	Sinus arrhythmia, atrial fibrillation	Sinus arrhythmia, atrial fibrillation, multiple or frequent premature atrial or ventricular contractions	Atrial fibrillation, multiple or frequent premature atrial or ventricular contractions, intermittent ventricular tachyarrhythmias

- When a single beat is dropped the blocked interval is twice the normal R-R interval, in contrast to sinus arrest, in which the interval is longer.
- SAB is uncommon and generally is considered a benign, vagally induced variation of normal.

Sinoatrial arrest
Sinus arrest results in variable-length periods of asystole. This is more likely to be associated with pathology than is SAB, so prolonged periods of atrial asystole of variable duration should be regarded with suspicion. Persistence of either arrhythmia at elevated heart rates (whether from exercise or parasympatholytic agents) is a likely indication of myocardial disease.

Atrioventricular Block
There are three types of atrioventricular (AV) block: first-degree; second-degree, or partial; and third-degree, or total, heart block. The first two are common, occurring in up to 44% of horses, with second-degree block being more common than first-degree block. Both first- and second-degree AV block may be found in the same animal, the first giving way to the second with relaxation. Generally, a horse must be relaxed to show either of these arrhythmias. Third-degree block is always of clinical significance.

First-degree AV block
With first-degree AV block, the heart rate usually is normal or low. The P-R interval is variable, becoming progressively longer (to a threshold of 0.425 to 0.47 seconds), then returning to normal. This block can be detected on auscultation by variation in the interval between the ACS (S_4) and S_1.

Second-degree AV block
The most consistent feature of second-degree AV block is dropped beats, in which the P wave is not followed by QRS-T.
- an ACS (S_4) can be heard as a soft "lu-" in the blocked cycle, but is not followed by S_1 or S_2
- There usually is variation in the P-R and P-P interval (sinus rate).
- Type, I or Wenckebach, block consists of a progressive lengthening of the P-R interval preceding the dropped beat; this is the most common type of second-degree block in horses.
- Type II block is characterized by dropped beats without any variation in the P-R interval.
- In most cases only one beat is dropped at a time, but occasionally two or more consecutive beats are dropped (more likely in horses with second-degree AV block at higher atrial rates).
- The clinical significance of second-degree AV block is a subject of debate.
  - Some clinicians consider it a benign physiologic variant, particularly if the arrhythmia subsides with exercise and does not reappear until heart rates approach resting values.
  - When severe, it is presumed to be pathologic, possibly indicating myocardial disease.

Third-degree AV block
In third-degree AV block, interruption of conduction between the atria and ventricles is complete and the structures beat independently, the atria at the inherent sinus rate of 28 to 40 beats/min and the ventricles at a lower, idioventricular rate of 10 to 20 beats/min.
- Possible causes include aortic aneurysms with hemorrhage into the ventricular septum, inflammation and degeneration of the AV node, pericarditis, myocarditis, and digoxin toxicity.
- Third-degree AV block can be continuous or intermittent.
- Consistent clinical signs are lethargy/weakness, reduced exercise tolerance, syncopal episodes, and bradycardia.
- Atrial contraction occasionally occurs during ventricular systole when the AV valves are closed, resulting in a prominent regurgitant wave in the jugular veins.
- The conformation of QRS varies.
  - QRS may be normal when ventricular systole is rhythmic.
  - QRS can widen and take on bizarre shapes when ventricular systole is irregular.

Treatment usually is not attempted; drug therapy is of little value and the prognosis for performance is poor. However, the possibility that the arrhythmia is a recent result of acute myocardial injury from which the horse may recover should be considered.

Atrial Fibrillation

Atrial fibrillation (AF) can develop in horses with preexisting heart disease or in otherwise healthy horses.

◆ It most often occurs in an uncomplicated form (i.e., no other detectable signs of heart disease) in fit, young racehorses.
  • Horses usually respond well to treatment and return to their previous level of performance.
◆ When AF appears in animals with signs of circulatory dysfunction, it indicates deterioration.
◆ AF carries the poorest prognosis for response to treatment (1) in larger, older horses; (2) when there are concurrent signs of heart disease; and (3) when it has been present for months.
◆ Horses with AV valvular (particularly left AV valve) regurgitation and subsequent atrial enlargement are predisposed; attempts to correct AF in these cases often are unsuccessful.

Clinical signs

Clinical signs vary with the animal's use and the presence or absence of heart disease.

◆ A sudden reduction in exercise tolerance is typical in otherwise healthy horses.
  • In cases of paroxysmal AF (see below), there may be episodes of poor performance interspersed with periods of normal performance.
  • Horses used for light exercise may show no obvious reduction in performance.
◆ Syncopal episodes are likely when AF accompanies another cardiovascular abnormality and when the resting heart rate is high or cardiac reserve low.
  • All horses with AF are potential candidates for syncope.
◆ Epistaxis has been described in several cases.

◆ Physical examination reveals the characteristic totally irregular rhythm.
  • Heart rate can be low, normal, or high (range, 17 to 120 beats/min); most uncomplicated cases lie in the normal range.
  • The rhythm waxes and wanes, with relatively long periods of asystole between rapid runs of several beats.
  • When the resting heart rate is normal or low, the arrhythmia can be mistaken for second-degree AV block (see p. 108).
  • There is marked variation in the intensity of heart sounds, S_1 being especially loud during a run of fast beats.
  • Pulse strength varies from almost imperceptible to strong, depending on cardiac output.
  • Pulse deficits may be encountered, especially when the heart rate is high or heart failure is present.
  • Jugular filling occurs during periods of ventricular inactivity.
◆ Cardiac rhythm during exercise is irregular, though less noticeably so, and a high ventricular rate may obscure f waves on the ECG (see below).
◆ Postexercise recovery generally is unremarkable.

Diagnosis

The diagnosis is suggested by the typical history and clinical signs, and is confirmed by ECG findings, which are quite characteristic.

◆ The baseline shows marked irregularity, with both coarse and fine f waves reflecting random atrial activity, along with total absence of P waves.
◆ The heart rate and R-R intervals vary widely.
◆ QRS complexes generally are unremarkable, although some variation in amplitude often is encountered; the T waves can also vary in amplitude.

Treatment

Approach to treatment depends on the cardiovascular status. Where there are other signs of cardiac disease, treatment is of limited value.

The primary objective in uncomplicated cases is cardioversion to support a return to useful work. Oral quinidine sulfate generally is used to induce cardioversion.

- The usual dose rate is 10 g PO q2h until cardioversion occurs, signs of toxicity are encountered, or a maximum dose of 60 g has been given (see p. 113).
  - A test dose of 5 g is given the day before to identify horses that are sensitive to quinidine.
- An ECG is taken immediately before each dose.
  - Response consists of elevation in heart rate (typically 60 to 70 beats/min) with increased coarseness and reduced frequency of f waves.
  - The heart rate usually falls immediately after cardioversion but does not return to normal for several hours.
- Horses that fail to respond to 2-hourly dosing or that show signs of toxicity before converting should be treated with an extended (q6-12h) dosing regimen at the same or reduced dosage.
  - If this approach is used because of quinidine toxicity, concurrent treatment with digoxin (low dose; see p. 117) should be used on the second day.
- Prior digitalization should also be considered in the following circumstances:
  - evidence of heart failure or reduced myocardial performance
  - high resting heart rates before cardioversion
  - history of marked tachycardia during previous attempts at cardioversion
  - evidence of significant organic heart disease, such as valvular regurgitation
- Total body potassium deficit may inhibit cardioversion, so, if necessary, oral potassium should be supplemented.
- Quinidine gluconate, dihydroquinidine chlorhydrate, and dihydroquinidine gluconate can be given IV to induce cardioversion, although toxicity is more likely than with oral dosing.

- Total reported dosages of dihydroquinidine gluconate range from 3.5 to 22 g, with rates of infusion of 0.1 to 0.68 g/min; cardioversion occurs in 15 to 120 minutes.
- The horse must be kept under close supervision and constantly monitored by ECG.
- Management after cardioversion depends on the degree of cardiovascular dysfunction.
  - Horses suspected of suffering from myocarditis require rest.
  - In uncomplicated cases, the horse can immediately begin 2 to 3 days of light exercise or paddock turn-out, then gradually return to full exercise over 2 weeks.

Prognosis

The younger the horse when the arrhythmia occurs and the shorter the time it is present, the better the prognosis for permanent cardioversion. Relapse can happen, sometimes immediately after cardioversion or months later. Horses with AF and no other cardiovascular abnormalities can continue to work, as long as they are not expected to perform intense effort. Prognosis in horses with signs of heart failure is poor.

Paroxysmal Atrial Fibrillation

In paroxysmal atrial fibrillation, the arrhythmia spontaneously appears and disappears. It is mostly an exercise-induced condition. Affected horses show a sudden decrease in performance during work, and the arrhythmia is discovered on postexercise examination. Paroxysmal AF can persist for minutes or days, followed by successful performance after spontaneous resolution. If the arrhythmia persists, the horse should be rested until a normal rhythm has been reestablished and maintained for several days.

Atrial Flutter and Atrial Tachycardia

Atrial flutter

Atrial flutter is a tachyarrhythmia in which the heartbeat is rhythmic and the atrial rate high.

- Atrial complexes (f waves) are regular and consistent in conformation, giving the baseline a saw-tooth appearance; they are large and rounded compared with normal P waves.

- The ventricular rhythm is regular, although the rate varies from very low to very high.

Atrial tachycardia

Atrial tachycardia is an arrhythmia in which rapid firing of an atrial ectopic focus results in a rapid, rhythmic ventricular rate (up to 200 beats/min).

- Atrial tachycardia must be differentiated from sinus tachycardia.
  - The rate is higher and the P waves are of unusual conformation with atrial tachycardia.
- The term *paroxysmal atrial tachycardia* is used when the arrhythmia is intermittent.
  - Syncope may occur and the pulse may be weak during such episodes.
- Atrial tachycardia usually indicates atrial myocardial disease.
- This arrhythmia should initially be treated with digoxin.
- Spontaneous conversion to atrial fibrillation makes management easier, because it allows treatment with quinidine sulfate.
  - Quinidine should be used with caution in horses with atrial tachycardia or flutter because it can dramatically increase the ventricular rate.

Premature Atrial Contractions

Premature atrial contractions (PACs) are characterized by a short P-P interval and change in the conformation of the P wave; QRS conformation usually is normal.

- Sinus arrhythmia with a wandering pacemaker can look similar.
- There may be a pause after a PAC.
- Single PACs usually are of limited clinical significance.
- Persistent or frequent PACs after exercise may reflect atrial myocardial disease.

Preexcitation or Wolff-Parkinson-White Syndrome

The ECG criteria for Wolff-Parkinson-White (WPW) syndrome are an abnormally short P-R interval during sinus rhythm and prolonged QRS with initial slurring (delta wave):

- This arrhythmia is not common in horses; when present, it is not always persistent, but may appear for several cycles then subside.
- Significant variation in QRS conformation is a frequent finding.
- This arrhythmia can be associated with poor performance and unsteadiness during racing, but in most cases it is an incidental finding.
- A predisposition to paroxysmal atrial arrhythmias may be anticipated.

JUNCTIONAL AND VENTRICULAR ARRHYTHMIAS

Ventricular arrhythmias usually are clinically significant. They tend to fluctuate, gradually or even suddenly changing from one type to another. Several clinical associations are common to all, and the approach to management often differs only in degree from one arrhythmia to another. Identification and removal of the underlying cause is always of primary importance.

Clinical Associations

Causes of ventricular arrhythmias

Ventricular arrhythmias frequently are encountered in association with myocardial damage, especially if the insult is acute, as in ionophore toxicity or viral myocarditis. Other possible causes include:

- severe electrolyte disorders, especially disorders of potassium balance
- drugs (e.g., certain anesthetics, digitalis)
- hypoxia (e.g., severe respiratory disease, severe anemia, acute blood loss)
- endocarditis involving the left side of the heart

When evaluating horses with ventricular arrhythmias, extracardiac factors should be ruled out first.

Effects on performance

Even in the absence of other signs of cardiac disease, horses with ventricular arrhythmias perform poorly. When the arrhythmia is intermittent, performance may be equally variable.

General ECG Characteristics

A characteristic common to ventricular arrhythmias is the QRS-T complex not accompanied by a P wave.

- Occasionally, retrograde conduction occurs, especially with junctional activity, and the P wave occurs during or even after the QRS.
- When activity in the atria and ventricles is totally dissociated, P waves and QRS-T complexes are both present but bear no consistent relationship to each other.
- Changes in QRS conformation may vary from beat to beat.
  - In most junctional arrhythmias, QRS conformation is normal.
  - QRS duration and conformation are frequently, but not consistently, abnormal in ventricular arrhythmias.
  - Less pronounced changes in QRS conformation can also result from electrolyte imbalance, certain drugs, and ventricular hypertrophy.
- A guide to clinical significance is the extent to which QRS varies in conformation; two or more different patterns usually indicate multiple foci, which carries a guarded prognosis.
- Close proximity between a premature ventricular contraction and the T wave of the previous cycle (R-on-T) also is serious, because it can precede ventricular tachycardia or fibrillation.
- When an ectopic focus captures the rhythm and beats at a high rate, the term *ventricular tachyarrhythmia* is used.
  - The same abnormal QRS appears repeatedly, sometimes at rates as high as 180 beats/min, although more typically at 100 to 140 beats/min.
  - During these runs of ectopic beats, the cardiac rhythm is regular, and rate rather than abnormal rhythm provides the clue to the problem.

Premature Ventricular Contractions

Premature ventricular contractions (PVCs) are characterized by their premature position in relation to normal sinus rhythm, absence of an associated P wave, and often bizarre QRS conformation.

- The resting heart rate usually is normal unless PVCs are occurring in association with systemic illness and/or myocardial disease, in which case the rate may be elevated.
- PVCs typically are accompanied by a loud S_1 and a soft, often imperceptible S_2, together with a pulse deficit if the ectopic beat occurs shortly after the sinus beat.
  - The ectopic beat often is followed by a pause.
- Single PVCs generally are of limited clinical significance, as long as they are infrequent, do not become more frequent with exercise, and have a consistent QRS conformation.
- Frequent PVCs, grouping of several PVCs, varying QRS conformation, and increased frequency during cardiac deceleration after exercise probably are clinically significant.

Ventricular Tachycardia

Ventricular tachycardia occurs when cardiac activity is taken over by an abnormal ventricular focus.

- QRS complexes are abnormal in conformation unless the ectopic focus is junctional.
- Regular atrial activity is at a slower rate and is independent of ventricular activity, but most P waves are obscured by overlying ventricular complexes.
- The T wave often is quite large and the S-T segment short, with QRS blending into the T wave; occasional capture beats may be seen.
- The heart rate usually is high, often >100 beats/min, and the rhythm is regular.
  - Where the arrhythmia is paroxysmal, the change in heart rate is sudden.
  - Episodes of syncope and respiratory distress may be seen at high heart rates.
- Heart sounds are pounding, and at high rates the pulse may be weak.
- Jugular pulsation may be seen when the right atrium contracts during ventricular systole.
- Persistent ventricular tachycardia can lead to myocardial failure.

Parasystole and AV Dissociation

These arrhythmias occur when there are two pacemakers, sinus and ectopic, each with its own intrinsic rate. They indicate probable myocardial distress (e.g., systemic disorders, myocardial disease). The nature of the resulting arrhythmia depends on the relative rates of these pacemakers.

Parasystole

In parasystole, the rate of ectopic discharge is slow, resulting in a more irregular rhythm than that found with AV dissociation. Parasystole is relatively benign.

AV dissociation

AV dissociation occurs when the ectopic focus has a higher intrinsic rate than the sinoatrial node and is responsible for the majority of ventricular activity.

- The atria and ventricles beat independently, and for most ventricular cycles there is no association between P waves and QRS complexes.
- Tachycardia is a consistent finding.
- Heart sounds vary in intensity according to the R-R interval, with a loud S_1 after a short diastolic interval; syncope is uncommon.
- Measurement of ECG intervals reveals the relatively constant rate of the ectopic focus.
  - Occasionally, both foci fire simultaneously and a fusion beat occurs.
- If untreated, AV dissociation can progress to ventricular tachycardia and even fibrillation.

Ventricular Fibrillation

This arrhythmia precedes death by seconds. It is characterized on ECG by coarse, low-frequency baseline undulations with no recognizable atrial or ventricular complexes. Pulse and cardiac impulses are absent. Little can be done, except perhaps when the horse is under anesthesia and ECG monitoring allows immediate recognition.

TREATMENT OF ARRHYTHMIAS

General Management

Removal of the underlying cause, particularly with ventricular arrhythmias, is the primary management approach and in many cases is all that is required. Where the underlying cause is extracardiac (e.g., electrolyte disor-

ders), the prognosis for response is excellent. Other therapies may include:
- antibiotics for infectious processes
- antiinflammatory medication for endocardial, myocardial, or pericardial inflammation
- restriction of physical activity, at least until the arrhythmia is under control
  - The horse should be rested for at least 60 days after all signs of active myocardial disease have subsided.
- correction of any electrolyte disturbances

Pharmacologic Management

When an arrhythmia is considered immediately life-threatening or permanent myocardial damage is likely, drug therapy is indicated. Specific antiarrhythmic therapy should also be considered in the following circumstances:
- for any ventricular arrhythmia
- for arrhythmias with multiform ventricular complexes
- when the resting heart rate remains at ≥90 to 100 beats/min, especially if the rhythm is irregular and there are pulse deficits
- for arrhythmias that cause significant reduction in cardiac output and syncopal episodes
- for persistent arrhythmias with an extracardiac pathogenesis that are unresponsive to primary-cause management

Antiarrhythmia therapy requires use of an ECG to confirm the diagnosis and monitor response.

Digoxin

Digoxin lowers the heart rate and improves myocardial perfusion by reducing the cardiac workload (via its positive inotropic effects).
- The main indication is treatment of supraventricular tachyarrhythmias.
- Prior digitalization often is essential when treating atrial arrhythmias associated with heart failure.
  - A single dose of 0.0022 mg/kg IV (heart rate >150 beats/min) or 0.011 mg/kg PO (heart rate 100 to 150 beats/min) is recommended.
- Dosage recommendations, response to treatment, and signs of toxicity are discussed in the section on heart failure, p. 117.

Quinidine

Quinidine is indicated for treatment of both supraventricular and ventricular arrhythmias; it is most often used to treat atrial fibrillation.

- The recommended IV dose rate is 0.5 mg/kg IV q10 min, up to a total of 4 to 6 mg/kg.
- The recommended oral dose rate is 20 to 22 mg/kg PO q2h, to a total dose of 60 to 80 g (88 to 132 mg/kg).
- There is wide variation in clinical response among horses; therapeutic plasma levels lie between 2 and 5 µg/mL.
- Idiosyncratic responses occasionally occur early in treatment and include collapse, urticaria, hyperesthesia, colic, and sustained tachycardia.
  - An oral test dose of 5 g is recommended before initiating therapy.
- Quinidine should be used with the caution in horses with signs of cardiac insufficiency.
- Horses with severe tachycardia require digitalization.
  - Concurrent use of digoxin and quinidine necessitates a lower dose of digoxin than that used alone to manage heart failure (see p. 117).

Toxic effects vary widely:

- Depression, increased frequency of defecation, and inappetence are common.
  - Nasal congestion is common and in severe cases may cause respiratory stridor.
  - These effects may presage other, more serious, signs, including marked hypotension, severe depression, unsteadiness/ataxia, sustained tachycardia, heart failure, colic, diarrhea, convulsions, laminitis, syncope, and sudden death.
- ECG indications of toxicity include an increase in QRS duration of >25% over the resting level, S-T segment changes, and tachycardia.
- A heart rate >100 beats/min is a clear sign of toxicity and may precede other signs.
- Acute quinidine toxicity can be treated with sodium bicarbonate (0.5 to 1.0 mEq/kg IV, repeated as necessary).

- Severe tachycardia or lack of response to bicarbonate may necessitate use of digoxin (at the single IV or PO dose rate given above).
- If signs of toxicity appear soon after the last oral dose, oral administration of activated charcoal should be considered.
- Horses showing signs of shock/hypotension require fluid therapy.

Procainamide

Procainamide is an antiarrhythmic drug with effects similar to those of quinidine, although it is more effective in ventricular than supraventricular arrhythmias. It may be of value in acute management of serious arrhythmias.

- Procainamide is given IV; reported dosages vary.
  - 0.25 to 0.75 mg/kg/min, diluted (for anesthetized horses)
  - 0.5 mg/kg q10 min to a total dose of 4 to 6 mg/kg
  - 19 mg/kg q6h
- It should be used only when continuous monitoring is possible, so that the dose can be titrated to response.

Propanolol

Propranolol is a β-adrenergic blocking agent with some quinidine-like actions at high dosages. The clinical response is dependent on prevailing sympathetic tone, so it is somewhat unpredictable. Propranolol might be used diagnostically to evaluate the role of sympathetic tone in an arrhythmia or to reduce the ventricular rate in cases of supraventricular tachycardia in which digoxin or quinidine has been unsuccessful.

- IV is the route of choice; reported regimens vary somewhat.
  - 0.22 mg/kg as a bolus (anesthetized horses)
  - 0.1 to 0.3 mg/kg q12h
  - 25-mg bolus q12h on days 1 and 2; 50-mg bolus q12h on days 3 and 4; and 75-mg bolus q12h on days 5 and 6
- In horses with heart disease, the initial IV dose should not exceed 0.1 mg/kg and should be given slowly over 1 minute.
- Bradycardia, hypotension, muscle weakness, and depression are common toxic effects.

- Dopamine or dobutamine (0.5 to 3.0 µg/kg/min IV) is recommended to treat overdosage.
- Atropine (0.45 mg/kg IV) may counteract excessive ventricular slowing or AV block.

Lidocaine
Lidocaine is a relatively safe antiarrhythmic agent that is used in the emergency management of life-threatening ventricular arrhythmias.

- Adverse reactions (including convulsions) can be minimized by giving the maximum dose of 2 to 4 mg/kg in aliquots of 0.5 mg/kg q5 min.
  - Diazepam (0.05 mg/kg) can be used to control lidocaine-induced seizures.
  - Never use the preparation of lidocaine that contains epinephrine.
  - Lidocaine has no effect on supraventricular arrhythmias.

Atropine and glycopyrrolate
Atropine and glycopyrrolate have been used for management of bradyarrhythmias in horses, but they may be more useful diagnostically for evaluating heart block. Vagally induced bradycardia responds to these agents, whereas idioventricular rhythms in third-degree heart block do not. Atropine can cause GI disturbances in horses, so its use is not recommended. Glycopyrrolate may be of value in the management of arrhythmias during anesthesia.

Potassium
Slow IV infusion of potassium chloride can convert some ventricular arrhythmias, although the response sometimes is slow.

- KCl is particularly appropriate when ventricular arrhythmias are due to digoxin toxicity.
- The maximum rate of IV administration is 0.5 mEq/kg/h.
- Ideally, dehydration and acid-base disturbances are corrected first and normal renal function established.
  - When a total-body K^+ deficit is likely to be contributing to the arrhythmia, an isotonic KCl solution should be given with an equal volume of isotonic dextrose.
- IV infusion of potassium can cause AV block and atrial, then ventricular standstill.

- ECG monitoring can be used to detect toxicity; obvious prolongation of QRS and disappearance of the P wave are indications to halt therapy immediately.

Magnesium
There is some evidence that ventricular tachycardia may be treated successfully with $MgSO_4$ at 1 to 2.5 g $MgSO_4$/500 kg/min IV to effect, not to exceed a total dose of 25 g.

Other Manifestations of Cardiovascular Disease

(pages 368-380)
Peter W. Physick-Sheard

SYNCOPE AND SUDDEN DEATH
Syncope
In syncope, temporary loss of blood supply to the cerebrum results in collapse or fainting. Causes can be cardiac or extracardiac.

- Arrhythmias (e.g., third-degree heart block, paroxysmal tachycardia) are the major cardiac cause.
  - Others include heart failure, pericarditis, and pulmonic stenosis.
- Extracardiac causes involving the cardiovascular system include obstruction to cerebral blood flow and neurologic disease associated with marked changes in autonomic tone (causing profound bradycardia).
- In foals, causes include hypoglycemia and severe respiratory or congenital heart disease.

Diagnostic approach
Every case should be investigated for predisposition to paroxysmal bradyarrhythmia or tachyarrhythmia. Investigation should include detailed cardiovascular and neurologic examinations, evaluation of cardiac rhythm at exercise, and, if available, 24-hour rhythm monitoring.

Sudden Death
Cardiovascular causes of sudden death are numerous and include rupture of an artery (e.g., aorta, pulmonary artery, uterine artery) or even an atrium or ventricle. Other conditions include endocarditis, parasite-

associated coronary artery obstruction, heart valve lesions, myocardial failure, and polyarteritis.

HEART FAILURE

Heart failure primarily indicates ventricular dysfunction and is the end result of most cardiac diseases. Nevertheless, it is uncommon in horses.

Acute vs. Chronic Failure

Acute heart failure

Possible causes of acute failure include:
- myocardial failure secondary to hypoxia in severe
- acute blood loss or respiratory disease
- acute myocarditis or toxic myocardial degeneration
- cardiac tamponade/pericardial effusion
- some cases of severe pleural effusion
- severe acute valve dysfunction, such as rupture of chordae tendineae
Pressure and/or volume overload lead to myocardial hypertrophy and eventual dilation.

Chronic heart failure

In chronic heart failure the primary lesion has been present for weeks or months, and several episodes of decompensation and compensation may have occurred. However, clinical manifestations of decompensation can be severe and rapid in onset.

Clinical Signs

Signs of acute left-sided heart failure (LHF) are fairly distinct, being a result of acute pulmonary edema, whereas those of right-sided failure (RHF) may develop more insidiously. Signs of both left and right failure often are found, but one side usually predominates.

Left heart failure

Failure of the left heart results in pulmonary congestion.
- In early cases, marked exercise intolerance and a tendency to cough are observed, although pulmonary edema is unlikely unless failure is acute.
  - Tachypnea and severe dyspnea may be the primary clinical signs in acute cases.
  - There may be froth at the nares.

- Weight loss is common and can progress to emaciation in chronic cases.
- With progression, weak or imperceptible pulses, cool periphery, pale mucous membranes, anxiety, and unsteadiness develop, and syncopal attacks may occur, particularly on exertion.
  - Cyanosis also is present in cases associated with congenital heart disease.
- Chronic pulmonary edema leads to diffuse pulmonary fibrosis; the resulting expiratory and inspiratory dyspnea can mimic severe chronic small airway disease.
  - Jugular vein distention may occur as a result of cor pulmonale.
- Auscultation may reveal a normal heart rate in early cases, but murmurs, arrhythmias, and a prominent cardiac impulse with evidence of cardiomegaly may be found.
  - A gallop rhythm at a resting heart rate suggests cardiac dilation or hypertrophy.
- Once the animal starts to decompensate, regurgitation of the AV valves is the norm, and widespread systolic murmurs are detected.
- Paroxysmal coughing, cyanosis, and appearance of froth at the nares and mouth are seen in terminal cases.

Right heart failure

Failure of the right ventricle causes:
- gradual jugular filling and pulsation (over 3 or 4 days)
  - Rapid development of complete, nonpulsatile jugular filling suggests obstruction to venous return, such as an intrathoracic mass or pericardial effusion, rather than RHF.
- ventral edema, initially in the sternal region and later on the ventral abdomen
  - Edema of the legs is not a prominent finding.
- diarrhea (equally likely with LHF)
  Cor pulmonale refers to a syndrome of RHF secondary to chronic respiratory disease. Except for the signs of severe lung disease and a tendency for respiratory excursions to obscure activity in the jugular veins, signs are typically those of RHF.

General Management of Heart Failure

Acute heart failure

Acute failure is initially managed by resolving the primary insult, if possible. Supportive therapy includes:

* stall confinement
* use of furosemide and bronchodilators (e.g., aminophylline) to assist ventilation
* discontinuation of supplementary salt
* maintenance of adequate hydration
  * NOTE: *Overzealous IV fluid therapy can have disastrous consequences.*

Antiinflammatory agents, such as flunixin meglumine, when myocarditis is suspected,

Digitalization (see below), if the primary insult cannot be corrected.

Chronic heart failure

Digitalization, diuretics, reduced salt intake, and controlled exercise are the main therapeutic approaches in chronic heart failure.

* If the problem is detected early, before signs of congestion are evident, digitalization and restricted exercise may be all that is required.
* In cases of severe left AV valvular regurgitation with respiratory signs, hydralazine (0.5 to 1.5 mg/kg PO q12h) is recommended.
* Furosemide (0.5 to 1.0 mg/kg/day PO or IV, in one or two doses) may be given as needed.
  * Horses on continuous furosemide therapy should be given oral KCl at 20 to 30 g/day.
  * Regular evaluation of electrolyte and acid-base status is necessary.

Digitalization

With cardiac glycosides, effective dosages and the level at which toxic signs are encountered vary widely among horses, sometimes making patient management difficult. The therapeutic index is narrow, and the drug is capable of causing a range of toxic signs, many of which may mimic or worsen the cardiac problem under treatment.

Dosage recommendations

* When the severity of signs indicates the need for rapid digitalization, or when attempting to control supraventricular tachyarrhythmias, an IV loading dose may be given.
  * Reported IV loading doses vary from 2.2 µg/kg to 15 µg/kg (see *Equine Medicine and Surgery V*).
  * The dose should be divided into three parts and given slowly at 1- to 2-hour intervals.
  * Facilities for close monitoring should be available.
* In most cases loading doses are not necessary; they should be avoided wherever possible.
* Oral maintenance doses vary from 11 µg/kg q12h to 35 µg/kg q24h.
  * Giving the drug twice daily in divided doses avoids wide swings in plasma levels.
  * Therapeutic plasma levels are achieved in 3.5 to 6 days.
  * Careful attention is essential to ensure that the horse has received the full dose.
* When concurrent furosemide therapy is used, digoxin doses at the low end of the range are adequate and reduce the potential for toxicity.
* When quinidine is administered concurrently, the lower dosages of digoxin should be used and serum levels monitored.
* If the horse becomes anorectic, serum digoxin levels should be measured to ensure that the presumed therapeutic range of 0.5 to 2.0 ng/mL has not been exceeded.

Response to treatment

Clinical response varies somewhat with the individual case.

* Encouraging signs include increased pulse strength, improved peripheral perfusion, and diuresis.
* The heart rate falls in most cases, especially when supraventricular tachyarrhythmias were present, and signs of congestion (cough, dyspnea, peripheral edema) gradually subside.
* Changes in demeanor are unpredictable and unreliable.

Failure to achieve a clinical response is an indication to increase the dosage, but only if there are no signs of toxicity.

Signs of toxicity

Overdosing, widely fluctuating serum levels, hypoproteinemia, dehydration, hypokalemia, reduced renal function, and concurrent use of quinidine sulphate or phenylbutazone predispose to digoxin toxicity.

- Early signs include depression, anorexia, and mild diarrhea.
  - These signs progress if treatment is continued at the same level, with the animal exhibiting obvious weakness.
- Bradycardia resulting from severe AV block can occur and results in hypotension.
  - Increased frequency of second-degree block and S-T segment deviation are early indicators of toxicity.
- Digoxin toxicity can also cause sinus tachycardia and a predisposition to conduction disturbances and ventricular ectopic activity.
  - These effects are of particular concern in cases of acute myocarditis and myocardial degeneration; digoxin should be used with great caution in such cases.
  - Cardiac glycosides should be avoided in horses exhibiting ventricular arrhythmias.

Diseases of the Endocardium and Valves *(pages 380-394)*
Peter W. Physick-Sheard

ACQUIRED DISEASES OF THE HEART VALVES

With regard to valvular lesions, the left heart is 3 to 8 times more likely to be involved than the right, and regurgitation is reported far more often than stenosis. The significance of valvular regurgitation depends on many factors, including the animal's use and the valve involved; severe regurgitation has obvious hemodynamic consequences, regardless of use. Murmurs are not a consistent guide to the presence of valve lesions.

Left AV Valvular Regurgitation

Left AV valvular (LAV) regurgitation is uncommon but usually is a problem when it is found, frequently causing signs of heart failure or atrial fibrillation. Signs generally are more severe with LAV regurgitation than with abnormal function of any other valve.

Clinical findings
Auscultable findings are as follows:
- The murmur is variable, but typically is soft and blowing, holosystolic, and band-shaped.
  - It is loudest on the left side, two-thirds of the way up from the elbow to the point of the shoulder, at the fourth to sixth intercostal space.
  - The murmur may radiate locally or be widespread.
  - When the valve is insufficient for only part of systole (e.g., with prolapse), the flow and murmur may be mid or late systolic.
- An intense S_3 ± an early diastolic murmur is often encountered in cases of moderate-to-severe LAV regurgitation.
- Decrescendo murmurs are heard in cases of severe regurgitation with left atrial/pulmonary venous hypertension.
- In cases of chordae tendineae rupture and LAV regurgitation, the murmur is intense and noisy and radiates dorsally and caudally.
  - The murmur is widespread on the left, easily heard on the right, and frequently accompanied by a palpable thrill.
  - Chordal rupture leading to acute onset of valvular regurgitation causes respiratory distress.

Decompensating cases of acute LAV regurgitation typically exhibit rapid onset of acute respiratory distress.
- Signs include severe dyspnea, tachypnea, cough, flaring of the nostrils, tachycardia, and severe exercise intolerance.
  - Profuse frothy, occasionally blood-stained nasal discharge is observed in very acute cases.
- Chordal rupture should be considered when respiratory signs are encountered.
- In peracute cases, acute pulmonary edema secondary to septicemia, toxemia, septic pulmonary embolism, or anaphylaxis should also be considered.

Diagnosis

Diagnosis, evaluation of compensatory change, and definition of prognosis are most easily achieved with echocardiography (two-dimensional, M mode, and Doppler). Left atrial and ventricular dilation confirms a hemodynamic effect and an increased risk of atrial fibrillation.

Treatment

Treatment of horses with mild LAV regurgitation is not indicated. Management of other cases depends on the severity of cardiac compromise.

+ Cardioversion may be attempted in horses with atrial fibrillation (see p. 113).
+ When regurgitation is due to progression of a chronic valve lesion and myocardial failure, digitalization may result in considerable improvement.
  • Positive inotropes can increase the regurgitant fraction, so clinical signs may not improve; hydralazine may reduce afterload in such cases (see p. 117).
  • The greatest response is likely to be seen with diuretics and stall rest.
+ Acute cases of chordal rupture also are best treated with total rest and diuretics.

Prognosis

Prognosis varies with the severity of cardiac dysfunction.

+ In horses not asked to perform maximally, mild regurgitation progresses slowly, if at all, and affected horses can have a normal life span and no noticeable reduction in performance.
  • Even moderate regurgitation may have no impact on longevity and little impact on performance in pleasure horses.
+ LAV regurgitation is a cause for concern in young horses intended for an athletic career.
+ Chordal rupture has a uniformly guarded prognosis for life and a poor prognosis for athletic performance; however, affected horses can survive for months or years.

Right AV Valvular Regurgitation

Regurgitation at the right AV valve (RAV) can result from cardiac failure secondary to LAV regurgitation; other causes include bacterial endocarditis and ventricular septal defect. Murmurs consistent with RAV regurgitation are frequently identified, but mild regurgitation at this valve may be normal. There is a higher prevalence of soft, holosystolic murmurs over the right AV valve in Standardbred racehorses.

Clinical findings

The murmur of RAV regurgitation is similar to that of LAV regurgitation, although rarely of the same intensity.

+ The murmur is best heard on the right side, from the second to fourth intercostal spaces, at a level midway between the elbow and shoulder.
+ It is soft, blowing, band-shaped, and holosystolic; in only a few cases does it radiate widely.
+ When pulmonary hypertension develops, the murmur may be grade IV or greater in intensity.
+ Clinical signs vary with the severity of regurgitation and accompanying cardiac abnormalities.
  • Mild-to-moderate RAV regurgitation may cause no signs and may not limit performance.
  • Jugular filling and pulsation may occur, but right heart failure and right AV valvular stenosis are far more likely causes.

Prognosis

The prognosis is far better than for LAV regurgitation, although a guarded prognosis is warranted when other signs of cardiac disease are present.

Aortic Valvular Regurgitation

Lesions of the aortic valve are reported more frequently than lesions of any other valve.

+ Aortic valvular regurgitation (AR) commonly is identified echocardiographically, but in many cases the flow is silent, both clinically and on auscultation.
  • There is a significantly higher prevalence in racehorses than in other horses.
+ AR can be found in both young and older horses, but clinical signs or echocardiographic evidence of left ventricular overload are seen only in older horses.

- When obvious signs of cardiovascular insufficiency are found, other factors most often are present (e.g., myocardial disease, atrial fibrillation, LAV regurgitation, endocarditis).

Clinical findings

Symptomatic but uncomplicated AR causes a murmur and minor circulatory changes.

- A prominent, bounding pulse may be felt in moderate-to-severe cases.
- The murmur typically is a decrescendo sound that lasts throughout diastole; it is best heard at the left heart base but radiates toward the apex of the left ventricle.
  - The sound can vary from barely perceptible to grade VI and may radiate to the right side.
  - A systolic murmur may also be heard and reflects increased stroke volume.
- Louder and coarser murmurs tend to be clinically significant, particularly when they radiate widely or are associated with a bounding pulse.
  - Soft and high-frequency decrescendo sounds, particularly those that last through to S_1, are of limited clinical significance in most cases.

Aortic and Pulmonic Stenosis

Acquired stenosis of these valves is rare and is most often a consequence of active or healing endocarditis (see below). Most cases of aortic stenosis are either minor valve disruptions that simply cause flow disturbances during systole or relative stenosis in which the rate of flow during systole exceeds the flow capacity of the valve (such as can occur with left AV valvular regurgitation or large ventricular septal defects).

Clinical findings

The murmur of true stenosis is classically crescendo-decrescendo in shape.

- It starts after S_1 and occupies most of systole, peaking shortly after S_1 and ending before S_2.
- It varies from musical to harsh and vibrant and is best heard over the left heart base.

- An increase in intensity can be anticipated with exercise.
- Midsystolic murmurs are not associated with clinical signs in most cases.

ENDOCARDITIS

Endocarditis is rarely diagnosed clinically; cases occur sporadically and are unpredictable.

- Endocarditis is not consistently associated with any particular clinical entity (including thrombophlebitis), and may develop with no current or recent history of a septic focus.
- Cases are categorized as acute or subacute, bacterial or nonbacterial, and valvular or mural.
  - The most common organisms isolated from cases of bacterial endocarditis are streptococci (usually *S. zooepidemicus*), staphylococci, and *Actinobacillus equuli*.
  - The distribution of valvular lesions, in descending order of prevalence, is aortic, left AV, right AV, and pulmonic.

Clinical findings

Clinical signs depend on the speed of onset, location of the lesion, and underlying etiology. Most cases in horses are subacute.

- There is fluctuating pyrexia, weight loss, lethargy, and depression; lameness is common.
  - The pyrexia may respond to antibiotics, only to relapse when treatment is withdrawn.
- Endocarditis is not always accompanied by a detectable murmur; when present, the murmur can involve any valve and may be systolic, diastolic, or continuous.
- The clinical course may last from weeks to months, with obvious signs of cardiac disease being only a terminal event.
- In acute cases the clinical course is as short as several days, with severe pyrexia and depression, along with reluctance to move that may reflect thoracic discomfort or lameness.
  - Signs of cardiac insufficiency, such as edema and jugular filling, develop rapidly.

- Embolic episodes are common and reflect the side of the heart involved.
  - Embolic showers from the right side can cause pulmonary hypertension, which contributes to right heart failure and may precipitate pulmonary edema and toxic shock.
  - Left-sided lesions often cause emboli in the kidneys, myocardium, and joints, resulting in signs of renal dysfunction, arrhythmia, and lameness.
  - Embolism of the cerebral vasculature can occur with aortic valvular endocarditis and may lead to a wide range of neurologic signs.
- Endocarditis likely occurs subclinically (or the diagnosis may be missed), with spontaneous resolution following nonspecific treatment.

Diagnosis

Diagnosis is based on clinical, laboratory, and echocardiographic findings.

- The diagnosis should always be considered in cases of variable, recurrent pyrexia that is responsive to antibiotics; a murmur should not be expected.
  - The index of suspicion is increased with evidence of embolic showering and multiorgan involvement; in some cases the initial signs are referable to an organ other than the heart.
- Laboratory data are nonspecific, the picture being consistent with persistent inflammation.
  - Anemia and neutrophilia are common.
  - Fibrinogen is elevated, particularly in acute cases; hypoalbuminemia and hypergammaglobulinemia may also be present.
  - Other biochemical abnormalities reflect embolic involvement of specific organs.
- blood culture should always be attempted, although results frequently are negative.
  - Ideally, cultures are repeated 3 times at 8- to 12-hour intervals during a pyrexic episode, after antibiotics have been withheld for at least 24 hours.

- Better results may be obtained by culturing arterial rather than venous blood.

Treatment

Treatment should be attempted in cases with no evidence of heart failure.

- Initial treatment with high-dose penicillin (50,000 IU/kg IV q6h) combined with gentamicin is recommended until results of blood culture are available.
  - Appropriate antibiotics must be continued for at least 4 weeks.
- Response to therapy is assessed by monitoring body temperature and repeating hematology and echocardiography.
  - If pyrexia does not abate within 4 to 5 days, the choice or dosage of antibiotics must be reassessed.

Prognosis

The prognosis often is poor, even with an initial response to treatment. Relapse is common, and varying degrees of valvular dysfunction (chronic incompetence and/or stenosis) can be expected; exercise tolerance is likely to be reduced. However, mild lesions that respond to therapy may carry a good prognosis.

CONGENITAL DISEASES OF THE ENDOCARDIUM

Tricuspid Atresia

The complex of tricuspid atresia consists of atresia or absence of the right AV orifice, right ventricular hypoplasia, an atrial septal defect, and a ventricular septal defect. A patent ductus arteriosus may also been present. Clinical signs include poor growth, lethargy, severe exercise intolerance, and cyanosis. An intense, pansystolic, shunt type of murmur usually is present, loudest at the left heart base; a diastolic component may be noted. Echocardiography and contrast studies allow definitive diagnosis. The prognosis is uniformly poor.

Other congenital endocardial defects, including endocardial fibroelastosis, aortic valvular regurgitation, and other abnormalities of the outflow valves, are discussed in *Equine Medicine and Surgery V.*

Diseases of the Myocardium *(pages 394-405)*

Peter W. Physick-Sheard

CONGENITAL AND FAMILIAL DISEASES

Ventricular Septal Defect

Ventricular septal defect (VSD) is the most common congenital cardiac anomaly in horses, either alone or as a component of more complex anomalies.

Auscultable findings

The location and distribution of the murmur indicate the position and nature of the defect.

- The murmur is intense and harsh and radiates widely; both S_1 and S_2 may be obliterated.
  - There is no dependable correlation between murmur intensity and clinical significance; small defects can produce intense sounds with minimal clinical consequence.
- Simple defects that shunt L to R generate a murmur that is loudest on the right side.
  - The murmur may be quite localized and easily missed.
  - The sound can usually be heard well forward on the left side, but is less intense.
  - If the shunt reverses, the murmur is most intense on the left side, over the left ventricle.
- An ejection murmur at the left heart base may simply reflect increased flow through the pulmonic valve, but an intense, shunt type of murmur at this location suggests the possibility of a complex anomaly of the great vessels (see p. 126).

Clinical signs and diagnosis

The clinical consequences of an isolated VSD vary enormously.

- The foal may be cyanotic and distressed at birth, or the anomaly may be an incidental finding in a mature, asymptomatic horse with no history of performance problems.
- Adverse effects are most likely when the defect is large (several centimeters) or when its location favors flow disturbance and L-to-R shunting.

- Even with relatively small defects, constant overcirculation of the lungs can lead to pulmonary hypertension and right ventricular hypertrophy.
- L-to-R shunting can also lead to right AV regurgitation (see p. 119).
- ◆ Definitive diagnosis is made by echocardiography and blood gas analysis.

Prognosis

The prognosis varies.

- ◆ With a small defect and no other abnormal findings, the prognosis is good.
  - With normal growth, the defect can become relatively smaller.
  - VSDs limit aerobic capacity but may still be compatible with some types of work.
- ◆ A guarded prognosis must be given for large defects, for defects complicated by other congenital anomalies or valve damage, and when there is concurrent respiratory disease.

Atrial Septal Defects and Persistent Foramen Ovale

True atrial septal defects as an isolated finding are uncommon in horses.

- ◆ Large defects cause volume overload of the right heart and lungs.
  - In time, pressure overload on the right heart reverses the shunt, resulting in systemic hypoxemia and volume overload of the left heart.
  - There is no auscultable murmur.
- ◆ Small fenestrations in the atrial septum may persist into adulthood and are asymptomatic.
- ◆ Persistent foramen ovale is often diagnosed postmortem in neonatal foals, but should more properly be described as probe patency, because anatomic closure lags behind functional closure by several days or weeks.

NUTRITIONAL DISEASES

Nutritional Myopathy

Selenium and/or vitamin E deficiency causes muscle degeneration and necrosis, including myocardial damage.

- ◆ Extensive myocardial involvement may cause sudden death, often

during exercise, or rapid onset of weakness, tachycardia, and dyspnea (heart failure and pulmonary edema).
* Arrhythmias are not uniformly present and should not be depended on for diagnosis.
* Postmortem findings include pale streaking of the myocardium, sometimes with calcification.

TOXIC DISEASES
Ionophore Toxicity
Ionophores are antibiotics that are primarily used as coccidiostats in poultry and to enhance feed conversion in cattle. Equine intoxication most often involves monensin, but can also occur with salinomycin. Lasalocid is another ionophore that could cause toxicity in horses. The acute toxic effects of ionophores involve skeletal and cardiac myopathy, renal and hepatic damage, and intravascular hemolysis.

Clinical findings in acute intoxication
Signs in acutely intoxicated horses can include:
* muscle weakness, ataxia, intermittent profuse sweating, difficulty rising, and recumbency
* abdominal pain, ileus, and/or diarrhea; these may be the prominent findings in less severely affected horses
* severe dyspnea (cardiogenic pulmonary edema ± compromised diaphragmatic function)
* arrhythmias and sudden death during exercise
Death occurs anywhere from 12 hours to several days after ingestion of the ionophore, although in acute cases most deaths occur within 24 to 36 hours.

Clinical findings in subacute intoxication
Findings in horses that survive the acute episode and in less acute cases of intoxication are more insidious.
* Signs include depression, reduced feed intake, cardiac arrhythmias, tachycardia and heart failure, and hyperventilation.
* Sudden death may occur without prodromal signs, presumably as a result of arrhythmias.

* Some horses simply show chronic disability, manifest as unthriftiness, cardiac dysfunction (tachycardia, arrhythmias such as ventricular ectopy and atrial fibrillation, S-T segment changes, and heart failure), and reduced exercise tolerance.
* Death or onset or recurrence of clinical signs may occur weeks after the acute episode.

Diagnosis
Diagnosis is based on the combination of history, including the pattern of herd involvement and recent diet change, clinical signs, and laboratory findings.
* Immediate dietary evaluation and analysis are indicated.
* Demonstration of an ionophore in the feed or stomach contents confirms the diagnosis.
* Laboratory findings in acute intoxication include transient (<24 hours) falls in serum calcium and potassium and elevations in urea, creatinine, and unconjugated bilirubin.
  * Magnesium and phosphorous may also decline; sodium shows little change.
  * Elevation in serum AP, primarily of bone origin, is seen.
  * Hemoconcentration is evident by elevations in PCV and serum proteins.
* Changes in AST, CPK, and LDH occur, with isoenzyme patterns in CPK and LDH indicating skeletal, cardiac muscle, and erythrocyte damage.
  * Changes in CPK and AST may be massive.
  * Muscle enzyme elevations may not be detectable in ambulatory chronic cases.
* ECG changes are nonspecific.
  * Initial flattening of the T wave with transient hypokalemia changes to a large T wave.
  * S-T segment depression and arrhythmias occur with extensive myocardial damage.
* Postmortem findings include pale or streaked myocardium, subcutaneous and pulmonary edema, congestion and hemorrhage, and pleural, abdominal, and pericardial effusions.

Treatment

Treatment is largely symptomatic: activated charcoal or mineral oil, volume replacement with polyionic solutions, IV supplementation with magnesium and phosphate, and stall rest. Digoxin should not be used.

Prognosis

The prognosis depends on the particular ionophore involved and the amount consumed.

* Ingestion of large amounts of monensin or salinomycin carries the worst prognosis.
* When the ionophore is present in lower concentrations and the horse eats little of the feed, prognosis for survival is fair to guarded.
* Residual myocardial damage prevents athletic horses from returning to their previous level of performance.

Other Toxic Myopathies

Any type of toxemia can cause myocardial necrosis, including intestinal clostridiosis and cantharidin poisoning (see Chapter 10, Alimentary System). Arrhythmias are encountered, though ECG abnormalities may reflect electrolyte and acid-base disturbances as well as toxic myocardial damage.

MULTIFACTORIAL DISEASES

Myocarditis

Myocarditis implies active inflammation of the myocardium. Its origin may be parasitic, viral (e.g., influenza, African horse sickness), or bacterial (e.g., strangles, acute endocarditis, septicemia); rarely is it primary.

Clinical signs and diagnosis

Findings are nonspecific and could reflect cardiac insufficiency of any cause.

* Signs include exercise intolerance, dyspnea on exertion, syncope, tachycardia disproportionate to fever, murmurs, gallop sounds, arrhythmias, signs of congestive heart failure, and sudden death.
* The principal diagnostic modalities are serum biochemistry, ECG, and echocardiography.
  * A strong association exists between elevated (>250 IU/L) serum

hydroxybutyrate dehydrogenase (HBD) and active myocarditis
  * ECG abnormalities include S-T segment and T wave deviations, slurring and prolongation of QRS, electrical alternans, and prolongation of P-R and Q-T intervals.
* Lesions usually are focal and widely scattered and may not be obvious at postmortem examination unless necrosis is severe.

Fibrosis, Infarction, and Coronary Arterial Disease

Myocardial fibrosis represents the end stage of myocardial cell loss, regardless of the primary insult. Possible causes either affect the coronary arteries or the myocardium directly, and include parasitic thromboendarteritis of the proximal aorta, endocarditis involving the left side of the heart, catecholamines, endotoxin, acute hypoxia during maximal exertion, potassium deficiency, equine infectious anemia, hyperlipemia (ponies), and exhaustion. Atrial and ventricular aneurysms are possible sequelae to myocardial infarction and/or fibrosis.

Equine Rhabdomyolysis Syndrome

Equine rhabdomyolysis syndrome (see Chapter 15, Musculoskeletal System) occasionally involves the myocardium. Progressive loss of myocardial functional capacity can be a consequence of repeated episodes. ECG changes include arrhythmias, tachycardia, and S-T segment changes.

Diseases of the Pericardium and Thoracic Cavity

(pages 405–409)

Peter W. Physick-Sheard

MULTIFACTORIAL DISEASES

Pericardial Effusion and Pericarditis

Benign pericardial effusion (transudation) may occur with congestive heart failure or hypoproteinemia, but most cases involve inflammation. Possible causes include trauma (e.g., rib fractures, penetrating chest wounds, foreign body protrusion through the esophagus or stomach), extension from myocardial or endocardial infection, neoplasia, systemic viral or bacterial disease, primary mycoplasma *(Mycoplasma felis)* infection, and extension of pleural and pulmonary inflammation.

Clinical findings

Findings reflect pressure on the heart and cardiac displacement.

- Tachycardia with a weak pulse, muffled heart sounds, and venous hypertension are classic.
  - Extensive ventral edema and jugular venous distention result.
  - Jugular pulsation may initially be evident, although severe distention of the pericardial sac (cardiac tamponade) may later result in fully distended, nonpulsatile veins.
- Prolonged capillary refill time and cool extremities indicate circulatory compromise.
- Depression and lethargy usually are observed, and colic is seen in some cases.
  - Pyrexia is not a consistent finding.
- Mucous membranes may be congested/hyperemic or cyanotic, and most affected horses are dyspneic.
  - Mucosal congestion and cyanosis likely reflect toxemia or respiratory compromise.
- Auscultation usually reveals muffling ± dorsal displacement of the heart sounds.
  - Clear heart sounds and friction rubs may be heard early in the course of disease (before extensive fluid accumulation) or after pericardiocentesis and drainage.
  - Horses with primary pleural effusion also have relatively clear heart sounds.

Diagnosis

Diagnosis is best confirmed by echocardiography and is further aided by pericardiocentesis (see discussion of treatment).

- The nature of the pericardial fluid varies with the primary insult.
  - In cases of bleeding into the pericardial sac, the fluid is bloody or serosanguineous.
- In idiopathic cases, the effusion usually is aseptic, but mildly inflammatory, sometimes containing significant numbers of eosinophils or histiocytes.
- Involvement of *M. felis* should be pursued in cases of idiopathic pericarditis, particularly when macrophages and healthy-appearing neutrophils are present.
- Septic effusions should be cultured, but often are culture-negative.
- Hematologic and serum biochemical findings are nonspecific and of limited value in diagnosis; elevated serum fibrinogen can be anticipated.

Treatment

Treatment is primarily aimed at draining the pericardial sac and controlling inflammation and sepsis when present.

- Pericardiocentesis is most safely performed with a polyethylene IV catheter
  - A 14 gauge, 12-cm (4.75 inch) catheter usually is adequate.
  - Aseptic technique must be used, even if a septic process is suspected.
  - Rapid drainage is contraindicated, especially in acute and severe cases.
  - Pericardiocentesis can be performed blindly (directly over the heart, in the fourth intercostal space), but laceration of a coronary artery with fatal cardiac tamponade is a definite risk.
  - Preferably, all pericardiocentesis should be performed under ultrasound guidance.
  - The catheter is inserted, bevel forward, between the ribs and oriented in a horizontal plane, pointing 30 degrees ahead of the transverse plane.
  - The catheter is withdrawn slightly if it is felt to grate against the heart, and should be withdrawn completely if an initially yellowish fluid becomes bloody.
- NSAIDs are indicated to relieve pericardial inflammation; corticosteroids may be used when culture is negative and antibiotics are given concurrently.

- Broad-spectrum antibiotic therapy is advised.
- Tetracyclines should be considered in cases of mycoplasma infection.

Prognosis

The long-term outcome may ultimately depend on the extent to which fibrin is laid down and organized. Survival of months or years after treatment has been reported. When a foreign body or mixed bacterial infection is involved, the prognosis is poor.

THORACIC MASSES

The most common thoracic masses are pulmonary abscesses/loculation and neoplasia. Pulmonary abscesses that interfere with cardiac function usually are located within the right ventral or cranioventral lung field. Except when the mass is large enough to interfere with cardiac filling, cardiac involvement is limited to caudal displacement and some change in the relative intensity of heart sounds, which may be heard over a wider area than normal.

Neoplasia

Mediastinal tumors can be large and may put pressure on the great veins, atria, or major airways, causing a clinical syndrome not readily distinguishable from right heart failure or pericarditis. Masses most often form in the cranial mediastinum and initially cause selective obstruction of cranial venous drainage.

Mediastinal lymphosarcoma

Mediastinal lymphosarcoma occurs in mature horses (mean age, 6 to 10 years).

- It may be accompanied by both pleural and pericardial effusion.
- Affected horses may be anemic because of bone marrow involvement; weight loss occurs in more chronic cases.
  - Peripheral lymphadenopathy is occasionally observed.
- Diagnosis is based on clinical signs and cytology.
  - Fluid can be obtained by thoracocentesis or by fine-needle aspiration of lymphoid masses.
  - Typically, the fluid is sanguineous and contains lympho-

cytes with marked variations in size and morphology, together with large, immature pleomorphic lymphoid cells.
- Corticosteroids effect short-term improvement in some cases, but the prognosis is extremely poor.

Diseases of Arteries and Veins *(pages 409-424)*
Peter W. Physick-Sheard and Lucy M. Edens

CONGENITAL AND FAMILIAL DISEASES

Persistent Ductus Arteriosus (PDA)

A continuous, or machinery, murmur associated with patency of the ductus arteriosus often is detectable within the first 24 hours in newborn foals (see p. 100). The vessel may remain anatomically patent for several days after birth or may close within 3 days, depending on the circumstances surrounding parturition and gestational age at birth. Thus a diagnosis of persistent ductus arteriosus (PDA) should not be made until the foal is >4 to 5 days of age. True PDA is rare in horses; most cases are associated with other cardiac anomalies. Signs include exercise intolerance and cardiovascular insufficiency.

Persistent Right Aortic Arch

Anomalies of the aortic arch are rare. The few reported cases involve the right fourth arch or left ductus arteriosus. Esophageal obstruction and regurgitation with inhalation pneumonia were observed. Thus this anomaly should be considered in cases of nasal regurgitation in foals, although it is a far less common cause than other congenital problems, such as cleft palate.

Persistent Truncus Arteriosus

If the septa that divides the truncus arteriosus fails to develop, the result is both ventricles being drained by a single vessel, a persistent truncus arteriosus (PTA). A ventricular septal defect accompanies this anomaly. Affected foals experience hypoxemia (PaO_2 <50 mm Hg), dyspnea, and some degree of cyanosis, and they have an intense machinery (continuous) murmur. Antemortem diagnosis requires echocardiography. The prognosis for survival is poor.

Pulmonic Atresia

In atresia of the pulmonary trunk (pseudotruncus arteriosus), the pulmonic valve is vestigial or absent and the pulmonary artery consists of a thin cord. All reported cases were accompanied by a ventricular septal defect and had a single large outflow vessel. A PDA is present in most cases. Clinical signs are typical of congenital heart disease involving R-L shunts and abnormality of the outflow tracts: lethargy, weakness, ill thrift, exercise intolerance, cyanosis, and a pansystolic murmur with a point of maximum intensity at the left heart base. Affected foals are symptomatic from birth and have a poor prognosis for survival.

Tetralogy of Fallot

Tetralogy of Fallot classically consists of: (1) stenosis of the pulmonic ostium, (2) dextrorotation of the aorta, (3) a ventricular septal defect, and (4) right ventricular hypertrophy. Pulmonic atresia may also be present. A harsh pansystolic murmur, loudest at the left heart base and radiating widely, is consistently reported. Most cases have an associated thrill on palpation, with tachycardia and reduced exercise tolerance. Cyanosis is not a consistent finding. The murmur is particularly intense and may take on a crescendo decrescendo shape, in contrast to the coarse, band-shaped sound typically associated with congenital shunts.

ARTERIAL THROMBOSIS

Aortoiliac Thrombosis

Aortoiliac thrombosis is an idiopathic thrombotic disease of the terminal aorta and its major branches. It is characterized by exercise-associated lameness or stiffness that disappears with rest. The primary lesion appears to be formation of a mural thrombus in the terminal aorta, just ahead of the origin of the external iliac ar-

teries. Lameness is associated with peripheral embolism as pieces of thrombus detach and block arteries that supply major muscles. The actual cause remains undetermined. Most recent reports involve young performance horses.

Clinical signs

Signs may initially be subtle, consisting of vague hind limb or back lameness. As larger areas of muscle become involved, characteristic signs become evident.

- The horse performs normally up to a "threshold" speed (which varies with each case), at which point stiffness in the affected limb(s) becomes evident.
  - Thoroughbreds may show a tendency to "bunny-hop" and Standardbreds to break gait.
  - If the horse is made to continue working, it may knuckle over, stumble, and possibly fall.
- Once exercise is stopped and the horse is rested, pain subsides within 15 to 20 minutes.
- Other signs include uncharacteristic irritability and a tendency to kick, hold the leg up, or stamp a hind foot after exercise
- The condition may involve one or both hind limbs, although almost invariably signs are asymmetric.
- Examination immediately after exercise usually reveals coolness of the hind limb and sometimes a regional absence of sweating.
  - Reduced skin temperature is most evident, and most reliable, around the gaskin.
- Asymmetry of muscle mass is seen in some cases.

Diagnosis

Diagnosis is primarily based on clinical findings.

- Palpation of the peripheral pulses can be a sensitive means of detecting abnormalities, even in horses with early signs.
  - Pulses should be palpated in the fully rested animal, rather than after exercise.
  - The coccygeal, saphenous, dorsal metatarsal, and digital arteries should be assessed.
  - The pulse contour distal to the site of obstruction is collateral

(flattened, weak, and prolonged); proximal to the obstruction, the pulse may be normal or increased.

- Obstruction often occurs at the level of the stifle, so a collateral pulse in the dorsal metatarsal and digital arteries and a normal or full pulse in the saphenous artery are typical.
- Asymmetry between the hind limbs or exaggerated pulse in the saphenous artery are especially useful findings.
- Discrete and localized obstruction of only arteries supplying muscle may not alter palpable peripheral pulses.

- Rate of filling of the saphenous vein immediately after exercise can also be useful.
  - Normally, the vein fills within 10 seconds after exercise ends.
  - With aortoiliac thrombosis, the time taken for filling depends on the extent of arterial obstruction and can be >90 seconds.

- Rectal evaluation is used to compare the quality and strength of the pulse in the major branches of the aorta.
  - Badly obstructed vessels may be greatly enlarged and firm.

- Transrectal ultrasonography using a routine pregnancy diagnosis probe can be rewarding.
  - Doppler ultrasound is necessary to demonstrate flow and localize the obstruction.

- Clinical laboratory data are of little diagnostic value; muscle enzymes are not elevated after an episode of exercise-induced lameness, unless muscle necrosis has occurred.

Treatment

Therapy mostly is symptomatic.

- Sodium gluconate may have some efficacy in dissolving recent (<24 hours), unorganized thrombi; however, in subacute and chronic cases, thrombolysis is unlikely with any therapeutic agent.
  - Aspirin therapy is rational in recent, active cases and may be capable of limiting further thrombus development.
  - Deworming is not likely to be helpful.

- Surgical correction using a thrombectomy catheter has recently been described.
  - Correction to the point of allowing race-intensity performance is improbable, and, because residual arterial damage is likely, the potential for ongoing thromboembolism remains.

- The only management approach of value thus far is regular exercise, as long as it does not cause the animal significant discomfort.
  - Regular, moderate exercise stimulates and maintains collateral flow.
  - If affected horses are not kept in light work, they should be turned out, not stall-rested.

Prognosis

Clinical deterioration may be slow in mildly affected horses that are kept in steady work. In other cases deterioration may be rapid, with horses becoming incapable of even light exercise in a matter of weeks. In any degree, the condition is not compatible with race-intensity exercise. In stallions, infertility may result from obstruction or shunting of blood away from spermatic arteries, and obstruction of the dorsal artery of the penis may cause impotence.

IATROGENIC THROMBOPHLEBITIS

Thrombophlebitis, the complete or partial obstruction of blood flow secondary to intravascular clot formation and accompanying mural inflammation, may be either septic or nonseptic. Serious, even life-threatening complications can result.

Causes include:

- mechanical trauma to the vascular intima associated with catheter insertion or repetitive motion of continuous indwelling IV catheters (see Chapter 4, Principles of Therapy)
- injection of irritating chemicals
  - Drugs most commonly implicated include glycerol guaiacolate, thiopental, phenylbutazone, and oxytetracycline.
  - The incidence of thrombophlebitis increases with repeated injections.

- Perivascular injection of irritating medications can also precipitate thrombophlebitis.
- hemostatic dysfunction in horses with systemic illness (especially endotoxemia) or a primary hypercoagulable syndrome
- bacterial colonization of IV catheters, especially in septicemic neonates

Clinical signs
Signs include:
- focal or generalized swelling of the vein, venous distention proximal to the site of thrombosis, and, if complete occlusion has occurred, regional edema
- pain on palpation of the site; the vein feels firm and cordlike, and if sepsis is present, the affected area is warm
- reluctance to move the head and neck
- purulent exudate draining or readily expressed from the venipuncture site, if bacterial infection is present
- pyrexia, depression, and anorexia, with septic thrombophlebitis
- extensive edema of the head and laryngeal area, if bilateral jugular thrombosis has occurred before the development of collateral circulation
  - Dysphagia and respiratory distress may result.

Diagnosis
Diagnosis is based on the history and clinical findings.
- Early signs of catheter-induced thrombophlebitis include difficulty infusing through the catheter, swelling at the site of catheter entry into the skin, pain on palpation over the catheter, and unexplained pyrexia.
- An inflammatory leukogram with hyperfibrinogenemia may be detected, particularly if the thrombus is septic.

ULTRASONOGRAPHY
- A thrombus appears as an echogenic area within the hypoechoic or anechoic lumen of the vein.
  - With partial obstruction, a circumscribed anechoic area can be imaged between the thrombus

and the vessel wall and followed along the course of the thrombus.
- With septic thrombophlebitis, the thrombus is less uniformly echogenic, containing anechoic or hyperechoic areas.
  - Discrete anechoic areas located centrally within the thrombus (cavitations) represent areas of fluid accumulation secondary to necrosis or bacterial infection.
  - Anaerobic infections are identified by numerous hyperechoic areas (acoustic shadows from gas bubbles).
- Recanalization is identified as an anechoic area between the thrombus and vessel wall.

CULTURE
Aerobic and anaerobic cultures should be performed on the catheter tip, any exudate draining or expressed from the catheter site, fluid retrieved from cavitary areas by fine-needle aspiration, and, if the animal is febrile, an aseptically collected blood sample (blood culture).

Treatment and prognosis
Treatment and practical guidelines for preventing catheter-induced thrombophlebitis are discussed in Chapter 4. Nonseptic thrombophlebitis usually resolves within several weeks, although recanalization may take several months. Septic thrombophlebitis also resolves over time, provided that appropriate therapy is administered and severe complications do not develop.

PULMONARY THROMBOEMBOLISM

Obstruction of the pulmonary artery by thrombi is a predictable consequence of iatrogenic thrombophlebitis. Other causes include surgery-induced tissue trauma, local hypoxia, and shock. Consequences depend on the size and extent of the thrombus. Although uncommon, rapid reduction in the cross-sectional area of the pulmonary arterial tree causes pulmonary hypertension, which may lead to cor pulmonale and death. A more common consequence is pulmonary abscessation and pneumonia.

PARASITIC ARTERITIS

Strongylus vulgaris infestation is responsible for a wide range of cardiovascular lesions and clinical problems, the most consistent being cranial mesenteric arteritis (see Chapter 10, Alimentary System). Aberrant parasite migration may also cause:

- tracts throughout the thoracic and proximal abdominal aorta, and tracts, endarteritis with thrombosis, and fibrous nodules in the bulb of the aorta
  - Lesions may lead to valvular endocarditis with regurgitation or stenosis, aneurysm and rupture of coronary arteries, coronary obstruction and myocardial infarction and, occasionally, sudden death.
- renal infarction
- parasitic embolism of the brain, resulting in encephalomalacia or encephalomyelitis
- tracts into the spinal cord, with varying degrees of locomotor dysfunction

VASCULAR NEOPLASIA

Vascular neoplasms are uncommon in horses. Tumorous vascular lesions may be loosely classified into benign angiomas and malignant angiosarcomas.

Angiomas
Hamartomas

Many angiomas are hamartomas, or developmental malformations of vascular tissue, rather than neoplastic processes. Hamartomas may be found at any site and often are present at or shortly after birth. They tend to develop as the animal grows and, like all vascular masses, may be pulsatile on palpation. Local infiltration is not a feature, so these masses can be excised.

Angiomas and hemangiomas

True angiomas or hemangiomas are classified as benign tumors of endothelial cells:

- They are most commonly found in the skin of the legs, head, and flank in young animals.
- These tumors generally are slow growing and nonulcerative, and vary from soft, fluctuating, fluid-filled structures to hard nodules.

- They usually are discrete, although they vary from sessile or pedunculated, localized lesions to cordlike, elongated masses.
- Their presence may be more a blemish than a clinical problem.
- It can be difficult to differentiate the lesion from angiosarcoma on biopsy, and local infiltration or recurrence after excision may prove problematic.

Angiosarcoma

Angiosarcoma (hemangiosarcoma) is a malignant tumor of endothelial cells.

- It occurs in mature horses (>5 years of age), but is uncommon.
- Metastasis is common and can involve various organs and tissues, including spleen, heart, lungs, brain, liver, bone, and skeletal muscle.
- The neoplastic masses are nodular, red, and vary in size up to several centimeters and in consistency from soft to hard; skin involvement is not a feature.
- Clinical signs include weakness, dyspnea, pallor, anorexia, and weight loss; icterus is a prominent finding in some horses.
  - Cases with skeletal muscle involvement have some degree of fluctuant external swelling.
- The clinical course is short (days or weeks) once signs become evident.
  - A common cause of death is hemorrhage from the masses.

VASCULAR ACCIDENTS
Rupture of the Aorta

Rupture of the aorta has been associated with a range of problems, including myocarditis, endocarditis with chronic aortic valvular regurgitation, and necrosis of the arterial media. Aortic rupture is uncommon.

Aneurysm/rupture
and aorticopulmonary fistula

Rupture most frequently occurs in the aortic root, just above the valve.

- In many cases sudden death results from hemorrhage into the pericardium (cardiac tamponade) or thoracic cavity.
  - Formation of a dissecting aneurysm can also occur.

- An aorticopulmonary fistula may develop when rupture extends into the pulmonary artery.
  - The fistula usually is associated with a murmur that is continuous and reminiscent of a patent ductus arteriosus, although it waxes and wanes, being loudest in diastole.
- Acute thoracic pain and distress may be evident at the time the aneurysm first develops; signs of heart failure subsequently develop.
  - Some aortic aneurysms are asymptomatic.

Aortic ring rupture

Aortic ring rupture occurs most often in stallions and involves separation between the aorta and its insertion at the fibrous annulus of the heart.

Hemorrhage can dissect into the right ventricle, interventricular septum, or left ventricle. When hemorrhage dissects into the right ventricle, the horse may progress rapidly to right heart failure or may survive for weeks or months and may even continue to undertake moderate physical effort, although all cases eventually terminate in heart failure. A diastolic murmur, loudest on the right side, may be heard.

Uterine Artery Rupture

Rupture of the middle uterine artery, uterine branch of the ovarian artery, or external iliac artery sometimes occurs in periparturient mares. This condition is discussed in Chapter 13, Reproductive System: The Mare.

9

Respiratory System

Examination of the Respiratory System

(pages 440-447)

**Frederick J. Derksen and
Mary Rose Paradis**

HISTORY

Pertinent questions include:
* duration since the presenting problem was first observed
* presence and nature of any nasal discharge or cough
* exercise tolerance
* vaccination history, especially strangles, rhinopneumonitis, and influenza

PHYSICAL EXAMINATION AT REST
Observation
Observation of horses with respiratory disease should include:
* evaluation of general condition
* respiratory rate and pattern—normal respiratory rate in adult horses at rest in a quiet environment is 10 to 40 breaths/min; inspiratory and expiratory times are equal
  * Tachypnea may be the result of respiratory disease, anxiety, or pain.
  * Dyspnea on inspiration usually is indicative of upper airway disease; dyspnea on expiration typically is a result of lower airway or pulmonary disease.

Physical Examination
Physical examination of a horse with respiratory disease should start at the head.
* Any discharge around the nares and eyes is noted.
* The amount of air exiting the nares is evaluated, as is the muscular tone of the nares.
* The paranasal sinuses are percussed.
* The mandibular and retropharyngeal lymph nodes are palpated.
* The larynx is palpated for atrophy of the intrinsic muscles.
* A thorough oral examination is advisable—sinus disease can be caused by problems with the roots of the upper cheek teeth.
* The cervical trachea and jugular furrows are palpated.

AUSCULTATION AND PERCUSSION
Auscultation
Following are some practical guidelines for auscultation:
* The caudoventral border of the auscultable lung field is delineated by a curved line from the seventeenth intercostal space at the level of the tuber coxae, the eleventh intercostal space at the level of the point of the shoulder, and the point of the elbow.
* In normal horses, breath sounds can be accentuated with exercise or a rebreathing bag.
* *Abnormal lung sounds are not pathognomonic for any disease.*

◆ Crackles (short, nonmusical, sharp sounds) are uncommon in adult horses but may be heard with pulmonary edema, atelectasis, diffuse fibrosis, and interstitial pneumonia.
  • They are most commonly heard in foals with bacterial pneumonia.
◆ Wheezes (musical, high-pitched sounds) are heard with obstructive lung diseases, including bronchopneumonia and chronic obstructive pulmonary disease.
◆ Tracheal sounds reflect the sounds generated in central airways without attenuation by pulmonary parenchyma; thus they provide information about the lung parenchyma.

Thoracic Percussion

Percussion is accomplished using either a rubber hammer (plexor) and a flat instrument (pleximeter) or the first two fingers of one hand as the plexor and one finger of the other hand, firmly pressed between two ribs, as the pleximeter. The technique allows delineation of aerated lung and detection of large space-occupying lesions, such as abscesses and pleural fluid.

EXAMINATION AFTER EXERCISE

Evaluation is not complete without examination during or after exercise, although horses in respiratory distress should not be made to exercise. This examination allows assessment of:

◆ exercise tolerance.
◆ respiratory noise production
◆ respiratory pattern during exercise
  • *Fixed* upper airway obstructions (e.g., pharyngeal cysts) cause dyspnea during inhalation and exhalation; *dynamic* obstructions (e.g. laryngeal hemiplegia) primarily cause inspiratory dyspnea.
◆ rate of recovery following exercise

EVALUATING FOALS FOR RESPIRATORY DISEASE

History

The history may indicate that the respiratory system is compromised.

◆ Premature birth or induced parturition can produce a foal with immature lungs.

◆ The lungs of foals delivered by cesarean section are likely to contain more fluid than normal.
◆ Premature placental separation or rapid expulsion after delivery may cause prenatal asphyxia.
◆ Meconium aspiration should be suspected if the foal has yellow staining.
◆ Prenatal colostrum leakage can predispose the foal to septicemia or bacterial pneumonia.

Physical Examination

Clinical signs of respiratory problems in newborn foals can be subtle.

◆ The normal respiratory rate is about 70 breaths/min at birth and about 40 breaths/min by 1 hour postpartum.
  • Tachypnea can be caused by hypoxia, hypercapnia, fever, or metabolic acidosis.
◆ Paradoxical medial movement of the rib cage with expansion of the abdomen on inspiration is a sign of severe respiratory disease.
◆ Auscultation is important but does not correlate well with the severity of pulmonary disease.
  • For the first 15 minutes of life, soft wheezes and crackles may be auscultated in normal foals.
  • Crackles and wheezes may also be heard in the dependent lung in a foal that has been in lateral recumbency.
◆ The foal's mucous membranes should be carefully examined.
  • Blue-tinged membranes indicate cyanosis and severe arterial hypoxemia (PaO_2 <40 torr); a cardiovascular examination should be performed to rule out congenital heart defects.

ANCILLARY DIAGNOSTIC AIDS

Endoscopy

Endoscopy allows identification of the source of nasal discharge and, in many instances, the source of respiratory noise. Ideally, endoscopy is performed before and after exercise. If possible, horses should not be tranquilized before evaluation. A thorough and systematic examination from nasal passages to distal trachea should be performed every time.

Evaluating laryngeal function

The arytenoid cartilages are assessed for symmetry and degree of abduction and adduction.

* Laryngeal function is observed at rest, after nostril occlusion for 20 to 40 seconds, and during induced swallow.
* Examination may be repeated following exercise, when the laryngeal muscles are fatigued.

Movement of the left arytenoid cartilage may be graded on a scale from 1 to 4.

Grade 1: normal. Arytenoid movements are symmetric, and abduction and adduction of the left and right cartilages are synchronous.

Grade 2: There is some asynchronous movement of the left arytenoid cartilage; however, full abduction can be maintained during swallowing and nasal occlusion.

Grade 3: Asynchronous movement of the left arytenoid cartilage is present, and full abduction cannot be induced or maintained during swallowing or nasal occlusion.

Grade 4: There is no substantial movement of the left arytenoid cartilage during any phase of respiration.

Laryngeal function can be further evaluated via endoscopy during treadmill exercise (see discussion of laryngeal hemiplegia).

Radiography and Ultrasonography

Radiography

* The head and neck can be radiographed with portable equipment, allowing evaluation of the nasal passages, paranasal sinuses, guttural pouches, pharynx, larynx, and trachea.
* In foals, radiographic evaluation of the thorax also is possible under field conditions.

Ultrasonography

* Ultrasonography is useful for evaluating the pleural space, revealing even small amounts of fluid and fibrinous material.
* Lung abscesses or areas of consolidation adjacent to the visceral pleura may also be detected.

Collection of Airway Secretions

Transtracheal aspiration

Transtracheal aspiration is useful for bacteriologic and cytologic evaluation of the lower airways. The technique is performed as follows:

1. A 5-cm^2 area is clipped on the ventral midline of the midcervical region (where the trachea is easily palpable) and aseptically prepared.
2. Local anesthetic is infiltrated subcutaneously, and a stab incision is made through the skin.
3. A 12-gauge trocar is inserted between adjacent tracheal rings; a catheter inserted through the cannula is directed down the trachea, and 50 mL of saline is injected into the catheter and immediately aspirated.
4. The aspirate is submitted for bacteriologic culture and cytologic evaluation.

Results of bacterial culture must be interpreted with caution as the equine trachea normally contains microorganisms reflective of those in the horse's environment:

* <10 colony-forming units likely reflects environmental contamination.
* ≥100 colony-forming units probably is clinically significant.
* Regardless, bacterial cultures must always be interpreted in light of other clinical data.

Bronchoalveolar lavage

Cell counts obtained by bronchoalveolar lavage (BAL) correspond well with histopathologic evaluation of the lung. The procedure is performed as follows:

1. The horse is tranquilized, and a 180-cm long endoscope or BAL tube is passed via the nostril into the trachea.
2. The instrument is gently wedged in a bronchus, and 3 × 100-mL aliquots of saline at body temperature are infused and gently aspirated.
3. A differential count of 500 cells is performed using a Wright's-Giemsa–stained preparation (see Table 9-1).

Thoracocentesis

Thoracocentesis is indicated when pleural disease is suspected. Pleural

Table 9-1
Total white blood cell counts and differential counts in bronchoalveolar lavage fluid of normal horses

	>Mean	Range
Neutrophils	8.9% ± 1.2%	1%-17%
Macrophages	45% ± 2.8%	28%-63%
Lymphocytes	43% ± 2.7%	25%-61%
Eosinophils	≤1.0%	<1.0%
Mast cells	1.2% ± 0.3%	0%-3.2%
Epithelial cells	3.5% ± 0.7%	0%-8%
Total WBC/L ($\times 10^6$)	182 ± 35	0-390
Volume recovered (mL)	150 ± 24	50-250

disease commonly is bilateral, so both sides of the thorax should be tapped.

* In the *right* hemithorax, thoracocentesis may be performed level with the point of the elbow, in the seventh intercostal space.
* In the *left* hemithorax, thoracocentesis is performed 4 to 6 cm (1.5 to 2.25 inches) dorsal to the point of the elbow, in the eighth or ninth intercostal space.
* Alternatively, a site is chosen using ultrasonography.

The procedure is performed as follows:

1. The area is aseptically prepared; following desensitization of the skin and underlying musculature, a stab incision is made through the skin.
2. An 8-cm (3 inch) teat cannula or blunt catheter attached to a three-way stopcock is inserted into the thoracic cavity, along the cranial border of the rib; pleural fluid is aspirated with a syringe.
3. The site is covered with an antiseptic cream and bandaged.

Other Diagnostic Procedures

Following are some specialized procedures that may be available at referral practices or institutions:

* *arterial blood gas analysis:* This is a useful quantitative test of pulmonary function.
  * Blood from the facial, carotid, or greater metatarsal artery is collected into a heparinized syringe.
  * Blood gas tensions remain constant for several hours if air is expelled from the syringe immediately after collection, the syringe is sealed, and the sample is stored on ice.
  * The normal $PaCO_2$ is 40 to 45 torr; an increase suggests hypoventilation.
  * At sea level, the normal PaO_2 is >85 torr (lower at higher elevations); in the absence of cardiovascular shunts or hypoventilation, a decrease indicates pulmonary disease.
* *percutaneous lung biopsy:* This procedure should be performed only if a diagnosis is essential in management of the case and when less invasive methods of evaluation have failed.
* *upper airway function tests:* Tests such as generation of flow-volume loops in exercising horses allow grading of the severity of lesions and evaluation of treatment efficacy.
* *pulmonary function tests:* These tests assess the mechanical properties of the lung, lung volume, and gas exchange; most are not useful in detecting subclinical lung disease.

DIAGNOSTIC TESTS FOR NEONATAL FOALS

An accurate assessment of a foal's respiratory system can be made using the following tools:

* *thoracic radiography:* Foals >4 hours old should have aerated caudodorsal lung fields; a thymic shadow may be seen cranioventral to the heart;

circular 0.5- to 2-cm (0.20 to 0.75 inch) lucencies are inconsequential.

♦ *ultrasonography:* A 7.5- or 5.0-MHz probe is used to image the heart and lungs.

♦ *arterial blood gases:* Values in normal foals depend on the position (lateral recumbency lowers the PaO_2) and excitement of the patient.

• PaO_2 in normal term foals ranges from 60 to 100 torr; $PaCO_2$ is 31 to 55 torr.

• Average values at 4 hours of age are PaO_2 of 80 torr and $PaCO_2$ of 45 torr.

• Respiratory distress syndrome is characterized by PaO_2 <60 torr and $PaCO_2$ >55 torr.

♦ *bacterial culture:* This is particularly important in septic foals with bacterial pneumonia.

• A sample could be obtained by transtracheal aspiration or BAL.

• In septicemic foals, blood cultures sometimes are helpful and are less stressful to obtain.

Respiratory Therapy

(pages 458-463)
Frederick J. Derksen, Clifford M. Honnas, and Mary Rose Paradis

PRINCIPLES OF EMERGENCY RESPIRATORY THERAPY
Oxygen Therapy

Oxygen therapy is effective only when tissue hypoxia is the result of pulmonary disease; it is not effective for hypoxia caused by upper airway obstruction, anemia, or decreased cardiac output (e.g., shock).

Practical considerations

♦ In the field, compressed oxygen may be delivered via a tube placed in the horse's nose; if the patient is recumbent, the trachea should be intubated.

♦ In an adult horse, the oxygen flow rate should be at least 10 L/min.

Temporary Tracheostomy

Emergency tracheostomy is performed to relieve severe dyspnea caused by an upper airway obstruction.

Technique

Tracheostomy can be performed in either standing or recumbent horses. The optimal site is the midcervical ventral midline, where the sternocephalic muscles diverge and the trachea is readily palpable.

1. The site is surgically prepared, and the skin and deeper tissues infiltrated with local anesthetic.

2. A 4- to 6-cm (1.50 to 2.25 inch) longitudinal incision is made on the midline, through the skin and subcutis; the sternothyrohyoideus muscle is separated to expose the trachea.

3. The annular ligament between adjacent tracheal rings is incised *transversely,* being careful to avoid the jugular veins and esophagus.

4. A tracheostomy tube is inserted into the tracheal lumen and secured in place.

Management of the tracheostomy site

♦ The site is inspected frequently to ascertain that the tube is patent and in place.

♦ The tracheostomy tube should be changed and the surgical site cleaned at least once daily.

♦ Once the airway rostral to the tracheostomy is patent, the tube should be removed and the wound allowed to heal by second intention (usually takes 14 to 21 days).

MEDICAL RESPIRATORY THERAPY
Bronchodilator Therapy

Sympathomimetic agents

Sympathomimetic drugs with specific affinity for β_2-receptors are the most common bronchodilators used in horses. Several of these drugs are effective when given via aerosol. Regardless of the route, large doses can cause trembling, excitement, sweating, ileus, colic, and tachycardia.

♦ *ephedrine:* The empiric dose is 0.14 mg/kg q12h IM.

• Drug tolerance develops after a few days, so progressively more drug is needed to maintain bronchodilation.

♦ *clenbuterol:* a specific β_2-receptor agonist and expectorant

• It is well absorbed orally, and twice-daily administration main-

tains blood levels in the therapeutic range.
- The recommended dose of 0.8
  µg/kg has little effect on the GI
  tract or heart.
- Progressively increasing dosages
  up to 3.2 µg/kg may be necessary
  to maintain a good response.
- Currently, clenbuterol is not
  available in the United States.
- *fenoterol:* A dose of 2 to 4 µg/kg via
  nebulization effectively provides
  bronchodilation in horses with recurrent airway obstruction.
- *pirbuterol and albuterol:* Inhaled
  doses of 1 to 2 µg/kg cause bronchodilation for 1 hour.

Anticholinergic drugs
- *atropine:* An effective bronchodilator, but its side effects of
  ileus, tachycardia, mydriasis, and
  excitation preclude its routine use
  as a bronchodilator in horses.
- *ipratropium bromide:* When administered via ultrasonic nebulizer at a
  dose of 2 to 3 µg/kg, it causes significant bronchodilation that lasts 4 to 6
  hours, with minimal systemic effects.

Phosphodiesterase inhibitors
Theophylline (aminophylline) is the
most commonly used bronchodilator
in this group:
- It is an effective bronchodilator
  when blood concentrations reach
  about 10 µg/mL; however, excitement occurs at 15 µg/mL.
- Absorption is erratic after oral administration, making the drug difficult to use clinically.

Hypoxemia
Hypoxemia is a common complication
of bronchodilator therapy, and apparently is due to ventilation-perfusion
mismatching. Especially in patients
with PaO_2 <64 torr (e.g., foals with
pneumonia), bronchodilators may decrease PaO_2 to critically low levels. In
these cases, oxygen therapy is indicated
in conjunction with bronchodilators.

Mast Cell Stabilizing Drugs
Sodium cromoglycate at a dosage of
80 to 200 mg q24h delivered via
aerosol can be effective in treating
small airway disease. In one study, clinical signs of recurrent airway obstruction were prevented for 24 days, after
only four consecutive daily treatments.

Corticosteroid Therapy
When delivered by aerosol, systemic
effects of corticosteroids can be
avoided. Aerosol administration of
beclomethasone using an Aeromask
at a dose of 3.75 mg/horse q12h for
2 weeks improves pulmonary function in horses with recurrent airway
obstruction.

PRINCIPLES OF THERAPY FOR FOALS
A foal in respiratory failure with a
persistent PaO_2 <50 torr and $PaCO_2$
>60 torr may require mechanical
ventilation for survival. A hypoxemic
foal with a normal $PaCO_2$ may need
only supplemental oxygen via nasal
insufflation.

Ventilatory Support
Mechanical ventilation
Mechanical ventilation of a foal is extremely labor intensive and often is
limited to intensive-care facilities.
However, short-term ventilation may
be required when transporting an affected foal to an intensive-care facility:
- A nasotracheal tube is placed (in
  most foals, a large-dog size endotracheal tube suffices).
- Assisted ventilation is accomplished by manual compression of
  a self-inflating 1-L resuscitation bag
  or by use of a demand valve attached to an oxygen source.

Oxygen supplementation
Supplemental oxygen can be delivered in various ways:
- face mask
- intranasal tube: A small feeding
  tube is placed into the nasal passage and sutured to the nostril.
- transtracheal catheter: A large-gauge
  silastic catheter is inserted between
  the tracheal rings in the midcervical
  region.
  Oxygen initially is delivered at 5 to
  10 L/min. Oxygen delivered in this
  manner should be humidified by
  bubbling it through a canister of
  sterile saline.

Nursing Care
General nursing care is very important in neonatal foals with respiratory
problems.

- The foal should be kept warm (but not overheated) with radiant heat lamps, hot water blankets, and heating pads.
- Adequate hydration and nutrition are essential.
  - Care must be taken not to overhydrate a foal that is already at risk of developing pulmonary edema.
  - Severe dyspnea can increase the foal's caloric needs 150% to 200%.
- Coupage (rapidly slapping the foal's chest with a cupped hand) gently loosens tenacious bronchial secretions.

Respiratory Diseases Affecting Multiple Sites

(pages 463-480)
Corrie Brown

INFLAMMATORY, INFECTIOUS, AND IMMUNE DISEASES
African Horse Sickness

African horse sickness is an acute/subacute systemic viral disease of equidae that currently is limited to Africa.

- Horses are most susceptible, with mortality rates approaching 100%.
- The virus causes loss of vascular integrity, so petechiation (diagnostic when found on the underside of the tongue), scleral injection, and conjunctival edema are common, together with signs of pulmonary edema ± hydropericardium; fever is a consistent feature.
- Diagnosis is difficult; the most reliable method is virus isolation from heparinized blood or a piece of spleen; testing is performed at the Foreign Animal Disease Diagnostic Laboratory, Plum Island, N.Y.

Equine Influenza
Tim Mair

Equine influenza is an acute, highly contagious, febrile respiratory disease that spreads rapidly in groups of susceptible horses.

- Infected horses shed virus during the incubation period (1 to 3 days) and for at least 5 days after clinical signs begin.
- Horses of all ages are susceptible, but young horses (<4 years of age), racehorses, and show horses are most at risk.

Clinical signs

- Onset typically is sudden, with development of a harsh, dry, nonproductive cough.
- Fever (39° to 42° C [100.5° to 107.5° F]), which may be biphasic, develops early and persists up to 5 days (longer if secondary bacterial infection develops).
- Affected horses are depressed and inappetent during the febrile stage.
- Submandibular and retropharyngeal lymph nodes frequently are tender and occasionally are enlarged.
- Serous nasal discharge develops initially; secondary bacterial infection often results in a mucopurulent discharge.
- Other common signs include tachypnea, tachycardia, epiphora, limb edema, muscle soreness, and stiffness.
- In partially immune, vaccinated, or recovered horses, signs often are mild or subclinical; in vaccinated racehorses, the predominant sign often is exercise intolerance.

Diagnosis

Diagnosis often is based on clinical signs, epidemiologic features, and hematologic examination (mild-to-moderate anemia, leukopenia, and lymphopenia, and later, monocytosis). Confirmation requires virus isolation, serology, or immunologic detection of the virus.

- ***Virus isolation*** may be attempted from nasal or nasopharyngeal swabs or tracheal aspirates, taken early in the course of infection.
- ***Serology*** should be performed during the early stages of disease and 2 to 3 weeks later.
  - Infection is indicated by a fourfold or greater increase in titer.
  - Some vaccinated or partially immune horses become infected and shed virus without showing an antibody rise of this magnitude.
- ***Rapid immunologic tests*** to detect virus antigens use either ELISA or fluorescent antibody.

- The laboratory-based ELISA has greater sensitivity for nasopharyngeal samples with low antigenic content than does the "field" assay.
- Immunofluorescent staining of nasal scrapings or tracheal wash fluid is a highly sensitive technique that gives results within 24 hours.

Treatment

Treatment is largely symptomatic.

- complete rest for 3 to 4 weeks in a clean, well-ventilated stable with minimum-dust management
  - A useful guide is to allow 1 week of rest for each day that the horse was febrile.
- general nursing care and good nutrition
- antibiotic therapy if secondary bacterial infection has developed
- NSAIDs for horses with high fever, inappetence, or stiffness

The typical clinical course and possible complications are outlined below:

- In uncomplicated cases, improvement is seen within 1 to 6 days, and complete clinical recovery occurs in 2 to 3 weeks.
  - In severe cases a recovery period of 3 to 4 months may be necessary before the horse is fit to resume training.
- Impairment of normal mucociliary clearance persists for about 4 weeks and predisposes to secondary bacterial infection; airway hyperreactivity (e.g., COPD) is a possible sequela.
  - In severely affected adults and in young foals with poor maternal immunity, secondary bacterial infection may result in bronchopneumonia.
- Guttural pouch empyema and sinusitis occasionally develop as longer-term complications.
- Myocarditis and cardiac arrhythmias may occur in very young and very old animals and in horses that are not rested during the acute phase.

Control of an outbreak

Following are some practical guidelines for control of disease during an outbreak:

- Immediately isolate all horses showing clinical signs; quarantine sick animals for 3 to 4 weeks.
- Quarantine exposed premises for at least 4 weeks after the last case.
- Limit movement of personnel assigned to sick animals, and use separate cleaning and grooming equipment for sick animals.
- Clean all exposed stalls, equipment, and transport vehicles with a virucidal product.
- Vaccinate all unaffected animals that have been previously vaccinated.

Prevention

Routine vaccination is the basis for prevention of equine influenza.

- Initially, two vaccinations are given 8 to 12 weeks apart, followed by a third 6 months later.
  - Revaccination is recommended every 6 months, except in situations in which there is massive virus challenge, in which case horses should be revaccinated every 3 to 4 months.
  - Vaccination may begin at any age, but foals <5 months of age respond poorly.
  - New horses should be isolated for 2 to 3 weeks and vaccinated (unless immunized within the previous 2 to 3 months) before introduction to the group.
- A transient reaction (fever, depression, edema, injection site pain, coughing, nasal discharge) occurs postvaccination in some horses.
- Inactivated subunit vaccines containing HA and NA antigens incorporated into an immune-stimulating complex (ISCOM) provide the most effective and long-lasting protection.

Equine Herpesvirus 1 and Equine Herpesvirus 4

Equine herpesvirus 1 (EHV-1) and EHV-4 are ubiquitous viruses.

- EHV-1 is associated with respiratory disease, abortion, and neurologic disease.
- EHV-4 is primarily associated with respiratory disease.
- Respiratory disease caused by EHV-1 or EHV-4 occurs enzootically among young horses on breeding farms and at assembling points (e.g., sales, training facilities).

- Outbreaks are common in the fall and usually involve EHV-4.
- Immunity following infection is short-lived, but subsequent infections usually are mild or subclinical.
- Both viruses can establish latent infections that may be reactivated by a variety of stimuli.

Clinical signs

Respiratory diseases associated with EHV-1 and EHV-4 are clinically indistinguishable.

- The incubation period is 2 to 10 days.
- Signs are more severe in young horses; infection frequently is subclinical in older horses.
- Fever (39.0° to 41.5° C [102° to 106° F]) may be biphasic and lasts 4 to 5 days.
- Serous nasal discharge later becomes mucoid and then mucopurulent; coughing, if present, usually is mild.
- Foals <4 months of age usually are only mildly affected, provided they have normal levels of passive (colostral) immunity.
  - Foals with failure of passive transfer may develop fulminating pneumonitis.

Diagnosis

- Clinical diagnosis is difficult because the overlap of signs associated with EHV infections and those of other infections, such as equine influenza and equine viral arteritis.
- Infection in young horses and foals may be confirmed by virus isolation and serology.
  - Virus isolation can be performed on nasopharyngeal swabs or whole blood (citrated or heparinized).
  - There is a serologic test that allows distinction between EHV-1 and EHV-4 infections.
- Confirmation of infection in older horses may be difficult because latent infections are common, and prior exposure or vaccination lead to high levels of serum antibody.

Treatment

Treatment is symptomatic, as described for influenza. Rest and a gradual return to work are most important.

Control of an outbreak

The major sources of viral contamination are nasal discharges and aerosolized respiratory secretions and the surfaces they contact.

- Horses exhibiting respiratory signs should be kept in isolation until 2 to 3 weeks after infection.
- Contaminated stable equipment and clothing should be disinfected.
- Booster vaccinations may protect previously vaccinated horses not yet exposed.

Prevention

- Several EHV-1 and EHV-4 vaccines are available.
  - Their efficacy is limited by the short duration of immunity and by virus latency.
  - Nevertheless, vaccination limits the severity of EHV-associated respiratory disease.
- Primary vaccination consists of two doses, 2 to 3 weeks apart.
  - Boosters are repeated at intervals from 3 months to 1 year, depending on the product.
- Segregation of horses on a farm into age groups is helpful in limiting an outbreak.
- New horses should be isolated for 3 weeks, with daily monitoring of rectal temperature.
- EHV-1 and EHV-4 are readily destroyed by heat and disinfectants.
  - Stables and transport vehicles should be steam-cleaned and disinfected regularly.

Viral pneumonia in neonates

In utero infection with EHV-1 during the last trimester can cause viral pneumonia in neonatal foals.

- Most of these foals are normal at birth but develop respiratory distress, reddened mucous membranes, and intractable diarrhea during the first week of life.
- Absolute lymphopenia and neutrophilic leukocytosis develop during the course of disease.
- Currently, there is no specific treatment; supportive care with IV fluids, warmth, and nutrition is necessary for survival.
- The prognosis is grave.

Equine Herpesvirus 2

Conditions attributed to equine herpesvirus 2 (EHV-2) include pharyngitis, conjunctivitis, pneumonia, and lower airway infection, mostly in foals and racehorses.

Equine Viral Arteritis

Equine viral arteritis (EVA) is a contagious viral disease caused by the equine arteritis virus (EAV).

◆ Serologic evidence of infection is much higher in Standardbreds (70% to 90%) than in other breeds (2% to 3%).

◆ Outbreaks often are associated with the movement of horses, and widespread dissemination can occur at racetracks and breeding farms.

◆ The two most important routes of transmission are respiratory and venereal.

  • Aerosol transmission is the primary route of dissemination at racetracks.

  • Carrier stallions are a major reservoir of EAV in the horse population.

◆ Transplacental transmission of EAV in late pregnant mares can cause congenital infection.

  • Infected foals develop rapidly progressive, fulminating interstitial pneumonia and fibronecrotic enteritis.

◆ Except in young foals, mortality is very low.

Clinical signs

Many cases of EVA in adults are subclinical. Clinical disease usually is most severe in very young or very old horses and in horses debilitated for other reasons. Clinical signs of symptomatic infection are variable.

◆ The incubation period varies from 3 to 14 days.

◆ Signs range from mild pyrexia to severe disease with abortion.

◆ Typical cases present with pyrexia (up to 41° C [105.8° F]), depression, inappetence, ocular and nasal discharge, conjunctivitis, rhinitis, stiff gait, limb edema (especially the hind limbs), periorbital edema, midventral edema (including the scrotum and prepuce or the mammary glands), urticaria, and edematous plaques (especially on the sides of the neck and face).

◆ Less common signs include dyspnea, coughing, diarrhea, ataxia, photophobia, and corneal opacity.

Diagnosis

Definitive diagnosis cannot be made on the basis of clinical features because signs are variable and subclinical infections are common. Diseases that may mimic EVA include infection with EHV-1 and EHV-4, equine influenza, and EIA; African horse sickness; purpura hemorrhagica; and urticaria.

Confirmation of EAV infection in adult horses can be achieved by:

◆ **virus isolation:** Nasopharyngeal or conjunctival swabs, semen, urine, and blood (heparinized or in EDTA) are suitable specimens.

  • In young foals that die from suspected EVA, lymphoid tissue of the respiratory and alimentary tracts should be submitted for histopathology.

◆ **serologic diagnosis:** A rise in serum antibody titer of fourfold or greater is diagnostic.

  • Paired blood samples are taken 14 to 28 days apart.

Treatment

Treatment of EVA is symptomatic.

◆ Most infected horses make full, spontaneous recoveries, and treatment often is unnecessary.

◆ Stallions that become pyrexic and develop extensive scrotal edema should be rested and treated with NSAIDs and diuretics.

◆ Antibiotics may be indicated in horses with evidence of secondary bacterial involvement.

There is no effective way of eliminating the carrier state in stallions, other than surgical castration.

Control of an outbreak

◆ Movement of horses onto and off the premises should stop immediately, pending the results of virologic tests.

◆ Clinical cases and in-contact horses should be isolated and appropriate samples taken for virus isolation and serologic testing.

◆ It is particularly important to isolate healthy seronegative stallions from all other horses.

◆ All horses on the premises, including those that are apparently healthy, should be screened serologically.

  • Repeated serologic testing is carried out every 14 days until the outbreak is over.

  • Seropositive horses should be isolated for at least 1 month.

Prevention

- Imported horses and semen, especially when originating from countries where EVA is endemic, should be tested for EAV before leaving the country of origin.
  - The horse or semen should be verified EAV-negative before being used in a breeding program.
- Breeding stock should be segregated from racehorses and other performance horses.
- A modified live vaccine (ARVAC) is safe and effective in stallions and nonpregnant mares.
  - It is not recommended for use in pregnant mares, especially during the last 2 months of gestation, or in foals <6 weeks of age.
  - Vaccination protects against EVA for 1 to 3 years, but does not prevent virus infection, multiplication, or shedding; it does reduce the duration and amount of virus shedding via the nasopharynx.

Equine Adenovirus

Adenovirus infection generally is not a significant clinical problem in adult horses, although it can cause mild, self-limiting upper respiratory tract disease, ocular discharge, and soft feces in Thoroughbred racehorses. Adenovirus infection is an important cause of respiratory disease in immunodeficient foals, especially those with combined immunodeficiency syndrome (CID; see Chapter 19, Hemolymphatic System).
In these foals adenovirus infection predisposes to fulminant bacterial pneumonia.

Diagnostic tests for adenovirus:
- identification of viral inclusion bodies in conjunctival smears
- virus isolation from nasal swabs
- electron microscopy and immunofluorescence of nasal or conjunctival smears
- serology

Equine Picornaviruses

Up to 80% of horses >5 years old have serum antibodies against equine picornaviruses (equine rhinovirus 1, 2, and 3). In these horses, infection is subclinical, although it may be associated with loss of performance. Rhi-

novirus infections become clinically apparent only when the horse is stressed by other factors, such as concurrent infection with EHV-4, transport, and race training. Infection can cause fever, inappetence, and nasal discharge. Diagnosis is based on serology; the virus may also be isolated from nasal or nasopharyngeal swabs.

Diseases of the Nasal Cavity and Paranasal Sinuses *(pages 480-490)*
John P. Caron

DIAGNOSTIC AND THERAPEUTIC CONSIDERATIONS

Diagnostic Aids

The following diagnostic tools may be used in clinical practice:

- *endoscopy:* A standard (11-mm) colonoscope is used to examine the nasal cavity, although a pediatric (6-mm) bronchoscope is needed to examine the turbinates and middle nasal meatus (for drainage from the nasomaxillary opening).
- *radiography:* High-speed film and rare-earth screens are recommended.
  - Structures usually evaluated include the nasal septum, facial skeleton, tooth roots, nasal conchae, and paranasal sinuses.
- *percutaneous sinus centesis (Kral tap):* This can be performed in the standing horse using local anesthesia ± sedation and a sterile Steinmann pin.
  - A sample of the contents is obtained for culture and cytology.
- *surgical exploration:* Exploration can be performed via a trephined opening or facial bone flap.
  - Facial flaps provide superior exposure and postoperative cosmesis.
  - The sinus can also be examined with a 4-mm arthroscope.

Surgery of the Nasal Septum and Nasal Turbinates

Surgery is indicated whenever a lesion in the nasal cavity causes primary respiratory obstruction or is known to be progressive or invasive. Resection of the nasal septum is described in *Equine Medicine and Surgery V.* Hemorrhage is profuse, so compatible whole blood should be available before surgery. A temporary tracheostomy is necessary.

CONGENITAL AND FAMILIAL DISEASES

Choanal Atresia and Other Developmental Abnormalities

Congenital lesions of the nasal cavity are uncommon and include:

- choanal atresia (failure of perforation of the bucconasal membrane at the caudal extent of the nasal cavity), either unilateral or bilateral
- congenital thickening or deviation of the nasal septum as a result of cystic degeneration
- congenital overgrowth of normal tissues of the nasal septum (hamartoma)
- longitudinal deviation of the nasal septum ± lateral nasomaxillary deviation ("wry nose")

DISEASES WITH PHYSICAL CAUSES

Redundant Alar Folds

Flaccid or redundant alar folds may cause partial upper airway obstruction.

- "False nostril noise" is a biphasic fluttering noise that is most pronounced on expiration.
- To confirm that the alar folds are the source of the abnormal respiratory noise, a mattress suture is placed through the alar folds and over the bridge of the nose before exercise.
  - In horses with redundant alar folds, this procedure eliminates the respiratory noise.
- Redundant alar folds seldom impair exercise capacity, so other causes of reduced performance should be investigated before concluding that the alar folds are a problem.
- Treatment consists of bilateral resection (see text).

INFLAMMATORY, INFECTIOUS, AND IMMUNE DISEASES

Bacterial Rhinitis

Bacterial infections of the nasal cavity are uncommon. Staphylococcal granulomas occasionally are found on the nasal turbinates or septum. These lesions may be secondary to mucosal trauma.

Bacterial Sinusitis (Empyema)

Bacterial infection of the paranasal sinuses most often involves the maxillary sinus.

- Sinusitis often is secondary to dental disease, such as patent infundibulum, tooth fracture, and periodontal disease, most commonly involving the fourth cheek tooth (first molar).
- It also may develop secondary to strangles or equine influenza.

Clinical signs

Signs include:

- unilateral nasal discharge, most often mucopurulent
- dullness or pain on percussion of the affected sinus
- facial deformity and, occasionally, ocular discharge and mandibular lymphadenopathy

Diagnosis

A thorough oral examination is worthwhile.

- ***endoscopy:*** Purulent exudate is seen draining from the nasomaxillary opening (unless the nasomaxillary duct or foramen is occluded by debris).
- ***radiography:*** Findings include fluid lines and, when dental disease is present, loss of the normal radiodense "halo" (lamina dura) surrounding the tooth root and loss of crown detail.
- ***percutaneous sinus centesis:*** A sample should be submitted for culture and sensitivity.

Treatment

- With primary dental problems, the offending tooth is removed via facial bone flap and tooth repulsion.
- *Drainage is essential for resolution.*
  - It often is accomplished by removal of the diseased tooth.
  - In other cases it is necessary to surgically create a rostral nasomaxillary opening.
- *Lavage* is indicated, either as the primary treatment or as an adjunct to surgery.
  - The sinus is irrigated with sterile saline via an indwelling catheter once or twice daily until the solu-

tion no longer dislodges a significant quantity of debris.

- *Antimicrobial therapy* is based on sensitivity results.
  - With adequate drainage, the antimicrobial course can be relatively short, especially in acute sinusitis.
  - In more chronic cases, a 3- to 4-week regimen (or longer) may be required.

Prognosis

Sinusitis secondary to upper respiratory infection and without bone involvement generally has a good prognosis for complete resolution.

Chronic empyema with bone involvement and facial deformity has a much less favorable prognosis.

Fungal Rhinitis and Sinusitis

Mycoses can produce granulomatous lesions that reach a size sufficient to cause partial airway obstruction. Treatment involves removal of the abnormal tissue.

Cryptococcosis

- Cryptococcal infections of the upper respiratory tract generally are found only in immunosuppressed patients.
- The causative organism (*Cryptococcus neoformans*) is quite invasive, and infection often results in the formation of draining tracts through the facial bones.
- Diagnosis is made by cytologic examination of smears; the organism also is easily cultured.
- Cryptococcosis is of some public health significance, and it is recommended that infected horses be destroyed.

Rhinosporidiosis

- *Rhinosporidium seeberi* causes granuloma formation near the mucocutaneous junction of the nares, more often on ventral portions of the nasal cavity and septum.
- The organism is difficult to culture, so diagnosis requires biopsy.
- Treatment is by surgical removal, although masses frequently recur.

Coccidioidomycosis

- *Coccidioides immitis* causes both localized and generalized disease. Coccidioidomycosis occurs in semiarid climates but has been seen as far north as Canada.

- Diagnosis is based on demonstration of characteristic "spherules" on biopsy.
- If the granuloma is accessible, treatment is by excision.
- Itraconazole may be useful in the treatment of this condition.

Phycomycosis

Phycomycosis is infection caused by *Pythium insidiosum* (*Pythium* spp.) or *Entomophthora coronata* (*Conidiobolus coronatus*).

- Disease is most common in, but not restricted to, coastal lowland areas.
- It is characterized by a purulent nasal discharge and areas of exuberant granulation tissue that frequently contain cores of necrotic material ("leeches" or "kunkers").
  - Lesions are pruritic and often are traumatized.
- A favorable prognosis is expected with early surgical removal.
- Ancillary treatment involves amphotericin B (100 mg in 250 mL of DMSO) applied topically twice daily for 8 weeks.

Aspergillosis

- *Aspergillus* spp. cause fungal plaques in the nasal passages.
- Affected animals have a slight purulent nasal discharge ± intermittent epistaxis.
- Plaques are observed endoscopically, but definitive diagnosis is by microscopic examination of exudate or biopsy specimens.
- The condition has been successfully treated with daily topical natamycin (25 mg in 100 mL sterile water) and with oral itraconazole.

NEOPLASIA

Nasal and Paranasal Neoplasms

Neoplastic conditions of the nasal septum and turbinates are rare. The most common neoplasms are squamous cell carcinoma and fibroma; osteomas may originate in the paranasal sinuses. About 70% of these tumors are malignant. Onset of signs is insidious, so many tumors are not detected until they are advanced. Thus the prognosis often is poor.

IDIOPATHIC DISEASES
Nasal Amyloidosis
Amyloid deposits in the nasal cavity may accompany the cutaneous form of the disease or be restricted to the rostral nasal cavity.

+ Deposits frequently are localized but may become extensive and involve the entire nasal cavity, nasopharynx, guttural pouches, and larynx.
+ The disease is diagnosed by special staining of biopsy specimens.
+ Treatment includes excision of accessible focal lesions and, if possible, removal of the primary cause (e.g., chronic suppurative disease, hyperimmunization).
+ Reports of successful treatment are rare.

Atheroma (Epidermal Inclusion Cyst)
An atheroma is a fluid-filled, cystlike structure at the caudal aspect of the nasal diverticulum (false nostril).

+ These cysts are easily identified by palpation.
+ Rarely are they associated with impaired athletic performance, and they need not be treated.
+ For cosmetic reasons, the cyst may be resolved by drainage (lanced via the nasal diverticulum), obliteration with counterirritants (e.g., 2% tincture of iodine), or surgical removal (best for permanent resolution).

Nasal Septum Deformation
The nasal septum may be deformed congenitally or by trauma, infection, or neoplasia.

+ Airflow through one or both nostrils may be seriously restricted, although in most cases signs are subtle and evidenced only during strenuous exercise.
+ Diagnosis is made by palpating the rostral septum, endoscopically observing the deformity or narrowing of the ventral meatus, or dorsoventral radiography.
+ Treatment of deformations that restrict performance is by nasal septum resection.

Paranasal Sinus (Follicular) Cyst
Cystlike lesions in the maxillary sinus may be congenital, although signs often are not apparent until adulthood.

+ The hallmark is facial deformity; dyspnea may be observed with very large cysts.
+ Mucoid or purulent nasal discharge may also be seen.
+ Percutaneous sinus centesis yields thick, honeylike fluid.
+ Radiographs may show abnormalities of one or more tooth roots, in addition to a multiloculated cystic cavity within the maxillary sinus.
+ Treatment involves drainage and removal of the cyst via facial bone flap.
+ Prognosis is fair; persistent respiratory obstruction, chronic nasal discharge, and concomitant dental abnormalities may complicate recovery.

Ethmoid Hematoma
Ethmoid hematoma is a slowly progressive, expansive hematoma that develops under the respiratory mucosa of the caudal nasal cavity or paranasal sinuses.

+ The usual presenting complaint is scant, unilateral, sanguineous nasal discharge at rest.
+ The hematoma, which typically is greenish in color, can often be seen endoscopically in the ethmoid region.
+ Surgical removal carries a good prognosis, although recurrence occurs in about 40% of cases.
  · Early lesions can be removed transnasally with a snare.
  · Small lesions can be photovaporized using a transendoscopic Nd:YAG laser technique; this approach provides effective hemostasis and can result in permanent resolution.
  · More extensive lesions are treated by sharp or laser excision via a frontonasal bone flap.
+ A less invasive technique involves intralesional injection with 10 to 20 mL of 10% buffered formalin, under endoscopic guidance; repeated injection may be necessary.
+ Follow-up endoscopic examination is recommended, because recur-

rence can occur as long as 3 to 4 years after treatment.

Nasal Polyps

Nasal polyps are pedunculated inflammatory masses, attached to either the conchae or the nasal septum.

- Presenting signs include exercise intolerance and stertorous respiratory noise.
- Mild, intermittent epistaxis or mucopurulent nasal discharge may also be present.
- Treatment is by excision using a snare or using transendoscopic electrosurgery or Nd:YAG laser ablation.
- Histopathologic examination is advised following removal.

Diseases of the Pharynx

(pages 491-500)

Ryland B. Edwards

CONGENITAL AND FAMILIAL DISEASES

Pharyngeal Cysts

Pharyngeal cysts can be found in the subepiglottic region (most common), dorsal pharyngeal recess, pharyngeal walls, guttural pouches, and along the caudal border of the soft palate. The highest frequency of cases occurs in horses 2 years of age; 67% of affected horses are male. Pharyngeal cysts have been reported in foals as young as 3 months old.

Clinical signs and diagnosis

- Foals with pharyngeal cysts usually present with chronic cough, nasal discharge, and signs of aspiration pneumonia.
- Mature horses may present with exercise intolerance or poor performance, dysphagia, abnormal respiratory noise, and, less often, nasal discharge.
- Pharyngeal cysts are best diagnosed by endoscopic examination
  - Subepiglottic cysts may be accompanied by epiglottic entrapment (see p. 148).
- Radiography ± oral barium may be used to evaluate the extent of

subepiglottic cysts and those involving the soft palate.

Treatment and prognosis

- Complete removal of the cyst and its lining is necessary to prevent recurrence.
- Subepiglottic cysts may be approached orally (and removed with a snare or laser) or via laryngotomy or pharyngotomy; smaller cysts sometimes can be removed transnasally in standing, sedated horses.
- The prognosis is good with complete excision.

Palatoschisis (Cleft Palate)

Clinical signs and diagnosis

- In most affected foals, the condition is recognized soon after birth by the presence of milk exiting the nostrils after nursing.
  - Signs of aspiration pneumonia may also be present.
  - Occasionally, a cleft palate goes unnoticed until the horse is mature.
- A cleft hard palate may be diagnosed by oral examination using a light.
- Endoscopy allows complete examination and is required for cases in which only the soft palate is affected.

Treatment and prognosis

- Successful treatment requires surgical correction.
  - Mandibular symphysiotomy provides the best exposure for repair.
  - Surgery is not recommended in foals with a large defect in the hard palate.
- Preoperative examination should include thoracic radiographs; if aspiration pneumonia is present, transtracheal wash should be performed for culture and sensitivity.
- Potential complications include partial or complete dehiscence of the repair, osteomyelitis or nonunion of the mandibular symphysis, continued soft palate dysfunction, and persistent pneumonia.
- The prognosis for successful repair is good, unless there is a large defect affecting the hard palate; the prognosis for athletic function is guarded because of the potential for continued soft palate dysfunction.

DISEASES WITH PHYSICAL CAUSES
Foreign Bodies and Iatrogenic Trauma
Foreign bodies that may lodge in the pharynx include metallic objects, wood, and thorns. The most common causes of iatrogenic pharyngeal trauma are repeated nasogastric intubation and trauma to the soft palate during surgical correction of epiglottic entrapment.

Clinical signs and diagnosis
* Signs of a pharyngeal foreign body may include purulent or bloody nasal discharge, swelling or cellulitis in the throat latch region, dysphagia, and dyspnea.
* Signs of iatrogenic trauma can include ptyalism, nasal discharge (may be bloody with acute injuries), dysphagia, and reluctance to eat and/or drink.
* Diagnosis is made with endoscopy.
* Pain and contrast radiography may also be used to define the area of injury.
  * Emphysema within the tissue planes indicates mucosal rupture.

Treatment and prognosis
* The surgical approach for foreign body removal depends on the object's location.
* Mild iatrogenic trauma (edema and mucosal inflammation) may simply require treatment with NSAIDs and feeding of wet hay, pelleted feed, or gruel.
  * When cellulitis is present, broad-spectrum antibiotics should be added.
* Iatrogenic cleft soft palate is treated surgically.
* If pharyngeal trauma is severe, the horse may need to be fed through an esophagostomy tube.
* The prognosis depends on the degree of trauma, the area that is injured, and the presence of secondary problems such as aspiration pneumonia.

INFLAMMATORY, INFECTIOUS, AND IMMUNE DISEASES
Pharyngeal Lymphoid Hyperplasia
Pharyngeal lymphoid hyperplasia likely is caused or exacerbated by exposure to respiratory irritants, allergens, bacteria, or viruses. It is common in horses <2 years of age. Pharyngeal lymphoid hyperplasia is classified as follows:
* *Grade 1:* normal; a few small, whitish follicles on the dorsal pharyngeal mucosa
* *Grade 2:* several small, inactive follicles, with occasional hyperemic follicles extending down the lateral pharyngeal walls
* *Grade 3:* numerous active follicles that are close together and cover the entire dorsal and lateral walls of the pharynx
* *Grade 4:* large, edematous follicles that frequently coalesce into broad or polypoid structures

Clinical signs and diagnosis
* Grade 1 and 2 lesions do not appear to be clinically significant.
* Grade 3 and 4 lesions can cause abnormal respiratory noise and exercise intolerance.
* Diagnosis is made by endoscopic examination.

Treatment
Medical management consists of the following:
* vaccination at 60-day intervals against equine influenza and EHV-1 and EHV-4
* systemic NSAIDs and topical anti-inflammatory mixtures (applied bid for 10 to 14 days)
* rest until the inflammation subsides, in horses with grade 3 or 4 lesions

Horses with grade 4 lesions may be treated with topical 50% trichloracetic acid, electrocautery, or cryotherapy.
* Cryotherapy and application of trichloracetic acid may be performed in standing horses; electrocautery is performed via laryngotomy under general anesthesia.
  * Nd:YAG laser may also be of use with these lesions.
* These treatments should be undertaken with caution because pharyngeal cicatrix is a possible sequela.
* Exercise should be restricted for 6 to 8 weeks after treatment.

Prognosis
The prognosis is good, but recurrence or incomplete resolution is common until 4 years of age.

Nasopharyngeal Cicatrices
Clinical signs and diagnosis

- Abnormal respiratory noise and exercise intolerance are the most consistent signs.
- Endoscopy reveals a constriction involving either the soft palate alone or the soft palate and the walls and roof of the pharynx.
  - Other abnormalities may be present, including arytenoid chondropathy, epiglottic deformity, and deformity of the guttural pouch openings.

Treatment and prognosis

- Treatment depends on the degree of respiratory compromise, associated diseases or deformities, and the horse's intended function.
  - Transnasal incision using a bistoury under endoscopic guidance has been described.
- Treatment may relieve partial respiratory obstruction, but close inspection for concurrent diseases is important because they often dictate the prognosis for future activity.

IDIOPATHIC DISEASES
Dorsal Displacement of the Soft Palate (DDSP)

DDSP may be intermittent or persistent.

- *Intermittent* DDSP may be induced by pharyngeal inflammation, excitement, fatigue, excessive poll flexion, placing the tongue over the bit, caudal retraction of the larynx, and dysfunction of the supporting muscles of the soft palate.
  - When present, laryngeal hemiplegia and epiglottic abnormalities (hypoplasia, flaccidity, or entrapment) may contribute.
- *Persistent* DDSP can occur secondary to guttural pouch mycosis, severe epiglottic hypoplasia or flaccidity, nasopharyngeal cicatrices, subepiglottic cysts, epiglottic entrapment, and after treatment for intermittent DDSP.

Clinical signs

- When DDSP occurs during exercise it causes expiratory obstruction, a prominent respiratory noise, and almost immediate exercise intolerance.
  - Intermittent DDSP usually is recognized when the horse is worked at speed.
- Horses with persistent DDSP may cough when eating, have food and water exit their nostrils, make a rattling noise when they whinny, and often develop aspiration pneumonia and weight loss.

Diagnosis

- Diagnosis of intermittent DDSP usually is based on a compatible history and endoscopic findings at rest.
  - Not all affected horses readily displace their soft palates at rest, and normal horses may temporarily displace their palates during endoscopic examination.
- Endoscopic evaluation during treadmill exercise currently is the best method of diagnosis.
- It is important to thoroughly examine the pharynx and larynx for other abnormalities.
- The larynx should be radiographed and epiglottic length measured; if epiglottic hypoplasia is present, the horse may continue to suffer from DDSP despite surgical intervention.
  - Before taking radiographs, metallic markers of known length should be placed on either side of the mandible to establish the magnification factor.
  - Normal thyroepiglottic length is 8.76 ± 0.67 cm in Thoroughbreds and 8.74 ± 0.38 cm in Standardbreds.

Treatment

Conservative treatment should be tried before surgical intervention.

- Initial treatment should be directed at any other respiratory problems.
  - Pharyngeal inflammation or lower airway infection should be treated with the appropriate anti-inflammatory and antibiotic medications.
- If no other abnormalities are found, the horse should be trained with a tongue tie and figure-8 noseband to prevent it from opening its mouth and retracting its tongue.

Surgical procedures for correction of DDSP include:

- *partial staphylectomy:* The caudal border of the soft palate is trimmed via laryngotomy.

♦ *myectomy:* Portions of the omohyoideus and the sternothyroideus muscles are resected along the ventral aspect of the neck to prevent caudal retraction of the larynx.

♦ *combined staphylectomy, tendon transection, and myectomy:* Partial staphylectomy is combined with transection of the tendons of the sternothyroideus muscles at their insertion on the caudal aspect of the thyroid laminae, and resection of a 5-cm (2 inch) portion of the sternohyoid muscles as they cross the laryngotomy incision.

  • These procedures are accomplished through a single incision, which allows the horse to miss little or no training.

♦ *combined staphylectomy, sternothyroideus tenectomy, and epiglottic augmentation:* This combination may be indicated in horses with a hypoplastic epiglottis (see discussion of epiglottic hypoplasia).

Prognosis

♦ 60% of horses with DDSP and adequate epiglottic length improve with some combination of these treatments.

♦ Horses with epiglottic hypoplasia have a poorer prognosis for successful outcome.

Pharyngeal Collapse

Pharyngeal collapse may be caused by:

♦ increased negative pharyngeal pressure caused by obstruction rostral to the pharynx (e.g., space-occupying masses, inflammation, nasal deformity, and Horner's syndrome resulting in vascular engorgement of the nasal mucosa)

♦ dysfunction of the supporting musculature (e.g., myopathy, hyperkalemic periodic paralysis)

Clinical signs and diagnosis

♦ Signs include exercise intolerance and abnormal respiratory noise.

♦ Diagnosis is made by endoscopic examination at rest and/or during treadmill exercise.

♦ Regions rostral to the pharynx should be evaluated for a cause of nasal obstruction.

Treatment and prognosis

♦ Treatment depends on the cause.

• Surgical resection may be indicated for an obstructive nasal mass or deformity.

• Nebulizing or spraying the nasal passages with decongestants may relieve vascular engorgement of the nasal mucosa.

♦ The prognosis also depends on the cause.

• Horses with Horner's syndrome may regain sympathetic innervation with time.

• The prognosis in horses that do not have evidence of nasal obstruction is poor.

Diseases of the Guttural Pouches *(pages 501-512)*

Spencer M. Barber

SURGICAL APPROACHES TO THE GUTTURAL POUCHES

Surgical exposure of the guttural pouches is most often indicated for treatment of guttural pouch empyema or tympany. The anatomy of the guttural pouch region is complex and may be altered by pouch distention. Caution must be taken to avoid iatrogenic injury to neurovascular structures (carotid arteries and cranial nerves VII and IX through XII).

Invasive Surgical Approaches

There are three traditional surgical approaches.

♦ *hyovertebrotomy:* a lateral approach, primarily used for removal of chondroids and inspissated pus

• The incision is made parallel and just cranial to the wing of the atlas.

• This approach provides good exposure and access to the medial septum, but ventral drainage and access to the pharyngeal openings are poor.

♦ *Viborg's triangle:* a ventrolateral approach that provides good ventral drainage and can be done with the horse standing

• The three surgical borders are the tendinous insertion of the sternomandibularis muscle dorsally, the linguofacial vein ventrally, and the vertical ramus of the mandible rostrally.

- A horizontal skin incision is made dorsal to the linguofacial vein, and a plane of dissection is made immediately ventral to the external carotid artery.
- The ventral aspect of the medial compartment is entered, relatively distant from the various neurovascular structures.

♦ *modified Whitehouse:* a ventral approach to the medial compartment that provides excellent access to the pharyngeal openings and medial septum, and the best ventral drainage

- A ventral paramedian incision is made just ventral to the linguofacial vein.
- Drainage can be established with the horse standing if the pouch is greatly distended.

Minimally Invasive Techniques

Minimally invasive techniques include electrocautery and laser, guided by rigid or flexible endoscopy, via transcutaneous entry ports.

CONGENITAL AND FAMILIAL DISEASES

Guttural Pouch Tympany

Guttural pouch tympany is distention of the pouch with air, caused by dysfunction of the pharyngeal orifice. Most cases are congenital and are seen in young foals; there is a higher incidence in fillies than in colts.

Clinical signs

♦ A large, fluctuant, resonant, nonpainful swelling is found in the parotid/laryngeal area.
- The problem often is unilateral, but the external swelling usually appears bilaterally and may even be symmetric.
♦ Severe swelling can cause dyspnea and dysphagia (milk or feed exiting the nostrils).
♦ Aspiration pneumonia is a rare complication.

Diagnosis

♦ On endoscopic examination, the pharyngeal opening to the guttural pouch appears normal; the dorsal pharynx may be asymmetrically compressed in cases of unilateral tympany.
♦ Catheterization of the involved pouch deflates it, which helps differentiate unilateral from bilateral tympany before surgery.
- Percutaneous centesis may also be used for this purpose.
♦ Radiographs show a pouch that is enlarged and filled with gas.
- Accumulation of exudate may create a fluid line.

Treatment

Conservative treatment (antibiotics, antiinflammatory agents, decompression) usually is ineffective. Surgical options for unilateral tympany include:

♦ *excision of the plica salpingopharyngea:* trimming of the pharyngeal opening
♦ *salpingopharyngeal fistulation:* creating a fistula between the affected guttural pouch and the pharynx
♦ *fenestration of the medial septum:* creating a communication between the two guttural pouches through the medial septum

Surgical options for bilateral tympany include bilateral salpingopharyngeal fistulation, and fenestration of the medial septum combined with either unilateral salpingopharyngeal fistulation or excision of the plica salpingopharyngea.

Prognosis

♦ The prognosis is good for unilateral problems treated by medial septum fenestration.
♦ A guarded prognosis should be given for foals with aspiration pneumonia.
♦ Neurologic injury occasionally occurs with invasive approaches and can result in dysphagia and dyspnea; if these signs do not resolve a few days postoperatively, a grave prognosis is warranted.

INFLAMMATORY, INFECTIOUS, AND IMMUNE DISEASES

Guttural Pouch Empyema

Guttural pouch empyema can occur in horses of any age, but young adults are more often affected. It usually occurs secondary to upper respiratory tract infections, especially with β-hemolytic streptococci.

Clinical signs

- The most common sign is mucopurulent nasal discharge, often persisting after recovery from an upper respiratory tract infection.
  - Empyema usually is unilateral but causes a bilaterally asymmetric nasal discharge, heavier on the side with the infected pouch.
  - The discharge may be intermittent and usually increases when the horse lowers its head.
  - In chronic empyema, the exudate may become inspissated.
- Sometimes the enlarged pouch displaces the pharynx and soft palate or causes nerve damage, resulting in dyspnea and dysphagia.

Diagnosis

- *Endoscopy* may reveal mucopurulent discharge from the guttural pouch opening.
  - However, a mucoid discharge at the pharyngeal openings can be seen with pharyngitis and upper and lower respiratory tract infections, and guttural pouch empyema can occur without any discharge from the pharyngeal openings.
- *Aspiration* of the pouch contents confirms the diagnosis and allows culture and sensitivity.
  - With inspissated material, a sample may be obtained by lavage with sterile saline.
- *Radiography* reveals a distinct fluid line in the guttural pouch.
  - A pouch completely filled with exudate has the same density as soft tissue.
  - Chondroids may produce an irregular pattern to the fluid line.

Treatment

- Acute empyema may respond rapidly to systemic antibiotics.
- If drainage persists or the condition is chronic when diagnosed, lavage via an indwelling catheter is indicated.
  - Lavage is performed 2 or 3 times/day with 500 mL of fluid.
  - After lavage, the horse's head must remain in a lowered position to assist natural drainage; tranquilization or placing the horse's feed on the ground is effective.

- Irritating solutions must not be used because they may cause neurologic damage.
  - Concurrent systemic antimicrobial therapy is indicated.
- Surgical drainage is indicated if the discharge persists after several days of lavage.
  - Inspissated material and chondroids cannot be removed by lavage; transendoscopic removal has been reported.
  - Surgical drainage should also be considered if dyspnea, dysphagia, or cellulitis is present.

Prognosis

- The prognosis is good if the condition is diagnosed early and treated aggressively.
- The prognosis is poor if neurologic signs are present; reflux of water and ingesta from the external nares, coughing, aspiration pneumonia, reinfection of the guttural pouches, and chronic weight loss are likely.

Mycosis

Guttural pouch mycosis is a fungal infection of the pouch wall that often interferes with the associated neurovascular structures.

- It is commonly caused by *Aspergillus nidulans,* although other fungi have been implicated.
- Infection usually is unilateral and typically involves the roof of the medial compartment overlying the internal carotid artery.
  - Occasionally, infection involves the lateral compartment and external carotid artery.

Clinical signs

- Signs vary with the neurovascular structure(s) involved; some cases are asymptomatic.
- Epistaxis at rest is the most common sign.
  - Mycotic infection usually is unilateral but causes bilateral epistaxis, with most of the hemorrhage exiting the nostril on the affected side.
  - Bleeding can range from a few trickles of blood to severe hemorrhage resulting in exsanguination.
- Dysphagia is the second most common sign.

- It may occur suddenly or develop slowly.
- Other signs, in order of decreasing frequency, are parotid pain, abnormal head posture, nasal catarrh, head shyness, abnormal respiratory noise, sweating and shivering, Horner's syndrome, colic, and facial paralysis.

Diagnosis

- *Endoscopic examination* of the pouch interior is important in confirming the diagnosis.
  - The lesion appears as a brown, yellow, green, or black and white necrotic, diphtheritic membrane raised from the surface of the pouch wall.
  - Laryngeal hemiplegia, DDSP, or collapse of the pharyngeal roof caused by neurologic injury may also be present.
  - The external carotid artery should be examined as it passes over the lateral compartment.
- *Radiography* usually is not necessary for diagnosis, but bony lesions have been reported.
  - Angiography can be used to demonstrate aneurysms of either carotid artery.

Treatment

- Patient stabilization is the most important facet of treatment for severe hemorrhage.
  - The horse should be confined and observed closely while awaiting spontaneous remission of bleeding.
  - Volume replacement with fluids or whole blood may be necessary, particularly if surgical treatment is planned.
  - Antibiotics are indicated if feed or blood has been aspirated into the lungs.
- Topical and systemic antifungal agents have been tried.
  - Topical agents alone usually are not effective, although ketoconazole, itraconazole, fluconazole, and enilconazole are effective against *Aspergillus* organisms.
- Surgical treatment is recommended because of the high incidence of fatal hemorrhage.

- The preferred technique involves permanent placement of a balloon-tipped catheter distal to the mycotic lesion, with ligation on the cardiac side of the lesion.
  - Ligation on the cardiac side is inadequate in preventing fatal hemorrhage, because retrograde bleeding can occur from the circle of Willis.
  - Spontaneous remission of the mycotic lesion occurs following occlusion of the underlying carotid artery.

Prognosis

- When occlusion of the affected artery both proximal and distal to the lesion has been achieved, the prognosis for survival is good.
- In patients with signs of cranial nerve dysfunction before or after surgery, the prognosis for complete recovery is poor.

Diseases of the Larynx

(pages 512-522)

Ryland B. Edwards

CONGENITAL AND FAMILIAL DISEASES

Rostral Displacement of the Palatopharyngeal Arch

This congenital abnormality occurs secondary to malformation or agenesis of the laryngeal cartilages and associated muscles.

- Signs may include dysphagia and secondary aspiration pneumonia, respiratory noise, and exercise intolerance; occasionally, this condition is an incidental finding.
- Diagnosis is made on endoscopic examination.
  - The corniculate process of one or both arytenoid cartilages is partially or completely hidden by the displaced palatopharyngeal arch.
- There is no effective surgical treatment; resection of the palatopharyngeal arch can lead to stricture and worsening of the clinical signs.
- The prognosis for performance in clinically affected horses is poor.

INFLAMMATORY, INFECTIOUS, AND IMMUNE DISEASES

Arytenoid Chondritis

Arytenoid chondropathy or chondritis may result from trauma or from inflammation of the arytenoid cartilages secondary to mucosal damage. It most often is unilateral. Possible causes include foreign body ingestion, nasogastric or tracheal intubation, and irritation in horses with idiopathic laryngeal hemiplegia.

Clinical signs and diagnosis

* Affected horses may have a similar history and presentation to those with laryngeal hemiplegia: exercise intolerance, upper respiratory noise, and even respiratory distress if the inflammation is severe.
* Horses may be febrile during the acute phase of the disease.
* Diagnosis is made by endoscopic examination, which usually reveals a swollen and/or irregularly shaped arytenoid cartilage and incomplete arytenoid abduction.
  * Protuberances into the laryngeal lumen may also be seen.

Treatment and prognosis

* If the only finding is protrusion of granulation tissue with adequate arytenoid abduction, laser resection of the granulation tissue can be effective.
* Arytenoidectomy is indicated for malformation with reduced arytenoid abduction.
  * Partial arytenoidectomy (removal of the entire arytenoid cartilage, except for the muscular process) is the procedure of choice for performance animals.
  * This surgery does not restore normal upper airway mechanics; only about 50% of horses perform at their previous or expected level of performance.
  * At least 10% of treated horses develop an intermittent or persistent cough when eating.
* Severe bilateral cartilage damage with perilaryngeal soft tissue involvement may warrant permanent tracheostomy.

Epiglottitis

Possible predisposing factors include inhaled allergens or irritants, inflammation from respiratory tract infection, mucosal irritation secondary to DDSP, foreign bodies, and poor-quality hay:

* Signs include exercise intolerance, increased respiratory noise, coughing, and, less commonly, dysphagia and airway obstruction.
* Diagnosis is made by endoscopic examination.
  * Abnormalities include ulceration and reddening of the epiglottic mucosa; thickening, edema, and discoloration of the epiglottis and aryepiglottic folds; exposed epiglottic cartilage; and dorsal elevation by granulation tissue proliferation on the ventral surface.
* Treatment usually includes broad-spectrum antibiotics, systemic NSAIDs, and topical antiinflammatory solution.
  * For example, 750 mL Furacin, 2 g prednisolone, and 250 mL DMSO added to 1 L of glycerin; 10 to 20 mL is applied transnasally bid through a no. 10 French catheter
  * Tracheostomy may be required in horses with severe dyspnea.
* The prognosis is good, but secondary complications, including epiglottic deformity, intermittent or persistent DDSP, and epiglottic entrapment, occur in about 30% of cases.

Aryepiglottic Fold Collapse

Aryepiglottic fold collapse may result from incompetency of the intrapharyngeal ostium. The collapse most often is bilateral, and inspiratory obstruction worsens with exercise.

* Horses with this problem have exercise intolerance, often with little or no abnormal respiratory noise.
* Diagnosis requires endoscopic evaluation during treadmill exercise.
  * The aryepiglottic folds collapse axially on inspiration and in some cases almost completely obstruct the larynx.
* Two procedures have been used to reduce the size of the intrapharyn-

geal ostium and prevent collapse of the folds:

- Induction of fibrosis of the aryepiglottic folds (using a laser in standing horses or electro-cautery via laryngotomy in anes-thetized horses).
- Resection of the aryepiglottic folds (using a laser in standing horses); can be combined with caudal palatoplasty (via laryngo-tomy, under general anesthesia).
- The outcome has been favorable in the limited number of cases treated at this time.

Laryngeal Hemiplegia

Idiopathic laryngeal hemiplegia is caused by degeneration or damage to the laryngeal nerve(s), most commonly the left recurrent laryngeal nerve.

Clinical signs and diagnosis

- Horses with laryngeal hemiplegia or paresis usually present with exer-cise intolerance and an inspiratory noise ("roaring").
- If a marked degree of dorsal cricoarytenoid muscle atrophy is present, the muscular process on the affected side is more prominent on external palpation.
- Endoscopic examination is the stan-dard method for identifying horses with laryngeal hemiplegia (see dis-cussion of ancillary diagnostic aids).
- Endoscopic evaluation during tread-mill exercise allows further defini-tion of laryngeal function in horses with grade 3 laryngeal hemiplegia.
  - Some of these horses have normal laryngeal function when exercised, but others lose the ability to fully abduct their arytenoid cartilages during maximal exercise.
- Grading during exercise is as follows:
  - Grade A is maximal arytenoid ab-duction.
  - Grade B is partial loss of abduc-tion.
  - Grade C is arytenoid collapse during inspiration.
- Horses with *right* laryngeal hemi-plegia should be examined for evi-dence of Horner's syndrome be-cause the nasal mucosal congestion it can cause results in upper airway obstruction that is not relieved by surgical laryngeal abduction.

Treatment

Treatment options include:

- *ventriculectomy ± vocalcordectomy*
  - Ventriculocordectomy alone may be effective in racehorses in which the vocal cord collapses into the airway without signifi-cant arytenoid collapse, and in draft horses used for pulling; however, it does not alter the in-spiratory noise.
  - The procedure can be performed using a laser in standing horses, or via laryngotomy.
- *laryngeal prosthesis* (prosthetic laryngoplasty)
  - The prosthesis is placed such that full arytenoid abduction is maintained.
  - If the horse has some arytenoid movement or if dorsal cricoary-tenoid muscle atrophy is min-imal, the recurrent laryngeal nerve should be transected.
  - Laryngoplasty often is combined with ventriculectomy.
- *arytenoidectomy* (see discussion of arytenoid chondritis)
- *reinnervation* techniques involving the ventral branch of the first cer-vical nerve:
  - nerve implantation into the dorsal cricoarytenoid muscle
  - nerve-muscle pedicle implanta-tion (the first cervical nerve and a small piece of omohyoideus muscle is implanted into the dorsal cricoarytenoid muscle)
  - nerve-to-nerve anastomosis (first cervical to recurrent laryngeal nerve)

Prognosis

- 60% of horses treated with pros-thetic laryngoplasty and ven-triculectomy return to their pre-vious level of performance.
  - Horses used for athletic en-deavors other than racing have a significantly better prognosis than do racehorses.
  - About 10% of horses develop a chronic cough from overabduction.
  - Other complications include par-tial loss of abduction over time, complete failure when the suture breaks or pulls through the carti-lage, infection of the implant,

and inflammatory reaction to the synthetic sutures.

◆ Success with reinnervation is around 75%, although it takes 6 to 12 months.

Epiglottic Entrapment

Entrapment of the epiglottis by redundant mucosa beneath it causes expiratory obstruction during exercise. In 97% of cases, the entrapment is persistent.

Clinical signs and diagnosis

◆ Epiglottic entrapment often causes exercise intolerance and respiratory noise during exercise.

◆ Diagnosis is made by endoscopy at rest, although intermittent entrapment may be apparent only with endoscopic examination during treadmill exercise.

  • The normal triangular outline of the epiglottis is identified, but the vascular plexus on the dorsal surface and the normal scalloped margins are obscured by a membrane.

  • Ulceration, a subepiglottic cyst, and diffuse epiglottitis may also be seen.

◆ The larynx should be radiographed and epiglottic length measured (see discussion of dorsal displacement of the soft palate).

Treatment and prognosis

◆ If the entrapping membranes are inflamed, it is best to rest the horse and initiate treatment with an NSAID or topical antiinflammatory solution before surgical correction.

◆ Treatment for persistent entrapment usually involves transnasal correction using a bistoury, electrocautery, or fiberoptic laser, in either the standing or anesthetized horse.

◆ Intermittent entrapment is approached orally or via laryngotomy with the horse under general anesthesia.

◆ The prognosis is good, although 5% of cases re-entrap and 10% to 15% experience DDSP after surgical correction.

Epiglottic Flaccidity

Epiglottic flaccidity may be related to neuropathy or fatigue of the geniohyoideus muscle.

◆ Exercise intolerance and respiratory noise are the most common signs.

◆ Diagnosis can be made by endoscopic examination, but treadmill evaluation is recommended to verify the problem during exercise.

  • Some horses have endoscopic evidence of epiglottic flaccidity at rest but have normal epiglottic tone when examined during treadmill exercise.

  • In others the epiglottis appears normal at rest but displays flaccidity during exercise.

◆ Augmentation by submucosal injection of Teflon along the ventral surface of the epiglottis is the preferred treatment, and is performed via laryngotomy.

◆ Favorable results have been obtained, but complications include continued DDSP and formation of excessive granulation tissue or an abscess.

Epiglottic Hypoplasia

Epiglottic hypoplasia is an uncommon congenital problem.

◆ Signs generally are associated with epiglottic entrapment or DDSP.

◆ A preliminary diagnosis may be made on endoscopic examination; confirmation is made radiographically (for normal epiglottic length, see discussion of dorsal displacement of the soft palate).

◆ There is no technique described for lengthening the epiglottis.

  • If hypoplasia results in epiglottic entrapment or DDSP, treatment should be directed toward these conditions.

◆ The prognosis for athletic performance is guarded to poor.

Diseases of the Trachea

(pages 522-526)

Clifford M. Honnas

SURGICAL PROCEDURES

Permanent Tracheostomy

Permanent tracheostomy is indicated when primary obstructive disease of the upper airway is irreversible or requires an extended time for resolution. Tracheostomy can be performed with the horse either standing and sedated or anesthetized. Daily observation and cleaning are necessary, and the horse should be kept in a dust-free environment. The technique is described in *Equine Medicine and Surgery V*.

Tracheal Resection and Anastomosis

Tracheal resection and end-to-end anastomosis is indicated in horses with cervical tracheal stenosis or collapse involving <6 tracheal rings. The most common indication is tracheal stenosis following tracheotomy. Surgery is performed under general anesthesia.

DISEASES WITH PHYSICAL CAUSES

Tracheal Trauma

Blunt injury resulting in tracheal perforation without disruption of the skin may not be recognized until subcutaneous emphysema develops (a nonpainful swelling that is soft, mobile, and crepitant). The diagnosis usually can be confirmed by physical examination, endoscopy, and radiography. Thoracic radiographs should be taken to check for pneumomediastinum, which can predispose to pneumothorax.

Treatment depends on the extent of the injury

- Small tears can be managed conservatively and usually form a fibrin seal in 1 to 2 days.
- Large tears should be managed surgically as soon as the horse's condition allows.
  - They are approached through the wound after debridement of devitalized tissue.
- Once the tracheal defect is closed, subcutaneous emphysema resolves in 7 to 10 days.

Tracheal Foreign Bodies

Foreign bodies tend to lodge in the horizontal portion of the trachea and cause persistent, chronic coughing.

- Inhaled plant material can cause chronic coughing, intermittent fever, fetid breath, and intermittent

bilateral purulent nasal discharge that periodically is blood tinged.
- Tracheal endoscopy can be used to identify foreign bodies.
- It may be possible to remove the object using an endoscope biopsy instrument, but tracheotomy often is necessary.
- The tracheotomy incision should be allowed to heal as an open wound; antibiotics are given on the basis of culture and susceptibility results of transtracheal aspirates.

Tracheal Collapse

Tracheal collapse occurs most frequently as a result of trauma or emergency tracheostomy. In ponies >10 years of age, it may result from dorsoventral flattening of the trachea.

- Most affected horses exhibit inspiratory stridor, exercise intolerance, respiratory distress, and cyanosis; but some horses are asymptomatic.
- Diagnosis can be confirmed by auscultation (increased air turbulence), palpation (may reveal the lateral edges of the flattened trachea), endoscopy, and radiography.
- Treatment depends on the cause, length of trachea involved, and accessibility of the site.
  - An extraluminal prosthetic device, such as a syringe casing, can be effective.
  - Partial chondrotomy may be required on the ventral aspect of each collapsed tracheal ring.
- Long-term prognosis is variable; horses with dorsoventral collapse have a poor prognosis, especially if the thoracic trachea is involved.

Tracheal Stenosis

Causes of tracheal stenosis include tracheotomy (especially in foals), *Streptococcus equi* abscesses in peritracheal lymph nodes, and trauma. Surgical options include tracheal resection and anastomosis, extraluminal polypropylene prostheses, surgical drainage of peritracheal abscesses, and multiple tracheal ring chondrotomies with placement of retention sutures.

INFLAMMATORY, INFECTIOUS, AND IMMUNE DISEASES

Granulomas

Granulomatous nodules occasionally are observed in the trachea during endoscopic examination.

- They most often are found just caudal to the larynx.
  - Foreign body (e.g., grass awn) irritation and inappropriate passage of a nasogastric tube are possible causes; granulomas can also develop at tracheotomy sites.
- Tracheal granulomas usually are an incidental finding and often cause no clinical signs.
- Large granulomas can be removed using an endoscopically guided snare or via tracheotomy; cryotherapy via endoscopy is an alternative for smaller lesions.
- The prognosis generally is good.

Diseases of the Lung

(pages 526-553)

Dorothy M. Ainsworth, Jill Beech, Corrie Brown, Frederick J. Derksen, Mary Rose Paradis, Patricia J. Provost, and Richard A. Mansmann

CONGENITAL AND FAMILIAL DISEASES

Neonatal Respiratory Distress Syndrome

Respiratory distress syndrome is seen most often in premature foals, particularly those delivered by cesarean section. Surfactant deficiency is likely involved.

Clinical signs and diagnosis

- Most affected foals are premature (low birth weight, short silky hair coat, soft pliant ears).
- They may be active for the first 30 minutes of life but quickly tire and become distressed.
- The respiratory rate is elevated, but the most obvious sign of distress is increased respiratory effort with paradoxical breathing (see discussion of evaluating foals for respiratory disease).
- Thoracic radiographs generally show a diffuse alveolar pattern

with air bronchograms; edema increases the lung density as the disorder progresses.

- The PaO_2 usually is <60 torr and the $PaCO_2$ is >60 torr; arterial pH ranges from 6.9 to 7.3.
- Other causes of respiratory failure, including congenital heart defects, meconium aspiration, and in utero bacterial or viral pneumonia, must be ruled out.

Treatment and prognosis

- The primary objective is to improve oxygenation and ventilation.
  - Mechanical ventilation with supplemental oxygen is the most effective way.
  - Surfactant replacement may also be beneficial.
- Currently, respiratory distress syndrome in premature foals has a grave prognosis.

Meconium Aspiration

Fetal stress can result in expulsion of meconium into the amniotic fluid before birth. This material can be aspirated in utero.

Clinical signs and diagnosis

- Foals stained with yellowish-brown amniotic fluid at birth likely have meconium aspiration.
  - There may be a brownish nasal discharge that is bilirubin-positive on a urine test strip.
- Respiratory rate and effort are increased; lung sounds may be normal or increased.
- Blood gas abnormalities vary from normal to hypoxia with respiratory acidosis.
- A caudal granular infiltrate is seen on thoracic radiographs.

Treatment

- An attempt should be made to suction the material from the lungs as soon as possible.
  - A small feeding tube can be inserted transnasally into the trachea; mild suction is applied as the tube is slowly withdrawn.
- Ideally, respiratory support is directed by blood gas analysis.

Milk Aspiration

Milk aspiration and subsequent pneumonia usually is secondary to a soft palate defect or displacement.

- The first signs are milk at the foal's nostrils after nursing, along with a gurgling sound in the throat.
- Consolidation of the accessory lobe usually is seen on thoracic radiographs.
- Treatment for any dysphagic condition that results in milk inhalation should include prevention of nursing and placement of an indwelling nasogastric tube for enteral feeding.
- Broad-spectrum antibiotics are necessary to eliminate the mixed bacterial infection.
- Vitamin E–selenium deficiencies may contribute to the problem; supplementation is helpful in these cases.

DISEASES WITH PHYSICAL CAUSES
Smoke Inhalation
Horses that survive a barn fire may sustain life-threatening respiratory tract injury (both thermal and chemical) and extensive skin burns. Pulmonary damage often is underestimated initially, and pulmonary edema progresses over the first 18 to 24 hours, so continual reassessment is necessary. Pneumonia is a potential complication in every smoke inhalation patient.

Treatment and prognosis
The main goals of treatment are to:
- maintain a patent airway
- provide supplemental oxygen
  - Oxygen insufflation via tracheotomy is necessary in animals with laryngeal edema.
  - Insufflation is continued until the horse can maintain normal oxygenation on its own.
- Alleviate pulmonary edema and bronchoconstriction.
  - Use of humidified oxygen, acetylcysteine, bronchodilators, and furosemide are beneficial.
  - Butorphanol can be used to treat paroxysmal coughing.
- Manage impending pneumonia and secondary organ failure.

The prognosis varies; persistent lung changes can result, but are not inevitable.

Aspiration Pneumonia
Aspiration of food material can result from any condition that causes dysphagia, including esophageal obstruction, guttural pouch disease, pharyngeal foreign bodies or cysts, cleft palate, and laryngeal surgery. Subsequent pneumonia can be severe. Therapy is directed at preventing further aspiration. Broad-spectrum antibiotics are indicated, and because anaerobic organisms likely are pres-ent, therapy should include penicillin or metronidazole.

Aspiration of mineral oil
When mineral oil is inadvertently deposited into the lungs:
- Xylazine sedation should be used to lower the horse's head and promote drainage.
- Antiinflammatory drugs should be given for several days and possible secondary bacterial disease monitored using thoracic radiographs, hemograms, and transtracheal aspirate culture.
- The prognosis usually is unfavorable because mineral oil initiates a chronic and progressive granulomatous reaction.

INFLAMMATORY, INFECTIOUS, AND IMMUNE DISEASES
Streptococcus equi subsp. *zooepidemicus* Infection
Previously referred to as *Streptococcus zooepidemicus,* this bacterium is the most common organism isolated from the lower respiratory tract of horses with respiratory disease. It is an important secondary invader following viral respiratory infection or transport-associated stress. The resulting pneumonia may be diffuse or focal; pulmonary abscesses and pleuritis can also develop.

Clinical signs and diagnosis
- Signs depend on the severity of infection.
  - Depression, fever, anorexia, and mucopurulent nasal discharge are common.
  - Lymphadenopathy, dullness on sinus percussion, abnormal lung sounds (suggestive of consolidation or pleural effusion), and dullness on thoracic percussion are variably found.
- Diagnosis is based on the isolation of the organism from the site(s) of infection; sensitivity testing is advisable.

Treatment

- Ceftiofur is effective; other drugs that may be effective are chloramphenicol, trimethoprim-sulfa combinations, rifampin, erythromycin, and synthetic penicillins.
- NSAIDs may improve the horse's attitude and appetite, but their antipyretic action complicates body temperature monitoring.
- Stress, including transport, should be avoided in affected horses.

Streptococcus equi subsp. *equi* Infection (Strangles)

Strangles is a highly contagious disease, especially in horses 1 to 5 years of age. Clinical signs usually appear within 10 days after infection.

Clinical signs and diagnosis

- Signs are variable, being dependent on the horse's immune status and prior exposure.
- Fever, depression, anorexia, nasal discharge (initially serous, then mucopurulent), and abscessed submaxillary, mandibular, and retropharyngeal lymph nodes are characteristic.
  - Lymph node enlargement may obstruct respiration and disrupt swallowing.
  - Retropharyngeal lymph nodes may rupture and drain externally or internally (potentially leading to aspiration pneumonia or guttural pouch empyema).
- Neck pain may be apparent, and lactating mares may become agalactic; myocarditis has been reported.
- Signs may last from <1 week to >2 months.
- Diagnosis is based on a history of exposure and on culture of the organism from nasal swabs or samples of exudate; lymph node swabs are most likely to culture positive.
  - A selective transport medium, such as Strepswab, aids laboratory diagnosis.

Treatment

- The decision to use antibiotics depends on the severity of clinical signs, and numbers and ages of exposed horses.
  - Mild infections localized to the lymph nodes or upper respiratory tract usually do not require systemic antibiotics.
  - Pneumonia, pleuritis, sinusitis, synovitis, guttural pouch empyema, and other systemic manifestations may require long-term antibiotic therapy; horses with suspected *S. equi* subsp. *equi* pneumonia should be treated rigorously.
  - Both penicillin and ceftiofur are likely to be effective.
  - Current evidence indicates that antibiotic use does not predispose to "bastard strangles."
- Superficial abscesses should be hot-packed; surgical drainage may be needed for lymph node abscessation and associated guttural pouch empyema and sinusitis.
- Dyspneic horses may require tracheostomy.
- Good nursing care includes providing palatable and easily swallowed food and, with animals unable or unwilling to eat, feeding by nasogastric tube.
- Purpura hemorrhagica can be a severe complication, often requiring long-term therapy with antibiotics and antiinflammatory drugs (see Chapters 17, Integumentary System, and Chapter 19, Hemolymphatic System).

Control and prevention

- Control of the disease requires quarantine of affected animals and thorough disinfection.
  - Feed, water buckets, and areas contaminated with secretions from infected horses facilitate spread of the infection.
  - Infection may be maintained for at least 8 months within a group of horses; premises are said to harbor the infection for up to 1 year.
- Commercial vaccines are available, although none is completely effective in preventing the disease.
  - Both the M-protein extract (Strepvax) and the adjuvanted purified enzyme extract (Strepgard) *may* reduce the frequency of clinical disease.
  - Large challenge doses of the organism may overcome immunity.

- Yearly boosters are recommended, although immunity may not last 12 months.
- Vaccination of pregnant mares 1 to 2 months before foaling has been advised.
- An intranasally administered live avirulent vaccine (Pinnacle) is available.

Streptococcus pneumoniae Infection

Streptococcus pneumoniae, an α-hemolytic streptococcus, is a known upper respiratory pathogen in humans; 5% to 60% of humans are carriers. However, the importance of this organism in horses is undetermined. It is sporadically isolated from horses and foals with lower respiratory disease (e.g., pneumonia, pleuritis), and pneumococcal septicemia has been reported in one foal; often, other pathogens are isolated concurrently. Horses recover after treatment with appropriate antibiotics.

Rhodococcus equi Infection

Rhodococcus equi, formerly known as *Corynebacterium equi,* is an important cause of pneumonia in foals 1 to 6 months old. Most show signs between 2 and 4 months of age. *R. equi* can survive in soil for at least a year and withstands drying and direct sunlight. Dusty environments and dry weather increase the prevalence of the disease.

Clinical signs

- Some foals are asymptomatic and are simply found dead; necropsy reveals diffuse lung abscessation.
- Others suddenly develop respiratory distress, with a rapid respiratory rate, flared nostrils, heaving respiratory pattern, and fever; cyanosis is common.
  - Usually there is no nasal discharge; auscultation may reveal wheezes and crackles, but there may be only an increase in coarseness and loss of soft vesicular sounds.
  - These foals may die within several days, even if treatment is initiated.
- In other foals, the clinical course is more chronic (weeks or months).
  - Systemic signs (e.g., synovitis, diarrhea, uveitis) may accompany pneumonia; osteomyelitis, osteoarthritis, endocarditis, and myocardial dysfunction may also develop.
  - These foals are febrile, often dyspneic, and usually look unthrifty.
  - Nasal discharge and coughing are variable; when present, the cough is soft and deep.
  - Auscultation may reveal only coarse or large airway sounds, but wheezes and crackles may be heard.
  - Affected foals are severely exercise intolerant, and even minor stress can worsen their dyspnea and precipitate collapse.
- In North America, the intestinal form of *R. equi* infection (diarrhea, poor growth, weight loss, ± peritonitis) rarely accompanies the pulmonary disease.
- Adult horses with *R. equi* infection have weight loss, fever, coughing, and dyspnea; rapidly progressive pleuropneumonia and ulcerative lymphangitis have been reported.

Diagnosis

- Results of clinical laboratory tests are nonspecific (increased platelet counts, leukocytosis, and hyperfibrinogenemia).
- *Tracheobronchial aspirates* often are diagnostic, revealing gram-positive pleomorphic rods.
  - Aspirates usually are culture-positive for *R. equi,* but false-negative results can occur.
  - Other potential pathogens may also be isolated, which can confuse the issue.
- *Thoracic radiographs* are helpful when cultures are negative.
  - A prominent alveolar pattern with ill-defined regional consolidation is common; acutely or mildly affected foals may have only a prominent interstitial pattern.
  - Nodular pulmonary lesions and lymphadenopathy are almost pathognomonic in foals of this age; however, these findings may not be present on initial examination.
  - Tracheobronchial lymphadenopathy is more common in foals that do not recover.
- *Lymphocyte immunostimulation tests* are useful in foals <2 months of

age; affected foals in this age group have a very high stimulation ratio compared with normal foals.

♦ An ELISA has been developed to detect specific *R. equi* antibodies.
  • However, some studies show no correlation between titers and infection, and antibodies to *R. equi* may not develop despite severe disease.

Treatment

♦ Erythromycin (25 to 30 mg/kg PO q6h) combined with rifampin (5 mg/kg PO q12h) is the widely recommended treatment of choice.
  • The organism usually is sensitive to gentamicin, vancomycin, amikacin, rifampin, erythromycin, and less to trimethoprim-sulfa combinations, chloramphenicol, and tetracycline; often it is resistant to penicillin.
  • Anecdotally, enrofloxacin has been used with success; however, articular cartilage toxicity is a potential adverse effect in young animals.
  • Oral erythromycin can cause diarrhea and/or dyspnea, and has been associated with fatal hyperthermia in foals.
♦ Bronchodilators and aminophylline have no proven clinical benefit in these foals.
  • Erythromycin elevates blood levels of aminophylline and delays its clearance, thus potentiating its toxicity.
♦ Nursing care, adequate nutrition, and good ventilation are important.

Prevention

♦ Attempts should be made to house foals in well-ventilated, dust-free areas and to avoid dirt paddocks and crowded conditions. Foal manure is a rich source of *R. equi* organisms, and preventing the exposure of other foals to fecal material helps limit spread of this disease.
♦ Stress and drugs that decrease immune function should be avoided.
♦ Monitoring rectal temperature, CBC, and plasma fibrinogen may help detect infection before clinical signs develop; thoracic radiography may be warranted in valuable foals.

♦ Any foals that die should be necropsied.
♦ ELISA tests are available but are not USDA licensed and are not completely reliable.
♦ Hyperimmune plasma administration can reduce the spread of this disease on affected farms.

Miscellaneous Bacterial Infections

Although various bacteria other than streptococcal species may be cultured from lower airway secretions and can be pathogens, the frequency of lung infection is low. Other bacteria that can cause pneumonia include *Klebsiella pneumoniae*, *Escherichia coli*, *Pasturella* sp., *Actinobacillus equuli*, *Staphylococcus aureus*, and *Bordetella bronchiseptica*. *Pseudomonas* spp. commonly are isolated from horses with pleuropneumonia. *Salmonella* spp. occasionally cause pneumonia in foals.

Anaerobic Infections

Anaerobes are important lower respiratory tract pathogens, especially in cases of necrotizing pneumonia, lung abscesses, and pleuritis/pneumonia complex.

♦ Isolation requires special culture techniques; samples should be transported in appropriate media, such as Port-A-Cul (suitable for both aerobic and anaerobic cultures).
♦ Anaerobes most commonly isolated are *Bacteroides fragilis* and *Prevotella* spp., followed by *Clostridium* spp.
♦ A putrid odor is characteristic of anaerobic infections and warrants a poor prognosis in horses with pleuropneumonia, but absence of odor does not exclude anaerobes as the cause of disease.
♦ When an anaerobic infection is suspected, penicillin is a good choice and often is combined with a drug effective against gram-negative bacteria.
♦ Metronidazole (15 to 25 mg/kg PO q6h) is excellent for treating anaerobic infections and also is effective against β-lactamase–producing anaerobes that are penicillin-resistant.
♦ Anaerobic infections of the lower respiratory tract have a poorer prognosis than do aerobic infections.

162 *Respiratory System*

Melioidosis

Melioidosis is an acute bacterial disease affecting a wide variety of animal species and humans; it is characterized by the formation of multiple visceral caseating abscesses.

* The etiologic agent, *Burkholderia (Pseudomonas) pseudomallei,* is a gram-negative bacterium that resides in soil in tropical and subtropical areas (currently not endemic in North America).
* Clinical signs usually include fever and respiratory distress.
* Diagnosis is dependent on culturing the organism.
  * Samples should be sent to a national or state high-containment laboratory.
* The organism is resistant to multiple antibiotics, and treatment of individual animals is discouraged; affected animals should be destroyed to decrease the spread of this disease.

Glanders

Glanders is a contagious disease primarily of horses and donkeys (which suffer a more acute and fulminating form of the disease). It is caused by *Burkholderia (Pseudomonas) mallei,* a gram-negative aerobic bacterium. Glanders was eradicated from the United States in 1937 and currently is restricted to Asia and some parts of eastern Europe. Infection usually causes fever.

* Other signs reflect the site of primary involvement and disease severity; sites include the nasal sinuses (causing yellow-green nasal discharge), lungs, and the skin of the extremities (causing poorly encapsulated pyogranulomas that spread locally or along lymphatics).
  * Regional lymph nodes become enlarged and suppurative or pyogranulomatous.
* Diagnosis is based on identification of the organism or ancillary serologic tests.
  * The disease is reportable and potentially zoonotic, so culture should be attempted only in a high-containment laboratory (e.g., National Veterinary Services Laboratories, Ames, Iowa).

* The organism is sensitive to many antibiotics; however, in the interests of disease eradication, animals with glanders should be destroyed.

Bacterial Pneumonia in Neonates

Bacterial pneumonia in neonatal foals usually is associated with septicemia.

* The newborn may be infected in utero or during or following parturition.
* Complete or partial failure of transfer of maternal antibodies is common in foals infected postpartum.
* The most common pathogens are *E. coli, K. pneumoniae,* and *A. equuli.*

Clinical signs and diagnosis

* Clinical signs may be vague.
  * The respiratory rate and effort can be normal; lung sounds can range from quiet to increased, and a cough rarely is present.
  * Some septic foals are normothermic on presentation.
* The most common sign is some degree of weakness and lethargy.
* The diagnostic plan should include CBC, arterial blood gas analysis, thoracic radiographs, blood cultures, and measurement of blood glucose and serum IgG.
  * An increase in band neutrophils and toxic changes are suggestive of septicemia.
  * Affected foals are hypoxemic, hypercapnic, and acidotic.
  * Hypoglycemia is common in septicemic foals <24 hours old.
  * Some degree of failure of passive transfer almost always is present in these foals.
* Radiographic findings are similar to those in foals with immature lungs, including increased interstitial patterns and loss of vascular clarity; consolidation of individual lung lobes (accessory lobe) may be evident.

Treatment

* Oxygen supplementation is needed to correct hypoxemia.
* Broad-spectrum antimicrobials should be used until culture results are obtained.
* Fluid therapy should consist of 5% dextrose for hypoglycemia, plasma transfusions to correct failure of pas-

sive transfer, and lactated Ringer's solution for volume expansion.
- Sodium bicarbonate is commonly used to treat the metabolic acidosis but should be used with caution because it can cause hypercapnia.
- General nursing care is essential for successful treatment.

Pneumocystis carinii Infection

Pneumocystis carinii is a ubiquitous sporozoan that causes interstitial pneumonia in humans. There have been sporadic reports of infection in foals, in association with either *R. equi* or *B. bronchiseptica*. Clinical signs reflect the bacterial pneumonia. Diagnosis is often made only at necropsy, although lung and endobronchial aspirates could be helpful. The antimicrobial of choice is trimethoprim-sulfamethoxazole at 30 mg/kg bid. Aerosolized pentamidine could be beneficial. It is important to appropriately treat the primary disease.

Parascaris equorum Infection

Larvae of the roundworm *Parascaris equorum* migrate through the lungs of foals and young horses.
- Infection typically causes mild pneumonia and coughing in foals 2 to 4 months old, characterized by:
  - the presence of eosinophils but no evidence of sepsis in transtracheal aspirates
  - no exposure to donkeys, which are a potential reservoir of *Dictyocaulus arnfieldi*
  - favorable response to fenbendazole, 15 mg/kg daily for 5 days
- Foals infected at a young age cough, have a mucoid or mucopurulent nasal discharge for about 10 days, and sometimes are tachypneic; they remain afebrile unless secondary infection occurs.
  - Copious exudate may be seen on endoscopic examination of the trachea.
- Horses infected at 8 to 10 months of age develop a cough, hyperpnea, inappetence, depression, and a serous/mucoid nasal discharge, and they lose condition.
- Diagnosis is difficult and often is based on ruling out other causes of respiratory disease.

- The presence of eosinophils in transtracheal aspirates without evidence of sepsis support the diagnosis.
- Fecal examination for ascarid eggs may not be helpful, because clinical signs occur before egg laying begins.
- The disease usually is self-limiting, so treatment may not be necessary.
  - Ivermectin and larvicidal doses of fenbendazole (60 mg/kg) may be effective.

Dictyocaulus arnfieldi Infection

The equine lungworm, *Dictyocaulus arnfieldi,* causes respiratory disease that is clinically indistinguishable from chronic obstructive pulmonary disease (see below). Infection occurs in horses pastured with donkeys, mules, or asses. Signs in horses are seen in autumn, following midsummer exposure; the reservoir hosts remain asymptomatic.

Diagnosis
- Patent infections are uncommon in horses, so Baermann fecal flotation is unreliable (although it usually is reliable in donkeys, mules, and asses).
- Diagnosis often is based on clinical signs of severe coughing and obstructive lung disease that begin in late summer or autumn after exposure to one of the reservoir hosts.
- Eosinophils in a transtracheal aspirate are strongly suggestive, but not diagnostic, of parasitism; rarely, the larvae or adults may be found in the transtracheal wash fluid.

Prophylaxis and treatment
- Horses should be housed with donkeys, mules, or asses only when the weather is very cold.
- Thiabendazole (440 mg/kg/day for 2 days) is effective in horses, although side effects include transient anorexia and fever.
  - Oral mebendazole at 15 to 20 mg/kg/day for 5 days decreases worm burdens and larval counts in donkeys.
- Currently, ivermectin is the drug of choice.

Chronic Obstructive Pulmonary Disease

Chronic obstructive pulmonary disease (COPD) is a complex syndrome.

- Clinical signs range from exercise intolerance in performance horses to expiratory dyspnea, cough, and weight loss (i.e., chronic "respiratory cripples").
- COPD is common in climates where horses are stabled and fed hay for long periods; it is uncommon in young horses, and the incidence increases with age.
- The predominant lesion is widespread bronchiolitis.
- The etiology is complex and incompletely understood, but appears to primarily involve an allergic response to environmental antigens (e.g., hay dust and molds).
  - Development of COPD often follows a viral respiratory tract infection.
  - There may be a genetic predisposition for COPD.

Clinical signs

- Signs may be apparent only during exercise, with affected horses not performing adequately.
- In other horses, signs include chronic intermittent cough (dry or productive), intermittent purulent nasal discharge (especially after exercise), and expiratory dyspnea.
- Signs usually are intermittent but may become continuous as the disease progresses.
- Increased expiratory effort eventually results in abdominal muscle hypertrophy (heave line).

Diagnosis

- *Historic information* is important when evaluating horses with COPD.
  - In many cases, the disease is seasonal, increasing when horses are housed indoors and fed hay; in the southern United States, signs may worsen during the late summer (see discussion of summer pasture–associated obstructive pulmonary disease).
  - Signs may develop after feeding a new batch of hay or moving the horse to a new barn.
  - In some horses, signs become apparent following a viral respiratory infection from which the horse never fully recovers.
  - Exposure to aerosolized irritants, such as ammonia fumes, dust, or

pollutants, exacerbates airway obstruction in affected horses.
- In severe cases, a presumptive diagnosis may be based on the history and clinical signs.
- When COPD causes only a decrease in exercise tolerance, auscultation findings often are normal.
  - The earliest abnormalities often are louder than normal expiratory sounds and wheezing at the end of exhalation.
  - Auscultation is only qualitative; it is not indicative of the severity of lung disease.
- In advanced cases, percussion may reveal caudoventral enlargement of the percussible lung field and more resonant sounds, suggestive of pulmonary hyperinflation.
- *Endoscopic examination* is an important diagnostic aid, especially in mildly affected horses.
  - Usually, the upper airway is normal, although exudate from the trachea may coat the pharynx.
  - Introduction of the endoscope into the trachea may induce coughing, suggesting a hyperirritable airway; yellow viscous material often is present in the trachea.
  - When examined, the central airways do not appear inflamed but contain exudate.
- *Thoracic radiographs* simply reveal a mixed pattern of radiodensity throughout the lung field, but they can be helpful in ruling out other causes of dyspnea.
- *Transtracheal aspiration* has some value in distinguishing COPD from parasitic lung disease (in which the tracheal cell population contains a large percentage of eosinophils), but cytologic findings correlate poorly with the lower airway cell population.
- *Bronchoalveolar lavage* cytologic findings correlate well with histopathologic scores in horses with COPD.
  - Clinically affected horses have marked elevations in the neutrophil percentage (see discussion of collection of airway secretions), but this is not pathognomonic for COPD.

- Cytologic findings in horses and ponies in clinical remission may be normal.
- Measurement of arterial oxygen tension (PaO_2) is the simplest and often the most helpful test of pulmonary function (see discussion of other diagnostic procedures).

Treatment

- The most important aim of therapy is to prevent exposure to environmental allergens.
  - The optimal environment is a pasture with shelter against inclement weather.
  - If pasture is not available, the horse should be housed in a well-ventilated barn with access to the outside; improving ventilation alone is insufficient.
  - Hay and bedding are the main sources of airborne dust; pelleted feed or haylage should be substituted for hay, and horses should be bedded on moist wood shavings or clay.
  - *Drug therapy without these management changes inevitably has poor results.*
- In racehorses with mild COPD, rest is an important part of therapy.
- Corticosteroids reduce the inflammatory response and resolve signs of COPD.
  - However, side effects are potentially serious and may become apparent weeks after initiation of therapy; sudden withdrawal may result in adrenal insufficiency.
  - Prednisone is administered orally every other morning at 1 to 2 mg/kg; after 2 weeks the response is assessed and the dosage gradually reduced to the minimum effective level.
- Bronchodilators are most effective when delivered by aerosol.
- Cromolyn sodium (200 to 300 mg by aerosol) can be effective prophylactically, if given before exercise or exposure to allergens.

Summer Pasture–Associated Obstructive Pulmonary Disease

This condition is a recurrent disease that occurs in pastured horses during the summer months in the southern United States. Affected horses develop signs indistinguishable from those of COPD.

Clinical signs improve markedly during winter months, whether horses are fed hay or remain on pasture, but signs recur each summer. Treatment is directed toward preventing exposure to the offending environment. Horses should be stabled and fed a diet of hay or pelleted feed.

Granulomatous Pneumonia

Clinical signs of granulomatous pneumonia can be similar to those of COPD. Affected horses may have weight loss and fever; careful auscultation reveals wheezes and, possibly, dull areas (large fibrotic masses or pleural effusion). Unlike cases of COPD, the wheezes persist and do not decrease following bronchodilation with IV glycopyrrolate (Robinul, 2 mg per 450-kg horse). Thoracic radiography is most helpful in diagnosis, revealing focal increases in lung density. Treatment generally is unrewarding.

Chronic fungal infections

Coccidioidomycosis, histoplasmosis, cryptococcosis, and aspergillosis can each cause chronic pulmonary disease and cachexia. None of these conditions is common in horses. Coccidioidomycosis appears to be the most common in the United States. It is a multisystemic disease of desert areas. The most common signs are weight loss and chronic cough; other signs include musculoskeletal pain, superficial abscessation, intermittent fever, and abdominal pain. Thoracic radiographs often reveal increased interstitial density, pleural fluid accumulation and, in some cases, irregular pulmonary infiltrates or displacement of airways by soft tissue masses. Serology aids diagnosis.

NEOPLASIA

Pulmonary Neoplasia

Primary lung tumors are extremely rare in horses. The most prevalent is myoblastoma, which may be evident on endoscopic examination of the airways as a nodular mass. Tumors that may metastasize to the lung include squamous cell carcinoma, lymphosarcoma, and hemangiosarcoma. Clinical signs of pulmonary neoplasia are nonspecific and include weight loss, coughing, purulent nasal discharge, and dyspnea. Thoracic radiographs, bronchoscopy, and lung biopsy may be required for definitive diagnosis. Treatment usually is unrewarding.

IDIOPATHIC DISEASES
Exercise-Induced Pulmonary Hemorrhage

Exercise-induced pulmonary hemorrhage (EIPH) is bleeding from the pulmonary vasculature as a consequence of the cardiopulmonary changes during exercise. Currently, the most favored hypothesis involves "stress failure" of the pulmonary capillaries as a result of the high transmural capillary pressures generated during intense exercise. Other postulated causes or possible contributing factors include chronic lung disease, partial upper airway obstruction, defects in hemostasis, abnormalities in RBC deformability, parasitic infestation, blood-borne pathogens, and excessive mechanical stresses within the pulmonary parenchyma during exercise.

Incidence and impact

- Epistaxis is reported in only 0.25% to 2.5% of racehorses, but studies using endoscopy and/or bronchoalveolar lavage indicate that the incidence of EIPH approaches 100% in racehorses.
  - EIPH is evident cytologically in some yearlings, but it is more common once horses begin athletic training, and its frequency increases with age.
- EIPH also occurs in other horses that perform strenuous exercise, such as eventing and polo.
- The true impact of EIPH on athletic performance remains controversial.
  - Mild episodes apparently have little or no effect on race performance, but horses with epistaxis and those that pull up in a race clearly suffer a reduction in performance.

Diagnosis

- *Endoscopic evaluation* should be performed 30 to 120 minutes after exercise.

- Most "bleeders" have blood in the trachea by 60 minutes after exercise, but if no blood is found and EIPH is highly suspected, endoscopic examination should be repeated.
- *Tracheobronchial aspirates* contain hemosiderophages (macrophages with intracytoplasmic hemosiderin) in horses with EIPH.
  - However, hemosiderophages may also be found in cases of pleuropneumonia, pulmonary abscessation or neoplasia, and thoracic trauma.
  - Hemosiderophages can persist for at least 150 days following an episode of EIPH.
- *Radiography* is of little value; most affected horses show only a slight bronchointerstitial pattern and, occasionally, increased opacity in the dorsocaudal lung.
- *Scintigraphic evaluation* may be useful for determining the severity of ventilation-perfusion mismatching and thus the possible impact on athletic performance.

Treatment and prevention

Prophylactic strategies are aimed at improving "lung health" and reducing pulmonary capillary hypertension.

- Decreasing the environmental allergen load is important and is accomplished by increasing pasture turnout time, bedding stalls with shavings or paper, and feeding pelleted rations and/or haylage.
- Routine vaccination and deworming also help to minimize pulmonary disease.
- Furosemide currently is the most popular drug used for prevention and treatment.
  - Many racing commissions allow it to be administered at dosages of 150 to 300 mg IV several hours before a race.

Interstitial Pneumonia in Foals

Interstitial lung disease primarily affects foals between 3 days and 6 months of age.

- The cause is unknown, but may involve viral infections, pneumotoxins (such as *Perilla frutescens*, pyrrolizidine alkaloids, and endotoxin), or allergic disease.

• Interstitial pneumonia is characterized by marked respiratory distress.
  • Affected foals have both inspiratory and expiratory dyspnea, but appear bright and alert.
  • There is no purulent nasal discharge.
  • Heart rate, respiratory rate, and rectal temperature are elevated, and auscultation reveals loud breath sounds; crackles and wheezes develop as the foal responds to therapy.
• Thoracic radiography shows a modest, diffuse increase in interstitial lung density.
• Transtracheal lavage yields fluid with low cellularity and a normal differential cell count; bacterial culture fails to yield pathogenic organisms.
• Each of these findings (clinical, radiographic, cytologic, and bacteriologic) help to differentiate interstitial from bacterial pneumonia.
• Therapy mainly is supportive, although corticosteroids appear to be important for a successful outcome; some foals require oxygen therapy or mechanical ventilation.
• Secondary bacterial pathogens must be identified by tracheobronchial culture and treated accordingly.
• The prognosis always is very guarded; those that survive tend to be older foals with a more gradual onset of signs.

Diseases of the Pleura, Mediastinum, Diaphragm, and Thoracic Wall (553-560)

Ralph E. Beadle and Mary Rose Paradis

DISEASES WITH PHYSICAL CAUSES
Thoracic Wall Trauma
Thoracic wall trauma may result in subcutaneous emphysema, pleuritis, pneumothorax, hemothorax, pneumomediastinum, or diaphragmatic hernia. Skin and muscle lacerations are managed using standard surgical techniques; simple rib fractures can

be managed conservatively. "Flail chest" (multiple rib fractures, resulting in destabilization of the chest wall) can be stabilized using an external fixation device.

Management of penetrating wounds
Patient stabilization is the primary consideration with wounds that enter the pleural cavity:
• Air in the pleural space must be removed and further entrance of air prevented.
• Ideally, the pleural space should be surgically explored and flushed with balanced electrolyte solutions, under general anesthesia with positive-pressure ventilation.
  • Alternatively, the pleural space can be flushed in the standing horse.
• Broad-spectrum antibiotics should be given for at least 7 days.
• With thoracic trauma caudal to the sixth rib, the abdominal cavity should be carefully evaluated; depending on the injury, abdominocentesis, ultrasonography, laparoscopy, or exploratory celiotomy may be indicated

Diaphragmatic Hernia
Diaphragmatic hernia is uncommon in horses; it may be congenital or acquired.
• Colic is the primary presenting complaint.
• Often the history reveals either a previous bout of strenuous exercise or a traumatic incident, such as running into a stationary object or taking a hard fall.
  • Pregnant or recently parturient mares also are at risk for diaphragmatic hernias.
• Auscultation of the thorax may be unrewarding; borborygmi in the thorax is common in normal horses, and ventral dullness may or may not be present.
• Percussion of the thorax may not reveal abnormalities; hernias involving large amounts of viscera are more likely to cause percussion abnormalities.
• Radiography is an excellent way to detect viscera in the thorax, although in most field situations thoracic radiography is possible only in foals.

- Ultrasonography is rewarding only if solid viscera (liver, spleen) are against the chest wall.
- Thoracocentesis can be diagnostic when the entrapped viscera become devitalized.
- Diaphragmatic herniorrhaphy is difficult in adult horses, so horses with symptomatic diaphragmatic hernias do not have a good prognosis.

Pneumothorax in Adult Horses

Unilateral pneumothorax is well tolerated in most horses. However, the thin, fenestrated caudal mediastinum predisposes to bilateral pneumothorax, which is life-threatening. Air may enter the pleural space from severely diseased lung (e.g., gangrenous pneumonia, emphysema) or trauma.

Clinical signs and diagnosis

- Horses with small amounts of air on one side of the thorax may not show any signs.
- Those with larger amounts of air in the pleural space(s) show respiratory distress (tachypnea, nostril flaring, cyanosis).
- Auscultation reveals less pronounced sounds on the affected side.
  - Bubbling sounds may be heard if air is escaping ventral to a fluid line.
- Ultrasonography reveals that there is no lung tissue against the thoracic wall.
- Radiographs reveal collapse of the lung.
- Pneumothorax can be confirmed most easily by thoracocentesis.

Treatment

Severe pneumothorax is an emergency—air should be removed from the pleural space as quickly as possible.

- This can be accomplished with a needle attached to a stopcock and syringe or with a vacuum device attached to a large-bore trocar catheter.
  - Less severe cases can be treated by attaching a unidirectional airflow device to a thoracic drainage tube.
- The needle or catheter is advanced through aseptically prepared and desensitized skin, in the sixth or seventh intercostal space.

Pneumothorax in Neonates

Pneumothorax is uncommon in neonatal foals.

- It generally is a sequela to trauma during birth.
- The foal can appear normal at birth and stand and nurse without difficulty.
- Increased respiratory rate and effort may be the first signs of distress; the foal's breathing pattern may become irregular.
- Auscultation may reveal increased harshness over the cranioventral areas (atelectasis); sounds may be absent over the dorsal regions (free air).
- Diagnosis is based on auscultation and radiographic findings.
- Treatment involves thoracocentesis (in the caudodorsal corner of the lung field in the standing foal) repeated every 12 to 24 hours until the problem resolves.
  - Small air leaks usually seal within a few days.
- The prognosis is good if the condition is uncomplicated by other problems.

Hydrothorax

Hydrothorax can be caused by congestive right heart failure, hypoproteinemia, thoracic lymphosarcoma, rupture of the thoracic duct, or thoracic wall trauma.

- Horses with hydrothorax may not exhibit clinical signs.
- Auscultation and percussion reveal a fluid line if the effusion is voluminous.
- Thoracocentesis reveals an increased amount of pleural fluid with low cellularity and protein content.
- Treatment involves draining excess fluid from the pleural space and addressing the cause.

Hemothorax

Hemothorax is uncommon in horses. It most often results from trauma to the thoracic wall or lung; tearing of pleural adhesions can also cause hemothorax. Ventral compression atelectasis and hemorrhagic shock can result if large amounts of blood are lost over a short period.

Clinical signs and diagnosis

- Findings vary with the rate and amount of blood loss.
  - Horses with a ruptured major vessel such as the aorta have massive amounts of blood in the pleural space (and/or pericardium) and rapidly die.
  - Involvement of other vessels usually is less dramatic.
- Tachycardia and tachypnea may result from anemia; tachypnea without tachycardia results from compression atelectasis.
- Auscultation and percussion reveal a fluid line when moderate to large amounts of blood pool in the pleural space.
- Thoracocentesis confirms hemothorax.

Treatment

- Treatment should be directed toward correcting the cause of hemorrhage, if possible.
- IV balanced electrolyte solutions are used to treat hypovolemic shock (see Chapter 5, Critical Care Medicine).
- If large volumes of blood are lost (PCV approaching 10%), blood transfusion is necessary.
  - Provided it is uncontaminated, blood from the pleural space may be autotransfused.

INFLAMMATORY, INFECTIOUS, AND IMMUNE DISEASES

Bacterial Pleuritis

Pleuritis (inflammation of the pleura) may be acute or chronic and unilateral or bilateral. Pleural effusion often is associated with pleuritis, but it does not necessarily signify pleuritis. Horses with infectious pleuritis usually have a history of a recent stressful event, such as long-distance hauling, vigorous athletic activity, or general anesthesia. Most cases of pleuritis are secondary to, and an extension of, pneumonia (viral or bacterial). Some cases are idiopathic.

Clinical signs

- Early cases of pleuritis are characterized by pain from inflammation of the parietal pleura; affected horses restrict thoracic wall movement.
  - As effusion develops, pain subsides but compressive atelectasis interferes with respiration.
  - As the condition progresses, fibrinopurulent exudate accumulates and may organize into adhesions between the lung and parietal pleura, which also restricts ventilation.
- Severely affected horses are depressed, have an anxious facial expression, and resent thoracic palpation; some are cachectic and have edema in the pectoral region.
- Respiratory rate, rhythm, and character are variable.
  - Mildly affected horses with no pleural effusion may show no abnormalities.
  - Those with intense pleural pain but no effusion may have rapid, shallow respiration marked by limited thoracic wall movement and an enhanced abdominal component; they may grunt while breathing.
  - Those with marked pleural effusion also have rapid, shallow respiration but usually have freer thoracic wall movement and fewer signs of thoracic pain; their nostrils flare markedly during inspiration, but abdominal breathing is not so marked.
- Horses with intense pleural pain stand with their elbows abducted and are reluctant to move.
  - These signs may mimic laminitis, but hoof tester examination of the feet is negative (although laminitis may develop later in the disease).
  - Intense pleural pain may also manifest as colic.
- Mucous membrane color and perfusion usually are unchanged in early cases of pleuritis.
  - As the condition progresses, the mucous membranes can become either cyanotic or injected, and capillary refill time increases.
- Pulse rates usually are increased as a result of pain initially and hypoxemia later.
- Most horses with pleuritis have a fever.

Diagnosis

• *Auscultation* may be unremarkable in horses with little or no pleural effusion.
  • Pleural friction sounds are very uncommon but are most likely in noneffusive cases; their absence does not rule out pleuritis.
  • In horses with effusive pleuritis, auscultation often reveals distinct lung sounds dorsal to the fluid line but muffled or inaudible sounds ventral to this line; crackles or wheezes may be detectable dorsally.
• *Percussion* may reveal pain, most readily elicited dorsally, and loss of resonance ventrally.
• *Hematologic examination* may show neutropenia in peracute cases; subacute and chronic cases show neutrophilia ± left shift.
  • The PCV may be normal, elevated, or decreased, depending on the presence or absence of dehydration and anemia of chronic disease.
  • Plasma fibrinogen and monocyte counts usually are elevated.
• *Ultrasonography* is useful for evaluating the pleural space; pleural fluid volume, number and size of fibrin tags, amount of loculation, and abscess formation can be determined.
  • Free gas echoes within the pleural fluid (a sensitive and specific indicator of anaerobic infection) may also be detected.
  • Ultrasonography also is useful for identifying sites for thoracic drainage.
• *Radiography* is best used to detect pulmonary disease once excess pleural fluid is removed.
• *Pleuroscopy* is reserved for evaluation of horses with chronic pleuritis and extensive areas of organized fibrin within the pleural space.

Thoracocentesis is an important aid.

• Fluid can be collected at the sixth or seventh intercostal space, just dorsal to the costochondral junction, or elsewhere as indicated by sonographic findings.
  • Aseptic surgical technique and infiltration of the skin, intercostal tissues, and parietal pleura with local anesthetic should be used.
  • An IV catheter, teat cannula, or bitch urinary catheter can be used; a syringe and/or three-way stopcock are attached to the catheter or cannula.
  • The catheter should be placed just cranial to the rib to avoid intercostal vessels and the accompanying nerve.
  • *Both sides of the thorax should be tapped.*
• Collected fluid is observed for color, turbidity, and odor.
  • Normal pleural fluid is yellow and clear; increased turbidity suggests increased numbers of WBC and the presence of fibrin.
  • A fetid odor suggests anaerobic infection, necrotizing pneumonia, or abscessation.
• The fluid should be Gram's stained and cultured for both aerobic and anaerobic bacteria.
  • Culture from each side of the thorax is essential.
  • Antibiotic sensitivities should be determined for all isolates.
  • A tracheobronchial aspirate also should be cultured; sometimes organisms are recovered from the tracheobronchial aspirate but not from the pleural fluid.
• Cytologic examination and measurement of protein content should be performed on the fluid.
  • Total WBC counts and protein concentrations of pleural fluid from normal horses are <10,000/µL and <2.5 g/dL, respectively; infectious pleuritis causes these values to rise.
  • Neutrophils are the predominant cell and may be degenerate or contain bacteria.
• Measurement of glucose concentration, pH, and LDH can be useful in revealing the presence of bacterial infections in pleural fluid.
  • A glucose concentration ≤40 mg/dL, an LDH concentration >1000 IU/L, and a pH <7.1 indicate a septic exudate.

Treatment

Treatment is dictated by the severity and duration of the disease.

- Antimicrobial agents should be chosen based on culture and sensitivity results.
  - Penicillin and trimethoprim-sulfonamide or penicillin-gentamicin combinations give a good spectrum of coverage initially.
  - If specific therapy is needed for anaerobes, metronidazole can be given at 7.5 to 15 mg/kg PO q6h.
  - Rifampin at 5 to 10 mg/kg q12h is worth considering for both gram-positive cocci and gram-negative organisms.
- *Drainage of fluid from the affected pleural space is extremely important.*
  - Drainage can be accomplished by inserting a no. 28 French trocar catheter into the pleural space, being careful to avoid the lateral thoracic vein and major structures in the thorax.
  - Use of a Heimlich chest drain valve allows drainage and prevents aspiration of air through the catheter.
  - Intermittent drainage of fluid pockets using ultrasound guidance is helpful when the indwelling cannula stops draining fluid.
- IV fluid therapy is mandatory in many horses with pleuritis.
  - Total protein should be monitored frequently, because some patients become very hypoproteinemic.
- If pain is causing anorexia, NSAIDs, such as phenylbutazone and flunixin, should be used; however, these drugs mask fever and can cause renal damage in dehydrated horses.
- Systemic heparin may be used at 20,000 U q12h to decrease fibrin formation within the pleural space and protect against laminitis; efficacy is questionable, however.
- Lavage may be attempted if the pleural fluid contains large numbers of bacteria and free fibrin.
  - Sterile, warm, isotonic, pH-buffered, calcium-free fluid is infused through a sterile no. 28 French trocar catheter in the ventral aspect of the thoracic wall.
  - The rate of administration is best determined from changes in the respiratory pattern; when the respiratory rate is >40 breaths/min with inspiratory nostril flare, fluid administration should be discontinued and fluid in the thorax allowed to drain.
- Thoracotomy is a salvage procedure for horses with chronic pleuritis and associated abscesses.
- Good supportive care is essential for a successful outcome.
  - This includes providing good-quality feed and water, leg wraps, frog supports (front feet), and short walks several times a day.
  - Silastic or other long-term catheters should be used to decrease the incidence of thrombophlebitis.

Prognosis

- Horses with pleural pain but no pleural effusion have a good prognosis if they are rested and treated appropriately.
- The prognosis with pleural effusion is guarded, although early and aggressive medical therapy can result in excellent long-term survival rates.
  - Complications include abscess formation, cranial thoracic masses, bronchopleural fistulas, pericarditis, laminitis, and thrombophlebitis.
- Chronic bacterial pleuritis warrants a poor prognosis and is expensive to treat.
- A grave prognosis should be given to horses that are toxemic and develop laminitis.

Mediastinal Abscesses

Mediastinal abscesses are the result of bacterial seeding of mediastinal lymph nodes. β-Hemolytic streptococci frequently are involved in young horses.

Clinical signs and diagnosis

- Horses with mediastinal abscesses usually exhibit fever, inappetence, neutrophilia, and elevated plasma fibrinogen.
- Some affected horses are in good condition, but others become very unthrifty.
- Cranial mediastinal abscesses often cause swelling at the thoracic inlet and may impinge on the trachea, esophagus, and great vessels.

- Affected horses may show respiratory distress, signs of choke, or apparent right heart failure (jugular distention and pectoral, thoracic limb, neck, and head edema).
- Physical examination often reveals no abnormalities if the abscesses involve lymph nodes in the middle and caudal mediastinum.
- Thoracic radiographs reveal enlarged lymph nodes, which can be mistaken for lung abscesses.

Treatment

- Involved lymph nodes should be surgically drained, if possible.
- Culture and sensitivity results should be used to direct antimicrobial choice.

NEOPLASIA

Thoracic Lymphosarcoma

Lymphosarcoma is uncommon in horses.

- Most cases are seen in middle-age horses, but the condition has been reported in horses as young as 2 years of age.
- Thoracic lymphosarcoma usually causes pleural effusion.
  - Weight loss, anorexia, depression, pectoral edema, respiratory distress, jugular distention, and exercise intolerance are common signs.

- Other findings variably include fever, dysphagia, colic, and diarrhea.
- Disease progression usually is quite rapid once signs appear.

Diagnosis

- *Thoracocentesis* yields copious pleural fluid, which may be blood tinged.
  - The protein concentration is elevated, although lower than that seen with pleuritis, and lymphocytes usually are the predominant cell (rather than neutrophils).
  - Many of the lymphocytes may be bizarre and have mitotic figures.
- *Abdominocentesis* should be attempted if a diagnostic sample cannot be obtained from the thoracic cavity; lymphoblasts sometimes are obtained from the abdominal cavity but not from the pleural space in horses with thoracic lymphosarcoma.
- *Hematologic results* usually do not reveal lymphocytosis or abnormal circulating lymphocytes, but may show anemia, leukopenia, and neutrophilia.
  - Hypercalcemia has been reported in horses with lymphosarcoma.

Glucocorticoids and chemotherapy offer potential avenues for therapy.

10

Alimentary System

Examination of the Alimentary System

(pages 575-580)

Stephen B. Adams

PHYSICAL EXAMINATION

A thorough physical examination should be performed on each horse showing signs of gastrointestinal disease, and should include:

* *visual inspection* for obvious abnormalities such as icterus, jugular swelling (esophageal obstruction), abdominal distention, and fecal staining of the perineum and tail
* complete *oral examination* in horses with obvious oral abnormalities, facial or mandibular swellings, quidding, excessive salivation, dysphagia, hemorrhage from the mouth, head shaking, or malodorous breath

Auscultation

The abdomen should be ausculted on every horse exhibiting colic, diarrhea, bloat, anorexia, weight loss, or any other sign referable to the alimentary system. At least three areas on each side of the abdomen should be examined. Simultaneous auscultation and percussion can identify tympanitic (gas-filled) viscera.

Auscultable abnormalities

Following are some common auscultable abnormalities:

* Absence of the periodic "gushing" sound on the right side (fluid entering the cecum from the ileum) suggests small intestinal obstruction or cecal impaction.

* High-pitched tinkling sounds in the colon indicate tympany.
  * .High-pitched sound or "ping" may also be heard on simultaneous auscultation and percussion.
* Loud, rumbling borborygmi are associated with spasmodic colic.
  * Increased borborygmi may also be auscultated during the early stages of enteritis.
* Sand accumulation in the colon can sound like sand being poured onto a sand pile.
* Reduction or absence of peristaltic sounds may be caused by ileus, ischemic bowel damage, shock and poor intestinal perfusion, high sympathetic tone, or drugs that inhibit motility.

NASOGASTRIC INTUBATION

A nasogastric tube should be passed in all horses exhibiting colic, to remove fluid and gas that may have accumulated in the stomach. Passage of a nasogastric tube also is useful for detecting obstruction of the pharynx or esophagus (choke). Nasogastric decompression is discussed in the section on diseases of the stomach.

RECTAL EXAMINATION

Rectal examination is one of the most important procedures for evaluation of the gastrointestinal system in horses. It should be performed in all horses with colic, chronic diarrhea, or weight loss. The technique is described in *Equine Medicine and Surgery V.*

Normal Structures

Structures that usually can be palpated in healthy horses include:

- *rectum* (feces should be evacuated before proceeding further with the examination)
- *female genital organs or male accessory sex organs* (see Chapter 12, Reproductive System: The Stallion, and Chapter 13, Reproductive System: The Mare)
- *bladder*
- *inguinal canals:* located approximately 1 handwidth lateral to the midline and cranioventral to the pelvis
- *small colon:* contains fecal balls and lies centrally in the caudal abdomen; normally 5 to 8 cm (2 to 3 inches) in diameter, with prominent sacculations and antimesenteric band
- *left ventral and left dorsal colon:* the ventral colon has sacculations and bands; the dorsal colon often is medial to the ventral colon
- *pelvic flexure:* palpable in the left caudoventral abdomen or midline on the abdominal floor; it normally is soft and compressible
- *spleen:* palpable on the left side, against the abdominal wall at the level of the last rib; the caudodorsal aspect has a sharp caudal edge
- *nephrosplenic ligament and caudal pole of the left kidney:* the hand should pass unimpeded from the spleen across the nephrosplenic ligament to the caudal pole of the left kidney
- *root of the mesentery (containing the cranial mesenteric artery and its branches), aorta, and iliac arteries:* the mesenteric root is located medial and slightly cranial to the caudal pole of the left kidney
- *right dorsal colon:* may be palpable in small horses directly cranial to and to the right of the mesenteric root
- *cecum:* the ventral band is palpable on the right side as it runs obliquely from caudodorsal to cranioventral; the medial cecal band may also be identified in small horses

- The dorsal attachment of the cecum can be identified along the right dorsal body wall, but the hand cannot pass dorsal to the cecum.
- The base and body are most identifiable when the cecum is distended with gas or ingesta.

Loops of small intestine are not palpable in normal horses.

Abnormalities Detected by Rectal Examination

Following are the more common or important abnormalities that may be detected by rectal examination:

- *anus:* lacerations, neoplasms, parasites, rectal prolapse
- *rectum:* rectovestibular/vaginal lacerations, rectal tears, perirectal abscess
  - The feces should be examined for blood, mucus, and sand.
- *inguinal rings:* incarceration of small intestine (stallions)
- *small colon:* impaction, enteroliths, and fecoliths, volvulus, rupture of the mesocolon (causes blood-tinged, tar-colored mucus or rectal mucosa)
- *uterus:* uterine torsion (crossed broad ligaments are palpable)
- *small intestine:* distention with gas or fluid
  - Moderate fluid distention but no taut or painful mesentery suggests enteritis.
  - Infarcted sections of bowel often are thickened and edematous.
  - Intussusceptions can be palpated as bowel that is thick and turgid (feels like a sausage).
  - Impactions of the ileum can be palpated to the right of midline.
- *pelvic flexure:* impaction (firm, doughy mass that can be indented with finger pressure)
- *large colon:* sand impaction (often has a gritty texture), malposition/displacement, obstruction, volvulus or torsion (extreme gas distention and very taut bands)
- *spleen:* nodules and other surface irregularities, splenomegaly, caudal or medial displacement
- *nephrosplenic space:* entrapment of the left colons (left dorsal displacement)

- **root of the mesentery:** enlarged mesenteric lymph nodes (neoplasia, lymphadenitis, abscessation), verminous arteritis (thickened arteries, fremitus)
- **right dorsal colon:** impaction
  - Large enteroliths; enteroliths in the transverse colon sometimes can be bumped with the fingertips but not grasped with the hand.
- **cecum:** cecal impaction (firm, doughy mass), ileocecal intussusception
  - When a distended organ is felt in the right caudal quadrant, has a distinct tenia without vessels or mesocolon, and is attached to the dorsal body wall, it most likely is the cecum.
  - The ileum is difficult to palpate unless impacted or intussuscepted; ileal impaction feels like a firm tube that sweeps to the medial base of the cecum.
  - Distended duodenum may be palpated around the caudal base of the cecum.
- **peritoneum:** adhesions, nodules, roughening, gritty surfaces, painful

---

Ancillary Diagnostic Aids *(pages 580-590)*
Stephen B. Adams and Janice E. Sojka

ENDOSCOPY

Endoscopy is useful for identifying or investigating the following abnormalities:

- **nasopharynx:** dysphagia and nasal or oral discharge
- **esophagus:** esophageal foreign bodies, ulceration, inflammation, diverticula, stricture, and perforations
- **stomach:** gastric ulceration, parasitism, neoplasia, and pyloric stenosis
  - The opening of the common bile duct can sometimes be visualized within the duodenal ampulla, and duodenal biopsies may be taken.
- **rectum and terminal small colon:** rectal masses, tears, or other abnor-

malities palpated *per rectum;* endoscopy also is useful for taking biopsies of rectal mucosa

DIAGNOSTIC IMAGING
Radiography

Radiography is most useful in evaluating the teeth, oral cavity, and esophagus. Following are some abnormalities that may be evaluated radiographically:

- **teeth and skull:** tooth root abscesses, congenital anomalies, maxillary or mandibular fractures, bony tumors or cysts, pharyngeal or retropharyngeal abscesses
- **esophagus:** megaesophagus, choke, stenosis, traumatic rupture, diverticula
  - Lesions are best imaged when barium is given to delineate the esophageal margins.
- **stomach:** stenosis, ulceration, partial torsion
  - Positive (barium) and negative (air) contrast studies increase the diagnostic potential.
- **small and large intestine:** radiography is of limited value in animals >350 kg (770 lb) body weight
  - In neonatal foals, intestinal distention may indicate ileus or atresia.
  - Barium per os or per rectum helps identify intestinal atresia and meconium impaction.
- **ventral abdomen:** enteroliths located in the ventral abdomen, sand impaction

Ultrasonography

The liver, spleen, and gut wall may be imaged percutaneously and evaluated for location, size, shape, and texture. Other uses of abdominal ultrasonography include:

- identification and evaluation of fluid, fibrin, and masses in the abdomen
- guidance for abdominocentesis and percutaneous biopsy of the liver and abdominal masses
- evaluation of intestinal motility
- evaluation of umbilical structures in young foals

Intestinal tract

Ultrasonography of the intestinal tract generally is limited to the following instances:

* **gastric squamous cell carcinoma:** an area of homogeneous tissue separates the spleen and liver from the stomach lumen
* **gastric ulcer disease in foals:** the duodenum (seen between the right liver lobe and the right dorsal colon) may appear enlarged and fluid-filled
* **ileus:** lack of movement of either the intestinal wall or ingesta
* **adhesions:** may be indicated by a localized segment of immobile intestine
* **small intestinal intussusception in foals:** cross-section of a portion of thickened bowel reveals a "bull's eye" pattern of concentric circles
* **left dorsal displacement of the large colon in horses** (nephrosplenic entrapment)

Scintigraphy

Recently, scintigraphy has been used to identify delayed gastric emptying in horses. The radionuclide is administered via nasogastric tube or fed in sweet feed. Abdominal images are taken immediately and periodically for 3 hours after administration.

CLINICAL PATHOLOGY TESTS

There are few clinical pathologic findings that are specific for intestinal disease. Results must be integrated with the history, physical examination findings, and clinical course.

Complete Blood Count (CBC)

No changes in the CBC are specific for intestinal disease.

* PCV increases with dehydration (e.g., diarrhea, dysphagia, shock) and with splenic contraction.
* PCV decreases with anemia (e.g., GI blood loss, parasitism, neoplasia, chronic disease).
* The presence of occult blood in the feces may implicate the gut as a source of blood loss.
* Plasma protein concentration should be taken into account when interpreting the PCV.

Leukogram

* *Neutrophilia* is caused by inflammation, infection, or stress.
  * Inflammatory or necrotic lesions often result in a regenerative neutrophilia; lymphocyte and monocyte numbers usually are normal.
  * Stress often results in the classic "stress leukogram" of mature neutrophilia, lymphopenia, and eosinopenia.
* *Leukopenia* is defined as a WBC count $<5500/\mu L$ in older horses and $<7000/\mu L$ in horses <2 years of age.
  * GI diseases that cause *neutropenia* include severe enteritis (e.g., salmonellosis, equine monocytic ehrlichiosis) and the overwhelming sepsis that accompanies bowel rupture.
* Toxic neutrophil changes occur with uptake of endotoxin by neutrophils.
* *Eosinophilia* most commonly occurs secondary to parasitic disease, although parasitized horses may have normal circulating eosinophil counts.
* Eosinophilia may also occur with eosinophilic granulomatous enteritis.

Protein Concentrations

Changes in plasma protein concentration may involve specific components (albumin, globulin, fibrinogen) or all components.

* *Hyperproteinemia* commonly accompanies dehydration.
  * *Hyperglobulinemia* may occur secondary to chronic antigenic stimulation, hepatitis, and inflammatory or septic conditions.
* *Hypoproteinemia* may result from protein-losing enteropathy, acute blood loss, or parasitism.
  * *Hypoalbuminemia* is a component of hypoproteinemia and also occurs with starvation and severe liver disease.
* *Fibrinogen* concentration increases with acute inflammatory disease.
  * Serum fibrinogen >1000 mg/dL is a poor prognostic indicator for survival, regardless of the underlying disease.
  * Serum fibrinogen may be low (<200 mg/dL) in severe liver failure or DIC.

Chemistry Panel

Serum electrolytes

Serum electrolyte changes are not specific for gastrointestinal disease. Hyponatremia, hypochloremia, and hypokalemia resulting from intestinal losses often develop in animals with diarrhea; hyperchloremia may be found in animals with diarrhea and severe acidosis. Hypocalcemia and hypomagnesemia are common findings in cantharidin (blister beetle) toxicosis.

Blood glucose

Hyperglycemia may be the result of stress, cantharidin toxicity, tumor of the pars intermedia of the pituitary gland or diabetes mellitus, or severe intestinal strangulation/obstruction. With the latter, blood glucose values >250 mg/dL are associated with a poor prognosis. *Hypoglycemia* may be present in horses with advanced liver disease or β-cell tumors of the pancreas and in horses and foals with septicemia.

Serum enzyme activities and other metabolic products

- BUN may be low in horses with liver disease and in those with severe diarrhea or a marked catabolic state.
- Liver disease may cause increases in AP, GGT, AST (GOT), SDH, and LDH.
- Hyperbilirubinemia indicates liver disease, hemolytic disease, or both.
- Serum bile acids are increased when there is obstruction to hepatic biliary flow.
- Biochemistry abnormalities associated with liver disease are discussed on p. 235.

Acid-Base Balance

Acidosis is the usual trend with GI disease and may result from excessive intestinal bicarbonate loss during secretory diarrhea or intestinal obstruction or from accumulation of lactic acid in horses with severe dehydration and endotoxic shock. *Alkalosis* may occur secondary to gastric disease, proximal enteritis, or colonic disease, although it generally is mild.

Fecal Examination

Following are the more common tests conducted on fecal samples in horses:

- *fecal flotation using hypertonic salt solutions:* used to detect parasite ova, although a negative finding does not rule out parasitism
- *microscopic examination of the feces:* leukocyte numbers often are increased in horses with infectious enteritis
  - Ciliated protozoa should be present in normal equine feces.
- *bacterial isolation techniques:* can be used to identify specific pathogens, such as *Candida, Salmonella, Campylobacter,* and *Clostridium spp.*
- *electron microscopy:* may be used to identify virus particles

Absorption Tests

Lactose absorption test

This test usually is performed to document lactose intolerance in suckling foals.

- The foal is fasted for 4 hours, and lactose (1 g/kg, 20% solution) is given via nasogastric tube.
- Plasma glucose values normally increase 30 to 90 minutes after administration of oral lactose; a rise of at least 35 mg/dL over baseline is expected.

Glucose or D-xylose absorption tests

These oral absorption tests are conducted as follows:

- The horse is fasted for 12 to 18 hours before testing.
- Glucose (1 g/kg) or D-xylose (0.5 g/kg) is given as a 10% solution, via nasogastric tube.
- In normal horses, blood glucose increases at least 50% over baseline within 2 to 4 hours and often doubles.
- A serum D-xylose concentration of at least 15 mg/dL is expected 60 to 90 minutes after intragastric administration in normal horses.

When interpreting the results, it is important to consider the following:

- Decreased absorption of these sugars has several potential causes.
  - small intestinal disease
  - delayed gastric emptying or abnormal small intestinal transit
  - increased bacterial metabolism within the gut lumen
  - decreased blood supply to the small intestine

- High-energy diets decrease the absorption of both sugars.
- Younger animals reach higher peak xylose concentrations than do adults.

ABDOMINOCENTESIS

Abdominocentesis is regularly performed on horses with colic, weight loss, diarrhea, abdominal masses, or abdominal infections. Following is a summary of the recommended technique:

- Abdominocentesis is performed on the ventral midline of the abdomen, at the lowest point (or 8 to 10 cm [3 to 4 inches] caudal to the sternum in horses with a taut, sloping abdominal contour).
- The site should be surgically prepared.
- A 1.5-inch, 18-gauge needle is satisfactory for abdominocentesis in most horses.
  - Teat cannulas or other small blunt cannulas also are suitable; a small skin incision, made after local anesthesia, is necessary when using cannulas.
- The needle should be advanced slowly into the abdominal cavity.
- Abdominal fluid should be obtained by gravity flow.
  - Fluid may be difficult to obtain in dehydrated horses and those in circulatory shock.
- Contamination with peripheral blood during collection often causes streaking of the sample, whereas red discoloration caused by intraabdominal hemorrhage usually is homogeneous.
  - Peripheral blood will clot in the collection tube, whereas abdominal fluid from horses with hemoperitoneum does not clot, and erythrophagocytosis may be seen cytologically.
  - Splenic puncture produces dark red blood with a higher PCV than peripheral blood.

Interpretation of Abdominal Fluid Findings

Normal abdominal fluid is yellow and clear or slightly turbid.

- Total protein is <2 g/dL.

- RBC and WBC counts are each <8000 cells/µL.
- Neutrophils comprise 40% to 90% of the total WBCs, and may be hypersegmented but are not degenerative.
- The fluid is sterile.

Common abnormal findings

The generalized reaction of the peritoneum to trauma is inflammation, with elevations of total protein and WBC count.

- This response occurs with infection, exploratory laparotomy, enterocentesis, neoplasia, and severely inflamed or infarcted bowel.
- Bacterial peritonitis can raise the protein concentration and WBC count in the fluid as high as 7 g/dL and 600,000 cells/µL, respectively.
  - However, enterocentesis or exploratory laparotomy in healthy horses can cause a transient increase in WBC count in excess of 400,000 cells/µL.
  - Fluid should be submitted for culture in all horses with suspected bacterial peritonitis.
- There is a reliable correlation between degenerative changes in neutrophils and the presence of toxin-producing microorganisms.

Evaluating Fluid from Horses with Colic

Abdominal fluid findings should always be interpreted in light of all other clinical and laboratory findings.

Color

- Intestinal strangulation/obstruction causes the fluid to turn shades of pink or red.
  - >20,000 RBCs/µL is highly correlated with the presence of a surgical lesion.
  - Serosanguineous abdominal fluid (with a high WBC count) may also occur in horses with proximal enteritis.
  - Orange fluid has been noted with nonstrangulating intestinal infarction.
- Green and brown colors suggest the presence of bowel contents, either bowel rupture/leakage or enterocentesis.
  - Brown abdominal fluid indicates a very poor prognosis.

◆ Milky white color indicates a high WBC count and is suggestive of bacterial peritonitis.

Total protein concentration

Peritoneal fluid protein concentration often is increased in horses with colic and indicates inflammation, vascular obstruction with protein leakage, or bowel necrosis. Increased protein concentration with normal or near-normal WBC and RBC counts in horses with clinical signs of upper small intestinal obstruction suggests proximal enteritis rather than a strangulation/obstruction.

Cytologic examination

Abdominal fluid can be smeared on slides, air-dried, and stained in ≤5 minutes (centrifugation may be necessary to concentrate cells in fluid with low cellularity).

◆ Slides should be examined for the presence of bacteria.
◆ Bowel rupture is indicated by the presence of plant material and numerous free bacteria, RBCs, and WBCs.
◆ Extracellular and intracellular bacteria with severe neutrophil degeneration indicates loss of bowel integrity and suggests a poor prognosis for survival.
◆ Enterocentesis is indicated by the presence of plant material and bacteria but no RBCs or WBCs.

EXPLORATORY LAPAROTOMY

Exploratory laparotomy is often performed for evaluation of the GI tract in horses with acute abdominal crises. (Indications for laparotomy are discussed in the section on principles of abdominal surgery.) Exploratory laparotomy also is useful for evaluation of horses with chronic colic or weight loss of undetermined origin and masses identified by rectal examination or ultrasonography.

LAPAROSCOPY

Laparoscopy can be used to detect metastasis of primary neoplasms, evaluate rectal tears, and view masses in the dorsal abdomen. It offers direct guidance for biopsies and can be performed on the standing horse.

Medical Therapy for Gastrointestinal Diseases *(pages 603-620)*
Catherine W. Kohn

CONTROL OF PAIN
Gastric Decompression

Horses with intestinal obstruction, ileus, duodenitis/proximal jejunitis, and, occasionally, acute enterocolitis may have gastric distention, resulting in severe pain. A nasogastric tube should be placed immediately and the fluid siphoned off to relieve pain and prevent gastric rupture. When reflux is copious or persistent, the nasogastric tube should be secured in place and frequent priming efforts made to evacuate the stomach until reflux ceases.

Analgesics

Gastrointestinal obstruction and acute enterocolitis cause severe abdominal pain. Drugs with the least deleterious effects on a compromised cardiovascular system and on gut motility should be chosen, and minimal effective dosages should be used in ill horses. Recommended drugs and dosages are provided in Table 10-1.

Precautions

◆ With most of these drugs, repeated or large doses may reduce visceral

Table 10-1
Dosages of drugs commonly used to provide visceral analgesia

Drug	IV dosage (mg/kg)
Xylazine	0.5-1.0
Detomidine	0.01-0.04
Morphine	0.02-0.10
Meperidine	0.2-0.6
Oxymorphone	0.01-0.06
Pentazocine	0.4-0.8
Butorphanol	0.05-0.1
Flunixin meglumine	1.1
Dipyrone	11-22
Xylazine/morphine	0.5/0.2-0.6
Xylazine/butorphanol	0.5/0.01-0.04

Modified from: Kohn CW, Muir WW: *J Vet Intern Med* 2:85-91, 1988.

pain or mask cardiovascular deterioration so effectively that the seriousness of the disease is obscured.

- Patients must be monitored closely for evidence of disease progression.
- Xylazine, detomidine, and morphine decrease intestinal motility, which could potentiate ileus or exacerbate large colon impactions.
- Phenothiazine tranquilizers cause marked hypotension, even in small doses, and should be avoided in patients with shock, especially if general anesthesia is planned.

MODIFYING BOWEL MOTILITY
Drugs to Stimulate Gut Motility

Ileus is a major complication of intestinal resection or exploratory celiotomy, and may also complicate medical intestinal diseases such as duodenitis/proximal jejunitis. The following drugs have been used, with varying success, in the management of ileus:

- *cisapride:* (0.01 mg/kg) exerts its prokinetic effect on the stomach, jejunum, ileum, cecum, right and left dorsal colon, and small colon.
  - Side effects include mild, transient discomfort and increased bowel sounds.
  - Ileus resulting from endotoxemia or devitalized bowel is resistant to cisapride.
- *metoclopramide:* (0.25 mg/kg IV, given over 30 minutes) can restore coordinated gastric and small intestinal motility in cases of postoperative ileus, but it causes periods of restlessness
- *neostigmine:* (0.022 mg/kg IV) increases propulsive activity of the cecocolic area and pelvic flexure, but decreases motility in the jejunum and delays gastric emptying
  - It should be withdrawn if signs of abdominal pain develop.
- *bethanechol:* (0.025 mg/kg) enhances gastric emptying; it should not be used if physical obstruction of gastric outflow is suspected
- *erythromycin:* (0.1 to 1.0 mg/kg IV) has a prokinetic effect on the stomach and large colon; it can in-

crease gastric emptying, but not as effectively as bethanechol

- *naloxone:* (0.05 to 0.5 mg/kg IV) coordinates cecal contractions and motility in the proximal colon, but is too expensive to use in most patients
- α_2-*antagonists:* (yohimbine [75 µg/kg] and tolazoline [1 mg/kg]) can promote intestinal motility, particularly in cases of postoperative or endotoxemia-induced ileus

It is important to remember that *return of gut motility depends on successful treatment of the underlying disease* and its associated metabolic abnormalities (especially hypocalcemia and hypokalemia).

MODIFYING FECAL CONSISTENCY
Cathartics

Cathartics are used most frequently for treatment of fecal impactions of the large colon. They have been classified by their mechanism of action.

- *irritant:* directly stimulates smooth muscle in the bowel wall
  - Examples include cascara sagrada (0.02 to 0.04 mL/kg of a 20% solution), danthron (15 to 40 g/450 kg), aloe (33 to 89 mL/kg), and castor oil (0.5 to 2.2 mL/kg).
  - These agents are contraindicated in obstruction and enterocolitis, and they *should not be administered* when the type of bowel disease is undetermined.
- *saline:* motility is stimulated by fluid accumulation
  - Agents include sodium sulfate (Glauber's salt, 0.2 to 1.0 g/kg), magnesium sulfate (0.5 to 1.0 g/kg), and magnesium hydroxide suspension (2 to 9 mL/kg).
- *hydrophilic colloid:* fluid distention stimulates motility and soften impactions
  - Examples include psyllium (250 g in warm water), methylcellulose (0.4 to 1.1 mg/kg), and bran (1 to 2 kg/450 kg).
  - These agents can be added to the normal ration.
- *emollient:* bowel lubricants
  - Examples include mineral oil (9 mL/kg) and raw linseed oil (1.1 to 2.2 mL/kg).

- *surfactant:* detergent actions dissolve the impaction
  - 7% dioctyl sodium sulfosuccinate (DSS) is given at 10 to 60 mg/kg (200 mg maximum).
  - These agents are toxic in excessive quantities and can cause mild colic and diarrhea.
  - Mineral oil and DSS should not be given concurrently.

Protectants and Antidiarrheal Agents

Several products have been used with varying success to resolve diarrhea in horses.

- *Bismuth subsalicylate and mineral oil* may exert a coating, protective effect on irritated or inflamed bowel.
- *Kaolin-pectin* (2 to 4 L/horse), administered once or several times per day via nasogastric tube, resolves diarrhea in a some horses.
- *Loperamide* (0.2 mg/kg IV or PO) dries rectal and gut contents without delaying defecation; this antisecretory effect may be useful in some cases.
- *Phenoxybenzamine* reduces diarrhea in a limited number of cases.
  - Hypotension is a side effect, so this drug should not be used in dehydrated horses.

GASTRIC ACIDITY AND PROTECTING THE GASTRIC MUCOSA

Histamine Type-2 Receptor Antagonists

The H_2-receptor blockers available in the United States are cimetidine, ranitidine, famotidine, and nizatidine. Cimetidine is the least potent, and famotidine is the most potent at suppressing gastric acid secretion.

Dosages

Responses of individual horses and foals to H_2 blockers are highly variable; clinical signs may abate at dosages lower than those required for ulcer healing.

- The recommended dosage for *cimetidine* is 6.6 to 10.0 mg/kg PO q4-6h, or 1.1 to 2.2 mg/kg/h IV.
  - Cimetidine should not be given orally for at least 1 hour after antacid administration.

- The recommended dosage for *ranitidine* is 6.6 mg/kg PO, or 2 mg/kg IV, q8h.

Duration of therapy

Duration depends on the response to treatment and is best assessed by repeated gastroscopy. Therapy usually is given for 14 to 21 days, but some horses require 30 to 40 days of treatment. Poor clinical response and slow ulcer healing may occur when the horse continues to be stressed by chronic disease or continued race training.

Omeprazole

Omeprazole (a proton-pump inhibitor) suppresses gastric acid secretion for up to 24 hours. The recommended dosage is 3 to 4 mg/kg PO q24h. For effective oral therapy, it is essential that the enteric coating on the tablets remains intact.

Sucralfate

At very low pH (<2) sucralfate becomes a sticky, amorphous mass that adheres to the base of a gastric ulcer and protects the underlying tissue.

- It is as effective as ranitidine in preventing phenylbutazone-induced gastric and duodenal ulcers in foals.
- Sucralfate should not be used as the sole agent to treat ulcers, unless repeated gastroscopy can be performed to monitor progress.
- In foals, sucralfate is given at 2 to 4 g PO q6-8h.
- Treatment should be scheduled for 1 to 2 hours before ranitidine or cimetidine administration.

Antacids

Antacids such as magnesium and aluminum hydroxide neutralize gastric acid and decrease peptic activity; they also bind bile acids and enhance synthesis of endogenous prostaglandins, thus improving gastric mucosal defenses. The recommended dosage is 0.5 ml/kg PO q6h. In general, the duration of antacid effect is short (15 to 30 minutes with most products); it is best to administer antacids 1 hour or so after feeding.

Other Agents

Bismuth subsalicylate (Pepto-Bismol) binds to gastric ulcers and has been used to treat foals with gastric ulcers and associated diarrhea. *Misoprostol* (Cytotec) is a synthetic prostaglandin E_1 that has both cytoprotective and acid suppressive properties. Side effects include abdominal pain and diarrhea; it can also cause abortion and should not be used in pregnant mares.

TRANSFAUNATION

Imbalance or absence of normal intestinal flora may predispose to or perpetuate intestinal dysfunction, especially diarrhea. Reestablishment of a normal enteric environment may speed return to normal function:

*   The best source of viable microfauna is cecal or colonic contents, obtained at necropsy from a nonparasitized, preferably *Salmonella*-negative horse with a healthy GI tract.
*   Cecal or colonic ingesta is strained, and 2 to 4 L of the filtrate is given via nasogastric tube to the recipient as soon as possible after filtering.
*   Multiple transfaunations may be required before normal feces are passed.
*   Substitutes for fresh ingesta elixir are yogurt and products containing *Lactobacillus* spp.

ANTIMICROBIAL THERAPY

Antimicrobial selection in patients with salmonellosis, *Ehrlichia risticii* infection, or other causes of acute enterocolitis are discussed in the relevant sections.

Prophylactic Antimicrobials in Surgical Patients

Antimicrobials should be administered before surgery so that high tissue levels are present during surgical manipulation. Broad-spectrum combinations are recommended; Na^+ or K^+ penicillin (20,000 to 100,000 IU/kg IV) plus gentamicin (2 to 3 mg/kg IV or IM) is a good choice. Antimicrobial therapy following surgery is discussed in *Equine Medicine and Surgery V.*

ANTIENDOTOXIC THERAPY

Systemic absorption of endotoxin from compromised bowel accounts for many of the pathophysiologic changes associated with strangulation/obstruction, nonstrangulating infarction, and invasive enterocolitis in horses. Therapies currently include:

*   flunixin meglumine, at 0.25 mg/kg IV q8–12h
*   antiendotoxin antiserum
*   polymyxin B, at 6000 IU/kg q12h, diluted in 300 to 500 mL of 5% dextrose and administered slowly IV
*   bismuth subsalicylate
*   heparin, up to 80 IU/kg IV; a decremental dosage regimen is recommended when several days of treatment are required
*   pentoxifylline; however, oral absorption is erratic and poor, so it is unlikely that the preparation currently available will produce consistent clinical effects

Surgical Therapy for Gastrointestinal Diseases *(pages 620-635)*
Stephen B. Adams

Detailed discussions of surgical techniques are given in *Equine Medicine and Surgery V.*

INDICATIONS FOR SURGERY IN HORSES WITH COLIC

Selection Criteria

The decision for surgery should be based on information obtained from a complete history, physical examination, and laboratory evaluation of blood and abdominal fluid. When doubt still exists after thorough evaluation, laparotomy should be considered as a diagnostic procedure.

Onset and course of disease

Sudden onset of colic with severe pain and rapid systemic deterioration suggests a surgical lesion. Deterioration despite aggressive medical therapy also is an indication for surgery.

Rectal temperature

Most horses with colic requiring surgery have a rectal temperature

<38.5° C (101.3° F) (unless physical activity or high ambient temperature causes hyperthermia). Rectal temperature >39.5° C, not attributable to physical activity or high ambient temperature, suggests infectious disease. Surgery is contraindicated in these patients.

Pain and analgesics
Unrelenting pain is an indication for surgery; the most likely causes are mesenteric traction (e.g., displacements, volvulus), ischemia, and strangulation of the bowel. Failure of flunixin or butorphanol to relieve abdominal pain and the need for frequently repeated doses of analgesics suggest that surgery is necessary.

Severe abdominal distention
Abdominal distention in adult horses usually is caused by accumulation of gas in the large colon or cecum. Severe abdominal distention in the absence of flatus indicates that surgical intervention is needed; bloated horses passing gas often recover without surgery.

Intestinal sounds
Complete absence of borborygmi suggests infarction or other irreversible morphologic damage to the bowel, necessitating surgical intervention. Intestinal sounds should be reassessed after fluids and analgesics have been administered; horses in which borborygmi return after treatment usually are not candidates for surgery.

Nasogastric intubation
Reflux of ≥4 L of gastric contents is abnormal. Continued reflux suggests obstruction of the stomach or small intestine; many diseases causing gastric reflux require surgery. However, horses with proximal enteritis or adynamic ileus often exhibit profuse gastric reflux and may respond to medical therapy.

Rectal examination
Palpable abnormalities that support a decision for surgery include taut, painful mesenteric bands, distended small or large intestine, and, possibly, abdominal masses.

Abdominocentesis
Peritoneal fluid with a serosanguineous or orange color and total protein concentration >3.5 g/dL is an indication for surgery. A peritoneal RBC count >20,000 cells/μL is highly correlated with the presence of a surgical lesion. But when the WBC count is elevated in the absence of an elevated RBC count, nonsurgical diseases such as peritonitis and enteritis should be considered. Finding large numbers of extracellular bacteria of varying morphology is a *contraindication* for surgery.

Peripheral blood values
The peripheral WBC count in horses requiring surgical intervention often is normal or slightly elevated. Nonsurgical diseases, such as enteritis or peritonitis, often cause mild-to-severe leukopenia.

Medical Diseases That Can Mimic Surgical Colic

Medical diseases that can cause signs suggesting that surgery is necessary include:

- proximal enteritis
- peritonitis
- ileus
- primary gastric dilation
- endotoxemia
- enterocolitis

PROGNOSIS FOR HORSES WITH COLIC

Findings that indicate a poor prognosis for survival include:

- marked depression
- heart rate > 100 beats/min
- capillary refill time >4 seconds
- no palpable facial artery pulse
- hematocrit >60%
- prolonged clotting time
- systolic blood pressure <70 mm Hg
- venous blood lactate >100 mg/dL and/or pH <7.2
- anion gap >25 mEq/L

Absence of intestinal sounds has also been correlated with a poorer survival rate, although the effects of drugs that inhibit intestinal motility (e.g., xylazine, detomidine) must be taken into account. In a practice setting, evaluation of the hematocrit and the total protein concentration and color of abdominal fluid allows an accurate assessment of the prognosis.

Observations at the time of surgery also are used to predict survival: extensive small or large intestinal necrosis warrants a poor prognosis.

Postoperative Complications

Complications may develop during recovery from anesthesia, during the early postoperative period, or later, following discharge from the hospital. Complications include the following:

* *recovery from anesthesia:* postanesthetic rhabdomyolysis, paresis, long bone fracture
* *early postoperative period:* incisional infection, ileus, peritonitis, salmonellosis, abdominal hemorrhage, laminitis, thrombophlebitis, abortion, shock
* *later postoperative period:* abdominal adhesions, incisional hernias, malabsorption of nutrients

In general, the sicker the horse, the more likely it is that postoperative complications will occur.

The Equine Neonate: Special Considerations

(pages 636-640)
Guy D. Lester

PHYSICAL EXAMINATION

Many GI diseases in young foals occur secondary to other diseases (e.g., sepsis, prematurity) or coexist with disorders that could adversely impact short- or long-term survival. Thorough physical examination is essential.

Indications for Surgery

Severe, unrelenting pain that is poorly responsive or nonresponsive to analgesics often is a valid sole criterion for surgical exploration. However, the decision to explore the abdominal cavity in a newborn foal should not be taken lightly, because foals are more susceptible to adhesions.

DIAGNOSTIC TOOLS

Ultrasonography

Abdominal ultrasonography in young foals should include examination of:

* umbilical structures (arteries, vein, and urachus) and the bladder
* intestines
  * Fluid-filled loops of small intestine are consistent with ileus or enteritis.
  * Gas shadows within the intestinal wall are a feature of necrotizing enterocolitis.
  * Small intestinal intussusception often is seen as a series of concentric circles (target, or bull's eye, lesions).
* intestinal motion (subjective assessment)
  * Typically, the intestine is hypermotile with enterocolitis and relatively motionless with volvulus or ileus.

Radiography

Diagnostic abdominal radiographs in neonatal foals can be obtained using portable x-ray equipment (15 mAs and 80 to 100 kVp). Plain radiography is useful for:

* identifying intraluminal obstructions (e.g., meconium)
* differentiating small and large intestinal disease
  * Advanced obstructive disease of the small intestine produces characteristic hairpin or stacked intestinal loops.
  * A prominent small intestinal gas pattern is commonly seen with ileus or enteritis, although ileus can be difficult to differentiate from mechanical obstruction.
  * Meconium impactions usually cause gas distention of the colon.

Contrast radiography

Contrast radiography helps define problems related to gastric emptying and intestinal obstruction. For upper GI studies, barium sulfate (5 mL/kg) is given via nasogastric tube; normally, all of the barium should leave the stomach within 2 hours. Barium enemas help identify impactions or congenital abnormalities, such as atresia coli. Up to 20 mL/kg of a 30% suspension is administered via Foley catheter (cuff inflated).

Abdominocentesis

Because of the potential for serious complications, abdominocentesis should be reserved for foals in which the distinction between surgical and medical diseases is not clear. Complications can be minimized by identifying pockets of fluid ultrasonographically and by using a blunt instrument, such as a bovine teat cannula. The technique should be avoided in foals with large colon distention.

Diseases Affecting Multiple Sites *(pages 640-651)*

Stephen B. Adams, Corrie Brown, Elspeth Milne, and Janice E. Sojka

CONGENITAL AND FAMILIAL DISEASES

Ileocolonic Aganglionosis

White foals born from overo–overo paint breedings are susceptible to lethal white syndrome (ileocolonic aganglionosis).

- Affected foals are completely white or have very little pigmented hair; the irides are blue and the skin is pink.
- Most foals appear normal at birth, stand and nurse, but do not pass meconium.
- Signs of colic and GI distention usually appear within 12 hours after birth, and most affected foals die within 48 hours.
- If exploratory surgery is performed, areas of the colon may appear stenotic and thin-walled.

INFLAMMATORY, INFECTIOUS, AND IMMUNE DISEASES

Anthrax

Anthrax is a rapidly fatal bacterial disease caused by *Bacillus anthracis,* large gram-positive bacteria that form spores when exposed to air. Transmission is via contact with infective spores present in soil, decaying carcasses, bone meal, wool, or hides. Spores can persist in the environment for years. In the United States, outbreaks have been reported in the lower Mississippi Valley, coastal areas of Louisiana and Texas, and parts of the Great Plains.

Clinical signs and diagnosis

Anthrax causes a rapidly fatal septicemia, with extensive and necrotizing vascular lesions.

- Often the most prominent clinical sign in horses is colic.
  - There may also be large, edematous swellings, especially in the cervical area.
- Death ensues within hours.
- The carcass autolyzes very quickly and blood may be present at body orifices.
  - Other postmortem lesions include an enlarged, friable spleen and multiple swollen, edematous, hemorrhagic lymph nodes.
- *Every attempt should be made to diagnose anthrax before the carcass is opened.*
  - A blood smear taken from an ear vein and stained with methylene blue reveals massive numbers of bacilli with pink capsules.
- The organism can be cultured from many tissues.

Prevention

A vaccine is used in endemic areas and has proven effective, even in the face of an outbreak. Proper disposal of infected carcasses is critical; burning is recommended.

TOXIC DISEASES

Cantharidin (Blister Beetle) Poisoning

Cantharidin toxicity usually is caused by ingestion of baled alfalfa hay containing dead blister beetles. Hay from southern and southwestern states is infested most often; storage of hay does not decrease the toxic principle in the dried beetles. Cantharidin is a topical irritant that causes severe irritation with mucosal degeneration and necrosis throughout the GI tract. It is excreted in the urine and also causes renal damage.

Clinical signs

Onset and duration of signs vary from hours to days.

- Signs include anorexia, depression, and colic (can be severe).
- Frequent urination may be noted; occasionally, hematuria or passage of blood clots in the urine is seen.
- Ulcerative lesions can be found in the mouth; affected horses may

play with their water and submerge their muzzles in it.

♦ Physical examination reveals increases in pulse and respiratory rates and rectal temperature; profuse sweating and signs of cardiovascular collapse may also be found.

♦ Absence of abdominal sounds is common, and diarrhea may develop.

♦ Hypocalcemia can result in synchronous diaphragmatic flutter, muscle fasciculations, and a stiff gait.

♦ The clinical course can be acute, and sudden death may occur.

Laboratory findings

PCV usually is elevated, consistent with clinical dehydration that develops.

♦ Hyperglycemia and neutrophilic leukocytosis indicate a stress response.

♦ Serum calcium and magnesium levels decrease rapidly after cantharidin ingestion.

♦ Hypoproteinemia and elevated serum CPK are relatively common.

♦ Serum sodium, potassium, and chloride and acid-base status usually are normal.

♦ Hematuria is uncommon, but urine usually is positive for occult blood.
  • Renal damage is indicated by dilute urine (SG 1.003 to 1.006) despite dehydration.

Diagnosis

Establishing a definitive diagnosis can be difficult.

♦ Any remaining hay should be examined carefully for beetles.

♦ Cantharidin can be identified in stomach contents and urine.
  • The earlier in the disease the sample is collected, the better the chance of finding the toxin.
  • At least 500 mL of fresh urine and 200 g of solid stomach contents should be submitted.
  • Serum may also be submitted, although the test is much less sensitive using serum.

♦ Hypocalcemia and hypomagnesemia, while not pathognomonic, are not commonly associated with other diseases that cause colic.

Treatment and prognosis

Treatment is symptomatic.

♦ Mineral oil (4 L/450-kg horse) may prevent absorption of the toxin.

• All exposed horses, even if not showing signs, should be treated with mineral oil.

• Activated charcoal (1 to 3 g/kg via nasogastric tube) may also be helpful, although it should not be given concurrently with mineral oil.

♦ Affected horses should receive IV fluids to maintain hydration and establish diuresis.

♦ Treatment with calcium- and magnesium-containing solutions also is indicated.

♦ Diuretics may be beneficial early.
  • Furosemide (1 mg/kg) may be used, but it can exacerbate hypocalcemia.
  • DMSO (1 g/kg IV as a 10% solution in polyionic fluids), is advocated for its diuretic and antiinflammatory effects and can be repeated q12–24h.

♦ Analgesics (e.g., α_2-agonists ± butorphanol) often are necessary to control the pain.

♦ Intestinal protectants, such as sucralfate (20 mg/kg PO q6–8h), may be of benefit.

♦ If antimicrobial drugs are given, potential for nephrotoxicity must be considered.

The prognosis often is poor, but depends on the amount of toxin ingested, the stage of disease when treatment is implemented, and the quality of intensive care provided.

Nonsteroidal Antiinflammatory Toxicity

The toxic effects of NSAIDs are related to inhibition of the physiologic actions of prostaglandins (cytoprotection of the gastric mucosa and preservation of renal blood flow during dehydration). NSAID toxicity is characterized by:

♦ GI ulceration (especially of the glandular gastric mucosa and right dorsal colon)

♦ protein-losing enteropathy (secondary to mucosal ulceration)

♦ renal papillary necrosis (in dehydrated animals)

The effects of different NSAIDs probably are additive. Foals are more susceptible than adult horses. Right dorsal colitis can occur in horses receiving recommended doses of phenylbutazone that are stressed by frequent trailering or strenuous exercise.

Clinical signs

- Initial signs are anorexia and depression.
- Colic, diarrhea, dependent edema, and oral ulcers (especially with administration of oral phenylbutazone) may develop as the condition progresses.
- Signs of endotoxemia may be found subsequent to severe GI ulceration.
  - If an ulcer perforates, diffuse peritonitis and death rapidly ensue.
- Right dorsal colitis causes colic, diarrhea, anorexia, lethargy, and weight loss (see p. 219).

Diagnosis

- A history of NSAID administration is critical to diagnosis.
  - A daily phenylbutazone dosage >8.8 mg/kg (4 g/450-kg horse) for 2 days consistently causes toxicity in foals, ponies, and adult horses.
  - Toxicity develops when flunixin is given to foals at 1.1 mg/kg/day for 30 days.
- Laboratory findings include hypoproteinemia, increased BUN, and neutrophilia with a left shift.

Treatment

- NSAID administration should be stopped immediately.
  - Another class of analgesic (e.g., butorphanol, xylazine) may be substituted if necessary.
- Fluid therapy should be instituted if the horse is dehydrated.
- Broad-spectrum antibiotics are indicated if severe ulceration is suspected.
- H_2 antagonists (e.g., cimetidine, ranitidine) are indicated if gastric ulceration is suspected.
- A low-fiber, pelleted diet, sucralfate, and psyllium mucilloid have also been advocated for treatment of right dorsal colitis (see p. 220).

NEOPLASIA

Gastrointestinal neoplasms are rare. The most common are squamous cell carcinoma, lymphosarcoma, and lipoma.

Squamous Cell Carcinoma

Alimentary squamous cell carcinoma most often involves the stomach but has been reported in the mouth, pharynx, and esophagus. Squamous cell carcinoma occurs most often in older horses. Predominant clinical signs are chronic weight loss and exercise intolerance. With oral or pharyngeal forms, dysphagia and/or dyspnea may also be obvious. Colic is not a common feature of gastric involvement, although anorexia and low-grade fever that is unresponsive to antibiotic therapy are common. The prognosis is grave.

Diagnosis of gastric squamous cell carcinoma

- Metastatic masses often can be palpated *per rectum* on the ventral abdominal wall or within the mesentery.
- Hypercalcemia and indications of liver disease (e.g., icterus, increased serum liver enzymes) are found in some cases; normochromic normocytic anemia is common.
- In some instances, exfoliated neoplastic cells are identified in abdominal fluid.
- Ultrasonography may reveal splenic, hepatic, diaphragmatic, or body wall masses.
- Endoscopy may allow direct visualization of the tumor, and neoplastic cells may be recovered via gastric lavage.
- Exploratory laparotomy allows definitive diagnosis.

Lymphosarcoma

Lymphosarcoma is an uncommon tumor in horses. Four types are described: multicentric, alimentary, thymic, and cutaneous. Within the GI tract, lymphosarcoma most often affects the small intestine and mesenteric lymph nodes; it has also been reported in the soft palate, large colon, and cecum. The prognosis is grave.

Clinical signs

- Onset of signs may be acute or chronic; young animals often are affected.
- Weight loss and depression are the most consistent signs of intestinal lymphosarcoma.

- Tachycardia, fever, icterus, colic, and diarrhea have also been reported.
♦ Signs of palatine lymphosarcoma include dysphagia and epistaxis.

Diagnosis
♦ Mesenteric lymphadenopathy or abdominal masses may be present on rectal examination.
♦ Anemia and hypoalbuminemia (secondary to protein-losing enteropathy) are common; globulin levels may be normal or increased.
♦ Ultrasonography may reveal splenic, hepatic, or body wall masses.
♦ D-Xylose or glucose malabsorption (see p. 177) suggests small intestinal involvement.
♦ Diagnosis may be made when atypical lymphocytes are found in peripheral blood (rare), peritoneal fluid, or biopsied tissue.
♦ Exploratory laparotomy and biopsy of affected areas allows definitive diagnosis.

Smooth Muscle Tumors

Intestinal leiomyoma and leiomyosarcoma are most common in the small intestine, but have been reported at other sites. The most consistent sign is intermittent or acute colic resulting from intestinal stasis and luminal obstruction. In many cases, definitive diagnosis can be made only during exploratory laparotomy. Resection usually is curative, and the long-term prognosis is good.

Mesothelial Tumors
Mesothelioma
Mesothelioma is an uncommon tumor that may occur in the pleural or peritoneal cavity. Signs include chronic weight loss, ventral edema, and colic. Diagnosis usually is made when neoplastic cells are found in peritoneal or pleural fluid. The prognosis is grave.

Lipoma
Lipomas are benign tumors that are common in older horses. The tumors do not metastasize and rarely become very large. They often develop on long stalks and may cause intestinal strangulation/obstruction (see p. 207).

MULTIFACTORIAL DISEASES
Nonstrangulating Intestinal Infarction
Nonstrangulating intestinal infarction is associated with verminous mesenteric arteritis and thrombosis caused by *Strongylus vulgaris* larval migration. Signs include mild-to-severe colic, with heart rates ranging from normal to >100 beats/min, and reduced or absent borborygmi; depression is common in the later stages of disease. Abdominal fluid may be serosanguineous and the protein and WBC count may be elevated.

Treatment and prognosis
♦ Supportive care with fluids, NSAIDs, and antibiotics is warranted.
  - Antithrombotic drugs may also be given.
♦ Lesions should be resected when surgically accessible.
♦ The prognosis is poor because the disease often is progressive, and peritonitis is common.

IDIOPATHIC DISEASES
Ileus
Ileus is the lack of effective intestinal motility, leading to functional obstruction of the intestinal tract. It may be caused by exhaustion, intestinal distention, peritonitis, enteritis, abdominal surgery, septicemia, metabolic derangements (particularly hypocalcemia and hypokalemia), drugs that inhibit intestinal motility (e.g., atropine), and hypoglycemia (foals). Ileus is most common in horses after colic surgery.

Clinical signs and diagnosis
♦ Gastric reflux and absence of borborygmi are hallmark signs of generalized ileus.
  - Borborygmi may be ausculted when ileus is due to ineffective motility or when ileus is localized to one section of the intestinal tract.
♦ Abdominal pain often is intermittent and when caused by gastric distention is relieved by gastric decompression.
♦ Systemic deterioration occurs with persistent ileus.
♦ Rectal examination often reveals distended loops of small intestine.

Treatment

- Underlying abdominal disease, such as peritonitis or intestinal infarction, must be treated before ileus can resolve.
- Metabolic imbalances should be identified and corrected with appropriate fluid therapy.
  - Nasogastric intubation should be performed regularly to reduce the risk of gastric rupture.
  - Decompression of other segments of the intestinal tract requires laparotomy.
- Abdominal pain should be controlled with analgesics that do not suppress bowel motility.
  - Atropine, glycopyrrolate, xylazine, and detomidine should be avoided.
- Several drugs have been tried to stimulate intestinal motility (see p. 180).
  - Continuous low-dose IV infusion of metoclopramide at 0.04 mg/kg/h may be useful for postoperative ileus.
  - Neostigmine (0.02 mg/kg SC q1h) is less effective with severe intestinal distention; it may cause bowel spasm, so should be used with caution following intestinal anastomosis.
  - Cisapride is a more promising treatment.
- Walking the horse every hour and offering small amounts of water once gastric reflux is relieved are beneficial.
- A second laparotomy may be necessary when ileus is refractory to medical therapy.

Grass Sickness

Grass sickness (equine dysautonomia) is recognized in many northern European countries; an identical condition (*mal seco,* or dry sickness) occurs in Argentina and Chile. Grass sickness occurs in grazing horses and is predominantly a disease of young adult horses (2 to 7 years). The acute form is characterized by lethargy, inappetence, dysphagia, and colic; death usually occurs within 2 days. The chronic form is characterized by severe weight loss, dysphagia, rhinitis, and abnormal sweating. Diagnosis

and management are discussed in *Equine Medicine and Surgery V.*

Spasmodic Colic

Spasmodic colic is a result of intestinal hypermotility. Causes include exercise or excitement, enteritis, parasitism, and moldy feed. The disease is characterized by loud, gassy intestinal sounds and intermittent abdominal pain, with little or no systemic deterioration and normal rectal findings. Spasmodic colic rarely is life-threatening, and spontaneous resolution is common.

Treatment

- Analgesics or antispasmodics (e.g., dipyrone, flunixin meglumine) are recommended for horses that do not recover spontaneously within an hour or so; atropine is contraindicated.
- Many clinicians also administer mineral oil via nasogastric tube.

Diseases of the Lips, Mouth, Tongue, and Oropharynx *(pages 652-658)*
Patrick T. Colahan

CONGENITAL AND FAMILIAL DISEASES

Cleft Palate

Cleft palate is uncommon in horses. The defect involves either the soft palate (more common) or both the hard and soft palates. The primary sign is milk dribbling from the nares of a neonatal foal after nursing. Typically, affected foals cough, have difficulty nursing, fail to grow normally, may lose weight, and are depressed; many of these signs are attributable to aspiration pneumonia. Diagnosis and treatment are discussed in Chapter 9, Respiratory System.

Cysts of the Oropharynx

Oropharyngeal cysts include subepiglottic cysts (see Chapter 9, Respiratory System) and cysts in the dorsal pharyngeal wall and soft palate. These cysts generally develop slowly. Signs, which include dyspnea or dysphagia, may not be noticed until 2 years of age. Some cysts are evident on endoscopic examination of the nasopharynx, but others are found only on visual examination of the oral cavity or palpation of the oropharynx. Excision can be performed via laryngotomy or with peroral transendoscopic Nd:YAG laser.

DISEASES WITH PHYSICAL CAUSES
Foreign Bodies
Foreign bodies, such as pieces of wire and wood, can be very difficult to locate, particularly if they are lodged in the tongue or deep in the oropharynx. Nonradiopaque materials, such as wood and plant awns, are the most difficult to find. Radiography after infusion of contrast medium into draining tracts can help locate the object; ultrasonography can also be helpful. Following removal, systemic antibiotics are recommended to control the cellulitis that usually accompanies foreign body penetration.

Lacerations of the Lips and Tongue
Small, superficial lacerations of the lips and tongue heal readily without treatment. Large and deep lacerations heal more rapidly and with less scarring if they are sutured. For lacerations with extensive soft tissue damage, it is best to delay repair until the devitalized tissues slough and the remaining tissues have good circulation.
Partial glossectomy
Partial glossectomy may be necessary for severe trauma to the tongue. Removal of the apex of the tongue as far caudal as the frenulum linguae can be tolerated quite well. After debridement, the muscular tissue is sutured with as many layers as necessary to close the dead space. The dorsal and ventral mucous membranes are then sutured together over the muscular tissue.
Postoperative management
Postoperative care for horses with tongue and lip injuries includes:
* NSAIDs

* antibiotic therapy (probably provides little aid to healing in most cases)
* feeding high-quality hay with soft stems

Pharyngeal Injuries
Injuries to the oropharynx usually are caused by nasogastric tubes, dental floats, or balling guns.
* Lesions often are located in the dorsal pharyngeal recess, caudal pharyngeal wall, or piriform fossae lateral to the larynx.
* Treatment includes debridement, frequent lavage (if possible), and systemic antibiotics.
* Deep wounds of the pharynx are serious injuries that warrant a guarded prognosis.
  * Cellulitis, necrosis, and abscessation frequently complicate these wounds and lead to dysphagia, dyspnea, and aspiration pneumonia.

INFLAMMATORY, INFECTIOUS, AND IMMUNE DISEASES
Amyloidosis
Amyloid deposits can develop in the mouth and nasal cavity (see Chapter 9, Respiratory System). In the oral cavity, the swellings caused by amyloid deposits are tender and subject to frequent trauma; they often are ulcerated. The only effective treatment is to resolve the inciting cause (repeated immune stimulation). Even with treatment, the prognosis for resolution is guarded.

Epulis
Epulis is benign hyperplasia of the gingiva, presumably in response to chronic irritation from plant awns or dental tartar. Removal of the inciting cause and resection of the hyperplastic tissue resolves the problem, but recurrence is common.

Gastrophilus and Habronema Infestation
Gastrophilus or *Habronema* larvae can cause transient ulcers in the mouth, particularly on the lips. Treatment

with organophosphate anthelmintics or ivermectin is effective.

Hyperkeratosis

Neoplasia and chronic irritation of the oral cavity can cause the oral mucosa, particularly beneath the tongue, to become pale, roughened, and thickened. The hyperkeratotic lesions resolve with removal of the inciting cause.

Phemphigus Vulgaris and Bullous Pemphigoid

The fragile, pale vesicles and bullae that are the early lesions of these rare autoimmune diseases commonly are not seen. Usually, the lesions consist of crusts and collarettes in the mouth and on mucocutaneous junctions. Definitive diagnosis can be made by biopsy and immunohistochemical methods; response to steroid therapy usually is only transient.

Stomatitis

Bacterial stomatitis is rare in horses; causative organisms include *Pseudomonas* and *Rhodococcus* spp. Viral or mycotic causes include vesicular stomatitis, horse pox, and candidiasis (generally secondary to prolonged antibiotic use in foals)

Treatment

♦ Horses with stomatitis are treated symptomatically by frequent oral lavage with dilute potassium permanganate or povidone iodine solutions.

♦ Severely affected animals may also require systemic antibiotics and IV fluid therapy.

♦ Resolution usually requires successful treatment of the primary disease.

METABOLIC AND TOXIC DISEASES

Systemic Disease

Stomatitis can be a sign of systemic diseases, such as mercury toxicity, uremia, phenylbutazone toxicity, cantharidin (blister beetle) ingestion, hyperadrenocorticism, and photosensitization.

Caustic Ingestion

Creosote and disinfectants are the most common chemicals involved.

The degree of damage depends on the concentration of the chemical and the duration of exposure.

Lampus

Lampus is a benign soft tissue swelling on the palate, immediately caudal to the incisors. It is found in some horses during eruption of the permanent incisors. These horses may be reluctant to eat or may salivate excessively while eating. Lampus resolves without therapy, although offering less fibrous feeds is advisable until the condition resolves. NSAIDs facilitate recovery.

NEOPLASIA

Tumors of the lips, tongue, and oropharynx are rare. Reported neoplasms include squamous cell carcinoma, fibrosarcoma, malignant melanoma, hemangiosarcoma, rhabdomyoma, rhabdomyosarcoma, ossifying fibroma, and lymphosarcoma. Of these, squamous cell carcinoma, fibrosarcoma, and ossifying fibroma are the most common.

Squamous Cell Carcinoma and Fibrosarcoma

The most common signs of lingual, oral, or oropharyngeal neoplasia are fetid halitosis and difficulty eating; oral tumors that invade the nasal cavity may also cause dyspnea. Tumors of the lips usually are obvious and easily identified on physical examination. Diagnosis and prognosis depend on histologic diagnosis from biopsy specimens.

Treatment and prognosis

♦ Tumors of the lips and rostral tongue are more readily resolved because they are noticed sooner and are accessible to surgery and radiotherapy.

♦ Tumors of the palate and pharynx usually are large and invasive and may have metastasized to regional lymph nodes before diagnosis.

♦ Squamous cell carcinomas may be successfully treated with radiotherapy, cryosurgery, and laser excision; however, recurrence is common after resection.

• Fibrosarcomas are less radiosensitive and tend to recur after excision.

Ossifying Fibroma

Juvenile mandibular ossifying fibroma occurs in the rostral mandible of horses 2 to 14 months of age. The tumor usually is obvious as a mass on the mandible below the incisors. Treatment involves surgical excision with either hemilateral or bilateral partial mandibulectomy.

Diseases of the Hyoid Apparatus *(pages 658-660)*

Patrick T. Colahan and Barbara Watrous

EXAMINATION AND DIAGNOSTIC AIDS

The obvious sign common to diseases involving the hyoid apparatus is dysphagia, including flaccidity of the tongue and ptyalism. Bleeding from the mouth or nose can be seen if a hyoid fracture opens into the oropharynx or guttural pouch.

Diagnostic Imaging

Diagnosis of hyoid abnormalities primarily depends on radiography. Some stylohyoid fractures are visible on lateral projections. Arthrosis of the temporohyoid articulation usually is evident only on a dorsoventral view, with the horse under general anesthesia and its neck extended. Deformation or fracture of the stylohyoid may be visible on endoscopic examination of the guttural pouch; hyoid fractures that extend into the pharynx also are visible endoscopically.

DISEASES WITH PHYSICAL CAUSES

Fracture of the Hyoid

Hyoid fractures can be caused by trauma or excessive traction on the tongue; they can also occur secondary to osteomyelitis (see below). Fracture of the stylohyoid may accompany fracture of the ramus of the mandible or occur with a blow to the poll (e.g., rearing and flipping over backward).

Treatment

Hyoid fractures may be repaired by wiring. However, the serious sequelae (cellulitis, severe dysphagia, and aspiration pneumonia) accompanying fractures that open into the oropharynx warrant a poor prognosis. Tracheostomy and feeding via nasogastric tube are useful during recovery. Closed unilateral fractures can heal without surgical intervention in 8 weeks.

INFLAMMATORY, INFECTIOUS, AND IMMUNE DISEASES

The stylohyoid and temporohyoid articulations can become involved in inflammatory processes originating in the middle ear or guttural pouch. Fusion of the temporohyoid articulation may result, which predisposes to fracture of the temporal bone and in some cases the stylohyoid bone. Damage to the adjacent vestibulocochlear and facial nerves and sometimes the glossopharyngeal, vagus, and hypoglossal nerves, can result. Affected horses show acute vestibular signs, including a head tilt.

Treatment and prognosis

• Long-term therapy with broad-spectrum antibiotics and NSAIDs is indicated.
• The prognosis for survival is guarded; if only the peripheral vestibular system is involved, the prognosis is fair to good.
• Partial stylohyoidostectomy can be performed to control the signs of chronic otitis media (persistent head shaking, ear rubbing, teeth grinding) and thus prevent fracture of the petrous temporal bone.

Diseases of the Teeth

(pages 660-675)

Michael Q. Lowder

DIAGNOSTIC AND THERAPEUTIC CONSIDERATIONS

Tooth Eruption and Nomenclature

Table 10-2 presents the most common ages for tooth eruption in horses; teeth usually are in wear 6 months after they

Table 10-2
Estimated tooth eruption times in the horse

Tooth	Eruption
DECIDUOUS	**TEETH**
First incisor	(D1) birth or first week
Second incisor	(D1 2) 4-6 wk
Third incisor	(D1 3) 6-9 mo
Second premolar	(Dp 2) birth or first 2 wk
Third premolar	(Dp 3) birth or first 2 wk
Fourth premolar	(Dp 4) birth or first 2 wk
PERMANENT	**TEETH**
First incisor	(I1) 2½ y
Second incisor	(I2) 3½ y
Third incisor	(I3) 4½ y
Canine	(C) 3½ y
First premolar (wolf tooth)	(P1) 6-9 mo
Second premolar	(P2) 2½ y
Third premolar	(P3) 3 y
Fourth premolar	(P4) 3½-4 y
First molar	(M1) 9-15 mo
Second molar	(M2) 2-3 y
Third molar	(M3) 3½-4 y

erupt. Eruption times may vary as much as 6 months among horses.

Dental Examination and Diagnostic Techniques

Examination should include a complete history (including the horse's eating and riding habits) and physical examination, paying particular attention to the horse's head and oral cavity.

Dental examination

Most horses need to be sedated for a complete dental examination. A full-mouth speculum is required to palpate the caudal molars, although examination of the other teeth usually can be performed without a speculum. In addition to the teeth, the buccal surface of the cheeks and the tongue should be palpated for abnormalities.

Diagnostic imaging

Radiography can be an important component of the diagnostic process. Four views (lateral, dorsoventral, and two obliques) should be taken when evaluating horses with suspected dental disease. Injection of contrast media into draining tracts often aids identification of the affected tooth. Nuclear scintigraphy sometimes identifies dental abnormalities that may have been inapparent radiographically.

Floating

Incisor arcade

The incisor arcade may require attention in individual horses. Excessive incisor length occurs in some horses and may interfere with the normal occlusion and/or excursion of the incisors or molars. An incisor rasp or Dremel carbide-chip burr is used to float the incisors until the occlusal surfaces of the two opposing arcades are in even contact.

Canine teeth

The canines can be floated to (1) correct partial fracture or overgrowth of a canine tooth, (2) facilitate insertion and removal of the bit, (3) reduce the chance of injury during breeding, and (4) treat and prevent formation of large calculi in older horses. The tooth is reduced with canine teeth nippers or with a Dremel diamond cut-off wheel and floated to smooth the cut edges.

Cheek arcade

The premolars and molars commonly require floating. A straight-blade float, inserted into the buccal space at a 45-degree angle to the teeth, is used to float the teeth in the upper arcade. The lower arcade is floated in the same manner, except that the tongue is held out of the way and the float is positioned on the lingual surface of the arcade. A caudal molar float is used to remove rear hooks (downward projections) and ramps (upward projections). A short-shank, 30-degree angle float is used to float the premolars.

Tooth Removal

Incisor teeth

Indications for incisor tooth removal include retained deciduous teeth, malalignment, and fractured or diseased teeth.

- Proper sedation and restraint are essential and can be augmented by a facial nerve block via the infraorbital or mental foramen.

- The gingiva is incised directly over the tooth and undermined with a periosteal elevator.
- The tooth is slowly moved from side to side to loosen the periodontal ligament.
- It is important to ensure that the entire tooth is extracted, not just the crown.
- Aftercare is minimal; daily flushing with warm water for a few days should be adequate.
  - NSAIDs may be given, but rarely are systemic antibiotics indicated.

Canine teeth
The only indication for removal of a canine tooth is fracture of the tooth below the gingiva. Surgical extraction is similar to that described for incisor teeth.

Wolf teeth
First premolars (wolf teeth) usually are found only in the upper arcade in males, although they may develop in females and in the mandibular arcade. Indications for removal include fracture, malalignment, bitting problems, and failure to erupt. Removal usually is a simple procedure.

- A wolf tooth extractor or a periosteal elevator and a pair of forceps may be used.
- The cylindrical end of the extractor is positioned directly over the crown of the tooth, and pressure is applied as the extractor is rotated back and forth.
- If the tooth fractures, a periosteal elevator is used to elevate the gingiva and rongeurs are used to remove the embedded piece of tooth.
- The horse's mouth should not be bitted for several days after removal of the wolf teeth.

Cheek teeth
Indications for removal of a premolar or molar include infection, cementum hypoplasia, fractures, supernumerary or loose teeth, sinusitis, malposition or malalignment, and dental tumors. Removal can be simple or complex, depending on the age of the horse, degree of disease or bone necrosis, degree of attrition, and tooth position.

- Extraction is more difficult in young horses.
- In most cases, radiography and endoscopy are recommended before extraction to ascertain which structures are involved.
- Cheek teeth can be removed via intraoral extraction, lateral buccotomy, trephination, or sinus flap; techniques are described in *Equine Medicine and Surgery V.*

Dental Caps
Dental caps are deciduous teeth that have not been shed, despite eruption of the permanent tooth. Caps usually involve the premolars, although deciduous incisors can also be retained. Removal of premolar caps is indicated when the caudal tooth is permanent and when the edges of the deciduous tooth are slivered or loose or prevent eruption of the permanent tooth. Large forceps are positioned on the retained cap and slowly rotated from side to side. Retained deciduous incisors are removed using the same techniques described for removal of permanent incisors.

CONGENITAL AND FAMILIAL DISEASES

Maxillary Prognathism (Parrot Mouth)
Maxillary prognathism (parrot mouth, brachygnathias, overbite) is the most common congenital dental abnormality in horses. Far less common is mandibular prognathism (sow mouth, monkey mouth, brachycephaly, underbite). These defects may be heritable. Some horses have a small degree of maxillary prognathism and yet perform their duties and maintain their body condition.

Management of maxillary prognathism
Considerations when deciding whether to treat an individual animal include age, intended use, body condition, and severity of the defect.

- If the discrepancy is mild, conservative treatment (frequent rasping of the elongated incisor arcade) or corrective orthodontics ("braces") may be attempted.
  - Corrective orthodontics should only be performed on animals between 2 and 6 months of age,

with <3 cm (1.25 inch) of space between arcades.

• If the discrepancy between the arcades is >3 cm, treatment usually is not attempted.

Supernumerary Teeth

Supernumerary teeth (polyodontia) can occur in the molar or incisor arcades. In the incisor arcade, the extra tooth may be removed for cosmetic reasons or if it causes bitting problems. In the cheek arcade, the extra tooth is best left alone if it is not causing a problem.

Dentigerous Cysts

Most often, dentigerous cysts are located near the ear but occasionally are found in the cranial vault or maxillary sinus. The cyst usually has a fistulous tract draining either into the pinna or exiting directly over the cyst. These cysts should be removed with the horse under general anesthesia. Preoperative radiographs should be taken to determine the extent of the cyst and bone involvement. The prognosis is excellent, unless complications arise as the dental remnants are separated from the underlying bone.

Other Conditions
Oligodontia
Oligodontia (missing teeth) is common and might be considered normal in some individuals.

Overcrowding
Overcrowding and shifting of teeth are common in Miniature Horses and Arabians, which often have a curved mandible. In these horses the last cheek tooth erupts at an abnormal angle and does not meet its counterpart in the opposing arcade. This problem is managed by frequent rasping.

DISEASES WITH PHYSICAL CAUSES
Incisor Arcade

Malalignment of the incisor arcade commonly occurs in middle-age and older horses. The contour of the arcade may be that of a smile, a frown, a tilt, or a step.

• The smile contour is corrected by reducing the length of the middle and lateral incisors on the lower arcade and filing the central incisors on the upper arcade.
  • This malalignment often is accompanied by malalignment of the molar arcade, so the table surface of the molar arcade must be kept in mind as the central incisors are reduced.
• The frown contour is corrected using the same principles, by reducing the central incisors on the lower arcade and the middle and lateral incisors on the upper arcade.
• The tilted (side-to-side) arcade requires reduction of tooth length on both incisor arcades.
• The stepped arcade is corrected by reducing the length of the elongated tooth.

Canine Teeth

A "blind" (unerupted) canine tooth can cause a horse to toss or shake its head. Treatment involves incising the gingiva over the tooth to aid eruption.

Molar Teeth
Wave mouth

Wave mouth can occur in any age of horse, but it occurs most frequently in older horses. The wave usually is located at the fourth premolar and first molar. The wave can be reduced by floating (mild cases) or with a Dremel burr or motorized float (more severe cases).

Step mouth

Step mouth also is more common in older horses. It develops when one tooth extends beyond the table surface of the adjacent teeth because of lack of an opposing tooth. The tooth is cut just above the occlusal surface using molar cutters or Gigli wire (less likely to fracture the tooth); the tooth surface is then filed smooth. A motorized Dremel tool can also be used to correct step mouth.

Smooth mouth

Smooth mouth affects older horses in which most, if not all, of the crown surfaces of the teeth are worn away. Typically, affected horses function well when fed a complete pelleted ration and any sharp points on the remaining teeth are floated. Smooth mouth in younger horses often is the result of improper floating. Feeding a soft ration allows the teeth to reshape with time.

Shear mouth

Shear mouth is characterized by an acute slope from the lingual to buccal surface of the upper cheek teeth and from the buccal to the lingual surface of the lower cheek teeth. It is associated with malocclusion of the incisors and narrowing of the intermandibular space and can lead to lacerations of the tongue, cheek, and palate. Frequent floating is the only effective treatment.

INFLAMMATORY, INFECTIOUS, AND IMMUNE DISEASES

Periodontal Disease

Periodontal disease is a major component of dental disease in older horses. With continual eruption, spaces can develop between adjacent teeth, allowing accumulation of food particles. Gingivitis and periodontal disease result and can eventually lead to tooth loss. Currently, there are no techniques available to prevent periodontal disease. Systemic antibiotics may be indicated when periodontal disease causes localized sepsis and halitosis.

Periapical Infection

Periapical infections are most commonly encountered in young horses when teeth are erupting.

- The diseased tooth should be examined radiographically to determine the extent of bone lysis and to evaluate the eruption space.
- If a retained deciduous tooth (cap) is present, it should be removed and, if necessary, the adjacent teeth filed to provide sufficient room for the erupting permanent tooth.
- Any draining tracts should be curetted and lavaged with antiseptic solution and systemic antibiotics and NSAIDs administered.
- If the area becomes inflamed again, the tooth will either require endodontic therapy (root canal surgery; see *Equine Medicine and Surgery V*) or need to be removed.

Patent Infundibulum

A patent infundibulum (dental caries, infundibular necrosis) develops when the infundibular cementum decays.

Patent infundibula usually are identified during careful oral examination.

- A blackish or brown spot (food particles and/or tooth decay) is seen in the center of the tooth.
- Some horses have halitosis, sinusitis, nasal discharge, and swelling over the affected tooth.
- Contrast radiography identifies any connection between the infundibulum and pulp cavity.
- It may be necessary to remove either part of the tooth (if the pulp cavity is not affected) or the whole tooth (if the pulp cavity is involved).

NEOPLASIA

Odontoma

Odontopathic tumors in horses are rare. Most are congenital and usually are identified when the horse is young. The most commonly reported odontoma in horses is ameloblastic odontoma of the maxilla. Most of these tumors are benign, but because of facial deformity and tumor size, useful life expectancy, even with treatment, is limited.

Ameloblastoma

Ameloblastomas primarily affect the mandible and usually affect older horses. They distort the mandible locally and appear radiolucent (cystic) radiographically. Benign osteomas, ossifying fibromas, and fibrous dysplasia each have a predilection for the mandible. Juvenile mandibular ossifying fibroma should be considered in the differential diagnosis (see p. 191).

Diseases of the Salivary Glands *(pages 676-677)*

James N. Moore

DISEASES WITH PHYSICAL CAUSES

Trauma to the Salivary Gland and Ducts

The parotid duct may be traumatized by a kick to the mandible, laceration, or guttural pouch surgery. Damage to the duct often results in a salivary fistula; the flow of saliva is most noticeable when the horse eats.

Management

♦ Most wounds to the salivary gland itself heal by second intention.

♦ Many wounds involving the parotid duct result in leakage of saliva for a short time but then heal by second intention.

♦ When the flow of saliva is sufficient to prevent wound healing, a salivary fistula develops.

♦ Surgery to reconstruct or destroy the duct is indicated for persistent fistulae.

♦ Another option is chemical destruction of the parotid gland using formalin (see *Equine Medicine and Surgery V*).

♦ Trauma to the sublingual salivary gland most often results in formation of a mucocele on the floor of the mouth, lateral to the frenulum; marsupialization into the mouth is effective.

Salivary Calculi

Salivary calculi are uncommon. Clinical findings may include swelling along the duct or acute inflammation of the gland. Treatment involves excision of the calculus.

INFLAMMATORY, INFECTIOUS, AND IMMUNE DISEASES

Sialoadenitis

Inflammation of the salivary glands is uncommon. The most common causes are trauma to the gland and obstruction of the salivary duct (e.g., with plant material). Sialoadenitis generally responds favorably to symptomatic therapy ($\pm$ antibiotics) and removal of any obstruction.

NEOPLASIA

Neoplasms rarely affect the salivary glands. Adenocarcinomas, acinar cell tumors, melanomas, and mixed tumors have been reported. Affected horses usually are aged. Clinical signs include pain, edema, and palpable enlargement of the gland. Diagnosis involves histologic examination of biopsy specimens. Generally, benign mixed tumors and acinar cell tumors are locally invasive and tend to recur; wide excision is required. Adenocarcinomas and malignant melanomas usually have metasta-

sized by the time a mass is evident, so treatment often is unsuccessful.

Diseases of the Esophagus *(pages 677-698)*
John A. Stick

DIAGNOSTIC AND THERAPEUTIC CONSIDERATIONS
Clinical Manifestations

Esophageal obstruction (choke) may be manifested by:

♦ ptyalism or regurgitation of food, water, and saliva from the mouth and nostrils

♦ dysphagia

♦ coughing

♦ repeated extension of the head and neck, retching

♦ other signs of distress or agitation
Electrolyte imbalances (hyponatremia, hypochloremia, and progressive metabolic alkalosis) and dehydration accompany cases of long duration. Aspiration pneumonia frequently follows esophageal obstruction, sometimes as early as 1 day after the onset of choke.

Diagnostic Tools
Radiography

Esophageal radiography is diagnostic in most instances. Plain films reveal obvious abnormalities, such as feed impaction and foreign bodies. Oral barium paste (85% w/v with water, 120 mL) localizes the obstruction and any disruption of the esophageal wall.

Endoscopy

Endoscopy can better define esophageal lesions diagnosed by radiography. The normal mucosa is white to light pink; reddening indicates mucosal disease. Swallowing produces luminal changes that give the appearance of diverticula or strictures. An inability to insufflate the esophagus and flatten the longitudinal mucosal folds usually indicates disease.

Manometry

Manometry can be used to further define certain esophageal problems.

Surgery

Techniques for esophageal surgery are described in *Equine Medicine and*

Surgery V. Despite meticulous surgical technique, complications can occur, including:

* dehiscence, leading to dissecting infections, fistulae, or stricture formation
* acid-base and electrolyte alterations
  * Daily oral administration of NaCl usually is all that is required; potassium requirements are met in feed, and alkalosis is corrected by the kidneys.
* laryngeal hemiplegia
* carotid artery rupture

CONGENITAL AND FAMILIAL DISEASES
Intramural Cyst
Esophageal cysts are uncommon.

* Clinical findings include dysphagia, regurgitation, a palpable soft tissue mass in the neck, and resistance to passage of a nasogastric tube.
* Diagnosis is confirmed when a filling defect is observed with contrast radiography.
* Endoscopically, the esophageal lumen may appear partially occluded, but significant gross changes usually are not observed because the mucosa appears normal.
* The cyst may be removed surgically.

Megaesophagus
Megaesophagus is dilation and muscular hypertrophy of the esophagus oral (proximal) to a constricted distal segment. Idiopathic dilation (congenital ectasia) can be treated conservatively with a mash diet (pellets mixed with warm water) fed from a trough elevated above the animal's withers. Access to roughage, including bedding, must be prevented.

DISEASES WITH PHYSICAL CAUSES
Diverticulum
Esophageal diverticula usually are acquired lesions and only occasionally cause esophageal dysfunction.

* Diagnosis is made by barium swallow esophagram.
* Traction diverticulum (outpouching of the esophagus by periesophageal fibrous tissue), even when large, produces few clinical signs and seldom requires treatment.

* Pulsion diverticulum (protrusion of mucosa through a defect in the muscularis) has a tendency to enlarge, so that risk of obstruction and rupture increases with time.
  * Surgical repair is indicated (see *Equine Medicine and Surgery V*).

Impaction
The most common type of esophageal disease is impaction with ingesta or bedding. Passage of a nasogastric tube and warm-water lavage usually are successful in relieving the obstruction; gentle external massage helps break up the mass. Xylazine sedation to lower the horse's head reduces the risk of aspiration. Alternative techniques if this method is unsuccessful include:

* lavage under pressure, using a cuffed nasogastric tube and dose syringe or stomach pump; if necessary, treatment is repeated in 8 to 12 hours
* lavage following esophageal relaxation by administration of atropine (0.02 mg/kg)
* lavage with the horse under general anesthesia, with the head lowered

Refractory impactions
Impactions that do not respond to conservative therapy should be evaluated radiographically and endoscopically and, if amenable, relieved by longitudinal esophagotomy. Surgery is preferable to repeated use of the nasogastric tube as a probang, which can cause severe trauma to the larynx and esophagus.

Aftercare
One aftermath of simple impaction is esophageal dilation, which predisposes to reobstruction. The condition resolves in 24 to 48 hours, provided the dilated area is kept free of ingesta. Following are guidelines for care following relief of esophageal impaction:

* Food should be withheld or only small quantities of a soft diet fed for 2 days.
* Glucose-electrolyte solutions should be provided in addition to fresh drinking water.
* Broad-spectrum antimicrobial therapy is indicated for 5 to 7 days because of the potential for aspiration pneumonia.
* Posttreatment endoscopic evaluation (± radiography) is warranted for obstructions that were present

for several days or were refractory to initial treatment.

♦ Circumferential mucosal ulceration is common and usually results in esophageal stricture.

Dilation

Dilation, or acquired megaesophagus, usually is the result of impaction, but can be caused by a distal constricting lesion (e.g., vascular ring anomalies in foals, or stricture). Once the primary lesion has been identified and corrected, dilation should not be a persistent problem, providing it is not of long duration.

Foreign Body

Small pieces of wood, wire, and medication boluses can become esophageal foreign bodies. They may perforate the esophageal wall, resulting in cellulitis or abscessation. The swelling that results usually obstructs the esophageal lumen and causes an impaction. Diagnosis is made by radiography and/or esophagoscopy.

Treatment

♦ Endoscopic retrieval of small, sharp foreign bodies is possible but difficult; general anesthesia is recommended to prevent swallowing during manipulation.
♦ Blunt or round foreign bodies may be treated similar to feed impactions, but gentle manipulation is mandatory to avoid esophageal rupture.
♦ Surgery is preferable to manipulations that could induce further esophageal trauma.
♦ Longitudinal esophagotomy with primary closure results in minimal complications when performed in a region of normal esophagus (see *Equine Medicine and Surgery V*).

INFLAMMATORY OR INFECTIOUS DISEASES

Ulceration and Esophagitis

Mucosal ulceration and esophagitis commonly occur secondary to long-standing impactions. Other causes in foals include phenylbutazone toxicity and severe gastroduodenal ulcer disease with reflux esophagitis (see p. 203). Diagnosis is best made by endoscopy.

Treatment

Goals of therapy are to minimize further mucosal damage, reduce inflammation, and control infection. Treatment includes:

♦ a low-bulk, minimally abrasive diet (mash)
  • The patient should be muzzled between feedings or all bedding should be removed.
♦ NSAIDs (if not implicated as causative agents)
♦ broad-spectrum antimicrobial therapy
♦ reexamination every 10 to 14 days
♦ H_2 blockers to reduce gastric acidity

Perforations, Lacerations, and Rupture

Causes of esophageal rupture include long-standing obturation, repeated or aggressive nasogastric tube passage, foreign body perforation, and external trauma to the cervical area (usually a kick). Swallowed air escapes from the rupture and causes subcutaneous emphysema, and cervical swelling usually prevents passage of a nasogastric tube. Contrast radiography reveals escape of barium into surrounding tissues.

Treatment

Ruptures that cannot drain through the skin result in leakage of saliva and ingesta into the adjacent tissues, where severe infection develops.

Establishment of drainage, preferably on the ventral midline, is necessary.

♦ Perforation or lacerations accompanied by minimal escape of saliva and ingesta can be repaired surgically, if treated within 12 hours of injury.
  • The horse should receive systemic antibiotics and be offered only drinking water; electrolyte and nutritional requirements should be met by tube feeding.
♦ Esophagostomy and insertion of a feeding tube distal to the defect allows feeding while the damaged area heals.
♦ Resection of the esophagus after rupture is warranted if the muscular layer is obviously necrotic and if the proximal and distal segments can be anastomosed without tension.

Stricture

Strictures most often are a result of mucosal trauma. Circumferential ulcers >2.5 cm wide may result in stricture formation within 30 days. Strictures are best demonstrated by positive-pressure contrast esophagograms. Conservative management is aimed at dilation of the stenotic segment:

- Early lesions can be dilated with frequent feeding of small quantities of soft food.
  - A low-bulk diet and antiinflammatory and antimicrobial therapy are recommended.
- Chronic strictures (>60 days old) may be corrected by esophagomyotomy, partial or complete resection and anastomosis, or patch grafting (see *Equine Medicine and Surgery V*).

Fistula

Esophageal fistulae should be considered when cervical swelling, fever, and dysphagia are present, a nasogastric tube can be passed to the stomach, and endoscopic findings are normal. Contrast radiography, using liquid barium administered under pressure, best demonstrates the lesion. Once ventral drainage is established, fistulae almost always heal spontaneously. If healing does not occur, resection of the sinus tract and closure of the stoma may be necessary.

NEOPLASIA
Squamous Cell Carcinoma

Neoplasms that cause esophageal obstruction are rare; squamous cell carcinoma is the most common neoplasm involving the esophagus. Biopsy and cytologic examination of brush samples obtained via endoscopy may provide an early diagnosis. The value of resection is questionable.

Diseases of the Stomach

(pages 699-715)

Alfred M. Merritt and
Martha Campbell-Thompson

DIAGNOSTIC AND THERAPEUTIC CONSIDERATIONS
General Diagnostic Approach

Gastric disease in horses usually causes nonspecific signs of intermit-

tent anorexia and abdominal pain. Weight loss, weakness, and fever may be seen with chronic conditions. Yawning, teeth-grinding, and "dog-sitting" (to relieve the pain of gastric dilation) are seen in some cases. The diagnostic approach generally should include the following:

- passage of a nasogastric tube (except in foals with gastroduodenal ulcer disease)
- rectal palpation (to rule out other abdominal disorders)
- CBC and serum chemistry panel
- peritoneal fluid collection and analysis
- oral glucose or D-xylose absorption tests (to identify delayed gastric emptying)

Gastroscopy

Gastroscopy is valuable in diagnosing gastric disease.

- Foals usually are fasted for at least 6 hours, and adults for at least 10 hours before gastroscopy.
- Normally, the squamous mucosa appears as a white, glistening, fairly smooth surface.
  - Some crater-like erosions may be seen where *Gastrophilus* larvae have been attached.
  - Thin pieces of desquamated epithelium often are seen dorsal to the margo plicatus in foals <1 month old.
  - The lesser curvature should be examined for early indications of squamous ulcer disease.
- The glandular mucosa is dark pink and appears more folded than the squamous mucosa.

Radiographic Examination

Contrast studies with barium sulfate (30% to 50% solution at 3 to 5 mL/kg) and/or air insufflation can be used to diagnose gastroduodenal ulcer disease and pyloric or duodenal stenosis in foals and gastric tumors and stenosis in adult horses. Gastric emptying can also be evaluated using scintigraphy.

Medical Therapy
Relief of gastric distention

Gastric distention must be relieved as quickly as possible by passing a nasogastric tube.

- If resistance to passage of the tube is encountered at the cardia, infusion of 5 to 10 mL of lidocaine may relax the cardia enough to allow intubation.
- Gas and fluid flow can often be induced by filling the tube with water and gently aspirating with a large dose syringe.
- Alternatively, 1 L of water is pumped into the stomach and siphoning induced by positioning the proximal end of the tube below the level of the horse's stomach.
  - The tube is moved back and forth several times to increase the chances of positioning the distal end in a fluid or gas pocket.
  - Siphoning is repeated several times.
- Reflux volume should be measured and the pH of the fluid checked; the nasogastric tube generally is left in place and taped to the halter.
- With gastric impactions, lavage with a large-bore tube may be attempted.

Prokinetic drugs

Before using prokinetic drugs to stimulate gastric motility, it is important to ensure that there is no physical obstruction to gastric emptying. The most promising agents with the fewest undesirable side effects are bethanechol (0.025 mg/kg IV slowly) and erythromycin (0.1 to 1.0 mg/kg IV slowly). Other agents with prokinetic potential include lidocaine, metoclopramide, fenoldopam, cisapride, and NSAIDs.

Antiulcer therapy

There are three basic pharmacologic approaches to gastric ulceration.
- Maintain an intragastric pH >4 with H_2 antagonists (e.g., cimetidine, ranitidine) or omeprazole.
- Coat the damaged mucosa with an acid-resisting agent (e.g., sucralfate).
- Provide E-type prostaglandins or stimulate their production by the gastric mucosa.
  - PGE_2 analogs are indicated in horses at risk of NSAID-induced ulcer disease.
  - Feeding corn oil (20 mL/100 kg body weight) increases PGE in the gastric contents.

Dosages for the drugs mentioned in this section are given on p. 181.

CONGENITAL AND FAMILIAL DISEASES

Pyloric Stenosis

Pyloric stenosis may be congenital or acquired.
- Clinical signs include abdominal pain, salivation, teeth grinding, retching, gastric reflux, and relief of pain after removal of gastric contents.
  - In congenital cases, signs may first appear when the foal begins to eat solid food.
- Endoscopy reveals gastric reflux entering the distal esophagus, and distal esophagitis and gastric ulceration.
- Radiography shows gastric dilation; megaesophagus and aspiration pneumonia may be seen in severe cases.
- Initial treatment consists of fluid, electrolyte, and nutritional support, and antiulcer therapy.
- Surgical correction by pyloroplasty or gastroenterostomy may be necessary (see *Equine Medicine and Surgery V*).

DISEASES WITH PHYSICAL CAUSES

Gastric Dilation

Gastric dilation may be primary (only involving the stomach) or secondary to a more distal gastric outflow obstruction. Causes of primary gastric dilation include excessive feed consumption (grass, hay, or grain), rapid water intake (especially after exercise), aerophagia (cribbing), and parasitism. Secondary dilation is more common and usually results from either intestinal ileus or obstruction.

Diagnosis and treatment

- The primary clinical sign is acute onset of moderate-to-severe abdominal pain.
  - The horse may lean back or assume a "dog-sitting" position.
  - Ingesta may be seen at the nares; retching and vomiting can indicate a terminal event.
- Most affected horses have hemoconcentration, hypokalemia, and hypochloremia.
- *As a priority*, a nasogastric tube must be passed and gastric fluid siphoned out repeatedly.

- Medical therapy is supportive for fluid losses, pain, and secondary complications (aspiration pneumonia and endotoxemia).
- A thorough workup should be performed to determine whether or not the condition is secondary to ileus, proximal enteritis, or intestinal obstruction.

Gastric Impaction

Gastric impaction may result from:
- gastric atony; for example, adynamic ileus, peritonitis, enteritis, trauma, chronic distention
- ingestion of feed that swells if improperly masticated; for example, wheat, barley, persimmon seeds
- accumulation of dry ingesta or foreign material; insufficient water intake, poor dentition, and rapid eating predispose to impaction

Diagnosis and treatment
- Signs include acute or chronic abdominal pain, retching, salivation, and ingesta at the nares.
- Endoscopic and radiographic examinations are used to confirm the diagnosis.
- Treatment consists of nasogastric lavage, if possible, or laparotomy with infusion of fluid and massage to soften the impacted mass.
- *Attempts at stimulating gastric motility are contraindicated due to the risk of rupture.*
- In many cases the diagnosis is made at surgery.

Gastric Rupture

Gastric rupture is a potential complication of gastric impaction or dilation, even with an indwelling nasogastric tube.
- The severe abdominal pain of gastric distention suddenly abates and the horse appears calm; however, signs of shock quickly develop.
  - Affected horses have marked tachycardia, hypochloremia, and septic peritoneal effusion.
- Presence of gastric reflux is not a reliable indicator of gastric rupture.
- Rectal palpation may reveal gritty ingesta free in abdominal cavity and on serosal surfaces.
  - Food particles may be recovered by abdominocentesis.

- Radiography may reveal free air near the diaphragm and surrounding the kidneys; ultrasonography may show excessive abdominal fluid.
- Inaccessibility and excessive contamination of the peritoneal cavity preclude surgical repair.

INFLAMMATORY, INFECTIOUS, AND IMMUNE DISEASES
Gastric Parasitism

Parasites of the equine stomach include *Gasterophilus* spp., *Habronema* spp., *Draschia megastoma*, and *Trichostrongylus axei*. Infection is common but rarely results in clinical signs. Ivermectin is effective against all of these parasites.

TOXIC DISEASES
Nonsteroidal Antiinflammatory Drug Toxicity

NSAIDs, such as phenylbutazone, flunixin meglumine, and ketoprofen, can induce varying degrees of GI mucosal damage that may manifest as ulceration. Phenylbutazone is the most toxic, and ketoprofen is the least toxic.

Diagnosis and treatment
- Signs include oral ulceration, excessive salivation, depression, and diarrhea.
- Serum protein and albumin concentrations decrease if intestinal ulceration is severe.
- The most important therapeutic approach is cessation of NSAID therapy.
- Specific antacid therapy may be unnecessary.
- Daily feeding of corn oil (20 mL/100 kg) may be a practical approach to inducing endogenous gastric prostaglandin production. NSAID toxicity is discussed further on p. 186.

NEOPLASIA

Squamous cell carcinoma occurs in the squamous gastric mucosa, mostly in horses >6 years of age.
- Signs may include anorexia, progressive weight loss, and colic (especially after a meal).

- Anemia, dysphagia, pleural effusion, and salivation also are seen in some cases.
♦ The diagnosis is supported by finding anemia and neutrophilia on CBC.
♦ Radiography may demonstrate the tumor, and ultrasonography may reveal metastases in the liver, spleen, or visceral peritoneum; the latter may be palpable per rectum.
♦ Endoscopy or exploratory laparotomy with biopsy are used to confirm the diagnosis.
♦ The prognosis invariably is grave.

MULTIFACTORIAL DISEASES
Gastric Ulcer Disease

Gastric ulcer disease in horses may be divided into four general categories, based on the inciting cause and/or age or use of the horse.

"Stress-related" glandular disease
♦ Ulcers develop in the glandular mucosa, adjacent to the margo plicatus, in severely ill or traumatized foals and horses; they can be severe enough to cause a perforation.
♦ Affected animals usually show no signs of gastric ulceration.

Primary Erosion/Ulceration of the Squamous Mucosa
♦ Erosions and ulcers in the squamous mucosa are common findings in horses of all ages.
  - >80% of young (≤4 yrs) Thoroughbreds in race training have squamous mucosal lesions.
  - The most common site is the lesser curvature, near the margo plicatus.
♦ Lesions may be subclinical, although they can cause poor appetite and performance.
♦ Horses with symptomatic ulcer disease respond well to antiulcer therapy, particularly therapies that suppress acid secretion.
  - Lesions often recur after cessation of treatment in horses that continue in training.

Gastroduodenal ulcer disease
This disease occurs in sucklings and early weanlings and is a serious problem in intensive mare/foal operations.

♦ The syndrome can manifest as a herd outbreak, with the first, and sometimes outstanding, clinical sign being watery diarrhea.
  - Some foals refuse to nurse and show mild signs of colic and/or teeth grinding.
  - A few foals are found dead.
♦ The most severe, and probably primary, lesion develops in the upper duodenum.
♦ If clinical signs suggest the presence of endotoxemia and/or peritonitis, ultrasonography should be performed; excessive intraabdominal fluid is highly suggestive of perforation.
♦ Most affected foals survive and are well within 1 week after treatment with antiulcer medications and supportive care.

A few foals become progressively more ill despite treatment and develop "classic" gastroduodenal ulcer disease.
♦ Signs include drooling, teeth grinding, periodic bouts of colic (especially after nursing), and marked weight loss.
♦ Endoscopy shows erosive esophagitis and squamous gastritis (± frank ulceration).
  - Occasionally, the primary lesion can be seen within the proximal duodenum.
♦ If these signs persist for >1 week, it is a strong indication that duodenal scarring and stenosis is mechanically obstructing gastric emptying.
♦ Treatment involves gastrojejunostomy (see *Equine Medicine and Surgery V*).

NSAID-induced disease
This problem is discussed on p. 186.

Diseases of the Small Intestine *(pages 716-735)*
William P. Hay, P.O.Eric Mueller, and Janice E. Sojka

DIAGNOSTIC CONSIDERATIONS
Small Intestinal Obstruction

The most common clinical findings with small intestinal obstruction are:

- abdominal pain, often poorly responsive to analgesics
  - Pain generally is worst with strangulating obstructions (e.g., volvulus, incarceration).
- presence of nasogastric reflux
- decreased or absent borborygmi
- small intestinal distention, detected by transrectal palpation
  Severe abdominal pain despite nasogastric decompression is the single most important indicator for surgical intervention.

Malassimilation Syndromes

Many conditions can interfere with digestion, absorption, and/or metabolism of nutrients from the small intestine. Malassimilation syndromes are characterized by (1) negative energy balance, resulting in weight loss, and (2) low plasma protein. Diarrhea may be present, but is not a consistent feature. If >60% of the small intestine is permanently damaged or surgically removed, the long-term prognosis is poor.

Protein-losing enteropathy

Protein-losing enteropathy typically causes lethargy, weight loss, and dependent edema (pectoral region, ventral abdomen, and prepuce).

- Although all classes of proteins may be lost into the gut lumen, serum albumin generally is decreased in relation to globulins.
  - Total plasma protein may be normal, so both albumin and globulins should be measured.
- Presumptive diagnosis may be made by ruling out other causes of protein loss (e.g., renal disease) and by excluding the possibility of liver failure (see p. 234).
- Definitive diagnosis is made by administering ^{51}CR-labeled albumin parenterally and documenting fecal protein loss.
- Oral absorption of glucose or D-xylose may be normal.
  Diseases that can result in protein-losing enteropathy include verminous arteritis, acute salmonellosis or other infectious enteritis, congestive heart failure, mesenteric abscess (e.g., *Rhodococcus equi, Streptococcus equi*), GI ulceration, granulomatous enteritis, and alimentary lymphosarcoma.

CONGENITAL AND FAMILIAL DISEASES

Meckel's Diverticulum

Meckel's diverticulum is a congenital tubular structure extending from the antimesenteric surface of the ileum. Feed material may become impacted in the diverticulum, resulting in chronic colic. If not surgically resected (see *Equine Medicine and Surgery V*), the diverticulum may rupture, resulting in fatal peritonitis.

Mesodiverticular Band

Persistence of one of the vitelline arteries results in a fold of tissue that runs from the mesentery to the antimesenteric surface of the small intestine, forming a pocket that can potentially entrap intestine. Definitive diagnosis is made, and the condition corrected during exploratory celiotomy.

DISEASES WITH PHYSICAL CAUSES

Postoperative Adhesions

Intraabdominal adhesions are the most common cause of recurrent colic after small intestinal surgery.

- Clinical signs include weight loss and inability to return to a roughage diet without repeated colic episodes; severe adhesions can lead to complete obstruction or strangulation.
- Treatment often is unrewarding.
  - Horses with mild strictures may be able to consume low-residue feeds (e.g., complete pelleted rations, lush pasture) without recurrent colic.
- Horses with severe obstruction require repeat celiotomy (see *Equine Medicine and Surgery V*).
  - Horses that require repeat celiotomy >60 days after the original surgery are 8 times more likely to survive long-term than those requiring repeat celiotomy before 60 days.

Intestinal Stricture

Small intestinal strictures result from fibrous adhesions (secondary to abdominal surgery or peritonitis) or from severe mucosal ulceration (mostly seen in foals <4 months old with severe duodenal ulceration; see

p. 203). Strictures in adult horses usually are confirmed during exploratory celiotomy and corrected by resection or bypass of the strictured segment. The prognosis in both foals and adults is guarded.

Epiploic Foramen Hernia

The epiploic foramen is a narrow space between the caudate process of the liver and the right lobe of the pancreas. The foramen increases in size with age, so epiploic foramen herniation is more common in horses >7 yrs old.

- Clinical signs are extremely variable.
  - Horses may present with severe abdominal pain or with marked depression (especially once severe intestinal ischemia develops).
  - Most affected horses have small intestinal distention on rectal examination, and many have nasogastric reflux.
- Results of abdominocentesis are variable.
- Diagnosis and correction are made during exploratory celiotomy (see *Equine Medicine and Surgery V*).
- Prognosis depends on the duration before surgical intervention and the amount of small intestine involved; recent reports indicate a long-term survival rate of 60% to 70%.

Mesenteric Hernia

Congenital defects (e.g., mesodiverticular bands) and traumatic rents in the mesentery or greater omentum provide potential sites for internal herniation.

- Clinical signs are indicative of intestinal obstruction.
- Peritoneal fluid may be normal early, but the total protein and WBC count increase as the intestine becomes devitalized.
- Diagnosis and correction are made during exploratory celiotomy (see *Equine Medicine and Surgery V*).

Gastrosplenic Ligament Incarceration

The gastrosplenic ligament runs from the greater curvature of the stomach to the hilar area of the spleen and is continuous ventrally with the greater omentum. Defects in the gastrosplenic ligament may be congenital or acquired (traumatic).

- Clinical signs vary with the degree of intestinal compromise.
  - Horses may initially present with mild-to-moderate abdominal pain, normal peritoneal fluid, and no nasogastric reflux.
  - Those with complete intestinal obstruction present with marked pain, nasogastric reflux, and serosanguinous fluid on abdominocentesis.
- The lesion usually cannot be palpated per rectum because of its cranial location in the abdomen.
- Diagnosis and correction are made during exploratory celiotomy (see *Equine Medicine and Surgery V*).

Inguinal Hernia
Acquired inguinal hernias

Acquired inguinal hernias usually are unilateral and most often occur in adult stallions. A predisposition has been reported in Standardbreds, American Saddlebreds, and Tennessee Walking Horses. Inguinal herniation and eventration also is a potential complication of castration. Herniation leads to acute intestinal obstruction and severe intestinal compromise.

- Palpation of the scrotum usually reveals a swollen, firm, cool testicle on the affected side.
- Intestine can be palpated per rectum entering the internal inguinal ring.
- Correction requires surgical intervention (see *Equine Medicine and Surgery V*).
- Castration of the affected testicle is recommended, although if the testicle is viable, it can be left in place and the vaginal ring partially imbricated to decrease the chance of recurrence.
- The prognosis for survival is as high as 76% with rapid surgical correction.

Congenital inguinal hernias

Inguinal hernias sometimes occur in young male foals.

- Most of these hernias can be manually reduced, close spontaneously as the foal grows, and seldom cause clinical problems.
- If the hernia is relatively small, the colt can simply be confined to a box stall and observed.

- The owner can be instructed to manually reduce the hernia several times daily.
- Foals with larger hernias may benefit from confinement and a figure-eight inguinal bandage (see *Equine Medicine and Surgery V*).
- Inguinal hernias that persist beyond 6 months of age or in which an excessive amount of bowel herniates through the defect require surgical intervention (see *Equine Medicine and Surgery V*).
- Ocasionally, a hernia ruptures through the vaginal tunic into the subcutaneous space; this leads to intestinal compromise that requires immediate surgical intervention.

Strangulating Umbilical Hernia

Most umbilical hernias in foals are reducible and do not result in intestinal incarceration (see p. 232). Nonreducible hernias present as a firm, warm umbilical swellings that are painful on palpation and cause signs of intestinal obstruction. These hernias should be considered an emergency requiring immediate surgical intervention (see *Equine Medicine and Surgery V*).

Intussusception

Intussusception of the small intestine occurs when a section of bowel telescopes inside the lumen of the adjacent distal segment of bowel. Predisposing factors include enteritis, dietary changes, parasitism (ascarids, tapeworms), mesenteric arteritis, and intraluminal masses or foreign bodies. Small intestinal intussusception is most common in foals and horses <3 years old.

Clinical signs and diagnosis

- Signs vary with the location, extent, and duration of the obstruction.
  - Intussusception of large sections of intestine usually results in complete obstruction and acute abdominal pain that is poorly responsive to analgesics.
  - Intussusception of shorter segments may result in partial or intermittent obstruction and chronic colic lasting weeks or months.
- Small intestinal distention often is palpable per rectum, and occasionally the intussusception can be palpated as a firm, tubular structure.

- In foals, radiography may reveal distended loops of small intestine.
- Ultrasonography may reveal small intestinal distention and the classic "bull's eye lesion."
- Peritoneal fluid protein and WBC count often are elevated, but may be normal.

Treatment and prognosis

- Treatment requires ventral midline celiotomy (see *Equine Medicine and Surgery V*).
- The prognosis depends on the extent and duration of the lesion; reported recovery rates vary from 42% to 100%.

Volvulus

Volvulus occurs when a segment of intestine rotates >180 degrees around the long axis of its mesentery. It can be primary or secondary to other small intestinal conditions.

Clinical signs and diagnosis

- Volvulus causes acute, severe abdominal pain that is poorly responsive to analgesics.
  - Hemoconcentration and hypovolemia develop rapidly.
- Nasogastric reflux often is obtained and frequent nasogastric decompression is required to minimize the chance of gastric rupture.
  - In most cases, pain is not relieved by gastric decompression.
- Moderate-to-severe small intestinal distention can often be palpated per rectum, and it is sometimes possible to feel the rotation at the root of the mesentery.
- Peritoneal fluid may be normal initially, but there generally is an increase in protein (>3 g/dL) and WBCs (>10,000 cells/μL) as intestinal compromise progresses.

Treatment and prognosis

- Small intestinal volvulus requires surgical correction (see *Equine Medicine and Surgery V*).
- The prognosis depends on the length of intestine involved and the degree of compromise.
  - Devitalized intestine necessitating extensive resection carries a poor prognosis.

Pedunculated Lipoma

Pedunculated lipomas are benign fatty tumors that arise from the mesentery or serosa of the intestine. As the lipoma enlarges, its attachment may lengthen, allowing it to wrap around intestine and cause complete obstruction. The jejunum or ileum is the site most often affected, although the small colon is involved in some cases. This is a condition of older horses (mean age 16 years); geldings and ponies are at increased risk.

Clinical findings and outcome

- Signs vary with the site, amount of intestine involved, and degree of strangulation.
  - Horses often present with mild to-moderate colic and may initially respond to analgesics.
  - Most have palpable small intestinal distention per rectum.
- Peritoneal fluid may be normal initially; however, most horses with strangulating lipomas have increases in peritoneal fluid protein and WBC count.
- diagnosis and correction are made during exploratory celiotomy (see *Equine Medicine V*).
- The prognosis depends on the extent of intestinal compromise; reported long-term survival rates are 50%.

INFLAMMATORY, INFECTIOUS, AND IMMUNE DISEASES

Strongyloides westeri Infection

Strongyloides westeri (thread worm) infection affects foals <6 months of age.

- It does not appear to be an important cause of foal diarrhea.
- Diagnosis can be made by flotation of fresh feces.
  - The eggs are smaller than strongyle eggs and contain a vermiform embryo.
- Most anthelmintics at recommended dosages effectively eliminate these parasites in foals.
  - Giving mares ivermectin immediately postpartum decreases the incidence of foal infection.

Ascariasis

Clinical disease caused by *Parascaris equorum* (roundworm) is predominantly seen in foals between 3 and 12 months of age. It can be a severe problem on farms where overcrowding of foals leads to accumulation of eggs in the environment. The larvae remain in their shells and are extremely resistant to environmental conditions; eggs remain infective for up to 5 years.

Clinical signs and diagnosis

Initially, the predominant clinical signs are coughing and nasal discharge (see Chapter 9, Respiratory System); signs of intestinal infection become apparent 2 to 4 weeks later.

Intestinal ascarid infection causes rough hair coat, poor growth, weight loss, pendulous abdomen, lethargy/ depression, and inappetence/anorexia.

More severe manifestations include diarrhea, colic, and ascarid impaction, which may result in complete small intestinal obstruction, bowel rupture, peritonitis, and death.

Hypoproteinemia (in particular hypoalbuminemia) often exists.

Diagnosis of a patent infection is made by identifying the eggs on fecal examination.

Treatment

- Foals in contaminated areas should be dewormed at 6-week intervals until 6 months of age.
  - Adult ascarids are susceptible to a wide variety of anthelmintics, but no formulation is completely effective against migrating larvae.
- A benzimidazole product (e.g., fenbendazole) should be used when treating a heavily parasitized foal for the first time; a more effective product can be used later.
  - Use of ivermectin or piperazine predisposes to ascarid impaction and intestinal rupture.
  - Concurrent administration of mineral oil may be beneficial.
- Ascarid impactions that cannot be resolved medically (e.g., with mineral oil and analgesics) require surgical intervention.

Tapeworm Infection

Anoplocephala perfoliata is the most common tapeworm found in horses. It has a predilection for sphincters and orifices, and large numbers may be found at the ileocecal junction.

- Young horses most often are affected.

- Enteritis, mucosal erosions and ulcers, perforation, peritonitis, and intussusceptions have been attributed to tapeworm infection.
- Diagnosis is made by fecal examination; the proglottids are about the size of a rice grain.
  - The typical angular eggs may be found on fecal flotation.
- Pyrantel pamoate (13.2 mg/kg) and niclosamide (100 mg/kg) effectively kill tapeworms.

Cryptosporidiosis

Cryptosporidia can cause diarrhea in immunocompromised foals. Diagnosis is made by identification of oocytes in feces (the tiny oocysts take up acid-fast stain) or examination of histopathologic sections. Specific treatment is not available, although oral paromomycin (50 to 100 mg/kg PO q24h) and hyperimmune colostrum reduce the severity and duration of cryptosporidial diarrhea in calves.

Viral Enteritis

Viruses produce malabsorption and diarrhea by destroying enterocytes at the tips of the villi. In foals, rotavirus is the most common viral agent, although coronavirus, adenovirus, and parvovirus also are implicated as pathogens. Rotavirus is an ubiquitous virus and usually causes diarrhea only when a large infective dose is ingested or when other pathogens, such as *Salmonella* organisms, are present. Poor sanitation and overcrowding are contributing factors.

Clinical signs and diagnosis

- Affected foals usually are <1 month old; clinical disease rarely occurs in animals >2 months old.
- Depression and anorexia are noticed first; profuse, watery diarrhea follows in 12 to 24 hours.
- Fever and leukopenia are variable findings and indicate concurrent bacterial infection.
- Diagnosis is made by use of a commercial ELISA kit or by detection of virus particles in feces or gut sections using electron microscopy.
- A supportive history and environmental conditions are important for diagnosis.

Treatment and prevention

- Therapy is aimed at restoring and maintaining hydration and electrolyte balance.
- Antibiotics are indicated in debilitated or septicemic foals.
- In most cases, the diarrhea resolves in 7 to 14 days.
  - Lactase deficiency should be suspected in foals with prolonged diarrhea (see p. 209).
- Prevention involves good hygiene and avoiding overcrowding.
  - Phenolics, 10% povidone iodine, and formaldehyde fumigation are effective against rotavirus; hypochlorites, quaternary ammonium compounds, and chlorhexidine are not.
  - Adequate passive transfer of antibody should be ensured in all foals.

Infectious Granulomatous Diseases

Several infectious agents cause granulomatous small intestinal disease, including *Mycobacterium tuberculosis (avium)* and *Mycobacterium paratuberculosis, Histoplasma* spp., and *R. equi.* Clinically, they may be impossible to distinguish from other causes of granulomatous enteritis; histopathologic examination and gut or fecal cultures may be required for specific identification. *Mycobacterium* spp. may be susceptible to isoniazid (3 to 20 mg/kg/day) or rifampin (10 mg/kg q12h). There are no reports of successful treatment for the intestinal form of *R. equi* infection.

Clostridial Enteritis

Clostridium perfringens and *Clostridium welchii* can cause peracute hemorrhagic enteritis in foals. Affected foals may be found dead or moribund, and most die within 24 hours of the onset of signs (which variably include colic and severe diarrhea). Clostridial enterocolitis is discussed further in the section on diseases of the large intestine.

NEOPLASIA

Alimentary Lymphosarcoma

Alimentary lymphosarcoma tends to be a disease of young horses (2 to 11 years). It can cause protein-losing enteropathy and malabsorption.

- Findings may include weight loss, mild colic, diarrhea, fever, dependent edema, and icterus.
- Malabsorption can be confirmed with oral glucose tolerance tests (see p. 177).
- Diagnosis is made by finding atypical lymphocytes in blood or peritoneal fluid or by intestinal or mesenteric lymph node biopsy.
- The prognosis is grave; the disease often is widely disseminated at the time of diagnosis.

Other Intestinal Neoplasms

Tumors of the intestinal tract other than lymphosarcoma and benign lipomas are very rare. Horses with intestinal neoplasia may present with a history of chronic colic or weight loss. Peritoneal fluid analysis may reveal atypical cells; however, normal peritoneal fluid does not rule out neoplasia. Intestinal leiomyomas are focal, benign lesions, and affected horses should have a good prognosis after resection of the lesion. The prognosis for other tumors varies.

MULTIFACTORIAL DISEASES

Lactase Deficiency

Lactase deficiency can result from a primary enteric disorder (e.g., viral enteritis) in young foals.

- The principal clinical sign is severe diarrhea, with dehydration, acidosis, and loss of electrolytes in an unweaned foal.
  - These signs can be identical to those produced by the causative agent.
- Hypoglycemia may develop from lack of a glucose substrate.
- Diagnosis is by an oral lactose tolerance test (see p. 177).
- Treatment consists of temporarily or permanently removing milk from the diet.
  - If the foal is of sufficient age, weaning is recommended.
  - Younger foals should be muzzled to prevent nursing and given oral rehydration solutions containing glucose or dextrose.

IDIOPATHIC DISEASES

Ileal Impaction

Ileal impaction is the most common cause of nonstrangulating small intestinal obstruction in horses. Feeding Bermuda grass hay has been implicated as a cause; limited forage intake, heat, and stressful conditions can also predispose horses to ileal impaction.

Clinical signs and diagnosis

- Signs vary with the duration of impaction.
  - Initially, abdominal pain often is marked because of intestinal spasms.
  - After this initial response, the horse may appear more depressed than in pain, until progressive small intestinal and gastric distention result in recurrence of abdominal pain.
- Early on, the distended ileum may be palpable per rectum, but later small intestinal distention often prevents palpation of the impacted ileum.
- Large volumes of reflux are obtained after several hours of obstruction.
- Hematologic abnormalities reflect the degree of dehydration, which can become severe.
- Peritoneal fluid initially is normal, but mild-to-moderate increases in total protein are found after several hours of obstruction; increases in peritoneal WBC count are not common.

Treatment and prognosis

- When the diagnosis is made early and abdominal pain is not severe, ileal impaction can sometimes be corrected with IV fluids, repeated nasogastric decompression, and analgesics.
- Most affected horses require surgical reduction of the impaction (see *Equine Medicine and Surgery V*).
- Long-term survival following prompt surgical intervention is as high as 70%; this figure rapidly declines as the time between impaction and surgery increases.

Muscular Hypertrophy of the Small Intestine

Muscular hypertrophy can occur as a primary idiopathic condition or as a compensatory condition (e.g., in response to chronic caudal stenosis). The hypertrophy narrows the intestinal lumen, causing partial or complete obstruction.

- Affected horses generally have a history of chronic, intermittent colic and present with lethargy, anorexia, and mild-to-moderate abdominal pain that is responsive to analgesics.
  - Nasogastric reflux often is absent.
- Small intestinal distention is palpable per rectum in only 50% of cases; it is sometimes possible to palpate the thickened intestine.
- Laboratory data, including peritoneal fluid analysis, often are within normal limits.
- Diagnosis and correction are made during exploratory celiotomy (see *Equine Medicine and Surgery V*).
- The prognosis depends on the degree of intestinal compromise; horses that are treated before intestinal compromise has become severe have a good prognosis.

Granulomatous Enteritis

Granulomatous enteritis is most common in young adult horses (2 to 5 years). Standardbreds are affected more often than other breeds, and a familial incidence has been reported. Suggested causes include an unidentified bacterium, hypersensitivity to a common antigen, and immune dysfunction.

Clinical signs

- The most common sign is chronic weight loss.
- Horses are bright and alert initially, but become increasingly depressed with debility.
- Appetite may be increased, normal, decreased, or variable; generally it is increased initially.
- Diarrhea is uncommon; if present, large intestinal involvement should be suspected.
- Roughened hair coat, alopecia, dry flaky skin, and pruritus may be present, particularly with the eosinophilic form of the disease (see below).
- Dependent edema develops if the animal becomes hypoproteinemic.
- Enlarged mesenteric lymph nodes may be palpated on rectal examination.

Diagnosis

The CBC often is normal, but there may be neutrophilia with a mild left shift.

- Hypoalbuminemia is the most consistent laboratory finding.
  - Total plasma protein may be low or normal, depending on the globulin levels.
- Glucose or D-xylose absorption tests may indicate decreased small intestinal absorption.
- Peritoneal fluid findings usually are normal.
- Rectal biopsy can be diagnostic if the rectum is involved.
- Definitive diagnosis is made by intestinal biopsies taken via exploratory laparotomy.
- Duodenal biopsy, taken via endoscopy, may become a valuable diagnostic aid.

Treatment and prognosis

Therapy is aimed at modulating the host's immune response with immunosuppressive drugs.

- Some horses improve on parenteral prednisolone at 2.2 mg/kg/day.
- In most cases treatment generally is unrewarding, and the long-term prognosis is grave.
- Feeding a high-quality ration free choice is necessary.

Eosinophilic Gastroenteritis

Eosinophilic gastroenteritis causes chronic weight loss, protein-losing enteropathy, dermatitis, and sometimes diarrhea. A wide range of organs may be affected, including the skin, intestinal tract, pancreas, salivary gland, mesenteric lymph nodes, and lungs, although not all organs are affected in every horse. The cause is unknown, but may involve a sensitizing allergen.

Diagnosis and treatment

- Laboratory abnormalities include hypoproteinemia, hypoalbuminemia (protein-losing enteropathy), and, occasionally, eosinophilia in the blood and peritoneal fluid.
- Diagnosis is based on biopsy of affected sites; skin and rectal mucosa are readily accessible.
- Successful therapy has been reported with dexamethasone at 0.2 mg/kg daily for 5 days, followed by de-

creasing doses of oral prednisolone, starting at 0.55 mg/kg q12h.
* The dose should be decreased to the smallest amount necessary to control clinical signs.
♦ Affected horses may need lifelong corticosteroid therapy.

Duodenitis–Proximal Enteritis

Duodenitis–proximal jejunitis is also referred to as *proximal enteritis, anterior enteritis, gastroduodenojejunitis,* and *hemorrhagic fibrinonecrotic duodenitis–proximal jejunitis.* Most cases occur in adult horses. Clostridial or *Salmonella* infection has been proposed as a cause.

Clinical signs

♦ The syndrome is characterized by an initial fever and acute onset of colic (sometimes severe) followed by depression.
♦ Signs of dehydration are found with progressive disease, and endotoxic shock may develop.
♦ Borborygmi may be absent.
♦ Gastric reflux, often in voluminous amounts, can be obtained via nasogastric tube.
  * The gastric reflux often is orange-brown or blood tinged, fetid, and alkaline.
  * Once the stomach has been decompressed, colic signs usually abate and depression is the most prominent sign.

Diagnosis

♦ Rectal examination findings are variable, ranging from no significant changes to distended, gas- or fluid-filled small intestine.
♦ Laboratory findings often include increased PCV, leukocytosis with band neutrophils and toxic changes, elevated serum alkaline phosphatase, and azotemia.
  * Alkalosis may be present initially, but acidosis develops with hypovolemic shock.
♦ The peritoneal fluid usually is normal in appearance, but may become serosanguineous.
  * Peritoneal fluid protein usually is >3 g/dL, but the WBC count is <6000 cells/μL.

Proximal enteritis is likely if rectal palpation does not indicate a condition that requires surgery, the peritoneal fluid has normal cellularity, and colic dissipates after gastric decompression. Surgery should not be performed unless repeat evaluation demonstrates clear surgical indicators.

Treatment

Treatment is primarily supportive.
♦ The first priority is to prevent gastric rupture by nasogastric decompression.
  * Initially, large volumes of reflux may be recovered (up to 8 L/h), so it is best to leave the nasogastric tube in place and siphon at regular intervals.
♦ IV fluid therapy should be instituted to restore and maintain fluid and electrolyte balance.
  * Bicarbonate should not be given unless blood gas analysis indicates acidosis.
  * Nasogastric intubation and IV fluid therapy may be required for several days.
  * Broad-spectrum antibiotics should be administered.
♦ Flunixin meglumine (1 mg/kg) often is used as an analgesic and to prevent some of the effects of endotoxin.
  * NOTE: *It is important to ensure adequate gastric decompression **before** administering an analgesic if a horse with proximal enteritis demonstrates colic.*
♦ In cases with severe, prolonged gastric reflux, surgical bypass may be necessary.

Prognosis

Mortality in horses with proximal enteritis varies significantly. With prompt, vigorous medical therapy, the prognosis is good. Life-threatening complications include laminitis, pleuropneumonia, hepatitis, renal disease, and peritoneal adhesions.

Diseases of the Cecum

(pages 735-740)
Michael W. Ross

DISEASES WITH PHYSICAL CAUSES
Cecal Torsion

Cecal torsion generally occurs only under situations of adhesion or entrapment (e.g., accompanying large colon volvulus). Surgical correction is the only viable treatment.

Adhesion

Adhesion of the cecum to adjacent structures is unusual, except after exploratory celiotomy, in which the cecum may adhere to the site of abdominal incision. Intermittent mild colic could result. Rectal examination may reveal chronic malposition or tension on the ventral cecal band.

INFECTIOUS, INFLAMMATORY, AND IMMUNE DISEASES

Typhlitis

Typhlitis, or inflammation of the cecum, occurs with enteric salmonellosis (see p. 215). It generally is not a primary disease entity.

MULTIFACTORIAL DISEASES

Cecal Impaction

Cecal impaction with fibrous feed material is the most common disease of the cecum.

- Old age, poor quality feedstuffs, and poor dentition have been implicated, but younger horses often are affected, particularly those hospitalized for musculoskeletal or GI problems.
  - Parasites (including tapeworms), abrupt dietary changes, certain drugs, and general anesthesia can each alter cecal motility.
- Affected horses that are treated with analgesics and allowed to continue eating are at risk of cecal perforation.

Clinical signs and diagnosis

- Cecal impaction typically causes mild abdominal pain, inappetence, and depression.
- Gut sounds are depressed, and the periodic cecal emptying sound is absent.
- Fecal production is decreased, and feces may range from dry to "cow flop" in texture.
- Vital signs are normal, except during painful episodes.
- Rectal examination reveals a firm, digesta-filled viscus with a distinct ventral band; the hand may be passed to the right of, but not dorsal to the viscus.

- Laboratory data, including peritoneal fluid analysis, usually are normal.
  - PCV and plasma protein may be mildly elevated, reflecting mild dehydration.

Treatment

Medical treatment is advised when the cecum is only moderately distended.

- liberal IV and oral fluid therapy
- withholding food until the cecum is palpably normal
  - Addition of laxative feedstuffs (e.g., bran mash, fresh grass) or switching to a low-residue pelleted diet may help prevent recurrence once the horse's normal diet is reintroduced.
- flunixin meglumine (1mg/kg IV) for analgesia
  - Xylazine affects cecal motility and should be avoided.
  - Horses in severe pain and those requiring multiple doses of analgesics more potent than flunixin meglumine are candidates for surgical intervention.

Surgery should be considered if the cecum is greatly distended with firm digesta, or if the impaction is refractory to medical treatment. Techniques are described in *Equine Medicine and Surgery V.*

Prognosis

The prognosis is guarded because of the possibility of recurrence or perforation.

Cecal Perforation

Cecal perforation can have one of two presentations:

- a primary entity in periparturient mares
- a secondary disease in horses with cecal outflow dysfunction, leading to cecal distention
  - Horses that are hospitalized or being treated for other disorders are at risk of developing cecal impaction and subsequent perforation.

Clinical signs after perforation are characteristic of endotoxin shock (rapid cardiovascular deterioration and death). There is no effective treatment.

Cecal Tympany

Gas distention of the cecum most often is secondary to large colon abnormalities (e.g., displacement, volvulus).

- Findings include moderate-to-severe abdominal pain and right-side abdominal distention with a cecal ping on simultaneous auscultation and percussion.
- Rectal examination reveals a gas-filled cecum with marked tension on the ventral band.
- Mild tympany associated with spasmodic colic can be managed medically with analgesics, antifermentives, oral fluids, and fasting.
- Cecal tympany secondary to colonic displacement or volvulus requires surgical correction of the primary problem.
- With severe cecal distention, *trocarization* may be necessary for pain relief.
  - After aseptic preparation of the right paralumbar fossa, a 5-inch, 14-gauge needle or IV catheter is inserted through the body wall into the cecal base.
  - Possible complications include localized peritonitis and cellulitis.

IDIOPATHIC DISEASES
Cecocecal/Cecocolic Intussusception

Intussusception of the body of the cecum into its base or continuation into the right ventral colon is uncommon. Possible causes or contributing factors include tapeworms, organophosphates, and intramural abscess or other damage to the cecal wall.

Clinical signs and diagnosis

There are three forms of cecocecal/cecocolic intussusception.

- *acute:* Changes in vital signs and laboratory values, including elevated peritoneal fluid protein and WBC and RBC counts, are more pronounced than with the other forms.
- *subacute:* Signs include depression, intermittent abdominal pain, and reduced fecal output.
- *chronic:* Signs include weight loss, fever, and intermittent mild abdominal pain.
  - As the invaginated bowel becomes devitalized, the horse show signs of increased abdominal pain and cardiovascular deterioration.

An enlarged viscus may be felt on rectal examination, although the cecum is not palpable in some horses. Exploratory celiotomy often is necessary to establish the diagnosis.

Treatment and prognosis

- Surgical management is necessary for a successful outcome (see *Equine Medicine and Surgery V*).
- The prognosis is good if all of the diseased cecum can be removed.

Infarction

Cecal infarction is rare. It can occur at any age, but is seen more often in foals <1 year of age.

- Signs vary from acute, severe abdominal pain and cardiovascular collapse to low-grade colic, diarrhea, and evidence of peritonitis.
- Surgery (partial typhlectomy) may be successful if only part of the cecal body is affected.
- If the entire cecum is necrotic, the prognosis is grave.

Diseases of the Large Colon *(pages 741-768)*
Noah D. Cohen and Kenneth E. Sullins

DISEASES WITH PHYSICAL CAUSES
Colonic Impaction

Impaction of dry fecal matter may be promoted by reduced water intake, coarse roughage, poor dentition, ingestion of foreign material or sand, and colonic displacement.

Clinical signs and diagnosis

- Colic may develop acutely or be mild and intermittent at first, then gradually worsen.
- Intestinal sounds may be normal or reduced.
- The mass may be palpable per rectum if the pelvic flexure or left colon is affected.
- Transverse colon impactions or more isolated sand impactions are not palpable.
- Laboratory values, including peritoneal fluid indices, initially are within normal limits, but change with metabolic deterioration.

Treatment

Medical therapy consists of:

- IV fluids (20 to 50 L/day) and correction of any electrolyte imbalances
- analgesics
- mineral oil (2 to 4 L, ± warm water), magnesium sulfate (0.5 kg in warm water), or psyllium (for sand impaction) via nasogastric tube
- small amounts of good-quality hay or fresh grass to stimulate bowel motility

Surgical intervention is indicated when pain cannot be easily controlled, peritoneal fluid values indicate bowel deterioration, or signs of endotoxemia appear.

Enteroliths

Enteroliths are mineral concretions that slowly form in the colon and lodge in the transverse colon, small colon, or pelvic flexure (less common).

- More cases are seen in California and the southern United States than in other parts of the country.
- Most cases occur in horses >4 years of age; mean age of affected horses is ~ 10 years.
- Signs are similar to those of impaction, except that they may be intermittent and chronic.
- Surgery is indicated with rectal or radiographic confirmation of an enterolith or when there is intractable pain or other evidence of complete colonic obstruction.
- Prognosis for survival is excellent.

Colonic Torsion/Volvulus

Large colon volvulus is a life-threatening condition. Postpartum mares are most often affected.

Clinical signs and diagnosis

- Abdominal pain is acute, severe, and often difficult or impossible to control.
- Cardiovascular deterioration progresses rapidly.
  - As gaseous distention worsens, respiration becomes compromised.
  - Hemoconcentration may be masked by sequestration of blood in the colon; when this situation occurs, the prognosis is grave.
  - An increase in peritoneal fluid protein also is associated with a poor prognosis.
- Rectal examination reveals extreme distention of the large colon, which

may be oriented transversely across the pelvic inlet.

Treatment and prognosis

- Successful therapy depends on expedient surgical correction (see *Equine Medicine and Surgery V*).
- One study reports a survival rate of 36%; survival rates from practices in areas that have a lot of brood mares exceeds 80%.
- Colopexy (via celiotomy or laparoscopy) can be effective in preventing recurrence.

Right Dorsal Displacement of the Colon

This condition involves displacement of the left colons to the right of the cecum, with the pelvic flexure lying near the sternum.

- Signs vary from insidious pain to violent, uncontrollable colic, depending on the amount of gaseous distention and tension on the mesentery.
- Metabolic indicators also vary from normal to those of obstructive shock (uncommon).
- On rectal examination, the right colons are oriented transversely across the pelvic inlet, and the left colons may extend beyond reach into the cranial abdomen.
- Right dorsal displacement requires surgical correction (see *Equine Medicine and Surgery V*).
- The prognosis is good in uncomplicated cases.

Left Dorsal Displacement of the Colon

This condition involves displacement of the left colons dorsal to the renosplenic ligament; it is also referred to as *renosplenic* or *nephrosplenic entrapment*.

Clinical signs and diagnosis

- The pain initially is mild and intermittent, but gradually worsens and becomes unrelenting.
- Metabolic status and laboratory findings vary with the duration and severity of the condition.
- Abdominocentesis often produces blood because the spleen is displaced ventrally and axially.
- Rectal findings are diagnostic when the colon can be traced over the renosplenic ligament.

- Ultrasound is useful in some cases.

Treatment and prognosis

- Exploratory laparotomy often is indicated (see *Equine Medicine and Surgery V*).
  - Many clinicians advocate rolling the horse under short-term general anesthesia.
- The survival rate is >90%.

Complications are uncommon, but include bowel rupture during reduction, recurrence of the displacement, and strangulation or focal necrosis of the left colons.

Displacement of the Pelvic Flexure and/or Left Colons

The most common form of pelvic flexure displacement is cranial flexion of the left colons, causing the pelvic flexure to lie near the sternum.

- Usually this is a nonstrangulating displacement, but it can obstruct the flow of ingesta.
- Clinical signs are variable, the severity of pain and the metabolic status depending on the duration and amount of gaseous distention.
- Typically, the pelvic flexure cannot be located on rectal examination.
- Such displacements often self-correct with analgesics and supportive therapy.
- The prognosis for survival is good.

Intussusception of the Large Colon

Intussusception of the large colon generally is a disease of young animals.

- Typical signs are mild, recurrent pain with continued passage of soft feces.
  - More severe colic occurs when obstruction leads to gaseous distention.
- Mild tachycardia persists, with variable depression of intestinal sounds.
- Mild fever may be present.
- Leukocytosis in the peripheral blood and peritoneal fluid is often present.
  - Plasma fibrinogen and/or peritoneal fluid protein may also be increased.
- Treatment consists of surgical reduction and/or resection of the affected segment.
- The prognosis is good with timely recognition and correction.

INFLAMMATION, INFECTIOUS, AND IMMUNE DISEASE

Salmonellosis

Salmonellae are non–spore-forming, gram-negative, facultative anaerobic bacteria. They produce a cytotoxin that causes enterocyte death and an enterotoxin, similar to that of *E. coli*, which may cause intestinal secretion of fluid and electrolytes. Many of their effects are mediated by endotoxin.

Epidemiology

Salmonellosis is the most common cause of infectious enterocolitis in adult horses. Its prevalence increases in the warmer months. Risk factors include transportation, changes in diet, antimicrobial treatment, surgery, and GI tract disorders. The immune status of the host undoubtedly plays an important role.

The most common sources of infection are:

- other horses, either by direct transmission or environmental contamination
  - Salmonellae can survive in soil for >300 days, in water for at least 9 months, and in dry fecal matter for up to 30 months.
- contaminated feed (in which salmonellae can survive for protracted periods)
- autoinfection

Clinical findings in Salmonella-induced colitis

Salmonellosis can manifest as acute or chronic disease; asymptomatic shedders also may be identified. This section discusses acute *Salmonella*-induced colitis.

- Clinical signs include lethargy, anorexia, colic, and diarrhea.
  - Pain may vary from mild to severe and often precedes diarrhea by hours or even days.
- The diarrhea usually is profuse and watery, with malodorous, greenish-black feces.
  - Onset of diarrhea may be gradual (over several days) or acute and "explosive."
- Tachycardia, dark red or purple mucous membranes (sometimes with a pale, "toxic" line adjacent to the teeth), and abnormal intestinal sounds ± abdominal distention are present.

- Frequent high-pitched sounds may be heard, but often intestinal sounds are decreased.
- *Complications* include laminitis, bacteremia/septicemia, renal failure, thrombophlebitis, DIC, hepatitis, and fungal pneumonia.

Diagnosis

- Laboratory abnormalities generally are nonspecific.
  - Leukopenia with neutropenia typically is observed early in the disease, but occur with any cause of enterocolitis and attendant endotoxemia.
  - Hypoproteinemia is common and may persist for weeks or months.
- Horses with colitis often have low serum sodium, chloride, potassium, and ionized calcium; they also tend to be acidotic.
  - Prerenal azotemia is common, although severe colitis can result in hemodynamic renal failure; careful monitoring of renal function is warranted in azotemic patients.
  - Presence of fecal leukocytes helps attribute the colitis to an invasive pathogen.
- In most cases, culture is used to detect salmonellae.
  - 10 to 50 g of feces should be submitted for culture on at least five separate days.
  - Culture of rectal mucosa collected with uterine biopsy forceps may also be rewarding.
  - If the animal does not survive, cultures of the cecum, large colon, and ileum, mesenteric lymph nodes, and spleen usually are more sensitive than fecal culture.
- Polymerase chain reaction (PCR) is more rapid and considerably more sensitive than culture.

Treatment

Salmonellosis is difficult to manage successfully. The mortality rate in some circumstances approaches 90%. Therapy primarily consists of supportive care.

- *Fluid therapy* is aimed at correcting fluid deficits and electrolyte or acid-base disorders.
  - Maintenance needs and ongoing losses must then be addressed

(see Chapter 4, Principles of Therapy).

- Fluid therapy should include provision of oral fluids, unless small intestinal ileus is present.
  - Both electrolyte solutions and fresh water should be offered.
  - An oral electrolyte solution can be prepared by adding 120 g (4 oz) of the following mixture to 12 L of water:

    455 g (1 lb) table salt
    311 g (1 box) "lite" salt
    (67% KCl and 33% NaCl)
    336 g (³/₄ lb) baking soda

- *Flunixin meglumine* (1 mg/kg IV q12h) helps combat endotoxemia and may have antisecretory effects.
- Fresh-frozen *plasma* or *hyperimmune serum* may be of some benefit in horses that are hypoproteinemic (total protein concentration <4.5 g/dL) or have evidence of endotoxemia.
- Use of *antimicrobial drugs* in adult horses with salmonellosis remains controversial.
  - Antibiotics do not change the course of the enteric infection nor speed resolution of the diarrhea, and they may prolong the duration of bacterial shedding.
  - Antibiotics tend to be used only if there is evidence or suspicion of bacteremia, septicemia, or immunosuppression.
  - Specific antimicrobial treatment should be based on results of susceptibility testing because resistance is quite variable among isolates.
  - Ceftiofur, trimethoprim-sulfa combinations, ampicillin, and enrofloxacin have all been used to treat salmonellosis.
- Activated charcoal (1 to 3 g/kg as a slurry q12-24h), bismuth subsalicylate (2 to 4 L), or mineral oil (2 to 4 L) via nasogastric tube may have some palliative effects.
- Feeding or nasogastric administration of psyllium (50 to 120 g [2 to 4 oz] q6-8h) may increase fecal bulk and promote colonic healing.
- Frog support with pads or bar shoes often is used in an attempt to prevent laminitis.

- Other preventive therapies have included DMSO (1 g/kg IV as a 10% solution q12-24h), heparin (20 to 40 IU/kg IV or SC q8h), and topical glyceryl trinitrate (2% paste; 15 to 30 mg per digital vessel).
- A diet of pelleted feed may help "rest" the colon; other horses do better when fed hay.

Control and prevention

Efforts at control and prevention are essential, particularly in places where large groups of susceptible horses can be found (e.g., racetracks, hospitals, horse shows). Specific strategies, including isolation, hygiene, and disinfection, are discussed in *Equine Medicine and Surgery V.*

Clostridial Diarrhea

Clostridia are endospore-forming, anaerobic gram-positive rods. *Clostridium perfringens* and *C. difficile* are the most common clostridial pathogens in horses.

- Disease caused by *C. perfringens* is more prevalent in young foals (<7 days old).
  - It usually is sporadic, but multiple cases have been reported on some farms.
- *C. difficile* causes fatal, hemorrhagic necrotizing enterocolitis in neonatal foals.
  - It can also cause diarrhea in foals and adult horses.

Sources of clostridial organisms include feces, soil, water, feeds, and sewage. Factors that contribute to the development of clostridial enterocolitis include intestinal mucosal damage, age and immunity of the host, use of antimicrobial drugs or dietary changes that alter intestinal microflora, virulence and number of ingested organisms, and stress.

Clinical findings

Clinical signs vary with the age of the animal and the clostridial species involved.

- Foals are more frequently affected, with signs ranging from mild diarrhea, to severe, hemorrhagic diarrhea, to sudden death.
- In adults, signs range from moderate-to-severe diarrhea to fatal enterocolitis.

- Signs of colic often accompany clostridial enterocolitis.
- Affected horses and foals usually are severely dehydrated and have signs of shock.

Diagnosis

Diagnosis of clostridial enterocolitis can be difficult.

- Laboratory findings are similar to those described for salmonellosis, except for the common finding of hematochezia in foals.
- Specific diagnosis of *C. perfringens* diarrhea is based on isolation of the organism and demonstration of its toxin in feces or intestinal contents.
- Demonstration of *C. difficile* in feces may be sufficient to attribute diarrhea to the organism.

Treatment

Treatment of severe clostridial enterocolitis often is unrewarding.

- Supportive treatment similar to that for salmonellosis should be implemented.
- Metronidazole (10 to 15 mg/kg PO q6-12h; see *Equine Medicine and Surgery V*) may be beneficial.
- Crystalline penicillin (22,000 IU/kg IV q6h, or higher doses) sometimes is advocated.
- Administration of probiotics or yeast products (e.g., brewers' yeast) may be helpful.

Control and prevention

- Avoiding oral lincomycin, erythromycin, and clindamycin in adult horses is recommended
- Vaccinating mares with a *C. perfringens* toxoid developed for ruminants was effective in one report, although this product is not registered for use in horses.

Ehrlichial Colitis (Potomac Horse Fever)

Ehrlichial colitis (Potomac horse fever, equine monocytic ehrlichiosis) in horses is caused by the rickettsial organism *Ehrlichia risticii,* a gram-negative, obligate intracellular bacterium. The disease generally is sporadic, although a seasonal distribution has been observed, with highest prevalence in July, August, and September.

Clinical signs

- Signs may include fever, depression, anorexia, colic, diarrhea, laminitis, and abortion.

♦ Any of these signs may be observed alone or in combination, rendering diagnosis difficult.
  • The fever is biphasic, but the first febrile episode often is missed.
  • <60% of affected horses have diarrhea; when present, diarrhea is variable in severity and duration, although it rarely lasts >10 days.
  • Laminitis develops in 30% to 40% of horses.
♦ Signs of endotoxemia are observed in some horses.
♦ Case fatality can approach 30%.

Diagnosis
Diagnosis generally is based on serologic testing.
♦ Paired serum samples should be collected 5 to 7 days apart.
  • A titer ±1:80 generally is considered positive.
  • Detecting a rise in titer often requires initial sample collection before onset of signs.
♦ A single titer is not useful, except that a negative titer indicates a disease other than ehrlichial colitis is likely.
♦ False-positive results are relatively common.
  Preliminary success with PCR is reported.

Treatment
♦ Ehrlichial colitis can be successfully treated with oxytetracycline (6.6 mg/kg IV q24h).
♦ Response to treatment can be observed within 12 hours.
  • If no improvement is seen within 24 hours, another diagnosis should be considered.
♦ If treatment is implemented early in the disease, signs resolve by 3 days and tetracycline often can be discontinued after 5 days.
♦ Supportive treatment for colitis should be implemented, as described for salmonellosis.
♦ Secondary salmonellosis can develop, so it is advisable to isolate horses with ehrlichial colitis.
  Vaccines to prevent equine ehrlichial colitis are commercially available (see Chapter 4, Principles of Therapy).

Colitis X
Colitis X is a condition of acute or peracute colitis that is clinically and pathologically indistinguishable from some cases of peracute clostridial enterocolitis (see p. 217).

Larval Cyathostomiasis
Infective cyathostome larvae penetrate the cecal and colonic mucosa, where they molt and become encysted for a varying and sometimes prolonged period.
♦ Pathogenesis is largely attributed to synchronous emergence of encysted larvae.
♦ Clinical disease most often occurs in the winter and spring.
♦ The disease is more common in younger horses (<6 years).
♦ A history of recent deworming has been linked to larval cyathostomiasis.

Clinical signs
Larval cyathostomiasis can cause either acute or chronic diarrhea.
♦ The progression and severity of colitis are less profound than with other causes of infectious colitis; signs of endotoxemia are rare.
♦ Chronic diarrhea often is fluctuant.
♦ Recurrent colic, weight loss, and fever also have been associated with larval cyathostomiasis.

Diagnosis
Diagnosis can be difficult.
♦ The history may indicate a good deworming program, making parasitism seem less likely.
♦ Fecal egg counts are of little value because the damaging parasites are larvae.
  • However, a herd average >400 eggs/g should increase suspicion of a parasitic problem.
♦ Anemia, hypoproteinemia, eosinophilia, and neutrophilia are seen in some cases.
  • An increase in β_1-globulins sometimes occurs with small strongyle infection.
  • Eosinophilia in peritoneal fluid, although inconsistent, also suggests parasitism.
♦ Response to treatment can be of diagnostic value.
♦ Definitive diagnosis can be made by microscopic examination of cecal or colonic biopsy specimens; a scraping of rectal mucosa also may reveal immature cyathostomes.

Treatment

Treatment is directed at killing adult and larval cyathostomes, controlling colonic inflammation, and providing supportive care.

- Adult and luminal immature cyathostomes can be killed with most commercially available anthelmintics, except benzimidazoles.
- Effective treatment against encysted larvae is limited to fenbendazole (10 mg/kg/d for 5 days or 50 to 60 mg/kg/d for 3 days) and moxidectin (manufacturer's recommended dosage).
- Corticosteroids may limit colonic inflammation
  - Dexamethasone can be given at 0.04 to 0.05 mg/kg IV or IM q24h for 4 days then tapered.
  - Tapering doses of oral prednisolone (reduction every 5 to 7 days from 2 mg/kg/d, to 1.5 mg/kg/d, to 1 mg/kg/d, to 1 mg/kg every other day) also are effective.

Other Parasites

Giardiasis

Giardia spp. infection has been associated with chronic diarrhea. Diagnosis should be based on:

- exclusion of other causes of diarrhea
- detection of giardial cysts in feces by immunofluorescence (commercial kit) or by microscopic examination of feces following zinc sulfate centrifugal flotation
- response to treatment with metronidazole

Cryptosporidiosis

Cryptosporidiosis primarily affects young, immunocompromised foals. It is discussed in the section on diseases of the small intestine.

TOXIC DISEASES

Right Dorsal Colitis

Right dorsal colitis generally is caused by administration of NSAIDs, most often phenylbutazone, and often at dose rates that are well tolerated by most horses (see p. 186). Other possible causes include chronic impaction, mechanical irritation, and tuberculosis (see *Equine Medicine and Surgery V*).

Clinical signs

- The most common signs are recurrent episodes of anorexia, lethargy, and low-grade colic.
- Physical examination reveals few abnormalities.
- The feces usually have a normal to soft consistency, but diarrhea occurs in some cases.
- Occasionally, ventral edema develops secondary to protein-losing enteropathy.

Diagnosis

- Presumptive diagnosis is based on a history of NSAID administration and on clinical signs.
- Several laboratory abnormalities may be present, but none is specific for the condition.
  - Anemia and hypoproteinemia (especially hypoalbuminemia) are common.
  - The WBC count usually is normal, although leukocytosis and hyperfibrinogenemia (inflammation), or neutropenic leukopenia (endotoxemia) occur in some cases.
  - Hypocalcemia also is common.
  - Some horses have prerenal azotemia and hyperbilirubinemia.
- Occult blood can be present in the feces, but currently available tests are not highly sensitive.
- Peritoneal fluid rarely is abnormal.
- Gastroscopy should be performed if possible, because signs are similar to those associated with gastric ulceration (which may be present concurrently).

Treatment

Medical management consists of:

- discontinuing NSAIDs
- ensuring adequate hydration
- feeding a low-bulk diet (pelleted feed) combined with psyllium mucilloid
  - Feeding small amounts of concentrate 4 to 6 times/day and restricting roughage for 3 to 6 months is recommended.
- administering sucralfate (22 mg/kg PO q8-12h)

Despite early recognition and medical management, some horses develop colonic strictures. Horses that require surgical management tend to have a poor prognosis.

MULTIFACTORIAL CAUSES

Antibiotic-Associated Diarrhea

Clindamycin, tetracycline, lincomycin, tylosin, and oral penicillin V can cause diarrhea in horses. Other penicillins, ceftiofur, erythromycin, and pyrimethamine-trimethoprim/sulfonamide combinations also have be implicated as potential causes of diarrhea. The mechanism likely involves alterations in intestinal flora that favor superinfection with pathogenic organisms such as clostridia. Contributing factors include dietary changes, hospitalization, concurrent intestinal disease, fasting, and surgery.

Clinical signs and diagnosis

- Diarrhea usually develops within a few days of initiating antibiotic therapy.
- Diarrhea varies in severity from mild and self-limiting to rapidly fatal, toxic enterocolitis.
- Definitive diagnosis is difficult.
  - The history indicates antimicrobial administration and unexplained diarrhea.
  - Resolution of diarrhea after withdrawal of the drug supports the diagnosis.
- Culture of feces may identify potential pathogens (e.g., salmonellae or clostridia).

Treatment

Treatment includes discontinuing the implicated drug and providing supportive care.

- If *C. difficile* is identified, metronidazole can be effective.
- Transfaunation using a slurry of feces, or preferably cecal colonic fluid, is indicated.
  - Brewers' yeast and probiotics may also be of benefit.

Chronic Diarrhea

Chronic diarrhea most often occurs in adult horses, but can develop in weanlings and yearlings. Identifying the cause often is difficult; a definitive antemortem diagnosis is reached in only about 25% of cases. Multiple factors may play a role; possible causes include:

- cyathostomiasis
- sand ingestion
- granulomatous colitis
- hepatic disease

- colonic neoplasia (e.g., lymphosarcoma)
- food allergies
- fermentative disorders
- chronic salmonellosis (uncommon)

Clinical findings

- In most cases, vital signs and intake of feed and water are normal.
- Fecal consistency may vary from semiformed stool to watery diarrhea.
- Physical examination findings generally are unremarkable.
  - Concurrent weight loss indicates a large colon problem.
  - Ventral edema may be present if significant hypoproteinemia exists.
- Rectal palpation findings often are normal, although colonic impaction with sand, lymphadenitis, and colonic/rectal edema may be detected.

Diagnosis

The database should comprise the following:

- complete history, including diet, deworming, duration of diarrhea, weight loss, concurrent illness, and all drugs used before or after the onset of diarrhea
- thorough physical examination, including rectal palpation
- CBC and serum chemistry profile (including protein electrophoresis)
- fecal egg count
- peritoneal fluid analysis
- analysis of feces for occult blood, sand, clostridial organisms and their toxins, salmonellae, giardial cysts, cryptosporidial oocysts, ciliated protozoa, and WBCs
  - Failure to find sand does not exclude it as a potential cause.
  - Ciliated protozoa should be present in normal, fresh feces; their absence indicates a severe alteration of colonic flora.
  - Increased numbers of fecal WBCs indicate an active inflammatory disease, which raises the suspicion of an invasive bacterial disease.

Other tests that may be worthwhile in certain cases include:

- carbohydrate absorption testing (see p. 177)
  - Generally, diarrhea is caused by colonic disease, so carbohydrate absorption is normal.

- rectal mucosal biopsy to identify inflammatory bowel disease or exclude salmonellosis
- radiography of the ventral abdomen to identify sand
- exploratory laparotomy or laparoscopy to collect biopsy specimens

Treatment

Specific therapies include:
- anthelmintics for parasitic causes
- metronidazole (7.5 mg/kg PO q6h) for giardiasis
- psyllium mucilloid for sand accumulation
- dietary alterations for suspected food allergies

Empiric treatments that may be attempted in other cases include:
- transfaunation with 5 to 6 L of fecal slurry or, preferably, cecal or colonic contents from a horse with no intestinal disease (recommended in horses lacking normal fecal protozoa)
- metronidazole (useful in horses with clostridial overgrowth)
- iodochlorhydroxyquin (5 to 10 g/500-kg horse PO q24h)
  - May improve or normalize the feces, but some horses respond only transiently and others deteriorate with this treatment.
- psyllium mucilloid either in the feed or via nasogastric tube
- immunomodulation with Equimune (1.5 mL IV once weekly for 3 weeks) and enrofloxacin (2.5 mg/kg PO q12h for 3 to 4 weeks)
- corticosteroids, such as prednisolone (1 to 2 mg/kg PO q24h for 3 to 4 weeks)
- provision of both fresh water and electrolyte solution, and frequent small meals of a complete pelleted ration with roughage restriction

Granulomatous Colitis

Granulomatous colitis may result from infectious causes, such as parasites and tuberculosis, or from systemic granulomatous disease, which is characterized by a generalized dermatopathy and granulomatous inflammation of multiple organs (see p. 211). A similar condition has been associated with ingestion of vetch species (*Vicia* spp.). If a parasitic cause is identified, anthelmintic and corticosteroid treatment may be of benefit. In other instances, corticosteroid or other antiinflammatory treatment (e.g., azathioprine) may provide temporary improvement.

IDIOPATHIC DISEASES

Tympany

Rapid fermentation of feed can lead to accumulation of large amounts of gas, possibly causing functional obstruction of the colon. Flatulence and colic result. Changes in feed are the most common cause, especially excessive carbohydrate intake or ingestion of mown grass.

Clinical signs and diagnosis
- Signs vary with the duration and severity of tympany.
  - Horses with flatulent colic mimic those with impaction.
- Colonic distention is palpable per rectum; some horses have obvious abdominal distention.
- Metabolic status and laboratory findings depend on the severity of the condition.

Treatment
- Horses with mild-to-moderate tympany frequently respond to analgesics and fluid therapy.
- Mineral oil via nasogastric tube aids elimination of offending materials.
- If distention becomes excessive, trocarization may be required.
  - For colonic tympany, trocarization is performed in the right and/or left flank, depending on the location of the distention.

Diseases of the Small Colon *(pages 768-777)*

R. Reid Hanson

DISEASES WITH PHYSICAL CAUSES

Meconium Impaction

Meconium normally is passed within the first 24 to 48 hours of life. Predisposing factors for meconium impaction include birth asphyxia, other intestinal disease, and insufficient colostral intake. The narrow pelvic canal in male foals is a contributing factor.

Clinical signs and diagnosis

- The first signs are tenesmus, tail flagging, and repeated efforts to defecate.
- Colic and progressive abdominal distention result from persistent impaction.
- Digital rectal evaluation may reveal an impaction.
- If no meconium is palpated, a lateral abdominal radiograph may reveal a more proximal fecal impaction associated with gas and fluid build-up.
- Peritoneal fluid is normal.
- Differential diagnoses include ruptured bladder, urethral obstruction with straining, atresia coli, and other causes of small colon obstruction (e.g., ovarian ligament strangulation).

Treatment

Treatment varies with the severity and site of impaction.

- Exercise stimulates intestinal motility and may be all that some foals require.
- Careful digital extraction resolves the impaction in some cases, but can cause rectal trauma.
- Enemas may be administered via soft tubing (e.g., 30 French Foley catheter, inserted 2.5 to 4.5 cm [1 to 2 inches]).
  - Mild soap in warm water is gentle and often effective.
  - Dioctyl sodium succinate (DSS; 15 mL of 5% solution in 1 L of warm water) generally is effective, although even dilute solutions may irritate the rectum.
  - N-Acetylcysteine (4% solution, 4 to 8 oz) is very effective, and may be repeated in 1 hour with a larger volume if needed; 24 to 30 oz are required to reach the transverse colon.
- Laxative therapy via nasogastric tube can be helpful.
  - Common choices include mineral oil (200 to 400 mL), DSS (15 mL of a 5% solution diluted in water), and linseed oil (15 to 20 mL).
- IV fluids are helpful in reducing uncomplicated but long-standing impactions.

- Analgesics may be required until the impaction passes.
- Surgical intervention should be considered in foals that, despite medical therapy, have progressive abdominal distention with poorly controlled pain (see *Equine Medicine and Surgery V*).
  - Other diagnoses should also be considered.

Ingesta Impaction

Clinical signs and diagnosis

- Small colon impactions usually affect adult horses in the fall and winter.
- Most affected horses have reduced fecal output and decreased borborygmi.
- Abdominal distention may be severe in those with complete obstruction; heart rate and abdominal pain also are pronounced in horses requiring surgery.
- Rectal examination is useful in making the diagnosis.

Treatment

- Successful medical treatment involves IV fluid therapy, laxatives (e.g., magnesium sulfate, 110 g q12h) or lubricants (mineral oil, 2 to 4 L) via nasogastric tube, and flunixin meglumine.
  - Early, aggressive therapy is paramount to the success of medical treatment.
- Surgery should be considered when medical management fails, abdominal distention develops, or changes in peritoneal fluid indicate compromise of intestinal viability.
  - Common complications after surgery included fever and diarrhea; adhesions involving the small colon may develop, requiring a subsequent surgery or euthanasia.

Fecalith, Bezoar, Enteroliths, or Foreign Body Obstruction

Small colon obstruction can be caused by *fecaliths* (inspissated fibrous fecal material), *phytoconglobates* (concretions of undigested food fragments and foreign particulate matter), *bezoars* (combinations of magnesium ammonium phosphate crystals and plant fibers [phytobezoars] or hair [trichobezoars]), *enteroliths* (concretions of magnesium ammonium phosphate salts deposited concentrically around a foreign nidus), or *foreign material* (e.g., twine, rope, rubberized fencing material).

Clinical signs and diagnosis

+ Horses with small colon obstruction are dull, anorexic, and have mild abdominal pain.
+ They may exhibit tenesmus if the obstruction is near the rectum.
+ With complete obstruction, abdominal pain is persistent, tympany increases, and the patient's condition deteriorates.
  + The intestinal wall surrounding the obstruction may undergo pressure necrosis and eventually perforate, leading to fatal peritonitis.
+ Single or multiple loops of distended small colon may be felt per rectum.

Treatment and prognosis

+ These obstructions are best removed via small colon enterotomy.
+ The prognosis is good if the condition is recognized and corrected early.

Volvulus

Volvulus of the small colon is rare. It occurs either as a single event or in association with abnormalities and malpositioning of other organs (e.g., large colon volvulus, uterine torsion). Pain is more severe than that associated with simple intraluminal obstruction; the horse is less responsive to analgesics, and systemic signs of circulatory shock develop rapidly. Treatment involves surgical correction.

Incarceration

Causes of small colon incarceration include strangulation by a pedunculated lipoma, other tumor, or ovary and rents or openings in the mesocolon. Rupture of the mesocolon can cause segmental ischemic necrosis of the small colon. Clinical findings and management are as follows:

+ Signs usually are more pronounced than those associated with simple obstructions.
+ Mesocolon rupture should be considered in postfoaling mares that show clinical deterioration with increases in peritoneal fluid protein

and RBC and WBC counts, and a palpable impaction of the descending colon.
+ Treatment involves surgical exploration and correction (see *Equine Medicine and Surgery V*).
+ The prognosis is related to the condition of the affected bowel and necessity for resection.

Abscessation

Abscessation of the small colon or mesocolon may develop subsequent to rupture of a mesenteric lymph node (e.g., bastard strangles), enterotomy, generalized septicemia, or trauma to the abdominal wall or rectum.

+ Unless the lesion progresses to form an extraluminal obstruction, intermittent fever, anorexia, and weight loss usually are the only signs.
+ In most cases, a specific diagnosis can be made only during exploratory celiotomy.
+ If the abscess is accessible, attempts can be made to drain or resect the abscess and diseased tissue; however, the prognosis generally is poor.

Intramural Hematoma

Intramural or subserosal hematomas may develop during parturition, from mucosal ulceration, or as a result of rectal trauma. In most cases, partial small colon obstruction can be successfully managed with oral fluids, lubricants or fecal softeners, and dietary control. When the hematoma totally obstructs the lumen, surgical intervention is necessary.

Intussusception

Intussusception of the small colon is rare. Most cases involve protrusion of part of the small colon and/or rectum from the anus (see discussion of rectal prolapse).

Diagnosis and treatment

+ Signs include chronic, intermittent abdominal pain, anorexia, and lethargy.
+ Complete obstruction causes continuous, severe abdominal pain and distention.
+ Rectal examination reveals moderate distention of the large colon and cecum with a tense, painful

viscus in the ventral abdomen just rostral to the pelvic brim.

- Peritoneal fluid protein and WBC count are increased, with some neutrophil degeneration.
- Resection and anastomosis are necessary.

Diseases of the Rectum

(pages 777-790)

R. Reid Hanson

CONGENITAL AND FAMILIAL DISEASES
Atresia Coli

Atresia coli is a defect in which a segment of the large or small colon is missing, and the adjacent segments of bowel are blind-ending. Atresia recti and atresia ani are similar conditions, although atresia ani may simply consist of a plane of tissue occluding the anal orifice. Functional atresia coli can occur in association with the recessive lethal white gene in paint horses (see p. 185).

Clinical signs and diagnosis

- Foals with atresia coli show signs similar to those of meconium impaction, beginning shortly after birth, but no feces are identified on digital rectal examination.
- Atresia coli or recti can be confirmed with radiography (after barium enema), endoscopy, or exploratory surgery.
- Atresia ani is confirmed visually.
- The foal should be examined for other congenital abnormalities.

Treatment

- In foals with atresia ani and a complete rectal pouch (identified by palpation of meconium through the vaginal wall or lateral to the anus), the persistent anal membrane is incised.
- If the entire rectum or part of the colon is atretic, exploratory surgery allows evaluation, and, if feasible, correction (has a high failure rate and often is impossible).
- The owner should be discouraged from repeating the mating that resulted in an affected foal.

DISEASES WITH PHYSICAL CAUSES
Rectal Tear

Most rectal tears occur during rectal palpation, and a rectal tear should be suspected when a sudden decrease in the resistance is felt or when fresh blood is observed on the palpation sleeve. Rectal tears are graded by severity.

- *Grade 1* tears are restricted to the mucosa and submucosa. Rectal bleeding is noted, and a small roughening or defect can be palpated in the rectal wall.
- *Grade 2* tears involve only the muscular layer of the rectal wall; the mucosa and serosa remain intact, and there is no bleeding. These defects often are incidental findings.
- *Grade 3* lesions involve all tissue layers, except the serosa (grade 3A) or mesorectum (grade 3B). These are deep defects that often are filled with feces.
- *Grade 4* tears involve perforation of all layers of the rectum and fecal contamination of the abdominal cavity. *This is the most severe type of rectal tear and constitutes an emergency.*

Clinical signs

- Grade 1 tears may cause no signs other than fresh blood on the rectal sleeve after palpation.
- Grade 2 tears often are asymptomatic, although rectal impaction may develop.
- With grade 3 or 4 tears, signs of fulminant peritonitis and endotoxic shock (e.g., abdominal splinting, colic, sweating, tachycardia, fever) develop within 2 to 3 hours.

Diagnosis

Whenever a rectal tear occurs, *prompt action is necessary.* The location and extent of the tear must be carefully evaluated.

- Epidural anesthesia and/or sedation (e.g., xylazine and butorphanol) facilitate examination.
- *Gentle* palpation, either bare-armed or wearing a surgical or latex examination glove, usually suffices; most rectal tears occur dorsally in the intraperitoneal portion of the rectum.
- Peritoneal fluid changes occur quickly in horses with grade 3 and 4 rectal tears.

- Nucleated cell counts can exceed
  50,000 cells/μl within 30 minutes.

Treatment and prognosis

Horses with grade 1 tears are treated
with medical therapy, alone or in
combination with suturing (under
epidural anesthesia).

- Broad-spectrum antibiotics should
  be administered.
- A laxative diet (e.g., water-soaked
  alfalfa pellets), mineral oil, and oral
  or IV fluid therapy (as needed) are
  recommended.
- The horse should be monitored
  closely for 1 week, with CBC and
  peritoneal fluid analyses.
- Grade 2 tears usually are manage-
  able with dietary control aimed at
  keeping the feces soft.

Horses with grade 3 or 4 tears require prompt and aggressive medical
and surgical intervention.

- The immediate goal is to prevent
  enlargement of the tear.
  - The horse should be tranquilized
    and epidural anesthesia used to
    eliminate straining.
  - All feces are then manually re-
    moved from the rectum *(carefully)*.
  - The rectum is packed with moist
    cotton inside a well lubricated
    3-inch stockinette, such that the
    pack extends from the anus to 10
    cm (4 inches) cranial to the tear.
  - The anus is closed with towel
    clamps or a purse-string suture.
- Vigorous medical management
  should be instituted.
  - Atropine (0.044 mg/kg IM or SC
    once) decreases intestinal
    motility for up to 12 hours.
  - Broad-spectrum systemic antimi-
    crobials, tetanus toxoid, and min-
    eral oil are administered.
  - Balanced polyionic IV fluids are
    essential.
- Several surgical options are avail-
  able for repair of rectal tears (see
  Equine Medicine and Surgery V):
  - direct surgical repair per rectum
  - surgical repair after partial pro-
    lapse of the rectum
  - fecal diversion using a temporary
    colostomy or rectal liner
  - surgical repair via celiotomy
- Primary closure of grade 3 tears can
  yield good results, if performed

early; a poorer prognosis is associated with grade 4 tears.

- Horses given adequate first aid
  care before admission have a
  better survival rate.

INFLAMMATORY, INFECTIOUS, AND IMMUNE DISEASES

Perirectal Abscess, Stenosis, and Stricture

Perirectal abscesses, rectal polyps,
and strictures can sufficiently
narrow the rectal lumen that impaction colic results. Perirectal abscesses most commonly develop
secondary to rectal tears. Other
causes include bruising of the rectal
wall during foaling and injections
into the gluteals.

Clinical signs and diagnosis

- The most common signs are low-
  grade colic, depression, anorexia,
  reduced fecal production, and
  tenesmus; fever is noted in some
  cases.
- Diagnostic tests might include abdominocentesis, aspiration or
  biopsy of the rectal mass with impression smears and culture, and
  ultrasonography.
  - *Streptococcus zooepidemicus* and *E.
    coli* are the most common organ-
    isms isolated.

Treatment and prognosis

Perirectal abscesses:

- Treatment involves drainage and
  flushing under either epidural or
  local anesthesia.
- Adjunctive therapy includes systemic antibiotics (based on sensitivity results), NSAIDs, flushing
  with a dilute antiseptic solution, and
  administration of stool softeners.
- When abdominal organs are involved, exploratory celiotomy is indicated.
- The prognosis is good if surgical
  drainage is effective and complications (e.g., peritonitis, stricture) do
  not occur.

Strictures:

- Strictures that involve only the
  anus can be successfully treated
  with transection of the anus and
  dietary changes to keep the feces
  soft.

- Strictures that involve the rectal ampulla may require a diverting colostomy.

Pruritus Ani

Causes of irritation to the anus and tail head include:

- pinworms *(Oxyuris equi)*
- hypersensitivity to *Culicoides* organisms (not limited to the tail head; see Chapter 17, Integumentary System)
- learned vices
- persistent enteritis, diarrhea, or food allergy

NEOPLASIA

Squamous cell carcinoma and melanoma are the most common neoplasms of the perineal region.

- **Squamous cell carcinomas** are locally invasive and metastasize slowly; lesions are necrotic and foul-smelling.
- **Melanomas** in the perineal region and ventral surface of the tail are most common in gray horses >15 years of age; the black nodules may be solitary or multiple.
  - The treatment of choice is early, wide excision or cryotherapy.
- **Intestinal leiomyomas** or **leiomyosarcomas** are rare, pedunculated tumors that form mural masses and may protrude into the bowel lumen; surgical removal is advised.
- **Lipomas** of the mesorectum occasionally cause strangulating obstruction of the rectum; if recognized early, they can be successfully removed via colpotomy.

MULTIFACTORIAL DISEASES

Rectal Prolapse

Although rare, rectal prolapse can occur in horses of any age. Any condition that results in prolonged tenesmus, such as parturition, diarrhea, constipation, and rectal irritation, can lead to prolapse of the rectum. Horses in poor body condition are predisposed.

Rectal prolapse is divided into four categories:

- **Type I** involves only the rectal mucosa; the rectal musculature and serosal tissues are not displaced.
- **Type II** generally involves displacement of the entire rectal wall with occasional involvement of the rectal ampulla.
- **Type III** involves displacement of the entire rectum with invagination of the terminal small colon.
- **Type IV** involves intussusception of the peritoneal rectum and a variable length of small colon through the anus.

When the small colon prolapses through the anus (type III or IV rectal prolapse), tearing of the terminal mesocolon and disruption of the vascular supply often result in ischemic necrosis of the peritoneal rectum. This complication is more common in postparturient mares that experienced dystocia and causes the most severe clinical presentation. Resection and anastomosis usually is impossible.

Treatment

- Treatment of the inciting cause is important.
- *Types I* and *II* rectal prolapses usually respond to medical management.
  - Manual reduction is aided by topical emollients, lubricants, or hyperosmotic compounds (e.g., glycerin or 50% dextrose).
  - Epidural anesthesia may be administered to reduce straining.
  - Once reduced, a purse-string suture is placed in the anus so that the sphincter can be dilated only 4 to 6 cm to permit defecation; the suture should be removed in 48 to 72 hours.
  - Mineral oil can be administered via nasogastric tube.
  - Feeding a laxative diet along with administration of warm water enemas for the next 10 days lessens the chance of recurrence.
- Surgical intervention for type I or II rectal prolapse may become necessary if the prolapsed tissue becomes necrotic (see *Equine Medicine and Surgery V*).
- Treatment of type III or IV prolapse depends on the length of the intussusception, the duration, and the owner's wishes.
  - If treatment is requested, the prolapse should be evaluated by celiotomy to determine the most appropriate surgical therapy (usually colostomy).

• Affected horses require treatment for endotoxic shock.

Rectovaginal Tear and Fistula

Lesions between the rectum and vagina can range from a small perforation that is difficult to identify, to a large hole between the rectum and vagina, or a complete tear through to the perineum. These lesions are discussed in Chapter 13, Reproductive System: The Mare.

Diseases of the Peritoneum and Mesentery *(pages 790-808)*
Susan D. Semrad

DISEASES WITH PHYSICAL CAUSES
Intraabdominal Hemorrhage (Hemoperitoneum)

Bleeding or effusion of blood into the peritoneal cavity with no visible blood loss occurs infrequently. Possible causes include:

• blunt trauma, causing rupture of the spleen, liver, or blood vessels
• vascular accidents, such as ruptured aneurysm of the aorta or cranial mesenteric artery
• complications of abdominal surgery or castration
• intestinal accidents
• rupture of the uteroovarian, middle uterine, or large intraabdominal vessels during foaling
• coagulopathies

Clinical signs

Signs vary with the primary injury and the rapidity and amount of blood loss.

• Acute, severe blood loss (e.g., rupture of a major vessel or parenchymal organ) rapidly progresses to hemorrhagic shock and death.
• When bleeding occurs less rapidly, signs may be more subtle.
  • Lethargy, inappetence, reluctance to move, pale or icteric mucous membranes, dehydration, mild colic, and slight tachycardia, tachypnea, and fever may be seen.

♦ Hemorrhage during parturition can be difficult to distinguish from second- and third-stage labor.

Diagnosis

♦ Careful physical examination, including rectal palpation, should be performed.
♦ Laboratory evaluation may be of little value initially.
  • The PCV does not decrease for at least 8 hours after significant blood loss.
  • Total plasma protein decreases gradually, often before the PCV decreases.
♦ Abdominocentesis usually is required to confirm hemoperitoneum.
  • A large volume of bloody fluid can be obtained from multiple sites, erythrophagocytosis is seen on direct smear, and the PCV is similar to or less than that of peripheral blood.
♦ Ultrasonography may show fluid in the ventral abdomen.
  • The spleen and liver should be examined for size and presence of masses or tears.

Treatment

Management is difficult, because the underlying cause often is unknown.

♦ Supportive measures include treatment for shock and hypovolemia (see Chapter 4, Principles of Therapy).
♦ Laparotomy may be indicated in cases of splenic, hepatic, or uterine rupture.
  • Exploratory surgery should also be considered in horses with bleeding after previous surgery or with bleeding that cannot be controlled within 12 hours.
♦ When bleeding is less severe or hemorrhage following uterine vessel rupture is confined within the broad ligament, *conservative* measures should be undertaken.
  • Restoration of effective circulating volume with IV fluids is imperative.
  • Use of hypertonic saline remains controversial; it is contraindicated in animals with coagulation disorders and when hemorrhage is inadequately controlled (see Chapter 4).

- Plasma and/or whole blood transfusion is indicated when the plasma protein or albumin concentration and PCV decline to unacceptably low values (see Chapter 4).
- Pain relief (e.g., flunixin meglumine, ketoprofen, butorphanol) and maintenance of a positive energy balance are important.
- Broad-spectrum antimicrobials are indicated if abdominal contamination is suspected.
- Parenteral oxytocin has been recommended when rupture of a uterine vessel is suspected.

Prognosis
- The prognosis is grave after rupture of the spleen, liver, or a major blood vessel.
- In any case of intraabdominal hemorrhage, recovery may be complicated by peritonitis, intraabdominal hematoma or abscess, or laminitis.

Penetrating Abdominal Wounds

The abdominal cavity may be entered through wounds in the abdominal wall, rectum, vagina, or uterus. *Penetrating abdominal wounds are serious and require immediate attention.*

Clinical signs
- Signs of acute, severe abdominal bleeding are listed in the previous section.
- Intestinal perforation with gross contamination of the abdomen leads to overwhelming toxemia, septic shock, and death.
  - With minor, well-contained injury to the bowel wall, manifestations of peritonitis are slower to develop and are less severe (see p. 229).
- Intestinal herniation may induce severe pain and profound shock.

Diagnosis
- Diagnosis is based on the history and physical examination (e.g., entrance and exit wounds).
- Laboratory data reflect wound duration and degree of abdominal contamination.
- Abdominocentesis helps assess the degree of peritoneal contamination.
- In foals or small horses, free gas, fluid, or alterations in size or position of major abdominal organs

may be observed on abdominal radiographs.
- Definitive diagnosis and treatment often require surgical intervention.

Treatment and prognosis
- Immediate therapy is aimed at controlling life-threatening hemorrhage and shock and protecting any exposed viscera.
- After stabilization, exploratory laparotomy may be indicated to assess the degree of damage and attempt repair.
- *Until proven otherwise, perforation of the intestinal tract should be assumed* following a penetrating abdominal wound, and broad-spectrum antimicrobial therapy should be initiated.
  - Gram-negative, gram-positive aerobic and anaerobic organisms may be present.
- A grave prognosis is warranted for wounds accompanied by perforation of abdominal viscera, laceration of major blood vessels, or tearing of the mesentery and enclosed vessels.

INFLAMMATORY, INFECTIOUS, AND IMMUNE DISEASES
Peritonitis

Peritonitis may be classified according to origin (primary or secondary), onset (peracute, acute, chronic), extent (diffuse, localized), and presence of bacteria (septic, nonseptic). Peritonitis usually is acute, diffuse, and caused by contamination with intestinal bacteria.

Clinical signs

Signs vary with the primary disease, infectious agent involved, and duration.
- Common signs are reluctance to move, splinting of the abdominal wall and sensitivity to external pressure, groaning or grunting, colic, fever, anorexia, weight loss, diarrhea, and tachycardia; signs of ileus and dehydration may also be present.
- Horses with *peracute* peritonitis (e.g., after intestinal rupture) show profound toxemia and rapid deterioration; death may occur within 4 to 24 hours.
- *Acute diffuse* peritonitis causes abdominal pain, sweating, muscle

fasciculations, dehydration, depression, and anorexia; body temperature may be high, low, or normal.

◆ Horses with *localized, subacute,* or *chronic* peritonitis show intermittent colic, depression, anorexia, weight loss, intermittent fever, ventral edema, exercise intolerance, decreased or absent intestinal sounds, and mild dehydration.

  • In some cases, weight loss, depression, and inappetence are the only signs.

Diagnosis

Peritonitis should be suspected in a horse with a history of predisposing factors, suggestive clinical signs, and compatible laboratory data.

◆ In peracute or acute peritonitis, severe neutropenic leukopenia with a degenerative left shift is present.

  • Hypoproteinemia and an increased PCV reflect protein sequestration and dehydration.

  • Serum fibrinogen is increased if the process has been present for ≥48 hours.

  • Metabolic acidosis and electrolyte (Na^+, K^+, Cl^-) losses may be significant.

◆ In cases of acute peritonitis of longer duration and in localized or chronic peritonitis, the WBC count may be normal or there may be neutrophilic leukocytosis.

  • Other possible findings include a few band neutrophils, lymphopenia or lymphocytosis, and monocytosis.

  • Hypergammaglobulinemia causes hyperproteinemia, despite hypoalbuminemia.

  • Normocytic normochromic anemia, reflective of chronic disease, may be present.

Findings on *rectal examination* are inconsistent. When present, abnormalities may include:

◆ a "gritty" or "dry" feeling to serosal and parietal surfaces

◆ decreased fecal or dry fecal material in the intestine

◆ pain on palpation of the abdominal organs or parietal peritoneum

◆ intestinal impaction or distention secondary to ileus

◆ an abdominal mass (abscess or neoplasia)

Abdominocentesis confirms peritonitis but may not reveal the cause.

◆ The peritoneal fluid may be serosanguineous, turbid, flocculent, or purulent.

◆ Peritoneal WBC counts in horses with acute peritonitis (100,000/μL) usually are higher than in those with chronic peritonitis (20,000 to 60,000/μL).

◆ Early in the disease, the increase in WBC count primarily is due to an increase in neutrophils (degenerative or nondegenerative).

  • In more chronic cases, mononuclear cell and macrophage numbers increase.

◆ Mesothelial cells may become hyperplastic and mimic neoplastic cells in chronic cases.

◆ Peritoneal protein concentrations are increased.

◆ Bacteria may be seen free or phagocytized by peritoneal leukocytes.

  • *Failure to identify bacteria cytologically does not rule out septic peritonitis.*

  • Samples should be submitted for Gram's stain and aerobic and anaerobic cultures.

◆ Examination of the fluid for plant fibers, foreign substances, bile, and chyle also is valuable.

Treatment

Early, aggressive therapy is required. Treatment is based on three principles:

◆ stabilization of the animal's condition

  • Arrest endotoxic and/or hypovolemic shock; correct metabolic and electrolyte abnormalities, dehydration, and hypoproteinemia; and manage pain

◆ isolation and correction of the primary insult or underlying disease process.

◆ treatment of any infection

  • These infections typically are multimicrobial, involving both aerobes and anaerobes.

  • Bactericidal antibiotics are preferred (e.g., aminoglycoside plus penicillin or ampicillin).

  • Metronidazole may be effective against anaerobes resistant to penicillin.

  • Intermittent drainage of abdominal fluid via catheter or indwelling drain may be helpful.

Peritoneal lavage may be beneficial in horses with generalized peritonitis in which little response has been seen to antimicrobial therapy and fluid drainage.

- Two approaches are described.
  - retrograde irrigation through a ventrally placed ingress-egress drain (Foley catheter)
  - placement of ingress catheters in both paralumbar fossae for infusion of fluids, with placement of a drain along the ventral midline for removal of fluid and exudate
- Greater success may be achieved with peritoneal lavage during surgery. Therapy with heparin (20 to 40 U/kg IV or SC q8h, or in lavage fluid) has been recommended to prevent adhesion formation, although results are inconsistent.

Prognosis

- With early, aggressive therapy and rapid correction of the primary lesion, the prognosis generally is fair to good for localized and mild, acute diffuse peritonitis.
- In chronic cases and in cases with severe abdominal contamination, the prognosis is poor.
- Complications include abdominal adhesions or abscesses, laminitis, and organ failure.

Abdominal Abscesses

Abdominal abscesses can occur as a sequela to respiratory infections and/or septicemia; most are located in or around the mesentery. Abscesses have also been associated with umbilical infections, foreign body penetration of the small intestine, ascarid infection in foals, verminous arteritis, peritonitis, and foaling accidents. A mixed population of bacteria usually is present; the organisms most commonly isolated are *S. equi, S. zooepidemicus, R. equi, Corynebacterium pseudotuberculosis,* and *Salmonella* spp.

Clinical signs

- Depression and anorexia are consistent findings; increases in heart and respiratory rates, persistent or intermittent fever, and dehydration often are present.
- Chronic weight loss, sometimes resulting in severe emaciation, occurs in some horses.

- Some horses have intermittent or persistent colic that is unresponsive to medical therapy.

Diagnosis

- A history of recurrent or vague abdominal pain, weight loss, and intermittent or continuous fever is highly suggestive.
  - Previous illness as a result of septicemia or respiratory disease, or close association with horses with *S. equi* infections should increase the level of suspicion.
- Laboratory findings vary.
  - The CBC may be normal, but more often, neutrophilic leukocytosis, hyperfibrinogenemia, and mild normocytic normochromic anemia are evident.
  - A mild left shift, lymphopenia, or absolute monocytosis may be present.
  - Neutropenia with a degenerative left shift and toxic changes indicate abscess leakage.
  - Plasma protein and globulin concentrations are increased, whereas plasma albumin concentration is normal or decreased.
- Peritoneal fluid protein concentration and WBC count typically are normal or mildly increased.
  - Free and phagocytized bacteria may be seen if the abscess is leaking or perforated.
  - Fluid should be submitted for Gram's stain, cytology, and culture and sensitivity.
- Rectal examination may reveal no abnormalities or a mass within the mesentery.
- Abdominal radiographs may be useful in young foals and small horses.
- Ultrasonography may reveal an abdominal or umbilical abscess (foals).
- Laparoscopy or laparotomy sometimes is necessary for definitive diagnosis.

Treatment

Long-term (1 to 6 months) antimicrobial therapy is the mainstay of medical therapy.

- Penicillin and ampicillin are effective against some of the commonly implicated pathogens.
  - Trimethoprim-sulfadiazine, gentamicin, or amikacin is added for gram-negative coverage.

- Aminoglycosides or erythromycin (+ rifampin) are adequate for *R. equi* abscesses.
- Metronidazole is effective against anaerobes, especially *Bacteroides fragilis.*
- Recurrence of signs is common when antimicrobial therapy is prematurely withdrawn.

Other therapeutic or supportive measures include:

- drainage of the abscess using ultrasonographic guidance or during surgery
- maintenance of hydration and electrolyte balance with oral or IV fluids
- pain relief using analgesics
- maintenance of a positive energy balance

Prognosis

- Streptococcal abscesses often respond well to antimicrobial therapy if abdominal viscera are not extensively involved.
- Complications (e.g., abdominal adhesions, peritonitis, laminitis) may interfere with recovery.

Abdominal Adhesions

Adhesions can occur secondary to infectious, ischemic, inflammatory, or traumatic insults to the bowel, peritoneum, or other abdominal organs. Adhesions are a frequent complication of exploratory laparotomy, castration, or reproductive surgery and are a common cause of postoperative colic in horses with small intestinal lesions. Manifestations range from acute intestinal obstruction to chronic weight loss and poor performance.

Treatment and prognosis

- Mild or chronic colic often is responsive to analgesics and dietary management.
- Surgical intervention is required for adhesions that cause complete intestinal obstruction.
- The prognosis always is guarded because of the progressive nature and frequency of recurrence after surgical intervention.

NEOPLASIA

Neoplasia of the abdominal cavity is rare in horses. Several tumor types (squamous cell carcinoma, hemangiosarcoma, lymphosarcoma, mesothelioma, malignant melanoma) can spread throughout the abdominal cavity and may involve the peritoneal surface. Common signs include chronic weight loss, anorexia, depression, exercise intolerance, icterus, and chronic colic. In some cases an abdominal mass or mesenteric lymphadenopathy is identified on rectal examination. Except for lymphosarcomas, neoplasms usually do not exfoliate into the peritoneal fluid. Response to medical and surgical therapy generally is poor.

MULTIFACTORIAL DISEASES
Ascites

Ascites (serous fluid accumulation within the peritoneal cavity) usually results from transudation or exudation of fluid from the surfaces of the liver, gut, or mesentery.

- *Transudates* are colorless with a low cell count ($<9000/\mu L$), protein concentration (<3 g/dL), and specific gravity (<1.015).
  - Causes include chronic hepatic disease, renal disease, congestive heart failure, mediastinal tumors, and hypoproteinemia (e.g., parasitism, protein-losing nephropathy).
- *Exudates* are white, yellow, or pink, with a high cell count ($>9000/\mu L$), protein concentration (>3 g/dL), and specific gravity (>1.015).
  - The most common causes are inflammatory lesions of the GI tract.
- Chyloabdomen (resulting from impaired lymphatic drainage or erosion of the lymphatics) and uroperitoneum (resulting from rupture of the bladder, ureter, or kidney) are specific types of ascites.

Clinical signs

- In adult horses, ascites often is not evident until massive fluid accumulation is present.
  - Nonspecific abdominal distention with dyspnea suggests ascites.
- In foals and small horses, a fluid wave may be appreciated on ballottement of the abdomen.

- Ascites usually occurs secondary to a chronic debilitating disease, so anorexia, weight loss, weakness, lethargy, and dependent edema often are observed.

Diagnosis

- The history, clinical signs, and laboratory findings reflect the primary disease.
- Rectal examination may reveal no abnormalities, or the intestine may "float" in the abdomen
- Ascites is confirmed by abdominocentesis.
- Abdominal radiography may be helpful in foals or small horses.
  - A loss of contrast or a hazy, opaque appearance suggests fluid accumulation.
- Ultrasonography also allows identification of excessive fluid in the peritoneal cavity.

Treatment and prognosis

- Treatment and prognosis are determined by the underlying disease.
- Except for uroperitoneum, ascites usually warrants a guarded to grave prognosis.

Diseases of the Abdominal Wall

(pages 808-816)
Eric P. Tulleners

CONGENITAL AND FAMILIAL DISEASES

Umbilical Hernia

Umbilical hernias occur in <2% of foals. Most umbilical hernias are small (<5 cm) and uncomplicated.

Treatment

- Typical small umbilical hernias are nonpainful and completely reducible; a watch-and-wait attitude may be adopted, with daily reduction performed by owners.
- If the hernia is not resolved by 4 to 6 months of age, intervention is indicated.
  - Hernia clamps are favored by some practitioners for completely reducible hernias that are <5 cm in diameter (see *Equine Medicine and Surgery V*).

- If surgical closure is contemplated, it should be done when the animal is about 6 months of age (see *Equine Medicine and Surgery V* for a description of surgical techniques).
- Incarceration of intestine in an umbilical hernia occurs in 2% to 10% of cases, usually in foals ≥6 months of age with large hernias (see p. 206).
- Large (>5 cm) umbilical hernias occasionally are occur in older foals or secondary to disruption of previous herniorrhaphy attempts.
  - Unless infected, prosthetic reconstruction with synthetic mesh should be performed.

Inguinal Hernia

Congenital inguinal hernias are discussed on p. 206.

DISEASES WITH PHYSICAL CAUSES

Incisional Hernias with Acute Total Dehiscence

Disruption of an abdominal incision usually occurs in the first 3 to 8 days after surgery and is preceded by a brown serosanguineous discharge from the wound. Support may be provided by sterile compresses under an elastic bandage that encircles the abdomen; however, bandaging cannot prevent evisceration. Once incisional disruption is recognized, emergency reconstructive surgery is necessary (see *Equine Medicine and Surgery V*).

Traumatic Hernia

Traumatic hernias primarily occur from blunt trauma, such as a kick or collision. In many cases, the wound does not penetrate the abdominal wall and can be treated with local therapy and, if necessary, abdominal bandaging. After 30 to 60 days, residual defects in the body wall may be sutured or, if very large, repaired with synthetic mesh.

INFLAMMATORY, INFECTIOUS, AND IMMUNE DISEASE

Umbilical Cord Remnant Infection

Umbilical remnant infections are an infrequent but potentially serious problem in young foals.

- They often are caused by poor umbilical hygiene and a dirty environment.
- Most affected foals are <8 weeks old; examination reveals heat, swelling, pain, and discharge of urine or purulent material from the umbilicus.
- Ultrasonography is useful in determining which structures are involved and to what extent.
  - The urachus is involved in most cases; the umbilical vessels may also be infected.
- Bacterial septicemia with dissemination to other organs, particularly bone, joint, and lung, is a common and serious sequela; hence, surgical extirpation is recommended (see *Equine Medicine and Surgery V*).
  - Enteric gram-negative and streptococcal organisms commonly are isolated.

MULTIFACTORIAL DISEASES
Incisional Hernias
Large defects in the abdominal wall requiring prosthetic reconstruction are uncommon. These defects most often arise from partial incisional dehiscence after ventral midline celiotomy or after failed umbilical herniorrhaphy. Any infection should be eradicated before the defect is reconstructed with mesh (see *Equine Medicine and Surgery V*). The prognosis for recovery and future use is excellent.

Diaphragmatic Hernia
Diaphragmatic hernias, whether congenital or acquired (traumatic), are rare in horses.
- Affected adult horses may have a history of trauma.
- Most horses are presented in serious abdominal crisis.
  - Diagnosis is made and repair performed (if possible) during exploratory celiotomy.
  - Some large or dorsally positioned defects are inaccessible, precluding effective closure.
- In some horses, signs are limited to low-grade, chronic, recurrent abdominal pain; but occasionally the hernia is an incidental finding at necropsy.

Abdominal Wall Hernia and Prepubic Tendon Rupture in Pregnant Mares
Abdominal wall hernias and prepubic tendon ruptures are associated with twins, trauma, hydrallantois, and excessive ventral edema. They are more common in older draft mares.
Clinical signs and diagnosis
- Initially, affected mares show mild-to-moderate discomfort and progressive ventral abdominal enlargement with extensive pitting edema.
- Mares with prepubic tendon rupture have a stiff gait and are reluctant to move or lie down.
  - They may assume a sawhorse stance, with tipping of the pelvis and elevation of the tail head and tuber ischii.
- Mares with abdominal wall defects prefer to lie down and are willing to walk; elevation of the tail head or tuber ischii is not present.
- The accompanying edema can make it impossible to determine the exact site and extent of the defect by external palpation.
  - The caudal abdominal floor should be palpated per rectum to determine if it is intact and if herniation is present.
  - Ultrasonography can be useful in delineating the extent of the injury.
Treatment and prognosis
- Parturition should be induced in late-term mares with an abdominal wall hernia that are showing no signs of intestinal incarceration.
  - After delivery, the hernia is reduced and the defect supported with an abdominal bandage.
  - Reconstruction of the defect should be delayed until 1 to 2 months after parturition.
- Worsening of vital signs and abdominal pain that is unresponsive to analgesics indicate intestinal incarceration; emergency celiotomy may be necessary in these mares (see *Equine Medicine and Surgery V*).
- Parturition should also be induced in mares with prepubic tendon rupture.
- The prognosis after mesh reconstruction of abdominal wall hernias is fair to good.

Diseases of the Liver

(pages 816-833)

Catherine J. Savage

DIAGNOSTIC AND THERAPEUTIC CONSIDERATIONS

Clinical Signs of Liver Disease

Subclinical hepatic disease is common in clinically normal horses because of the liver's large functional reserve. Clinical signs consistent with hepatic disease include:

- *icterus:* This can occur for a variety of reasons.
  - inappetence (hyperbilirubinemia resulting from fasting usually is ≤5 mg/dL)
  - erythrolysis (easily recognized by a low PCV, often <20%)
  - extrahepatic problems (e.g., endotoxemia, large colon distention)
  - idiopathic (some horses, especially Appaloosas, appear mildly icteric at all times)
  - hepatic compromise
- *hepatoencephalopathy:* This occurs in horses with severe and advanced liver disease and usually indicates a poor prognosis; signs variably include the following:
  - depression, excessive yawning, somnolence, recumbency/coma
  - compulsive walking, circling, head pressing
  - maniacal behavior often interspersed with somnolence and stupor
  - seizures
  - inspiratory dyspnea caused by pharyngeal and/or laryngeal paralysis (more often seen with pyrrolizidine alkaloid toxicosis)
- *coagulopathy:* Production of clotting proteins is decreased in severe liver disease; platelet counts are normal.
  - Clinical signs include excessive bleeding and hematoma formation at blood sampling sites, epistaxis, hemarthrosis, hemoabdomen, and hemothorax.
- *edema and ascites:* Hypoproteinemia, specifically hypoalbuminemia, can be profound in cases

of liver failure; serum albumin <2.2 g/dL results in dependent edema and ascites.

- *colic and weight loss:* Cholelithiasis is the most common hepatic cause of chronic colic.
  - Septic cholangitis, cholangiohepatitis, obstruction of the common bile duct secondary to duodenal stenosis, and hepatic neoplasia also may cause abdominal pain.
  - Weight loss is seen with chronic liver disease and in cases involving infectious agents (e.g., cholangiohepatitis, hepatic abscessation).
- *dermatitis:* Photosensitization involving unpigmented skin can occur with liver failure.
  - The worst cases of hepatic photosensitization are seen with pyrrolizidine alkaloid toxicity.
- *fever, depression, and anorexia:* These nonspecific signs are seen with many conditions affecting the liver, including infective processes, acute hepatic necrosis, and neoplasia.

Clinicopathologic Abnormalities

Bilirubin and urobilinogen

Bilirubin may be increased in cases of inappetence, hemolysis, hepatocellular disease, and biliary obstruction.

- A concentration of conjugated bilirubin >20 % of the total bilirubin is significant.
- Biliary tract blockage increases both unconjugated and conjugated bilirubin; when conjugated bilirubin is increased, it can be detected in the urine on dipstick analysis.
- Complete blockage of the common bile duct also results in absence of urobilinogen (which normally is detectable) in the urine.

Bile acids

Measuring serum bile acids is the best test for evaluating hepatic (particularly biliary) function.

- The highest concentrations occur in horses with obstructive biliary disease (e.g., cholelithiasis) and in foals with portosystemic shunts (uncommon).
- It is not necessary to take fasting and postprandial samples in horses;

one sample will suffice at any time of the day.
♦ Total bile acid concentrations >20 µM/L indicate hepatobiliary disease.

Hepatic enzymes

Although some enzymes are better indicators of hepatocellular than biliary damage, hepatocellular damage soon leads to biliary damage, and vice versa. Thus a mixed pattern of serum enzymes commonly occurs.

♦ *aspartate aminotransferase (AST or SGOT):* increased in cases of hepatocellular damage
  • AST is also present in skeletal and cardiac muscle, so it is important to measure serum creatine kinase (CK) to differentiate hepatic and muscle disorders.
  • Plasma concentrations increase slowly and persist for 10 to 14 days.

♦ *L-iditol dehydrogenase (L-iDH, or sorbitol dehydrogenase [SDH]):* the most sensitive indicator of hepatocellular damage
  • L-iDH is unstable once collected and has a short plasma half life, so many laboratories do not offer this assay.

♦ *lactate dehydrogenase isoenzyme 5 (LDH-5):* a specific indicator of hepatocellular damage
  • LDH 5 is stable at room temperature for >24 hours and is measured by many laboratories.
  • Measuring total LDH is not useful, because it is not specific for the liver.

♦ *arginase:* one of the best indicators of hepatocellular necrosis
  • It can marginally increase with fasting.
  • The plasma half life is short, so serial sampling can be useful for evaluating disease progression or resolution.

♦ *γ-glutamyltransferase (GGT) and alkaline phosphatase (AP):* indicators of biliary damage, whether secondary to infection, stasis, obstruction, or inflammation
  • Horses in maximal exercise training (e.g., racehorses) often have increased plasma GGT.

Fibrinogen, leukogram, and erythron

Some liver disorders can cause the following abnormalities:

♦ *hyperfibrinogenemia:* indicates hepatic inflammation (e.g., cholangiohepatitis, neoplasia)
♦ *hypofibrinogenemia:* can occur secondary to liver failure (decreased production)
  • This indicates a poor prognosis.
♦ *leukocytosis with a left shift:* occurs in some cases of cholangiohepatitis
♦ *increased PCV:* may occur in horses with acute hepatic necrosis
  • Horses with persistent, nonresponsive polycythemia have a poor prognosis.
♦ *hemolytic anemic crisis:* may result from hepatic failure and usually is terminal

Clotting profile

Indicators of hepatic coagulopathy include increases in prothrombin time (PT) and partial thromboplastin time (PTT, APTT). Horses with biliary stasis and obstruction may have secondary vitamin K deficiency; these horses also have prolonged PT and PTT.

Prognostic Indicators

Findings supportive of a guarded to poor prognosis in horses with hepatic failure include:

♦ acute onset of signs indicating hepatoencephalopathy, colic, or coagulopathy
♦ low serum albumin, fibrinogen, glucose, and/or BUN
♦ increased blood ammonia
♦ low PCV (<18%) or profound polycythemia (PCV >55%)
♦ prolonged prothrombin and partial thromboplastin times

Hepatic Ultrasonography

The liver can be imaged on the right side from the fifth or sixth to at least the fifteenth intercostal space, provided there has been no right-side lobe atrophy. The liver can be only partially imaged on the left side, from the seventh to the ninth intercostal space.

Sonographic abnormalities

Following are some significant sonographic findings:

♦ right lobe atrophy: causes include aging, cirrhosis, acute hepatic necrosis, and chronic compression

associated with distension of the right colon and cecum
- Cirrhosis may result from hemochromatosis or pyrrolizidine alkaloid toxicity.

◆ changes in parenchymal density, such as focal masses, nodular patterns, diffuse increases in echogenicity (fibrosis, inflammation, fat infiltration)

◆ dilation of bile radicles along with either hepatomegaly or cirrhosis: indicates obstructive biliary disease (e.g., duodenal stenosis, infective cholangitis)

◆ dilated biliary radicles adjacent to portal vessels (double parallel portal sign): also highly suggestive of cholelithiasis

Liver Biopsy

Liver biopsy is useful for histologic evaluation and for bacterial culture and sensitivity.

◆ A clotting profile (including platelet count, fibrinogen, PT, and PTT) must be performed before biopsy.

◆ Percutaneous liver biopsy is best performed using ultrasonographic guidance.

Techniques are described in *Equine Medicine and Surgery V.*

THERAPY FOR SEVERE HEPATIC DISEASE AND HEPATIC FAILURE

Therapy for horses with hepatic failure should include the following:

◆ *tranquilization:* if the horse's behavior suggests hepatoencephalopathy
- Diazepam should be avoided; flumazenil (a benzodiazepine antagonist) may be useful.

◆ *IV fluid therapy:* dextrose (2.5% to 5 %) should be given as a constant IV infusion at 10 to 20 mL/kg/d.
- Lipemic animals may also benefit from parenteral nutrition (see Chapter 4, Principles of Therapy).
- Hypoalbuminemic animals may require IV plasma.
- Horses with coagulopathy may need transfusion with fresh, whole blood.
- Vitamin B should be added to IV infusions.

◆ *antimicrobials:* if an infectious process or endotoxemia is suspected (see below)

◆ *antiinflammatory drugs:* NSAIDs usually are given
- Prednisolone (0.4 to 1.0 mg/kg PO q24-48h) may be useful for chronic-active hepatitis.

◆ *dietary modifications:* low crude protein and supplementation with fat-soluble vitamins
- Diets based on grass hay and beet pulp are recommended.
- Alfalfa and most grains and pellets should be avoided.
- Vitamins A, D, E, and K should be added, especially in cases of biliary stasis/obstruction.
- Vitamin K_1 is especially important when a coagulopathy is suspected or confirmed.

◆ *intestinal modifiers:* oral neomycin and metronidazole can reduce bacterial proliferation, and hence ammonia production, in the gut; lactulose may also be effective

Dosage of tranquilizers, antiinflammatory drugs, and antimicrobials (penicillins, tetracyclines, erythromycin, chloramphenicol, and some cephalosporins) *that are metabolized or excreted by the liver should be reduced to avoid toxicity.*

Antimicrobials

Antimicrobial therapy is important in the management of cholangitis, cholangiohepatitis, hepatic abscessation, and acute hepatic necrosis. When ascending infection along the common bile duct is suspected, the antimicrobial choice should reflect the most common intestinal isolates (gram-negative organisms and anaerobes); however, broad-spectrum coverage is recommended.

Common antimicrobial choices include:

◆ procaine penicillin G (20,000 to 40,000 IU/kg IM q12h) + gentamicin (6.6 mg/kg IV or IM q24h) + metronidazole (15 mg/kg PO or per rectum q6h)
- K^+-penicillin (20,000 to 40,000 IU/kg IV q6h) can be substituted for procaine penicillin.

◆ ceftiofur (2.2 mg/kg IV or IM q12h) + metronidazole (as above)

- ceftiofur + gentamicin + metronidazole (all dosages as above)
- potentiated sulfa (e.g., trimethoprim–sulfadiazine at 15 to 30 mg/kg PO q12h)
- potentiated sulfa + metronidazole (both dosages as above)
- enrofloxacin (2.5 to 5.0 mg/kg PO q12h)
  - NOTE: *Enrofloxacin should be used only when specifically indicated; it is ineffective against* Streptococcus *spp. and anaerobes.*
- enrofloxacin + metronidazole (both dosages as above)

CONGENITAL AND FAMILIAL DISEASES
Portosystemic Shunts
Portosystemic shunts are rare in horses. Clinical and laboratory evidence includes:

- unusual and erratic behavior, starting at 2 to 4 months of age; signs may be intermittent
- hyperammonemia and hypoglycemia
- increased serum bile acids but normal hepatic enzyme concentrations

NEONATAL DISEASES
Tyzzer's disease
Tyzzer's disease is an acute or peracute, multifocal, coagulative hepatitis in foals. It is caused by the bacterium *Clostridium piliformis*, a motile, filamentous, spore-forming, gram-negative rod.
Clinical findings
Tyzzer's disease usually is peracute.
- Foals are susceptible between 7 and 42 days of age.
- Often, affected foals are found dead, without premonitory clinical signs.
- Others may show severe, acute illness with fever, depression, anorexia, diarrhea, seizures, and tachypnea; icterus often is absent in foals with very acute onset of disease.
- Laboratory findings indicate severe hepatocellular necrosis; unconjugated hyperbilirubinemia and increases in AST, SDH, AP, and GGT are common.
- Definitive diagnosis relies on necropsy and histologic evaluation, as culture is difficult.

Treatment and prognosis
No specific treatment exists; supportive care should include:
- IV correction of dehydration, shock, metabolic acidosis, and hypoglycemia; and provision of nutritional support
- tranquilizers and anticonvulsants (other than diazepam) as needed
- oxygen insufflation
- antimicrobials (susceptible in vitro to penicillins, tetracyclines, and erythromycin)

There are no reports of successful therapy.

Herpes Hepatitis
Foals infected in utero with EHV-1 usually are aborted. Occasionally, infected foals are born alive with severe pneumonitis, hepatitis, and GI disease. These foals do not survive, and necropsy reveals characteristic foci of hepatocellular necrosis with intranuclear (acidophilic) inclusion bodies in large numbers of hepatocytes.

Morgan Foal Hepatic Failure
Signs of hepatic failure, depression, and weight loss have been reported in Morgan weanling foals. The cause is unknown.

INFLAMMATORY, INFECTIOUS, AND IMMUNE DISEASES
Cholangiohepatitis and Cholangitis
Many horses with cholangitis/cholangiohepatitis present with inappetence, fever, and icterus.
- Affected foals may have a history of gastric and/or duodenal ulceration causing partial obstruction of the duodenum.
- Laboratory findings include increases in serum GGT, AP, bile acids, and possibly AST and L-iDH (especially with cholangiohepatitis).
- The most common bacteria are intestinal organisms, including *E. coli, Citrobacter* spp., *Aeromonas* spp., *Klebsiella* spp., *Salmonella* spp., and *B. fragilis.*
  - Antimicrobials should be selected accordingly.

Hepatic Parasites

Parasites that may damage the liver, even on an aberrant basis, include large strongyles, *Parascaris equorum,* liver flukes, and *Echinococcus granulosus.* In most cases, liver damage is subclinical.

Liver flukes

Fasciola hepatica occasionally infests horses and donkeys.

- Signs include fatigue, exercise intolerance, diarrhea, urticaria, and alterations in appetite.
- Large-volume fecal samples are necessary to detect ova.
- Oral oxyclozanide kills adult flukes; treatment should be repeated in 2 to 4 months.

TOXIC DISEASES

Pyrrolizidine Alkaloid Toxicity

Pyrrolizidine alkaloids are found in many plants in the United States, especially in the northwest regions. Plants most commonly incriminated are:

- *Senecio* spp. (e.g., ragwort, groundsel, tar weed)
- *Crotalaria* spp. (e.g., rattlebox)
- *Amsinckia* spp. (e.g., fiddleneck)
- *Heliotropium* spp. (e.g., common heliotrope)
- *Cynoglossum* spp. (e.g., hound's tongue)
- *Echium* spp. (e.g., salvation Jane)

Clinical signs and diagnosis

- Hepatic failure resulting from pyrrolizidine alkaloid toxicity manifests as icterus, depression, weight loss, anorexia, tachycardia, ataxia, dermatitis, and behavioral changes.
- Inspiratory dyspnea (a manifestation of hepatoencephalopathy) occasionally occurs.
- Serum GGT, AP, bile acids, and bilirubin usually are increased.
- Hepatic histology reveals giant hepatocytes (hepatic megalocytosis), although these cells may also occur with aflatoxicosis, portal fibrosis, and other hepatopathies.
  - Fibrosis develops in longer-standing cases, beginning in portal regions.
- At necropsy, the liver usually is small, firm, and tan or yellow.

Treatment and prognosis

No specific treatment exists.

- If horses have only mild hepatic damage, removal from the contaminated pasture or food source may be sufficient to halt disease progression.
- Once hepatic failure develops, the prognosis is poor; death usually occurs within 2 weeks.

Mycotoxicosis

There are at least two important mycotoxins in horses.

- *Blue-green algae* causes intoxication after the horse drinks from an infected pond or dam.
  - Toxicity is most common in late summer and early fall, especially if the water is alkaline and has a high organic material load.
  - Affected horses show signs of liver failure or diarrhea, or they are found dead.
- *Leukoencephalomalacia* (moldy corn poisoning, see Chapter 11, Nervous System) causes neurologic disease; however, a secondary hepatic syndrome has been identified.
  - Fumonisin B1 causes extensive hepatocellular and biliary damage, and acute liver failure.
  - No specific treatment exists; some horses survive with intensive supportive care.

Iron Toxicity

Iron toxicity has been diagnosed in neonatal foals given oral ferrous fumerate and in adult horses.

- Foals are more likely to develop hepatic failure if the iron supplement is administered before ingestion of colostrum.
- Diagnosis is made by evaluating hepatic tissue.
  - Histologically, fibrosis and cirrhosis, and excessive iron storage (using Prussian blue stain), may be present.
  - Hepatic iron concentration in normal horses is 100 to 300 ppm (mg/kg); it is dramatically increased (e.g., >6000 ppm) in cases of iron toxicity.
- Therapy is nonspecific.
  - Whole blood can be removed on a regular basis to diminish iron stores.

• IM administration of deferox-
amine mesylate has been used in
humans.

MULTIFACTORIAL DISEASES
Neoplasia
Primary hepatic neoplasia is uncommon in horses; metastatic dis-
ease involving the liver is much
more common.
• *Lymphosarcoma* is most often diagnosed and may be a primary or secondary manifestation.
  • It can occur in young horses.
  • Ultrasonographic images may be
    normal or may show single or
    multiple masses.
• *Hepatocellular carcinoma* also has
been reported in young horses.
  • Signs may include abdominal
    distention, abdominal pain,
    weight loss, weakness, and ery-
    throcytosis with normopro-
    teinemia.
• *Biliary (cholangiocellular) carcinoma*
is a tumor of the biliary tree, occur-
ring in older horses.
  • Clinical signs are nonspecific
    (e.g., inappetence, intermittent
    fever, depression, colic), and can
    be similar to those of cholelithi-
    asis (see p. 240).
  • Bilirubin, GGT, AP and other
    hepatic enzymes may be
    increased.

IDIOPATHIC DISEASES
Acute Hepatic Necrosis (Theiler's Disease, Serum Hepatitis)
Idiopathic acute hepatic necrosis is a
devastating disease affecting adult
horses.
• Proposed causes include administration of equine biologic products
(e.g., plasma, tetanus antitoxin),
viral infection, and type III hypersensitivity.
• Farm problems involving both clinical and subclinical cases have been
reported.
• Signs are suggestive of widespread,
severe hepatocellular damage, usually progressing to hepatic failure.

• Laboratory findings include increased serum bilirubin (especially
unconjugated) and hepatic enzymes,
sometimes with dramatic increases
in L-iDH, arginase, SDH, and AST.
• Ultrasonography usually reveals a
homogenous pattern and sometimes a dramatic decrease in liver
size over several days.
• Affected horses require intensive
supportive therapy, but usually the
prognosis is poor.

Cholelithiasis
Cholelithiasis is the most common
cause of biliary obstruction in horses,
yet it is rarely diagnosed, possibly because clinical signs are not obvious
until the common bile duct is obstructed. Initiating or contributing
factors may include parasite migration, ascending gram-negative infection, foreign bodies, and alterations
in bile composition.
Clinical signs and diagnosis
• Affected horses usually have a history of recurrent, mild colic ±
weight loss and fever.
• Severe icterus is common, and conjugated bilirubin often exceeds
20% to 30% of total bilirubin.
• Serum bile acids and LDH-5, AP,
and GGT often are increased.
• Leukocytosis, hyperfibrinogenemia,
and hyperglobulinemia also may
be noted.
• Ultrasonography may reveal biliary
periportal fibrosis (which can increase the liver's echogenicity,
often equaling that of the spleen).
  • Thickened, distended bile ducts
    and either echodense choleliths
    or acoustic shadowing may also
    be noted.
• Liver biopsy may reveal periportal
and portal fibrosis, distension of
biliary canaliculi, and biliary
hyperplasia.
Treatment
• Celiotomy with choledochotomy
or choledocholithotripsy (manual
breakdown of choleliths) can be
successful.
• Broad-spectrum antibiotic therapy
is always indicated.

Diseases of the Pancreas *(pages 833-838)*

Catherine J. Savage

DIAGNOSTIC AND THERAPEUTIC CONSIDERATIONS

Clinical Signs of Pancreatic Disease

Clinical signs of pancreatic disease are nonspecific.

- Colic and shock usually accompany acute exocrine damage.
  - Colic is caused by gastric distension (reflux from the inflamed and static small intestine), peritonitis, and hemoabdomen.
  - *Severe gastric dilation can result in rupture if left untreated.*
  - Acute pancreatic exocrine disease also predisposes to DIC.
- Horses with chronic pancreatitis may have weight loss, intermittent colic, and icterus.
- Most horses with diabetes mellitus present with polyuria and weight loss.
  - Some horses with secondary diabetes mellitus have hirsutism resulting from pituitary adenoma.

Clinicopathologic Abnormalities

Serum amylase and lipase

In horses with acute or chronic pancreatic disease, serum amylase and lipase concentrations can be normal or increased.

- Normal serum amylase in horses is 14 to 35 U/L.
- It may be useful to compare serum and peritoneal fluid amylase values; in acute pancreatitis, peritoneal concentrations (normally <14 U/L) may exceed serum concentrations.
- Other causes of increased serum amylase include some disorders involving the small intestine (e.g., duodenitis–proximal jejunitis) or kidneys and administration of narcotic drugs.
- Normal serum lipase in horses is 23 to 87 U/L; normal peritoneal fluid lipase is <36 U/L.

Lipemia

Gross lipemia, evident in a blood sample, can be a sign of hepatic disease or of pancreatic failure. Pancreatic disease should be seriously considered in lipemic horses, especially if one is *not* dealing with hyperlipidemia/hyperlipemia (see Chapter 18, Endocrine System).

Serum enzymes

Serum GGT and AST may be elevated in cases of pancreatic disease, which can make it difficult to differentiate between hepatic (more common) and pancreatic disease. The most prevalent isoenzyme of LDH in the pancreas is LDH-1.

Serum calcium

It is important to evaluate the serum calcium concentration and correct it for hypoalbuminemia.

- Horses with pancreatic problems, especially if acute and necrotizing, often have moderate-to-severe hypocalcemia.
  - Acute pancreatic disease must be differentiated from blister beetle toxicity (see p. 185).
- Sometimes horses with pancreatic disease have hypercalcemia.

Fibrinogen and globulins

Hyperfibrinogenemia may occur with pancreatitis; however, values can be difficult to interpret if severe disease precipitates DIC. Pancreatic inflammation can also cause hyperglobulinemia.

Diabetes mellitus

Pancreatic endocrine disease generally involves β-cell damage and thus causes type I primary diabetes mellitus (hypoinsulinism). Hyperglycemia and glucosuria invariably are present. Diagnostic tests for diabetes include:

- insulin concentration
  - An increase in plasma insulin 3 hours postprandially, with concurrent hyperglycemia supports a diagnosis of type II primary diabetes (insulin resistance) or secondary diabetes.
- glucose tolerance test
  - Blood glucose and insulin are measured before and q30 min for 3 to 5 hours after nasogastric administration of glucose (0.5 to 1 g/kg in 2 L of water).
  - Normal horses show an increase in insulin and a consequent reduction in blood glucose back

into the normal range within 1 to 2 hours.

- insulin response test
  - In horses with type I diabetes, hyperglycemia is normalized within 3 hours of administration of protamine zinc insulin (0.5 IU/kg IM, 1 hour before feeding).
- endogenous ACTH assay
- growth hormone assay

Diabetes mellitus is discussed further in Chapter 18, Endocrine System.

Ultrasonography

The pancreas can be imaged on the right side. Pancreatic tissue surrounds the portal vein and lies over the caudal vena cava at the craniomedial aspect of the right kidney.

Laparoscopy

The right lobe of the pancreas and the entrance of the pancreatic duct into the duodenum can be seen via laparoscopy.

Therapy for Pancreatic Disease

Therapy is only palliative.

- If the horse is showing signs of abdominal pain or gastric contents are seen at the nares, a nasogastric tube should be passed immediately.
- The circulatory system should be supported with IV polyionic fluids ± plasma.
  - Whole blood transfusion may be useful in cases of DIC.
- Heparin may be added to the plasma or whole blood, or can be administered separately.
- Analgesics and antimicrobial drugs may also be considered.

INFLAMMATORY, INFECTIOUS, AND IMMUNE DISEASES

Causes of pancreatitis include migrating parasites, bacteria (ascending or hematogenous), viral infections (e.g., VEE, EIA), and immune-mediated disease.

Acute Pancreatitis

Horses with acute pancreatitis cannot easily be differentiated from those with other causes of severe colic.

- If peritoneal fluid amylase is increased, and especially if it is greater than the serum amylase, a diagnosis of acute pancreatitis may be appropriate.
- No specific therapy exists; management should be supportive and intensive.
  - NSAIDs, opiates (e.g., butophanol), antimicrobial drugs, and copious volumes of IV fluids should be administered.
  - An indwelling nasogastric tube should be placed and the horse refluxed q2-4h.
  - Plasma calcium should be monitored regularly and calcium-containing fluids given.
  - Tetracyclines should be avoided.
  - Despite therapy, the prognosis is poor to grave.

Chronic Pancreatitis

Chronic pancreatitis rarely is definitively diagnosed antemortem. Verminous migration and chronic eosinophilic dermatitis/enteritis are possible causes. Weight loss usually is severe and progressive in these horses. From whatever cause, fibrosing lesions of the pancreas may lead to type I primary diabetes mellitus or to extrahepatic cholestasis and liver damage.

TOXIC DISEASES
Vitamin D Toxicity

Vitamin D toxicity causes weight loss, stiffness, and polyuria/polydipsia. Soft tissue mineralization occurs and may involve the pancreas. Therapy includes cessation of vitamin D administration; anecdotally, corticosteroids may be helpful.

NEOPLASIA

Pancreatic adenocarcinoma is rare. Peritoneal fluid may be cloudy, with an increased WBC count and protein concentration, and peritoneal and thoracic fluids may contain abnormal cells. Serum amylase and lipase, and peritoneal fluid amylase concentrations may be normal.

11

Nervous System

Examination of the Nervous System

(pages 865-880)

Caroline N. Hahn, I. G. (Joe) Mayhew, and Robert J. MacKay

The neurologic examination is a systematic search for neuromuscular abnormalities and asymmetries. Examination should start at the head and proceed caudally to the tail.

EXAMINATION OF THE HEAD
Behavior
Bizarre and inappropriate behavior, such as head-pressing, compulsive wandering, or circling (generally to the side of the lesion), is a sign of cerebral disease.

Mental Status
The animal's responsiveness to its environment is controlled by the brainstem and cerebrum. The response to visual, tactile, auditory, painful, olfactory, and gustatory (nursing) stimuli should be considered. Horses that are recumbent because of spinal cord disease usually are bright and alert, unless they are anorectic, dehydrated, exhausted, or unduly frightened. They can become frantic in their effort to rise.

Head Posture and Coordination
Head tilt or turn
Unilateral vestibular lesions, whether central or peripheral, often result in

a head tilt (lateral deviation of the poll, while the caudal neck and muzzle remain on the midline). In comparison, cerebral lesions that cause continual circling often result in turning of the head and neck to one side, but the head itself is not tilted. Musculoskeletal disorders must also be considered with any asymmetry or deviation of the head and neck.

Abnormal head movements
Animals with bilateral (peripheral) vestibular disease frequently show wide swinging movements of the head and neck. With cerebellar disease, fine control of head positioning often is lost, resulting in awkward, jerky movements (intention tremor).

Cranial Nerves
In general, when more than one cranial nerve is involved, a more central lesion should be suspected. Brainstem pathology typically involves multiple cranial nerves and also causes signs of central disease, such as depression and limb weakness.

CN I: olfactory nerve
Clinical deficit of smell (anosmia) is rare. Normal function is crudely evaluated by the patient's ability to smell its feed or the hand of the examiner.

CN II: optic nerve
The visual pathway is tested by the menace response.
- A threatening gesture of the hand toward the horse's eye elicits immediate closure of the eyelids.

- Neonatal foals and some stoic, depressed, or even excited animals do not respond normally.
- Animals with diffuse cerebellar disease may have bilaterally deficient menace responses.
  - A true visual deficiency may be detected while the animal moves about its environment or when objects are placed in front of it.

Lesions of the eye and optic nerve result in ipsilateral blindness, while lesions of optic tracts, lateral geniculate nucleus, and occipital cortex cause contralateral blindness. An ophthalmologic examination should be included in the neurologic evaluation.

CN III: oculomotor nerve

Oculomotor nerve function is assessed in part by observing a change in pupil diameter in response to light:

- The first observation to be made is the size and symmetry of the pupils, considering the amount of ambient light and emotional status of the patient.
- The response to light directed into the eye (pupillary light response) is then noted.
  - The normal response to light directed into one eye is constriction of *both* pupils.
- A widely dilated pupil in an eye with normal vision suggests a CN III lesion.
  - Such an eye is unresponsive to light directed into either eye.
- A dilated pupil in an eye with absent menace response indicates an optic nerve (CN II) lesion.
- Edema and space-occupying lesions in the forebrain can compress the brainstem and affect the oculomotor nerves.
  - Asymmetric cerebral swelling may cause unequal pupillary size (anisocoria), usually evident as ipsilateral pupillary dilation.
  - Progressive, bilateral pupillary dilation after cranial injury is an indication of severe brainstem contusion and suggests a grave prognosis.

CN III: oculomotor nerve, CN IV: trochlear nerve, CN VI: abducens nerve

The oculomotor nerve also innervates the extraocular muscles, along with the trochlear and abducens nerves.

The functions of these nerves are tested by observing the position of the eyes within the orbits and by observing eye movement:

- An abnormal eyeball position (strabismus) results when these nerves or muscles are damaged (not common in horses).
- Deviation of the eyeballs more commonly results from disturbance of the vestibular system.
  - Vestibular strabismus usually is ventral and may be medial, but, unlike true strabismus, which is rare, the eyes can be moved out of the abnormal position by moving the head.
- Periorbital lesions, particularly traumatic and neoplastic, can also cause eye deviations.
- Congenitally blind horses may have abnormal eyeball positioning and movement.

CN V: trigeminal nerve

The trigeminal nerve contains motor nerve fibers to the muscles of mastication and sensory nerve fibers from most of the head:

- Bilateral loss of motor function results in a dropped jaw, inability to chew, and subsequent sialosis; the tongue may appear to protrude.
  - After 1 to 2 weeks, the temporal, masseter, and pterygoid muscles atrophy.
  - Unilateral lesions result in unilateral muscle atrophy without dysphagia.
- Function of the sensory branches is assessed by lightly brushing the ears, eyelids, external nares, and lips and observing for movement of the part stimulated (facial reflexes) and a cerebral response (e.g., withdrawal and shaking of the head).
  - In stoic or depressed animals, sensation may be assessed by lightly pricking the internal nares and nasal septum.
- Unilateral lesions of the medulla oblongata can cause ipsilateral facial hypalgesia and hyporeflexia without atrophy of the masticatory muscles.
  - This may cause feed to become impacted in the rostral cheek pouch.

- Cerebral lesions can produce contralateral facial hypalgesia, especially of the nasal septum.

CN VII: facial nerve

The facial nerve is predominantly a motor nerve innervating the muscles of facial expression, as well as the lacrimal glands and certain salivary glands.

- It is the motor pathway of many of the reflexes tested previously.
- Initial evaluation involves inspection for symmetry of facial expression and observation of the menace, palpebral, and corneal reflexes and movement of the ears, eyelids, lips, and nose.
- Facial paralysis generally is seen as drooping of the ear and lips, retraction of the nose toward the unaffected side, slight protrusion of the tongue on the affected side, and ptosis of the upper eyelid.
  - When the only signs are weakness of the lips and a deviated nasal philtrum, only the buccal branch, or more likely the facial nerve along the side of the face, is involved.
- Depression, ataxia, and signs of other cranial nerve dysfunction indicate a central (e.g., medulla oblongata) rather than a peripheral lesion.
  - Facial nerve paralysis often accompanies vestibular signs with lesions of the middle and inner ear (see p. 270).
- With various focal thalamic and cerebral lesions, the facial muscles may become hypertonic and hyperreflexic, resulting in spontaneous and reflexively initiated "grimacing."
  - The facial reflexes are intact and may be hyperactive.
  - Irritative CN VII lesions, such as peracute encephalitides, can also cause grimacing.

Damage to the sympathetic nerves that innervate the eyeball results in Horner's syndrome.

- Signs include miosis (pupillary constriction), ptosis (drooping of the upper eyelid), and enophthalmos with protrusion of the nictitating membrane.
  - Vision and pupillary light response are unaffected.
- Additional signs include dilation of facial blood vessels, hyperemia of nasal and conjunctival mucosae, and sweating, especially from the base of the ear to about the level of the axis.
- These signs can be seen with lesions anywhere along the sympathetic pathway, including the brainstem, cervical spinal cord, thoracic inlet, cervical vagosympathetic trunk, and guttural pouches.

CN VIII: vestibulocochlear nerve

The cochlear (auditory) division of this nerve is involved in the sense of hearing, which can be very difficult to assess. The vestibular division supplies the major input to the vestibular system and thus controls balance. Signs of vestibular disease can be seen with lesions involving any part of the vestibular system.

- Nystagmus when the horse's head is in a normal position (spontaneous nystagmus) and/or with the head held steady by the examiner in various abnormal positions (positional nystagmus) indicates a disorder of the vestibular system.
  - In peripheral vestibular disorders, the fast phase of nystagmus is directed away from the side of the lesion and from the direction of head tilt.
- When lesions involve the central components of the vestibular system (medulla oblongata), spontaneous and positional nystagmus may be horizontal, vertical, or rotary.
  - Such lesions frequently affect adjacent structures, causing ataxia, paresis, and depression.
- Signs of peripheral vestibular disease often markedly improve within several days as the patient accommodates; in such cases blindfolding immediately exacerbates the signs.

CN IX: glossopharyngeal nerve, CN X: vagus nerve, CN XI: accessory nerve

The major role of these nerves is sensory and motor innervation of the pharynx and larynx:

- Function is tested by listening for normal upper airway sounds, observing swallowing of food and water, assessing the swallowing reflex by passage of a nasogastric tube, and if necessary, endoscopic examination of the larynx and pharynx.

- The thoracolaryngeal adductor response ("slap test") should also be assessed.

♦ The most important sign of an abnormality is paralysis of the pharynx and larynx, causing food and water to appear at the nares; stertorous breathing may also be noted.

♦ Lesions in the medulla oblongata usually affect adjacent structures, resulting in depression, ataxia, weakness, and signs of other cranial nerve involvement.

♦ These cranial nerves can be damaged in guttural pouch disease.

CN XI: accessory nerve

This nerve innervates the trapezius and the cranial part of the sternocephalicus. Loss of function is difficult to detect without electromyography.

CN XII: hypoglossal nerve

The hypoglossal nerve is the motor to the tongue.

♦ The tongue must be inspected for symmetry, normal movement, strength, and bulk.

♦ A unilateral lesion of the hypoglossal nucleus or nerve results in unilateral atrophy of the tongue and weak retraction when the tongue is pulled out.

♦ Bilateral involvement interferes with prehension and swallowing; the tongue protrudes and the horse cannot draw it back into the mouth.

EVALUATING GAIT AND POSTURE

The first observation to be made is which limbs have an abnormal gait and/or posture, and second, whether there is evidence of a musculoskeletal abnormality. Evaluation is done while the animal is walking, trotting, turning tightly (pivoting), and backing. If possible, the gait should be evaluated while the animal is walking up and down a slope, walking with the neck extended, walking while blindfolded, and running free in a field. Subtle signs become more obvious when the animal performs these more involved maneuvers and as the animal tires.

The essential components of a neurologic gait abnormality are:

♦ weakness or paresis (indicating interruption to motor pathways)

♦ ataxia (abnormal proprioceptive sensory pathways), classified as hypometria or hypermetria

Identifying these abnormalities can help localize a lesion within the nervous or musculoskeletal system (Table 11-1).

Weakness

Upper motor neuron (UMN) lesions often cause ipsilateral flexor weakness caudal to the lesion.

♦ Signs include dragging of the limbs, worn hooves, a low arc to

Table 11-1

Prominent gait and postural abnormalities present with neurologic lesion at different locations

Lesion Location	Gait and Postural Abnormalities				
	Postural Deficits	Paresis	Ataxia	Hypometria	Hypermetria
Cerebrum	+++	0	0	0	0
Brain stem	++	++	++	++	++
Vestibular	+++	0	++	++	0
Cerebellum	++	0	+++	+	+++
Spinal cord UMN	++	++	++	++	++
Peripheral nerve/LMN	++	+++	+	(++)*	(+++)*
Musculoskeletal	+	++	0	+	0

0 = Not usually expected.
+ = Mild if present.
++ = Usually present.
+++ = Quite characteristically present.
* = Usually only with selective sensory fiber involvement.

the swing phase of the stride, stumbling and knuckling, and possibly trembling or collapse during weight-bearing.
- Hind limb weakness is detected by walking beside the horse and pulling the tail laterally.

Profound extensor weakness in only one limb suggests a lesion of the spinal cord gray matter or peripheral nerve (i.e., a lower motor neuron [LMN] lesion) or in the muscles of that limb. With severe weakness in all four limbs but no ataxia or spasticity, neuromuscular disease must be strongly considered (see p. 283).

Ataxia

Ataxia, or proprioceptive deficit, is poor coordination in moving the limbs and body. It is seen as:
- swaying of the pelvis, trunk, neck, and sometimes the whole body
- weaving of the affected limbs during the swing phase of the stride
- circumduction of the outside limbs when turning and circling
- maintenance of abnormal limb posture when stopped after turning tightly
- pacing

It can be difficult to differentiate weakness from ataxia. Walking the animal on a slope and with its head elevated often exaggerates ataxia, particularly in the fore limbs.

Hypometria

Hypometria (spasticity or stiffness) is seen as stiff movement of the limbs with very little flexion of the joints. It generally indicates a lesion affecting the UMN or vestibular pathways to that limb. Spasticity may be the most obvious sign in animals with cervical spinal cord disease.

Hypermetria

Hypermetria describes an increased range of joint movement and is seen as overreaching of the limbs with excessive joint flexion. Hypermetria without paresis is characteristic of cerebellar disease but also is prominent in some peripheral nerves diseases, such as stringhalt.

Grading Gait Abnormalities

The degree of weakness, ataxia, and hypometria or hypermetria is graded for each limb. A scale of 0 to 4+ is used.

- A score of 1+ indicates signs that are just detectable, while 4+ indicates that the patient stumbles and may fall at normal gaits.
- With compressive lesions in the cranial cervical spinal cord or with focal brainstem lesions, signs generally are one grade more severe in the hind limbs than in the forelimbs.

EVALUATING THE NECK AND FORELIMBS

If a gait alteration is detected in the forelimbs and there are no signs of brain involvement, this part of the examination attempts to confirm involvement of the spinal cord from C1 to T2 and to localize the lesion within these segments:
- The neck should be manipulated to assess normal range of movement.
  - Reluctance to flex the neck or pain on flexion warrants careful assessment.
- Local cervical and cervicofacial responses are assessed by lightly tapping the skin dorsal to the jugular groove.
  - The normal response is ipsilateral flicking of the skin on the side of the neck, rostral flicking of the ear, blinking, contracture of the labial muscles ("smile"), and contraction of the brachiocephalicus, which may pull the shoulder forward.
  - Cervical lesions can suppress these responses.
  - Sensory perception over the neck and forelimbs can be assessed by continuing the skin tapping over the horse's shoulders and distally on the limbs.
- Regional sweating is a useful localizing sign.
- The sway reaction is tested by pushing against the horse's shoulder, both while it is standing still and while walking forward; weakness is seen as lack of resistance to lateral pressure.
- Pinching and pressing down with the fingers on the withers of a normal animal results in some ventral movement (lordosis) but then resistance or bracing.
  - An animal with forelimb weakness may not be able to resist this pressure and may buckle

• Hopping can be performed by lifting one forelimb at a time and pushing the horse with a shoulder to make it hop on the weight-bearing limb.
  • A weak limb may buckle and high-stepping can be present, with ataxia in the limbs.

Evaluating Recumbent Patients

If a recently recumbent horse cannot attain a dog-sitting posture, the lesion is likely to be in the cervical spinal cord (or brain). If only the head but not the neck can be raised off the ground, there probably is a severe cranial cervical lesion.

Muscle tone can be assessed by manipulating each limb.
• Flaccidity with no motor activity is typical of a LMN lesion.
• A severe UMN lesion cranial to C6 causes decreased or absent voluntary effort, but there is normal or increased muscle tone in the limbs (spastic paralysis).

Spinal reflexes

The following spinal reflexes should be assessed in recumbent patients. Some can be difficult to elicit in heavy adult horses. A spinal reflex can be intact without the animal perceiving the stimulus:
• *flexor reflex:* This involves pinching the skin of the distal limb with needle holders and observing for flexion of the fetlock, knee, elbow, and shoulder
  • If the flexor reflex is absent, the lesion likely involves the C6-T2 gray matter, peripheral nerves (median and ulnar), or flexor muscles.
  • Lesions cranial to C7 may result in an exaggerated reflex and, with severe UMN lesions, a crossed-extensor reflex (synchronous extension of the opposite limb) can be present.
• *triceps reflex:* Extension of the elbow normally results when the relaxed limb is held slightly flexed, and the triceps tendon is ballotted with a heavy plexor.
  • This reflex involves the radial nerve and spinal cord segments C7-T1.
  • If the reflex can be easily elicited in heavily muscled animals, a

UMN lesion cranial to the spinal cord segments likely is involved.

Skin sensation

Lesions of the peripheral nerves (e.g., suprascapular and radial nerves) cause characteristic gait abnormalities, paralysis and selective muscle atrophy, specific reflex loss, and sensory deficits (see p. 279).

EVALUATING THE TRUNK AND HIND LIMBS

If there are signs only in the trunk and hind limbs, any spinal cord lesion(s) will usually be between T2 and S3. Mild and particularly chronic cervical spinal cord lesions can present as a 1+ gait abnormality in the hind limbs with no forelimb signs. The examination proceeds as follows.
• The trunk and hind limbs are observed and palpated for malformation and asymmetry.
  • Muscle atrophy indicates a lesion of the thoracolumbar gray matter.
• Gentle pricking of the skin over the lateral trunk causes contraction of the cutaneous trunci muscle, seen as flicking of the skin over the trunk.
  • This reflex involves the segmental thoracolumbar spinal nerves (at the level of the site being tested), ascending thoracic white matter tracts, and spinal cord segments C8-T1.
• The sway reaction for the hind limbs involves pushing against the pelvis and pulling on the tail while the horse is standing and while walking.
  • Extensor weakness (notably with LMN lesions) results in little resistance to pushing or pulling the hindquarters while the horse is standing still.
  • With flexor weakness (notably with UMN lesions), the horse resists lateral pressure at rest but is moved off stride very easily while walking.
  • This test can help detect asymmetry in weakness and/or ataxia in the hind limbs.
• Pinching and pressing down with the fingers on the thoracolumbar or sacral paravertebral muscles causes a normal horse to fix the thoracolumbar spine and resist the ventral motion.

- A weak animal usually cannot resist the pressure and thus overextends the back and begins to buckle in the limbs.
- Running a blunt probe along the thoracolumbar and then the gluteal musculature allows evaluation of how well the horse can move its thoracolumbosacral vertebrae as it extends (lordosis) then flexes (kyphosis) its back, respectively.
  - A weak horse often buckles in the hind limbs when this is done.

Evaluating Recumbent Patients

A recently recumbent horse that uses its forelimbs well in an attempt to rise most likely has a lesion caudal to T2. The hind limb spinal reflexes should be evaluated in all recumbent animals and the amount of voluntary effort and muscle tone assessed. However, consideration must be given to possibly exacerbating a fracture. The absence of voluntary movement in a limb that is flaccid and areflexic strongly suggests an LMN lesion. The following reflexes are assessed:

- *patellar reflex:* performed by supporting the limb in a partly flexed position, firmly tapping the middle patellar ligament with a heavy plexor, and observing for stifle extension
  - This reflex involves the femoral nerve and spinal cord segments L4 and L5.
- *flexor reflex:* performed by pinching the skin of the distal limb with needle holders and observing for flexion of all limb joints.
  - A stronger stimulus may be necessary to elicit this reflex in a heavy horse that has been recumbent on a limb for some time.
  - This reflex involves the sciatic nerve and spinal cord segments L5-S2.

Skin sensation

As for the forelimbs, lesions of the peripheral nerves to the hind limbs, such as the femoral and peroneal nerves, cause specific motor deficits, though the precise sensory deficits can be difficult to define (see p. 280). Skin sensation must be assessed independent of reflex activity.

EVALUATING THE TAIL AND ANUS

A completely flaccid tail with no voluntary movement indicates a lesion of the sacrococcygeal segments or nerves. Decreased voluntary tail movements can be found with lesions cranial to the coccygeal segments, but usually the spinal cord lesion must be severe for tail weakness to be apparent. The perineal reflex is elicited by lightly pricking the skin of the perineum and observing reflex contraction of the anal sphincter and flexion (clamping down) of the tail. This reflex involves the perineal branches of the pudendal nerve (S1-S3). Lesions involving the cauda equina are discussed on p. 278.

NEUROLOGIC EXAMINATION OF FOALS

Neurologic evaluation of foals is similar to that of adults, with the following exceptions.

- Newborn foals normally hold the head flexed slightly more than adult horses and move it in a jerky manner, especially in response to visual or tactile stimuli.
- The eyeball position in newborn foals is ventromedial, and although foals appear to see by a few hours of age, they do not blink to menacing gestures until 5 to 15 days of age.
  - They do, however, blink at bright light and jerk their heads away from menacing gestures
- Spinal reflexes are hyperactive in newborn foals.
  - Up to approximately 1 month of age there are strong crossed-extensor reflexes in the forelimbs and hind limbs.
- "Wheelbarrowing" by lifting the forelimbs, then the hind limbs, off the ground and making the foal walk backward, then forward, respectively; hopping the foal to the left and right on each forelimb in turn; and hemistanding/hemiwalking are useful tests.
  - Brainstem, spinal cord, and peripheral nerve lesions cause postural deficits on the same side as the lesions; thalamic and cerebral lesions produce contralateral abnormalities.

Ancillary Diagnostic Aids *(pages 880-883)*

Caroline N. Hahn, I. G. (Joe) Mayhew, and Robert J. MacKay

CEREBROSPINAL FLUID ANALYSIS

Cerebrospinal Fluid Collection

Samples of cerebrospinal fluid (CSF) can be obtained from the lumbosacral area in standing horses and from the atlantooccipital (AO) and lumbosacral areas in anesthetized horses.

Atlantooccipital space

Following are guidelines for CSF collection at the AO space.

* A 3.5-inch, 20-gauge (90 × 0.9 mm) spinal needle is recommended, inserted 1 to 3 cm (0.5 to 1 inch) in foals and 5 to 8 cm (2 to 3 inches) in adults.
  * A 1.5-inch, 19-gauge (40 × 1.1 mm) disposable needle is preferred in young foals.
* The needle is inserted on the dorsal midline, in the center of an imaginary line drawn between the cranial borders of the wings of the atlas.
* Entrance to the subarachnoid space is felt as a sudden loss of resistance to needle passage.
* CSF is collected as a free catch or *slowly* aspirated, 10 mL in adult horses and 5 mL in foals.

Lumbosacral space

Sedation with butorphanol and an α_2-agonist greatly facilitates lumbosacral CSF collection in standing horses. The area for needle insertion is the palpable depression on the dorsal midline, just caudal to the spine of L6 (between the tubera sacrale).

* A 6- to 8-inch, 18-gauge (165 to 205 × 1 to 2 mm) spinal needle is required in large horses; a 3.5-inch, 20-gauge (90 × 0.9 mm) spinal needle is used in foals.
* A change in resistance may be felt when this space is entered; usually some response by the horse, such as a flick of the tail, indicates correct needle placement.

Sample Handling and Analysis

It is important to handle the CSF sample gently and have it analyzed as quickly as possible after collection.

Normal values

Normal CSF is clear and colorless.

* Total protein concentration is 20 to 80 mg/dL (0.2 to 0.8 g/L; absolute range, 5 to 115 mg/dL; 0.05 to 1.15 g/L).
* The WBC count is <6 cells/μL (<0.006 × 10^9/L); red blood cells (RBCs) are absent.
* The refractive index (measured with a hand-held refractometer) is 1.335.

Interpretation of abnormalities

Common abnormalities include xanthochromia (yellow discoloration) and opacity:

* Xanthochromia usually indicates trauma or vasculitis (leakage of plasma or RBCs from damaged vessels, as seen with equine herpes virus-1 [EHV-1] myeloencephalopathy).
  * If the first few drops of CSF are pink but subsequent fluid is clear, the RBCs likely are an artifact of collection.
* Total protein concentration >150 mg/dL and WBC counts >50/μL result in opacity.
  * Excessive numbers of white blood cells (WBCs) are seen with trauma, infections, neoplasia, and some degenerative, toxic, nutritional, immune-mediated, and metabolic diseases.
  * Bacterial meningitis results in CSF neutrophilia, whereas most viral CNS diseases produce a lymphocytic response.

Albumin quotient and IgG index

Leakage of blood or plasma into the CSF raises the protein content; this occurs in traumatic, vascular, inflammatory, and some degenerative diseases. Globulin production within the CNS can also raise the CSF protein content, although this usually is seen only in chronic infectious and possibly some immune-mediated diseases. Two indices are used to evaluate CSF protein:

* Albumin quotient = (CSF albumin/serum albumin) × 100
  * Mean values in normal horses are 1.4 ± 0.4 (AO) and 1.5 ± 0.4 (lumbosacral).
  * A CSF albumin concentration >56 mg/dL or an albumin quotient of >2.35 may indicate increased BBB permeability.

- IgG index = (CSF IgG/serum IgG) × (Serum albumin/CSF albumin)
  - An indicator of intrathecal IgG production; the mean in normal horses is 0.194 ± 0.05.
  - An IgG index >0.27 may indicate intrathecal IgG production.

RADIOGRAPHY

Plain radiography is vital to document fractures, luxation, malformations, and occasionally infections and neoplasms of the skull and vertebral column. Myelography should be done only when results could alter management of the case. The technique is described in *Equine Medicine and Surgery V.*

OTHER DIAGNOSTIC TOOLS

Other diagnostic tools that may be useful in specific cases include needle electromyography for localizing gray matter lesions and peripheral nerve diseases, electroencephalography to record the electrical activity of the brain, thermography and scintigraphy to detect changes in superficial blood flow, and peripheral nerve and muscle biopsy to confirm the presence of LMN disease.

Diseases of Multiple or Unknown Sites

(pages 884-903)
Caroline N. Hahn, I. G. (Joe) Mayhew, and Robert J. MacKay

VIRAL NEUROLOGIC DISEASES
Eastern, Western, and Venezuelan Encephalomyelitis

Within the United States, eastern equine encephalomyelitis (EEE) has been reported in all states on the eastern seaboard and Gulf coast and in a number of western states. Outbreaks of western equine encephalomyelitis (WEE) have occurred in the western and midwestern United States and in west central Canada, Mexico, and South America. No epizootics of Venezuelan equine encephalomyelitis (VEE) have been reported in the United States since 1971. These viruses are maintained in nature by sylvatic cycles involving mosquito vectors and bird, reptile, or rodent reservoirs. Epizootics of EEE and WEE tend to occur in mid to late summer.

Clinical findings

The clinical and serologic events after infection with EEE, WEE, or VEE virus are similar, differing only in detail and lethality. Infected horses respond in any or all of the following ways:

1. Inapparent infection with low-grade viremia and fever about 2 days after infection; mild lymphopenia and neutropenia usually are present
2. Generalized febrile illness (up to 41° C [106° F]), with anorexia, depression, tachycardia, diarrhea (VEE), and profound lymphopenia and neutropenia; some severely affected horses die
3. Clinical encephalomyelitis (the classic form of the disease)

Findings associated with *clinical encephalomyelitis* are as follows:

- Signs first appear about 5 days after infection, and most deaths occur 2 to 3 days later.
  - Biphasic febrile episodes often precede the onset of central nervous system (CNS) signs.
- CNS signs are referable to diffuse or multifocal cerebral disease.
  - Often the first sign is a change in behavior, such as irritability, aggression, or somnolence; self-mutilation, hyperesthesia, and hyperexcitability have been reported.
  - Food and water usually are refused.
  - Further signs of dementia often follow, including head-pressing, leaning, and compulsive walking.
- Brainstem and spinal cord involvement become more obvious as the illness progresses.
  - Blindness and lack of a menace response may be noted.
  - Other cranial nerve signs, including nystagmus, facial paralysis, and lingual and pharyngeal paresis, often develop, as do progressive ataxia and paresis.

Diagnosis

Presumptive diagnosis is based on clinical signs, especially in endemic areas, and confirmed with serology.

♦ A fourfold rise in antibody titer between acute and convalescent serum samples taken 7 to 10 days apart is considered positive.
  • A very high single titer in an unvaccinated animal probably is diagnostic.
♦ Comparison of serum hemagglutination inhibition titers for both EEE and WEE helps differentiate horses challenged with wild EEE virus from vaccinated horses.
  • A EEE/WEE titer ratio of 2:1 probably indicates vaccination, a ratio of 4:1 is suspect for EEE, and a ratio of ≥8:1 most likely represents EEE.
  • A specific ELISA can also distinguish between vaccinal (IgG only) and virulent virus-induced (IgG and IgM) titers.

Treatment

Treatment is largely supportive.

♦ Treatment for cerebral edema and inflammation should be instituted in horses that are rapidly deteriorating and can include the following drugs:
  • dexamethasone at 0.05 to 0.1 mg/kg IM or IV q6h for 1 to 2 days
  • flunixin meglumine at 0.5 mg/kg IM q12h
  • mannitol (0.25 to 0.5 g/kg IV as a 20% solution), DMSO (1 g/kg IV as a 10% solution in 5% dextrose q12h for up to 3 days), or furosemide (0.5 to 1 mg/kg IV)
♦ Seizures can be controlled with α_2-agonists, diazepam, or barbiturates (see Table 11-3).
  • Severe hyperthermia (40° C [104° F]) may contribute to seizures and should be treated with cold water or alcohol baths.
♦ Diligent nursing care is essential.
  • IV fluids may be necessary to maintain hydration.
  • An indwelling stomach tube can facilitate feeding of dysphagic horses.
  • Recumbent animals should be encouraged to remain sternal; any decubital lesions should be treated vigorously.
  • Intermittent bladder catheterization and manual evacuation of the rectum may be necessary.

A VEE outbreak requires quarantine of horses.

Prognosis

Mortality rates are 75% to 90% for EEE, 19% to 50% for WEE, and 40% to 90% for VEE. Death usually is preceded by a period of recumbency, during which the horse may be semicomatose and convulsing. Surviving horses gradually recover over a period of weeks but may have residual signs of CNS damage.

Control

Monovalent, bivalent (EEE and WEE), and trivalent vaccines (EEE, WEE, and VEE) are available, the choice for a particular area depending on the likely occurrence of the diseases.

♦ Horses should be given 2 injections 3 to 4 weeks apart, at least 1 month before the onset of mosquito activity, and then revaccinated at least annually.
  • The optimal time for vaccination is January and February in Florida and Mexico and May and June in Canada and the northern United States.
  • Revaccination at least once during the summer is necessary in areas with warm climates and long mosquito seasons.
♦ Foals of vaccinated mares should be given a series of 2 or 3 monthly vaccinations, beginning at 3 months of age; foals may be revaccinated at 12 months.

General control measures aimed at reducing mosquito populations significantly diminish but do not eliminate the risk of equine infection.

Rabies

Rabies has been diagnosed in horses in most parts of the world. The United Kingdom, New Zealand, Australia, Hawaii, and some Pacific and Caribbean islands are currently free of the disease. The presentation can be highly variable, so in endemic areas, rabies must be included as a differential diagnosis in any horse showing unusual neurologic signs.

Epidemiology

Rabies usually is transmitted by salivary contamination of a bite wound. The majority of wildlife vectors are small to medium size omnivores, such as skunks and raccoons in the United States and bats in South America. The incubation period in horses ranges from 2 weeks to several months.

Clinical signs

Signs, at least terminally, are those of diffuse or multifocal CNS disease. However, presenting signs and the clinical course are extremely variable.

- Signs can include, either singly or in combination, anorexia, depression, blindness, mania, hyperesthesia, muscle-twitching, lameness, paresis and ataxia, urinary incontinence, colic, and sudden death.
- Signs are predominantly encephalitic or referable to spinal cord disease.
- Horses with spinal cord involvement often have ascending flaccid paralysis, with retention of urine and feces and loss of spinal reflexes and sensation as signs advance.
  - Initial hyperesthesia and self-mutilation may be observed.
  - The horse progressively loses the ability to stand and finally to remain sternal.
  - There may be no disturbance of behavior or appetite until the final stages.
- Horses with the encephalitic form usually manifest early behavioral changes, such as profound depression ("dumb" rabies) or unprovoked excitement ("furious" rabies).
  - Other signs of brain disease, such as dysphagia, facial paresis, nystagmus, and altered vocalization, often are present.
  - Fever is common at some point during the course of the disease.
  - Tetraparesis and ataxia appear early and progress quickly to recumbency.
- Horses with either form become comatose or convulse and thrash violently before dying, usually within 3 to 10 days of the onset of signs.

Diagnosis

Clinical diagnosis of rabies may be difficult but should be considered in any horse showing rapidly progressive CNS signs, especially in areas where rabies is enzootic.

- Signs of severe gray-matter disease (flaccid limbs, tail paralysis, analgesia, and loss of spinal reflexes) strongly suggest rabies.
- CSF from rabid horses frequently is normal but may show moderate elevations in protein content and mononuclear cell numbers.
- Fluorescent antibody staining of the cornea or muzzle hair follicles of suspect horses may be a useful antemortem test, although false-positive and false-negative results occur.
- If rabies is suspected, the brain should be split in half and one half refrigerated (but not frozen) until it can be transported to a diagnostic laboratory.
  - The other half may be fixed in 10% formalin for later histologic examination if tests for rabies are negative.
  - The remainder of the carcass should be incinerated or buried at a depth deeper than 1 m (3 feet).

Prevention

Horses in high-risk areas may be immunized by annual vaccination, beginning at 3 months of age, with a commercial inactivated vaccine. If a previously immunized horse is bitten by a suspect rabid animal, it can be given 3 booster immunizations over 1 week and quarantined for at least 90 days. Postexposure immunization of animals not currently vaccinated is thought to be unsafe.

Equine Herpesvirus Myeloencephalopathy

The primary lesion of EHV-1 myeloencephalopathy is believed to be immune-mediated vasculitis (arteritis), with secondary hemorrhagic and ischemic infarction of neural parenchyma.

- EHV-1 myeloencephalopathy is most common where there are aggregations of horses, as in racing, breeding, or boarding establishments.
  - 100% morbidity has been reported in some groups of horses.
- Outbreaks may be temporally associated with respiratory illness or abor-

tion or may occur in the absence of other recognized EHV-1 syndromes.

• The paralytic form of EHV-1 infection is most frequently seen in mature horses with high levels of circulating antibodies.

Clinical signs

Signs of neurologic disease develop about 7 days after infection.

• Fever (up to 41° C [106° F]), with or without a cough and serous nasal discharge, often precedes neurologic signs by several days.

• Horses are either febrile or normothermic at the onset of neurologic signs, such as peracute paresis and ataxia; signs may be mildly asymmetric.

  • Typically, the hind limbs are more severely affected.

• Signs begin suddenly and progress rapidly over 48 hours but then stabilize quickly.

  • Early involvement varies from subtle clumsiness or stiffness during circling to "dog-sitting" or recumbency.

  • If recumbency occurs, it usually is within the first 24 to 48 hours.

• Affected horses usually are alert and have a good appetite.

• Bladder distention is common, sometimes accompanied by urinary incontinence.

  • Vulvar or penile flaccidity can be seen.

  • Tail elevation, decreased tail tone, and perineal hypalgesia are inconsistent findings.

  • Depression, nystagmus, eye deviation, and other signs of brainstem disease may be seen.

Diagnosis

Presumptive diagnosis is based on clinical signs and evidence of active EHV-1 infection.

• Confirmation requires either isolation of the virus from nasopharyngeal swabs and blood buffy coats or demonstration of a fourfold rise in antibody titer over 7 to 10 days.

• Xanthochromia and marked elevation of protein content (100 to 500 mg/dL; 1.0 to 5.0 g/L) in CSF samples are supportive; cell numbers usually are normal.

  • Serum-neutralizing titers in CSF are not consistently elevated.

Treatment

Any horse with suspected EHV-1 infection should be isolated until the diagnosis is ruled out. Affected horses that remain able to stand recover with adequate supportive care.

• Recumbent horses should be bedded well and encouraged to remain sternal.

  • Horses in lateral recumbency must be frequently rolled.

• Food and water may have to be offered by hand or given via nasogastric tube.

• Use of laxatives or enemas or manual emptying of the rectum may be necessary.

• Secondary bacterial infections of the urinary or respiratory tract must be treated vigorously.

• Glucocorticoids may be helpful, especially early in the disease.

  • Dexamethasone (or equivalent) may be given at 0.05 to 0.1 mg/kg IV q6h the first day and up to several days thereafter, depending on the response to treatment.

Prognosis

Most horses that remain standing recover completely. Time to recovery primarily depends on the severity of the initial signs and ranges from several days to 18 months. Many horses that become tetraplegic are euthanized, although there are reports of horses that stand again after being recumbent for several weeks.

Prophylaxis

Modified live and inactivated EHV-1 vaccines are commercially available, but their efficacy in preventing EHV-1 myeloencephalopathy has not been critically evaluated. In fact, there is some evidence that prior vaccination does not confer protection against this condition and in some instances may actually increase the risk of neurologic disease.

BACTERIAL NEUROLOGIC DISEASES

Listeriosis

Clinical disease caused by *Listeria monocytogenes* infection is rare in horses. A form of equine listeriosis with signs primarily referable to brainstem and cauda equina involvement has been reported. Listeric meningitis can occur in neonates. Treatment with high levels of potassium penicillin G or sodium ampicillin along with supportive care should be effective if used early.

Bacterial Meningoencephalomyelitis in Foals

Clinically recognizable meningitis usually is caused by hematogenous spread of bacteria to the meninges or by direct extension of suppurative processes in or around the head (e.g., brain abscess) or a penetrating wound to the skull. Bacterial meningitis most often is seen as a complication of failure of passive transfer and sepsis in neonatal foals.

Causative organisms

The bacteria involved are those most commonly causing neonatal septicemia:

- β-Hemolytic streptococci
- *Actinobacillus equuli*
- *Escherichia coli*
- *Klebsiella pneumoniae* and coagulase-positive staphylococci (both uncommon)

Salmonella spp., especially *S. typhimurium,* can cause meningitis in older foals. In adult horses, sporadic cases of meningitis have been associated with *Streptococcus equi* and *Actinomyces* spp.

Clinical signs

Signs and their progression in foals with bacterial meningoencephalitis are as follows:

- The bacteremic phase is characterized by fever, lethargy, and lack of affinity for the mare.
- Early meningeal involvement is indicated by behavioral changes, such as aimless walking ("wanderer"), depression ("dummy"), and abnormal vocalization ("barker").
  - Initially there is cutaneous hyperesthesia, muscular rigidity, and tremors.
- Signs rapidly progress to blindness, loss of the sucking reflex, multiple cranial nerve abnormalities, and ataxia and paresis.
  - Hyperesthesia is followed by diffusely diminished sensation and reduced spinal reflexes.
- If the foal is left untreated, recumbency, coma, seizures, and death quickly occur.

Diagnosis

Bacterial meningitis requires rapid and meticulous management, so early diagnosis is essential.

- The diagnosis is confirmed by finding bacteria, increased numbers of inflammatory cells (especially neutrophils), and high protein and low glucose concentrations in the CSF.
- Aggressive efforts should be made to identify the causative organism.
  - At a minimum, CSF and blood must be cultured aerobically and anaerobically and a Gram's stain test performed on the CSF sediment.

Treatment and prognosis

Antimicrobial therapy should be guided initially by CSF Gram's stain results and subsequently by bacterial culture and sensitivity tests.

- Table 11-2 lists drug choices and dosages, based on Gram's stain results.
  - Potentiated sulfa drugs are useful as initial treatment when the causative organism is unknown.
  - Ceftiofur may be the antimicrobial of choice for treatment of gram-negative meningitis
- Antimicrobial therapy should be continued for at least 14 days, or at least 7 days after resolution of clinical signs.

Supportive therapy also is important.

- Dehydration is avoided or corrected with oral or IV fluids.
  - Metabolic derangements such as azotemia, hyponatremia, hyposmolality, and hypoglycemia are common and should be identified and corrected.
- Severe hyperthermia is managed with alcohol baths, fans, and cold water enemas.
- Seizure control is as discussed for perinatal hypoxic/ischemic encephalomyelopathy (see p. 258).
- In rapidly deteriorating foals, DMSO (1 g/kg IV as a 10% solution in 5% dextrose) and/or corticosteroids (e.g., dexamethasone 0.05 to 0.1 mg/kg IV) should be considered.

The prognosis is poor. Even with appropriate and intensive treatment, >50% of affected foals die.

Table 11-2
Suggested initial antimicrobial therapy for bacterial meningitis in foals

Gram's stain	Antimicrobial	Dose (per kg)	Interval (hour)
Not available	Potassium penicillin G or	50,000 U	6
	sodium ampicillin	50 mg	6
	plus		
	Gentamicin sulfate or	6.6 mg	24
	amikacin sulfate	21 mg	24
	Trimethoprim-sulfa*	25 mg	12
	Enrofloxacin	5 mg	24
Gram-positive cocci	Potassium penicillin G	50,000 U	6
	Sodium ampicillin	50 mg	6
	Methicillin	25 mg	4
	Ceftiofur	10 mg	6
Gram-negative rods	Sodium ampicillin	50 mg	6
	Trimethoprim-sulfa*	25 mg	12
	Gentamicin sulfate	6.6 mg	24
	Amikacin sulphate	21 mg	24
	Ceftiofur	10 mg	6

*Supplement foal with folinic acid as described in text.

Borreliosis

Clinical signs of Lyme disease, or borreliosis, in horses include chronic weight loss, sporadic lameness, swollen joints, low-grade fever, muscle tenderness, anterior uveitis, and meningoencephalitis (see Chapter 11, Nervous System). Positive polymerase chain reaction (PCR) results from synovial fluid or CSF are considered diagnostic. Oxytetracycline is the drug of choice for borreliosis; third-generation cephalosporins may be useful if neuroborreliosis is suspected.

FUNGAL NEUROLOGIC DISEASE
Cryptococcosis

Cryptococcal meningoencephalomyelitis is caused by *Cryptococcus neoformans,* a saprophytic, yeastlike fungus commonly found in soil and feces. Meningeal and cerebral localization likely occurs after hematogenous or direct spread from a benign or clinical focus in the respiratory tract (nasal cavity, paranasal sinuses, and lungs).

Clinical signs and diagnosis
Signs may be acute or insidious in onset but usually progress slowly.

- The clinical picture is typical of diffuse meningitis, with dementia, blindness, dysphagia, initial hyperesthesia, and rigidity.
  - These signs progress to ataxia, weakness, recumbency, convulsions, coma, and death
- Antemortem diagnosis may be made by the following means:
  - finding the encapsulated organisms in an India ink preparation or routine laboratory stain of CSF sediment
  - positive culture
  - positive latex-agglutination test for cryptococcal antigens in the CSF
- Clinical evidence of a primary cryptococcal infection should be sought, including culture and India ink preparations of any nasal or tracheal exudates.

Treatment
A suggested but unproven regimen for a 450-kg horse is 100 to 150 mg of amphotericin B IV in 4 L of 5% dextrose on alternate days for at least 6 weeks, plus 5 to 15 mg of amphotericin B intrathecally (under anesthesia) once weekly for at least 4 weeks. Possible side effects are nephrotoxicity and neurotoxicity.

PROTOZOAL NEUROLOGIC DISEASE
Equine Protozoal Myeloencephalitis

Equine protozoal myeloencephalitis (EPM) is caused by *Sarcocystis neurona*. The organism is confined to North, Central, and South America; however, cases have been documented all over the world in exported horses, often many months after arrival. Horses of all ages may be affected, but most are 1 to 6 years old at the onset of signs.

Clinical signs

EPM can cause lesions of widely varying size and severity in any part of the CNS and thus can mimic almost any neurologic disease.

- Onset of signs commonly is peracute or acute.
- Gait abnormalities, often interpreted as lameness, may be seen early in the course of disease.
- Ataxia, weakness, recumbency, muscle atrophy, and occasionally behavioral changes are other primary signs.
- Sensory deficits, focal sweating, single-limb paralysis, reflex loss, and cranial nerve dysfunction may also be seen.
- Signs can be symmetric in all limbs, but markedly asymmetric signs are common.

Diagnosis

CSF collection and analysis is key to antemortem diagnosis.

- Occasionally CSF is abnormal, indicating inflammatory disease.
- Western blot detection of antibodies in CSF is highly correlated with histopathologic lesions.
- PCR for *S. neurona* antigens in CSF is quite accurate in confirming a diagnosis of EPM.
- Predictive values of CSF immunotesting can be disappointing in some circumstances (e.g., survey of young stock for presence of disease).

Electromyography can support the diagnosis of EPM, as may response to specific antiprotozoal therapy and worsening of signs with glucocorticoid administration.

Treatment and prognosis

Treatment is based on use of antiprotozoal drugs that inhibit folic acid synthesis.

- Current recommendations include pyrimethamine at 1 mg/kg PO once daily, in combination with sulfadiazine or trimethoprim-sulfadiazine at 20 to 25 mg/kg PO q12h.
- Treatment should be continued until the CSF tests negative by Western blot.
  - An alternative though less successful regimen is to treat for a minimum of 4 weeks beyond complete resolution of signs, or 4 months, whichever is longer.
- Treated horses should be monitored with WBC counts every 2 to 4 weeks; antiprotozoal therapy must be reduced or discontinued if leukopenia develops.
- Other antiprotozoal drugs such as diclazuril may soon be available for use in horses

In severely affected horses with acutely progressive neurologic signs, drugs that decrease inflammation and edema should be given as needed until signs stabilize.

- DMSO may be given once daily at 1 g/kg slow IV in 3 to 4 L of 5% dextrose solution.
- Dexamethasone at 0.05 to 0.1 mg/kg given 1 to 4 times over 24 hours may be helpful in the short term, although prolonged corticosteroid use may favor protozoal proliferation.

PARASITIC NEUROLOGIC DISEASE
Verminous Meningoencephalomyelitis

Verminous meningoencephalomyelitis is an extremely variable clinical entity.

- A spectrum of signs is possible, ranging from a nonprogressive, localized neurologic deficit to rapidly fatal, diffuse encephalitis.
- The disease usually occurs sporadically.
- Anthelmintics may be effective early in the course of disease.
  - *Strongylus vulgaris* migration can be treated with fenbendazole (60 mg/kg PO, repeated in 48 hours).
  - *Hypoderma* spp. (warble or cattle grub) migration can be treated with trichlorfon (40 mg/kg PO, repeated in 1 to 3 days).
  - Avermectins are probably the drug of choice, although it can take a few days for the worms to be killed with these drugs.
- Antiinflammatory therapy with flunixin meglumine (1.1 mg/kg/day IV)

and/or dexamethasone (0.05 to 0.1 mg/kg IV q6h) should begin during the acute phase of the disease.

TOXIC DISEASES
Chemical Intoxications
Important nervous system toxicoses are discussed elsewhere in this chapter. The following syndromes are rare but occasionally have local or regional significance:

* *mercurialism:* Chronic ingestion of contaminated feed causes cerebellar and spinal cord neuronal degeneration, with signs of ataxia, hypermetria, muscle tremors, and coarse head nodding.
* *urea:* Early signs are aimless wandering and incoordination, followed by severe depression, head pressing, convulsions, and death.
* *monensin:* Clinical signs include depression, anorexia, and hind limb incoordination and weakness (see Chapter 8, Cardiovascular System).
* *carbamates and organophosphates:* Toxicity usually results from overzealous application of insecticides, acaricides, or anthelmintics or accidental contamination of food or water.
  * Signs include anxiety, hyperexcitability, colic, frequent urination, sweating, and muscle.
* Tremors that may be generalized.
  * Muscle hyperactivity and stiffness may be followed by weakness, recumbency, and death from respiratory insufficiency.
  * Organophosphate toxicity can be treated with atropine (0.1 mg/kg, half slow IV and half IM) and 2-PAM (20 mg/kg IM).
* *metaldehyde:* Accidental ingestion of slug bait causes generalized sweating, muscle fasciculations and chronic spasms, incoordination, and rapid respiratory and heart rates.
  * Death can occur within 7 hours.
  * Heavy sedation and anticonvulsant therapy are all that can be tried.

Plant Intoxications
The following plants contain neurotoxins of clinical significance in horses.
* *Datura* spp. (thorn apple, jimsonweed), *Atropa belladonna* (deadly

nightshade), and *Dubosia* spp. (corkwoods) are unpalatable but may be inadvertently included in hay or grain.
  * Signs include anorexia, depression, excessive urination and thirst, diarrhea, mydriasis, muscle spasms, and convulsions.
  * Physostigmine is the treatment of choice and should be used to effect.
* *Solanum nigram* (black nightshade) causes colic, ataxia, weakness, tremors, and convulsions; treatment with atropine should be helpful.
* *Oenanthe crocata* (hemlock water drop root), *Circuta* spp. (water hemlock), and *Daucus carota* (wild carrot) grow in wet or swampy areas.
  * Signs of poisoning include salivation, mydriasis, colic, delirium, and convulsions.
* *Laburnum anagyroides* (laburnum) is very toxic to horses; it causes excitement, incoordination, sweating, convulsions, and death.
* Ingestion of hay heavily contaminated with *Lathyrus hissolia* (grass vetchling) can cause severe attacks of ataxia provoked by moving or handling of affected animals.
  * Recovery follows removal of the contaminated feed.
  * Peripheral neuropathy has also been associated with *Lathyrus* spp. ingestion; the most prominent signs are laryngeal paresis and a stringhalt type of gait.
* *Robinia pseudoacacia* (false acacia, black locust tree) causes anorexia, depression, weakness, and paralysis when horses eat the bark or sapling sprouts.
* *Eupatorium rugosum* (white snakeroot) and *Aplopappus heterophyllus* (rayless goldenrod) cause "trembles" in horses, sheep, and cattle.
  * White snakeroot grows in moist areas around ditches and streams in the midwestern and eastern United States; rayless goldenrod is primarily found in the southwestern United States.
  * After ingestion of these plants for several days, horses exhibit depression, weakness, tremors, and dysphagia; labored breathing and urinary incontinence also are seen.

- Recovery occurs gradually after removal of horses from the offending plants.
- *Descurainia pinnata* (tansy mustard) can cause blindness and tongue paralysis.
- *Stipita robusta* (sleepy grass) is a tall perennial needlegrass found in Colorado, New Mexico, and Texas.
  - Signs range from mild stupor to recumbency and deep sleep; a catatonic syndrome may be seen in which severely affected horses are "frozen" in unusual positions.
  - Recovery occurs over several days.
- *Cycas circinalis* (cycad) nuts cause ataxia and spinal cord degeneration when fed to horses.

Snakebite and Tick Paralysis
Snakebite
The venom of elapine snakes is mainly neurotoxic, with minimal local effects. This group includes cobras, mambas, and coral snakes of India, Africa, Asia, and Central and South America, and the tiger snake, brown snake, and death adder of Australia. Horses bitten by elapine snakes pass through an initial period of excitement and hyperesthesia, followed by generalized weakness manifested as depression, mydriasis, dysphagia, and tremors. Treatment with specific antivenin is effective.

Tick paralysis
Ixodes holocyclus ticks can cause generalized flaccid paralysis in foals, resembling botulism. Recovery quickly follows removal of the offending tick(s). The ear tick, *Otobius megnini,* has been associated with severe muscle cramping, intermittent prolapse of the third eyelid, sweating, pawing, and muscle fasciculations. Signs recur until the ticks are removed.

IDIOPATHIC DISEASES
Perinatal Hypoxic/Ischemic Encephalomyelopathy (Neonatal Maladjustment Syndrome)
Neonatal maladjustment syndrome is a noninfectious syndrome of cerebral signs in newborn foals. It results from hypoxic and ischemic events occurring around the time of delivery:

- Category 1 foals are normal at birth, with onset of clinical signs 6 to 24 hours later.
- Category 2 foals often have a history of an abnormal delivery and/or exhibit abnormal behavior immediately after birth; they have a much poorer prognosis.

Clinical findings
Signs are abrupt in onset and referable to diffuse cerebrocortical impairment.

- Sudden stiff, jerky movements of the head and body progress to extensor spasms of the neck, limbs, and tail.
- Often there is complete loss of the sucking reflex.
- If able to stand, the foal may wander aimlessly, oblivious to its surroundings.
- Hyperexcitability, teeth grinding, lip retraction, exaggerated chewing/sucking movements or "gulping" of air, and abnormal vocalization ("barking") have also been noted.
  - Many of these signs are caused by partial or mild generalized seizures.
- The rate of progression varies, but affected foals often become recumbent and semicomatose, with clonic convulsions.
  - Close observation may reveal constricted or dilated, asymmetric pupils, and there may be abnormal respiratory patterns and sounds.
- Unless there is concurrent sepsis, the hemogram is relatively normal.

Treatment and prognosis
Management is aimed at maintaining the foal's body temperature, hydration, caloric intake, electrolyte and acid-base balance, and blood glucose concentration (see Chapter 6, Neonatal Evaluation and Management). If needed, oxygen may be provided by nasal insufflation. The adequacy of passive transfer of immunity also should be assessed. Other specific measures include:

- avoiding unnecessary stimuli, such as bright lights and loud noises
- seizure control as necessary
  - Mild partial or generalized convulsions can be controlled with light manual restraint.
  - If convulsions are severe enough to cause recumbency, hyperthermia, or distress, immediate

control can be provided with 5 to 10 mg diazepam IV as needed.
- For long-term control, phenobarbital can initially be administered at 10 to 20 mg/kg IV, diluted in saline and given over 15 to 20 minutes, followed by 5 to 10 mg/kg IV or PO q12h.
- Phenytoin at 5 to 10 mg/kg IV followed by maintenance doses of 1 to 5 mg/kg q6-12h may control seizures; phenobarbital should be tried first.
- DMSO (0.5 to 1 g/kg IV in 1 L of 5% dextrose)

With reasonable care, at least 80% of category 1 foals without signs of sepsis recover over several hours to several weeks.

Diseases of the Forebrain *(pages 904-913)*

Caroline N. Hahn, I. G. (Joe) Mayhew, and Robert J. MacKay

DIAGNOSTIC AND THERAPEUTIC CONSIDERATIONS

The hallmarks of disorders of the cerebral hemispheres include behavioral changes, altered states of consciousness, central blindness, and seizures.
- Failure to recognize familiar companions, continual yawning, facial twitches (partial seizures), and drifting to one side when blindfolded may be indicative of a subtle lesion.
- Circling toward the affected side, depression, head pressing, and generalized seizures indicate more severe disease.

Seizures

Generalized seizures reflect diffuse cerebral disturbance. Continual seizures (status epilepticus) should be controlled with α_2-agonists or sodium pentobarbital before proceeding with further evaluation (Table 11-3). Diazepam often is effective for short-term control of seizures.

CONGENITAL AND FAMILIAL DISEASES
Hydrocephalus

Hydrocephalus is rare in horses. It has a wide variety of causes, both congenital and acquired; an inherited defect has been proposed in some cases. Neonates with hypertensive obstructive hydrocephalus have an enlarged calvarium with open sutures. However, normal neonatal foals, especially premature and Arabian foals, also have domed foreheads. CNS signs include lack of affinity for the dam and reduced or absent desire or ability to nurse. If signs progress, the foal may

---

Table 11-3
Drugs used to treat seizure disorders in horses*

	Drug	50-kg Foal	500-kg Horse
Initial therapy	Diazepam†	5-20 mg IV per dose	25-100 mg IV per dose
	Pentobarbital	150-100 mg IV to effect	To effect
	Phenobarbital	250-1000 mg slowly IV	2000-mg doses
	Phenytoin	200-1000 mg IV per dose	
	Xylazine	25-50 mg IV per dose	300-500 mg IV per dose
	Detomidine	0.5-4 mg IV	5-40 mg IV
	Romifidine	2-5 mg IV	20-50 mg IV
Maintenance	Phenobarbital	100-500 mg PO bid	1-3 g PO, bid
	Potassium bromide	1-2 g PO sid	5-14 g PO sid

*Although these drugs have been used with success, several are not licensed for use in horses. These doses should be regarded as guidelines only, and drugs should be given to effect. Smaller doses may be equally effective. It is most appropriate to monitor blood concentrations of all anticonvulsant drugs during maintenance therapy.
†Do not leave in plastic container or syringe for more than a few minutes or drug may become inactivated.

develop blindness and profound depression. Specific medical or surgical treatment is not recommended.

DISEASES WITH PHYSICAL CAUSES
Cerebral Trauma
Signs referable to cerebral damage most frequently occur after trauma to the frontal or parietal regions of the head.

- There may be an initial period of unconsciousness of minutes or hours.
- Subsequent neurologic signs tend to vary with the degree of intracranial pressure.
  - Signs typically include depression, circling toward the side of the damaged cerebral hemisphere, blindness, and sometimes decreased facial sensation contralaterally.
  - There may be asymmetry and fluctuation of pupil size, with a tendency toward miosis.
  - Apart from depressed menace responses and lingual paresis, all other cranial nerve responses should be intact.
  - Gait abnormalities suggest progressive involvement of other parts of the brain.
  - Seizures indicate a forebrain lesion.
- Severe swelling of the cerebral hemispheres can result in herniation against the midbrain, causing dilated, unresponsive pupils and tetraparesis; this is a serious sign.

Treatment and prognosis
Initial management of cerebral trauma is supportive, with the main objective of reducing or minimizing brain swelling.

- Seizures may be controlled with 5 mg (foal) to 100 mg (adult) of diazepam as necessary.
  - Intractable seizures or unmanageable thrashing may require sedative or anesthetic doses of thiamylal sodium or sodium pentobarbital (see Table 11-3).
  - α_2-Agonists must be used cautiously, because they may exacerbate CNS hemorrhage.
- Dexamethasone (or equivalent) at 0.1 to 0.25 mg/kg should be given

within 6 hours of the traumatic incident and may be repeated every 4 to 6 hours for 1 to 4 days.
- Furosemide and other renal diuretics may be useful in conjunction.
- Horses presented in a coma or semicoma may be given DMSO 1 g/kg as a 10% solution in 5% dextrose as a slow IV infusion, repeated every 12 to 24 hours for up to 4 days.
  - Mannitol (0.25 mg/kg as a 20% solution by slow IV infusion q6-12h for up to 24 hours) may be used; theoretically it can exacerbate intracranial (especially subdural) bleeding.
- Recumbent horses should be rolled often to minimize ventilation-perfusion abnormalities.
  - Humidified 100% O_2 may be given via nasal tube or mask.
  - If possible, the horse's head should be kept at heart base level or higher.
- Other supportive care includes maintenance of hydration and correction of electrolyte and acid-base abnormalities.

Constant reevaluation is necessary to assess response to treatment. If there is improvement within 6 to 8 hours, treatment should be repeated. If there is deterioration or no improvement, more aggressive medical therapy or surgical intervention, such as exploratory craniotomy and decompressive procedures, should be considered. If a comatose patient does not improve or continues to deteriorate for 36 hours after injury or surgery, euthanasia usually is indicated.

Intracarotid Injection
A violent reaction typically occurs within 5 to 30 seconds of intracarotid injection.

- Initial signs range from apprehension with a wide-eyed expression and sudden facial twitching, head shaking, kicking, and running, to recumbency and loss of consciousness.
  - Marked cardiovascular changes, such as bradycardia, arrhythmias, and blood pressure fluctuations, may accompany CNS signs.
- With xylazine, detomidine, butorphanol, acepromazine, and other

water-soluble drugs, horses usually regain consciousness within an hour and completely recover within a week.

- Consistent findings during recovery are decreased facial (nasal septum) sensation, blindness, and deficient menace response, all contralateral to the injection side.
- Intracarotid injection of procaine penicillin, phenylbutazone, and other oil-based or insoluble drugs warrants a much worse prognosis.
  - Intractable seizures, coma, or stupor often necessitate euthanasia in such cases.

Treatment

Treatment is largely symptomatic and includes:

- use of protective padding and sedation
- dexamethasone, DMSO, and anticonvulsant therapy
  - Mannitol may be contraindicated.
- atropine (0.04 mg/kg IV) for severe bradycardia and arrhythmias from rapid injection of α_2-agonists.

INFLAMMATORY, INFECTIOUS, AND IMMUNE DISEASES
Cerebral Abscess

Cerebral abscesses are rare in horses and are most commonly associated with epizootics of *Streptococcus equi* infection (strangles).

Clinical signs

Onset of neurologic signs may be acute or insidious, and the clinical course often is characterized by marked fluctuations in the severity of signs.

- Consistent early signs are contralateral blindness, deficient menace response, and decreased facial (especially nasal septal) sensation.
- Most obvious are behavioral changes such as depression, head-pressing, aimless wandering, and sudden, unprovoked excitement.
- Affected horses may circle or stand with the head and neck toward the affected side.
- Later there may be signs of brainstem compression, such as asymmetric pupils, ataxia, and weakness.
- Signs can progress to episodes of unconsciousness, recumbency, and seizures.

Diagnosis

Diagnosis is largely based on a history of prior strangles infection and the clinical signs.

- Other possible causes of asymmetric cerebral disease include protozoal myeloencephalitis, trauma, aberrant parasite migration, parasitic thromboembolism, and cholesterol granuloma.
- CSF changes depend on the degree of meningeal or ependymal involvement.
  - Xanthochromia and moderate elevation in protein content are common.
  - Elevations in inflammatory cells (particularly neutrophils) are found only when there is associated diffuse meningitis or ependymitis.

Treatment and prognosis

If signs are acute, severe, and rapidly progressive, corticosteroids should be given until the signs stabilize. Otherwise, therapy is based on prolonged use of large doses of antimicrobial drugs.

- For a cerebral abscess caused by *S. equi,* potassium or sodium penicillin can be given at 25,000 to 100,000 IU/kg IV q6h for 1 to 2 weeks, followed by procaine penicillin 22,000 IU/kg IM q12h for at least 4 weeks.
  - Addition of rifampin (5 to 10 mg/kg/day PO) is worth considering.
- Results in horses have been poor; an alternative approach is surgical evacuation of the lesion after localization by computed tomography or intraoperative ultrasonography.

Recovered horses may have residual deficits, such as impaired vision and decreased facial sensation contralaterally.

METABOLIC DISEASES
Hepatoencephalopathy

Hepatoencephalopathy is characterized by abnormal mentation in horses with severe hepatic insufficiency. The more common causes of liver failure are pyrrolizidine intoxication, hyperlipemia in ponies and donkeys, acute hepatic necrosis (Theiler's disease), and *Bacillus piliformis* hepatitis (Tyzzer's disease) in foals. Liver disease is discussed in Chapter 10, Alimentary System.

Clinical signs and diagnosis

Signs of hepatoencephalopathy are referable to diffuse cerebral impairment.

* Depression and inappetence typically are the first signs, although there can be an abrupt onset of abnormal behavior.
  * Affected horses may stand for hours with their heads hanging, periodically jerking the head upward for no discernible reason.
  * There is repeated yawning, grimacing, or twitching of the muzzle and lips.
* Somnolent periods, marked by head pressing or leaning against a wall, may alternate with periods of compulsive walking, during which the horse is oblivious to its surroundings.
* As the disease progresses, diminished menace responses, visual impairment, and upper respiratory stridor caused by laryngeal paralysis are common.
* Generalized seizures and coma occur terminally.
* The diagnosis usually is suspected from the history and clinical signs and can be confirmed by laboratory findings indicative of liver failure.

Treatment and prognosis

The prognosis is poor to hopeless. Usually there is irreparable liver damage at the time of onset of CNS signs. Nevertheless, occasional recoveries are recorded. Treatment generally is supportive.

* Hypoglycemia should be corrected with IV glucose.
* It may be worth minimizing gut absorption of protein breakdown products by giving mineral oil or oral neomycin (10 g/450-kg horse q6h).
  * Metronidazole (15 to 20 mg/kg PO q12h) could be considered in conjunction.
  * Lactulose and sorbitol are used in humans and small animals.
* If the horse survives, it should be fed a palatable diet that is low in protein and high in carbohydrates (e.g., grass hay with citrus or beet pulp and milk products such as yogurt).

Hypoglycemia

Blood glucose levels of <40 to 50 mg/dL (<2 to 2.5 mmol/L) can result in weakness, depression, and ataxia; signs may progress to loss of consciousness. Seizures associated with hypoglycemia are uncommon in adult horses but sometimes occur in foals. Hypoglycemia is encountered most often in neonates, usually as a complication of sepsis or prematurity (see Chapter 6, Neonatal Evaluation and Management). Horses with end-stage liver failure or Addison's syndrome also may have blood glucose levels of <40 mg/dL (<2.0 mmol/L) after withdrawal of corticosteroids.

Leukoencephalomalacia

Contamination of feed, particularly corn products, by *Fusarium* spp. fungi is the usual cause of leukoencephalomalacia (moldy corn poisoning). These fungi produce fumonisin toxins, which are hepatotoxic and neurotoxic. Cool, humid conditions favor growth of *Fusarium* spp., so most cases of leukoencephalomalacia occur from late fall to early spring.

Clinical signs and diagnosis

Toxicosis frequently has components of both leukoencephalomalacia and hepatic necrosis, with the relative importance of brain or liver lesions depending on the dosage and duration of intake. Signs of leukoencephalomalacia are seen acutely 2 to 24 weeks (average 3 weeks) after initial ingestion of moldy corn.

* Initial signs include depression, unresponsiveness, head pressing, circling, aimless wandering, blindness, and, occasionally, unprovoked excitement and frenzy.
  * Signs frequently are asymmetric.
* Further progression may be associated with pharyngeal paralysis, incoordination, and, finally, recumbency, paddling, coma, and death.
* It is usually fatal, with overall mortality rates in outbreaks varying from 40% to 84%.
* The clinical course usually is 1 to a few days but is much longer in horses that recover.
* Affected horses usually are afebrile, which helps distinguish this disease from arboviral encephalomyelitides (EEE, WEE, VEE).

- Results of CSF analysis may be normal but can include neutrophilic pleocytosis.
- Gross necropsy lesions usually are diagnostic and consist of focal areas of liquifactive hemorrhagic.
- Necrosis in the white matter of one or both cerebral hemispheres.

Treatment

Treatment is only supportive.

- Contaminated feed should be removed and an effort made to eliminate toxin already in the alimentary tract by use of laxatives and activated charcoal.
- Corticosteroids and nonsteroidal antiinflammatory drugs (NSAIDs) probably should be given.
- Anticonvulsant therapy is indicated to control seizure activity.

NEOPLASIA

Neoplasms of the nervous system are rare in horses. Lymphosarcoma is the most common secondary neoplasm affecting the nervous system. Melanomas occasionally invade the CNS of gray horses.

MULTIFACTORIAL DISEASES

Juvenile Epilepsy

This condition occurs in otherwise normal foals from several weeks to several months of age. It is more common in Arabians. Seizures begin without warning and recur for days or weeks.

- Mild generalized seizures with lip retraction, jaw-clamping movements, and sudden, deranged physical activity may progress to severe generalized seizures with loss of consciousness, opisthotonus, abnormal head and eye movements, and clonic convulsions.
- Affected foals typically pitch forward during an attack and traumatize the mucosae of their retracted lips; this finding can be a useful diagnostic aid.
- Asymmetric localizing signs are indicative of acquired rather than juvenile epilepsy.
- Usually seizures abate with or without treatment, although status epilepticus can ensue.

Treatment

Affected foals usually "grow out of" juvenile epilepsy without treatment, but anticonvulsant therapy should be instituted at the first signs and maintained for several weeks (see Table 11-3). Any underlying problem that may initiate seizure activity (e.g., fever) should be corrected. Postictal blindness may last up to a week in young foals.

Acquired Epilepsy

Epilepsy in adult horses is assumed to be acquired. An epileptogenic site (or sites) may become active after the horse has recovered from a cerebral insult, but the interval between brain disease and onset of seizure activity often is months or years. In some horses, there is no history of brain damage or evidence of current disease; these cases are referred to as idiopathic epilepsy.

Clinical signs

Seizures can occur without warning or may be preceded by a transient change in the horse's behavior (e.g., apprehension, vocalization).

- Similar changes are likely before each attack.
- Seizures may be partial, with signs localizing the lesion to one side, such as unilateral facial or limb twitching, or they may be generalized.
  - Partial seizures may progress to generalized seizures.
- Seizures generally last no more than a minute, and in the case of generalized seizures the animal regains its feet within several minutes.
- Transient postictal signs range from slight depression to stupor and blindness, usually lasting a few hours.

Treatment

Diseases causing seizures or seizurelike signs must be ruled out by a proper diagnostic workup. Management depends on the severity of the seizures.

- If seizures are mild, infrequent, or declining in frequency, no treatment may be necessary.
- Activities that induce seizures (e.g., feeding, changes in lighting) should be avoided or modified.

- With estrus-associated seizures, progesterone treatment or ovariectomy may be palliative.
- When epileptic seizures cannot be avoided by management changes or are severe or frequent, antiepileptic treatment may be instituted in deference to euthanasia (see Table 11-3).
  - After at least 3 months without attacks, the drug dose can be reduced gradually over another 3 months, with increases as necessary if seizures recur.

It generally is recommended that the horse not be ridden until it has been seizure-free, without anticonvulsant medication, for 6 months.

IDIOPATHIC DISEASES
Cholesterol Granuloma

Cholesterol granulomas (cholesteatomas) are found in the choroid plexuses of 15% to 20% of old horses. Most of these masses remain clinically silent, but some grow large enough to compress the brain tissue.

- Clinical signs typically are insidious in onset.
- Signs may be intermittent but usually are progressive, asymmetric, and referable to impaired cerebral cortical function.
  - Altered behavior, depression, somnolence and reluctance to move, generalized seizures, ataxia, weakness, and unconsciousness have been reported.
- Xanthochromia and elevated protein content usually are found on CSF analysis.
- Temporary improvement may be expected with corticosteroid treatment.

Behavioral Problems

(pages 914-931)

M.D. Marsden

Stereotypes and other behavioral abnormalities are well covered in *Equine Medicine and Surgery V*. The rationale for specific husbandry changes and indications for various drug therapies are discussed in detail.

Diseases of the Brainstem and Cranial Nerves (Autonomic and Somatic) *(pages 931-941)*

Caroline N. Hahn, I. G. (Joe) Mayhew, and Robert J. MacKay

Disorders of the brainstem can produce a range of clinical signs, from severe depression and ataxia to disturbances of homeostasis and dysfunction of specific cranial nerves.

DISEASES WITH PHYSICAL CAUSES
Brainstem and Temporal Bone Trauma

Injury to the brainstem usually is associated with trauma to the poll caused by rearing and hitting the head or falling over backward to strike the head on the ground. Three neurologic syndromes may result, either alone or in combination: optic nerve injury, midbrain syndrome, and the most frequent, medullary/inner ear syndrome.

Optic nerve injury

Stretching or shearing of the optic nerve results in sudden onset of blindness in one or both eyes. Pupillary dilation and suppressed menace responses are immediately apparent, and generalized retinal degeneration and optic nerve atrophy develop within 2 to 6 weeks. Posttraumatic optic nerve atrophy, which may complicate any head injury case, is irreversible.

Midbrain syndrome

Closed head injuries (i.e., without skull fracture) can result in midbrain compression from hemorrhage and edema. Profound neurologic signs and a poor prognosis accompany such injuries.

- Marked depression follows an initial period of coma; ambulatory horses have ataxia and weakness
- Extensive midbrain injury causes recumbency and "decerebrate" posturing with generalized extensor rigidity.
- Affected horses may have vision, but pupillary light responses are sluggish or absent.

- The pupils may be "pinpoint-sized" and fluctuant or dilated and fixed.
- Progression from miosis to bilaterally dilated, unresponsive pupils in a recumbent patient is a grave sign.
- Strabismus and abnormal vestibular nystagmus also may be seen.
- Bizarre respiratory patterns, cardiac arrhythmias, and bradycardia may occur with severe midbrain lesions.

Medullary/inner ear syndrome

Trauma to the back of the head may cause hemorrhage around the medulla and/or into the middle/inner ear. Preexisting osteochondroarthrosis and ankylosis of the temporohyoid joint(s) predispose to fractures of the hyoid bone and the osseous bulla and adjacent petrous temporal bone. The resulting neurologic signs often are asymmetric and quite variable.

- Hemorrhage into the middle and inner ear cavities causes vestibular and facial nerve signs, such as head tilt, circling, and leaning toward the affected side; ipsilateral facial paralysis; and spontaneous horizontal or rotary nystagmus.
  - Vestibular nystagmus may be abnormal or absent.
  - Bleeding may extend into the external ear and guttural pouch.
- Hemorrhage in or around the medulla and into the CSF causes additional signs, such as depression, ataxia, weakness, recumbency, and other vestibular and cranial nerve signs.
- Horses with acute vestibular signs often thrash and struggle violently in an effort to stand.

In horses exhibiting inner ear syndrome without medullary involvement, the prognosis is fair for complete recovery. With associated skull fractures, the outlook is guarded to hopeless.

Treatment

Supportive and medical treatment is as described above for treatment of cerebral trauma. Mannitol and other hypertonic solutions should be used cautiously because they can exacerbate intracranial bleeding.

Facial Nerve Trauma

Proximal facial nerve trauma usually is caused by fractures of the petrous temporal bone (after a blow to the head), the stylohyoid bone (usually as a consequence of temporohyoid osteoarthropathy), or the ramus of the mandible. Hemorrhage into the middle/inner ear, otitis media/interna, guttural pouch mycosis, and parotid lymph node abscessation can also involve the adjacent facial nerve. Distal facial nerve damage usually is due to direct injury from a blow or lateral recumbency, often as the nerve crosses the mandible and/or zygomatic arch.

Clinical signs

Injury to the facial nerve proximal to the ramus of the mandible causes full facial paresis.

- Complete unilateral facial paralysis is evident as deviation of the nose toward the normal side, reduced flaring of the ipsilateral nostril during inspiration, and ipsilateral drooping of the lip, eyelid, and ear.
  - Lip, eyelid, corneal, menace, and ear reflexes are reduced or absent; facial sensation remains intact.
  - Bilateral facial nerve paralysis causes dysphagia, evident as dropping of feed and accumulation of feed between the teeth and cheeks.
  - Chronic facial nerve paralysis causes muscle atrophy and fibrous contracture of the face.
- Damage within the facial canal often is associated with concurrent signs of vestibular nerve damage, such as head tilt, nystagmus, and circling.

Distal facial paresis usually involves only the nose and lips.

Prognosis

There is a fair chance of recovery with facial nerve deficits caused by trauma to the caudal aspect of the head. In the absence of severe skin laceration, the prognosis for distal facial paralysis is good, although recovery takes from several days to several months.

INFLAMMATORY, INFECTIOUS, AND IMMUNE DISEASES

Tetanus

Tetanus is a highly fatal, infectious disease caused by the toxin of

Clostridium tetani, a gram-positive, anaerobic, spore-forming bacillus. The disease causes muscular rigidity, hyperesthesia, and convulsions. Average case mortality is 75%. The most common route of infection is by wound contamination with *C. tetani* spores, especially puncture wounds and wounds with considerable necrosis, impaired blood supply, foreign bodies, or pyogenic bacterial infection. But any break in the skin or mucous membranes is a potential portal of entry for *C. tetani*. The incubation period usually is 1 to 3 weeks but may range from several days to several months.

Clinical signs

The severity and rate of progression of clinical signs depend on the dose of toxin and the size, age, and immune status of the affected animal.

- In many cases, a slightly stiff gait is the initial sign; some horses are reluctant to feed off the ground because of spasm of cervical muscles.
  - Overreaction to normal external stimuli is another early sign.
- Facial muscle spasms result in an anxious expression with retracted lips, flared nostrils, and erect ears; retraction of the eyeball results in prolapse of the nictitating membranes.
  - Spasm of the muscles of mastication may cause difficulty in eating ("lockjaw").
  - External stimuli, particularly a hand clap or tap on the forehead, or attempts at eating, often provoke further spasms of cervical, facial, masticatory, and extraocular muscles.
- Other muscles are progressively affected, causing a stiff, stilted gait with rigid extension of the neck, limbs, and tail ("sawhorse" stance).
  - Spastic paralysis of pharyngeal muscles sometimes results in regurgitation or aspiration of food, and inability to posture appropriately causes retention of urine and feces.
- Once an affected horse falls, it generally is unable to regain its feet.
  - In lateral recumbency, increased extensor tonus results in rigid extension of the extremities,

neck (opisthotonus), and back (lordosis).
- Even slight stimulation can cause prolonged generalized muscle spasms.

Death usually occurs after 5 to 7 days and is often caused by asphyxia that is due to spastic paralysis of respiratory muscles, laryngospasm, or aspiration pneumonia. In surviving horses, signs usually stabilize after about a week.

Treatment

Treatment generally is symptomatic and supportive, with particular emphasis on good nursing care. The main objectives of therapy are:

1. **Destruction of C. tetani organisms**
- Wound debridement, lavage, and large doses of penicillin are recommended.
  - Potassium penicillin G at up to 50,000 IU/kg q6h is recommended for the first 2 to 4 days.

2. **Neutralization of unbound toxin**
- Tetanus antitoxin (TAT) may be given IV, IM, or SC.
  - IV or IM dosages of 5000 to 10,000 IU probably are adequate to neutralize circulating toxin. in most cases, although most often larger doses are used
- Intrathecal (subarachnoid) administration of TAT may halt disease progression and improve survival rates if performed early (i.e., before recumbency); this is unproved.
  - 1000 to 5000 IU of homologous TAT are given at the cisternal or lumbosacral site after slow removal of an equivalent volume of CSF.
  - Seizures may result from this procedure.
- Tetanus toxoid should also be administered (at a separate site) because protective humoral immunity is not induced by natural disease.

3. **Control of muscle spasms**
- The horse should be kept in a quiet, dark environment and cotton plugs inserted into the ears.
- IV promazine (0.5 to 1.0 mg/kg q4-6h), chlorpromazine (0.4 to 0.8 mg/kg q4-6h), and acepromazine (0.05 to 0.1 mg/kg q4-6h) each provide effective muscle relaxation and sedation while allowing the horse to remain standing.

* Glycerol guaiacolate, with careful titration of its effects by slow IV drip, can produce adequate relaxation without recumbency.
* Methocarbamol (10 to 20 mg/kg IV q8h) relieves muscular pain and rigidity in mild cases and can be safely used in combination with a variety of sedatives.
* Diazepam (50 to 200 mg IV q4-6h) can be used alone or in combination with α_2-agonists (the dose of diazepam is reduced accordingly).

4. *General nutrient and metabolic support and good nursing care*

* Animals that can eat should be fed and watered from containers placed off the ground.
  * Dysphagic horses can be fed through an indwelling nasoesophageal tube or surgically created esophageal fistula.
* An indwelling IV catheter should be placed and used for all appropriate injections.
* Serum electrolyte concentrations and the hemogram should be monitored regularly and any abnormalities corrected.
* Infections such as aspiration pneumonia and cystitis must be treated vigorously.
* Manual rectal evacuation and bladder catheterization may be necessary.

Complete paralysis with curariform drugs and total respiratory and nutritional support may be considered for valuable foals.

Prognosis

Horses presented in lateral recumbency have very little chance of recovery; euthanasia should be considered. Recovery in horses that survive is gradual, taking at least 6 weeks in most cases, and usually is complete. Recovered animals are not protected from further episodes of tetanus.

Prophylaxis

Active immunization against tetanus is reliably achieved with commercial toxoids.

* The usual recommendation in adult horses is two injections 3 to 4 weeks apart, followed by annual revaccination, with boosters after lacerations or other tetanus-prone wounds.

* Tetanus antitoxin is widely used in unvaccinated horses after injury; however, acute fatal hepatic necrosis (Theiler's disease) has rarely developed 1 to 3 months after administration.
* All foals of mares unvaccinated in the last 30 days of gestation, and foals that have not acquired sufficient antibodies from colostrum should receive tetanus antitoxin at birth.
  * Tetanus *toxoid* should be given at 3, 4, and 6 months of age and then annually.

Guttural Pouch Diseases

Diseases of the guttural pouches are discussed in Chapter 9, Respiratory System. The following is a list, in approximate order of importance, of the significant neurologic abnormalities that may be associated with guttural pouch mycosis.

* dysphagia, ranging from occasional coughing during eating to regurgitation of feed, water, and saliva through both nostrils (damage to cranial nerves IX and X)
  * Inhalation pneumonia is a common complication in severely dysphagic horses.
* abnormal respiratory noises caused by soft palate paresis and displacement (IX, X) and/or laryngeal paresis (X)
* Horner's syndrome (sympathetic trunk and cranial cervical ganglion)
* facial paralysis (VII)
* lingual paresis or hemiplegia (XII)

Persistent dysphagia associated with guttural pouch mycosis warrants a guarded to poor prognosis. Complete recovery is possible but uncommon, although many horses can survive with persistent low-grade dysphagia. Other signs (e.g., laryngeal hemiplegia, facial paralysis, Horner's syndrome) are unlikely to improve.

TOXIC DISEASES

Nigropallidal Encephalomalacia

Prolonged ingestion of yellow star thistle *(Centaurea solstitialis)* or Russian knapweed *(Acroptilon cepens)* produces this neurologic syndrome in horses. Yellow star thistle poisoning has been reported in California, southern Oregon, Argentina, and Australia. Russian knapweed poisoning has occurred in western Colorado, eastern Utah, and eastern Washington.

Clinical signs

Signs are peracute in onset and reflect bilateral dystonia of the muscles of prehension and mastication:

- Affected animals hold the mouth partly open, with the lips retracted and the tongue partially protruded, resulting in a peculiar "wooden" expression.
  - There frequently is tremor of involved muscles.
- Despite a normal appetite, most affected horses are unable to move food back to the pharynx to be swallowed; weight loss and debility quickly follow.
  - Many affected horses can drink water by totally immersing their muzzles.
- Behavioral abnormalities, such as circling, depression, yawning, or frenzied activity, are common during the first few days but can be seen at any time.
- Usually the gait is normal, though at rest the limbs may be placed in inappropriate postures.

Treatment and prognosis

There is no effective treatment; most affected horses are euthanized or die. Mildly affected horses sometimes can accommodate sufficiently to eat pelleted complete feeds or grain.

Lead Poisoning

Chronic lead poisoning causes peripheral neuropathy, apparent as pharyngeal and laryngeal paralysis, with dysphagia, abnormal respiratory noises ("roaring"), and inhalation pneumonia. In most reports, affected horses live within the fallout or "smoke" zone of metal mining or smelting industries and are poisoned by eating pasture or hay contaminated by aerial fallout of lead.

Clinical findings

The earliest signs may be an abnormal inspiratory noise during exercise or coughing during feeding, with persistent "choke" and reflux of food through the nostrils.

- Pneumonia often occurs as a result of food inhalation.
- Other signs include dysmetria of the lips and tongue, facial paralysis, limb weakness and ataxia, and paralysis of the anal sphincter.
  - Anorexia, depression, weight loss, and a poor hair coat soon follow.
- Other variable signs include transient colic, lameness, protein-losing nephropathy with ventral edema, and a blue "lead line" along the gingival margins of the teeth.
- Anemia is common and occasionally is accompanied by immature RBCs and basophilic stippling.

Diagnosis

Diagnosis usually is based on the history and clinical signs, but lead assays of blood and urine may be diagnostic.

- Because 90% of lead in blood is bound to RBCs, blood lead levels in anemic or hemoconcentrated animals should be interpreted cautiously.
- Tissue levels of lead are consistently elevated in horses with chronic lead poisoning; the best tissues for analysis are bone, liver, and kidney.

Treatment

Chelation of the lead in soft tissues with calcium versenate appears to be most effective:

- 2% Ca-versenate is given at 50 to 100 mg/kg as a slow IV drip daily for 3 days
- Treatment is repeated after an interval of 4 days.
- Concurrent use of acidifying agents may promote resorption of lead from bone.

MULTIFACTORIAL DISEASES
Sleep Disorders (Narcolepsy-Cataplexy)

Narcolepsy is characterized by excessive daytime sleepiness and pathologic manifestations of rapid eye movement (REM) sleep. Cataplexy is a REM sleep abnormality in which the patient has episodes of muscle weakness with full consciousness. There appear to be two different syndromes of narcolepsy-cataplexy:

- a persistent form affecting horses of many breeds, and possibly familial

in some Miniature Horses and Suffolk, Shetland, and Fell ponies
* a fairly common and transient condition affecting foals and yearlings
  * Light horse breeds are most often affected.
  * Usually, affected foals have only one or a few episodes and then "grow out of it."

Clinical signs

Signs range from drowsiness with hanging of the head and buckling at the knees to sudden and total collapse and may vary from one attack every few weeks to more than 10 a day:
* When forced to walk, affected horses may appear uncoordinated.
* Some form of stimulation, such as grooming or petting, washing with a hose, or leading the horse out of a stall, often precedes an attack.
* Between attacks there is no neurologic abnormality.
* The condition usually does not worsen, though some aged mares have relentless progression of signs to the point of frequent and abrupt periods of collapse.

Diagnosis and treatment

Attacks can be induced with physostigmine (0.06 to 0.08 mg/kg IV), although lack of a positive response does not rule out a diagnosis of narcolepsy, and side effects, particularly diarrhea and colic, frequently accompany its use. Atropine (0.08 mg/kg IV) resolves signs of narcolepsy-cataplexy for up to 30 hours. For longer-term control, imipramine (1 to 2 mg/kg IV or IM q8-12h) may be useful. Signs are relieved for 5 to 10 hours without side effects.

IDIOPATHIC DISEASES

Temporohyoid Osteoarthropathy

Temporohyoid osteoarthropathy can result from otitis media/interna (see p. 270). Extension of the proliferative process can cause signs of peripheral vestibular and facial nerve disease. Sudden mechanical force applied to this ankylosed joint may result in bony fractures, usually through the petrous part of the temporal bone, often causing further damage to the vestibular and facial nerves. Other cranial nerves, especially IX and X, or adjacent areas of the medulla also may be affected, causing additional neurologic abnormalities, such as dysphagia and depression. Infection of the fracture site may lead to secondary otitis media/interna and leptomeningitis.

Diseases of Vestibular and Cerebellar Structures *(pages 941-945)*

Caroline N. Hahn, I. G. (Joe) Mayhew, and Robert J. MacKay

The function of the vestibular system is to maintain appropriate orientation of the trunk, limbs, and eyes with respect to the position and movements of the head. Therefore vestibular disease results in disturbed equilibrium and ataxia, usually without paresis. Vestibular disorders tend to be unilateral or asymmetric and are caused by either peripheral or central lesions.

CONGENITAL AND FAMILIAL DISEASES

Cerebellar Hypoplasia

Congenital or hereditary malformation/hypoplasia of the cerebellum is extremely rare in horses. Cerebellar syndromes and degenerative lesions have been reported in newborn Thoroughbred and Paso Fino foals. Signs of dysmetria and ataxia are evident as soon as the foal attempts to stand and walk.

Cerebellar Abiotrophy

Syndromes of familial cerebellar abiotrophy have been reported in Arabian and Oldenberg horses and Gotland and Eriskay ponies. Signs of cerebellar disease may be present at birth but usually develop during the first 6 months of life.
* Affected foals develop a spastic, ataxic gait and pronounced dysmetria ("goose-stepping"), especially of the forelimbs.
  * They may stand base-wide, with rhythmic swaying of the trunk and neck.

- Signs are exaggerated during walking or excitement; blindfolding has no effect.
- There usually is a head tremor, exaggerated by voluntary movements.
- The menace response is absent or suppressed bilaterally, although vision is unaffected.
- Progression of signs is variable but often slow or inapparent after initial rapid deterioration.
- There is no effective treatment, but some animals improve to varying degrees.

INFLAMMATORY, INFECTIOUS, AND IMMUNE DISEASES
Otitis Media/Interna

Otitis media/interna is rare in horses and is mostly seen in foals. The middle ear can be involved by direct spread of infection from the pharynx, guttural pouch, or external ear, or by hematogenous spread.

Clinical signs

Otitis media/interna causes vestibular signs of head tilt, circling, and ataxia.

- Head shaking may be a presenting complaint in cases of primary otitis media.
- Concurrent ipsilateral facial paralysis is common, and signs of facial nerve damage may precede vestibular signs.
- Rupture of the tympanic membrane occasionally causes discharge from the external ear.
- There may be fever and a hemogram indicating bacterial infection.

Diagnosis

Diagnosis often involves endoscopy, radiography, and culture.

- Endoscopic examination may disclose pharyngitis or guttural pouch disease.
- Ventrodorsal skull radiographs usually show sclerosis of the affected tympanic bulla, even in acute cases.
  - There may also be thickening and sclerosis of the stylohyoid and petrous temporal bones and fusion of the temporohyoid joint on the affected side.
- Flushing sterile fluid through the middle ear via tympanocentesis can be performed to confirm the presence of sepsis.

- Any ear, guttural pouch, or pharyngeal exudates or abnormal CSF should be cultured.
  - β-Hemolytic streptococci, penicillin-resistant staphylococci, and *Actinobacillus equuli* have been cultured from middle ear infections.
  - Other organisms, including *Aspergillus* spp., may be cultured with lesions extending from the guttural pouch.
- CSF may be normal or there may be elevations in protein and, with secondary fractures or infection, RBCs and WBCs.

Treatment

Prolonged antimicrobial therapy is justified in all cases.

- If streptococcal infection is suspected or if signs improve with penicillin therapy, high levels of penicillin should be maintained for 2 to 6 weeks.
  - Other appropriate drugs are ampicillin, sulfonamides, and trimethoprim-sulfa combinations and oxacillin for penicillin-resistant staphylococci.
- Short-term (12 to 48 hours) use of corticosteroids may be indicated for acute otitis interna.
- Surgical drainage of tympanic bulla empyema should be considered in cases resistant to medical therapy.
- To minimize the mechanical stresses resulting from ankylosis of the temporohyoid joint, consideration should be given to surgically removing a section of the affected stylohyoid bone.

Prognosis

The prognosis for functional recovery is fair, even though facial nerve and compensated vestibular dysfunction may remain. Central accommodation often occurs over a period of weeks, and affected animals may even return to racing.

TOXIC DISEASES
Rye Grass Staggers, Dallis Grass Poisoning, and Other Tremorgenic Mycotoxicoses

Several "staggers" syndromes in horses are caused by ingestion of tremorgenic mycotoxins.

- Rye grass staggers affects horses grazing perennial rye grass *(Lolium perenne)* in the summer or fall and horses fed rye grass hay in winter months.
  - It is most common in New Zealand but has been seen in the United States, Britain, and Australia.
  - The mycotoxin (lolitrem B) is produced by fungal endophytes in rye grass plants and seeds.
- Dallis grass poisoning (paspalum staggers) also occurs in New Zealand, Australia, the United States, and Europe.
  - Signs are caused by a toxin contained in the sclerotia (ergots) of *Claviceps paspali,* parasites found in Dallis grass *(Paspalum dilitatum).*
- Less well defined are "staggers" outbreaks in horses fed coastal Bermuda grass hay.

Clinical signs

In each case, signs are those of a vestibulocerebellar disorder with evidence of diffuse spinal or peripheral nerve involvement.

- Initially there is diffuse, intermittent, mild muscle tremor that progresses to ataxia, with a head nod, swaying, an uncoordinated gait, and a wide-based, rocking stance.
- Severely affected animals may stumble and fall, with severe tetanic muscle spasms.
  - If left undisturbed, recumbent horses usually recover and regain their feet in a short time.
- Excitement or blindfolding markedly exacerbates signs.

Treatment and prognosis

Removal of affected horses from the contaminated feedstuff results in resolution of signs in a few days to several weeks. Affected animals should be placed in a flat area that is free of obstacles and handled as little as possible until they recover. If chemical restraint is necessary, diazepam (50 mg IV in a 450-kg horse) may be the drug of choice.

Locoism

Locoweed toxicity (locoism) is a chronic, progressive neurologic disorder of horses, cattle, and sheep grazing the range lands of western North America. It is caused by prolonged ingestion of certain species of *Astragalus* and *Oxytropis* legumes (locoweeds). Outbreaks occur when normal forage is scarce, such as in conditions of overgrazing or drought.

Clinical signs

Clinical signs begin abruptly and indicate a diffuse CNS disorder.

- There are periods of depression alternating with frenzied excitement when disturbed.
- Variable visual impairment, headnodding, and dysphagia with lingual and labial paresis also are observed.
- Gait abnormalities may be severe and characterized by high-stepping, toe-scuffing, stumbling, and swaying; these signs are exacerbated by excitement.
- Weight loss occurs quickly and often progresses to emaciation and death.

Treatment and prognosis

Mildly affected horses recover within 1 to 2 weeks if promptly removed from the source of locoweeds. However, there is no treatment for or recovery from chronic locoweed poisoning.

IDIOPATHIC DISEASES
Idiopathic Vestibular Syndrome

Horses occasionally show acute signs consistent with unilateral peripheral vestibular disease, with no other neurologic sign and no history or evidence of trauma. This may be the result of a transient disease of the vestibular nerve, possibly viral or immune-mediated neuritis or labyrinthitis. Irrespective of therapy, signs resolve completely in 1 to 3 weeks.

Diseases of the Spinal Cord *(945-972)*

Caroline N. Hahn, I. G. (Joe) Mayhew, Robert J. MacKay, and Alan J. Nixon

CONGENITAL AND FAMILIAL DISEASES
Occipitoatlantoaxial Malformation

Occipitoatlantoaxial malformation describes a group of congenital disorders involving the occipital bones, atlas, and axis. The basic malformations include fusion of the atlas to the occiput, hypoplasia of the atlas and/or dens, and modification of the atlantoaxial joint surfaces. There may also be ventral luxation of the axis. The condition may have a simple autosomal recessive mode of inheritance in Arabians, the most commonly affected breed.

Clinical signs and diagnosis

Affected animals may manifest a wide variety of syndromes.

- Foals may be born dead because of severe parturient brainstem and spinal cord compression.
- With mild CNS compression during parturition, foals may show tetraparesis or tetraplegia.
  - A clicking noise may be heard when the foal's head is moved, presumably because of luxation-relocation of the axis.
- The atlas is palpably abnormal (the wings are small, bony pegs) and atlantooccipital movement is reduced.
  - These horses usually have an abnormal head and neck carriage, with the neck extended.
- Some cases are presented as wobblers, with progressive ataxia and tetraparesis in weanlings or yearlings.
- Diagnosis can be confirmed by radiography.

Management

Treatment is not attempted. Breeding affected animals and rebreeding their parents should be discouraged.

Myelodysplasia and Vertebral Anomalies

Myelodysplasias (congenital or developmental spinal cord anomalies) often are accompanied by gross malformations of the axial skeleton, such as spina bifida (failure of fusion of the dorsal vertebral arch), but congenital vertebral anomalies may occur with or without myelodysplasia. Thus congenital deviations of the axial skeleton can occur as part of the "contracted foal syndrome" (see p. 277). Myelodysplasia may be apparent at birth or manifested soon after as stable (but occasionally progressive) neurologic abnormalities such as paraparesis.

DISEASES WITH PHYSICAL CAUSES

Spinal Cord Trauma

Cervical vertebral trauma/fracture is the most common cause of spinal cord injury. The occipitoatlantoaxial region is most often involved. Foals that pull back against the halter and those that fall over backward are more likely to injure the occipitoatlantoaxial region. Any horse that rears up and falls may sustain head and cranial cervical trauma; this is also the likely mechanism for sacrococcygeal fractures that damage the cauda equina (see p. 278).

Clinical signs

Signs vary with the site and severity of spinal cord injury.

- Fractures of C1-T2 may result in tetraplegia or tetraparesis with ataxia.
  - A recumbent horse with trauma at C4-T2 should be able to lift its head and cranial neck.
  - A recumbent horse with a lesion at C1-C3 has difficulty raising its head off the ground.
- Fractures of T3-L6 may cause paraplegia or paraparesis and ataxia.
  - A paraplegic horse that "dog-sits" usually has a lesion caudal to T2.
- Fractures of the sacrum may produce urinary and fecal incontinence and sometimes muscle atrophy and a hind limb gait abnormality.
- Some degree of asymmetry may be present, but signs are almost always bilateral.
- There may also be other signs of injury, such as lacerations, hemorrhage, and distress.

Classically, neurologic signs appear suddenly at the time of injury. There may be a brief period of recumbency, followed by staggering and then recovery over hours or days. In some cases, onset of neurologic signs is delayed for hours, days, or even months, presumably as a result of vertebral instability, progressive hemorrhage, callus formation, and/or degenerative joint disease involving the articular processes. But it is worth noting that not all horses with a vertebral fracture develop signs of spinal cord damage.

Diagnosis

Diagnosis is based on the history, clinical signs, and radiography.

* A complete physical examination should be performed, using sedation if necessary.
* Rectal examination should be performed whenever possible to assess retention of urine and feces and to palpate the pelvis, sacrum, and caudal vertebrae.
* A thorough neurologic examination should allow localization of the lesion(s).
  * Hyporeflexia, hypotonia, sensory defects, and sweating are helpful localizing signs.
* Radiography is useful in confirming vertebral damage and deciding whether or not surgery is indicated.
* CSF analysis sometimes is useful in ruling out other causes of peracute spinal cord disease, such as EHV-1 myeloencephalitis, larval migration, and protozoal myeloencephalitis.
  * Evidence of subarachnoid hemorrhage may be found in horses with spinal cord trauma; however, results of CSF analysis in such animals often are normal.

Treatment

Optimal treatment of spinal cord trauma remains controversial.

* In the peracute stages, dexamethasone (0.1 to 0.2 mg/kg IV) may be given up to 4 times daily for 2 to 4 days.
  * After the first 24 to 48 hours, the benefit of corticosteroids probably is reduced, and problems with infection, laminitis, and delayed bone healing can become significant.
  * Megadose (160 mg/kg in the first 24 hours) methylprednisolone sodium succinate begun within 8 hours of injury can reduce long-term neurologic deficits in humans and dogs with spinal trauma.
* If continued bleeding is suspected or systemic blood pressure is elevated, one to two standard doses of furosemide may be useful.
* The horse must be kept calm or sedated with α_2-adrenergic agonists, acepromazine, pentobarbital, or other agents.
* DMSO (1 g/kg as a 10% solution in 5% dextrose, given slowly IV at 12-hour to 24-hour intervals for up to four doses) may be tried.

* Antibiotics are indicated to manage concurrent skin lesions, cystitis, and pneumonitis in recumbent patients.

External manipulation, external and internal fixation, and surgical decompression and fusion may be options in some patients. Surgery is indicated if the horse's neurologic condition deteriorates despite appropriate medical therapy and decompression of the spinal cord and stabilization of luxations or fractures is feasible.

Prognosis

The prognosis for return to use is guarded to poor, particularly in recumbent patients. However, final judgment should be withheld for 1 to several hours, provided the horse is not suffering unduly. Thorough and repeated neurologic examinations help in arriving at a prognosis and evaluating progress of the animal. Unfortunately, healing often results in some degree of vertebral malalignment, callus formation, and degenerative changes in adjacent articulations, resulting in permanent spinal cord compression.

INFLAMMATORY, INFECTIOUS, AND IMMUNE DISEASES
Vertebral Osteomyelitis

Infection of the vertebrae or intervertebral disks may result in compression of the spinal cord and paraparesis or tetraparesis. The causes and associations of vertebral osteomyelitis are the same as those for infections of the appendicular skeleton (see Chapter 15, Musculoskeletal System). Causative organisms vary somewhat with the animal's age.

* In neonatal foals, the most likely agents are β-hemolytic streptococci, *Actinobacillus equuli,* and *E. coli.*
* In older foals, *Rhodococcus equi, Klebsiella* spp., *Corynebacterium pseudotuberculosis,* or *Salmonella* spp. also may be implicated.
* Any of these organisms may cause the disease in adults, in addition to coagulase-positive staphylococci, *Actinobacillus lignieresii, R. equi, Mycobacterium bovis, Brucella abortus,* coccidiomycosis, *Eikenella corrodens,* and *Aspergillus* spp.

Clinical signs and diagnosis
Signs vary with the stage of disease.
- As sepsis becomes established, there is localized pain, manifested as resistance to palpation, stiffness, and reluctance to move the affected vertebrae.
  - Fever, neutrophilia, and elevated plasma fibrinogen also may be expected at this stage.
- Compression fractures of weakened vertebral bodies cause acute onset of neurologic signs, indicative of the spinal cord segment affected.
  - Spread of infection into the epidural space can also cause neurologic signs, which may begin insidiously.
- Radiography is an important aid to diagnosis, although radiographic changes may not be present at the first sign of disease.
- If meningitis develops, pleocytosis and elevated protein may be expected on CSF analysis; more often, CSF findings are normal or consistent with spinal cord compression.
- Tests for *Brucella abortus* and tuberculosis should be considered in adult horses.

Treatment and prognosis
Every effort should be made to obtain aerobic and anaerobic cultures before treatment.
- Samples may be collected via needle aspiration, percutaneous biopsy or excision of infected bone, and aspiration of paravertebral or other abscesses.
  - Blood and urine samples could also be submitted for culture.
- Appropriate antimicrobial therapy should be continued for at least 6 weeks.
- If neurologic signs have been rapidly progressive or if there is profound spinal cord compression, surgical exploration and drainage could be attempted.

The prognosis is guarded to poor unless patients are treated before neurologic signs are marked.

TOXIC DISEASES
Bracken Fern and Horsetail Poisoning
Ingestion of *Pteridium* (bracken fern) or *Equiperdum* (horsetail) spp. causes neurologic disease as a result of thiaminase-induced thiamine deficiency.
- Most cases of poisoning are due to incorporation of bracken fern or horsetail into hay.
- Signs begin insidiously several weeks after ingestion begins and may even develop after removal of the contaminated hay.
- The most obvious abnormality is ataxia, which may be severe and involve all four limbs.
  - Anorexia, bradycardia, and a "tucked-up" appearance are common.
  - Signs of forebrain disease, such as head-pressing and blindness, occasionally are seen.
  - Convulsions and opisthotonus occur terminally.
- Thiamine at 0.5 to 1 g PO q12h results in rapid resolution of signs.

Grove Poisoning
Grove poisoning is a syndrome of ataxia and convulsions that is reported in adult horses in south Florida. It occurs in areas of intensive horticultural activity, and has been associated with *Indigofera* spp. Signs fluctuate in severity but are progressive over time and usually result in recumbency and death. Ulceration and congestion of the gums and corneal edema and ulceration are other manifestations. Diazepam, atropine, saline purgatives, and alfalfa cubes and gelatin slurry given via stomach tube have helped in some cases.

MULTIFACTORIAL DISEASES
Equine Motor Neuron Disease
Equine motor neuron disease (EMND) is characterized by destruction of lower motor neurons in the brainstem and spinal cord, leading to characteristic signs punctuated by weakness.
- The majority of cases occur in the northeastern United States, although EMND has been reported in Europe, Japan, and South America.
- Quarterhorses, Appaloosas, and Standardbreds are more likely to develop the disease.
- Older horses (peak age, 16 years) are at a higher risk than young animals.
- The vast majority of cases have had little or no access to grass.

The cause is not known, although deficient antioxidant activity in the CNS likely is involved, as is the case in the comparable acquired form of the human disease (Lou Gehrig's disease).

Clinical signs

Findings depend on the stage of the disease.

- Weight loss in the face of a good or increased appetite, increased recumbency, and muscle tremors are consistent findings in early cases.
  - Weight loss often is noticed by owners several weeks before the onset of trembling.
- Affected horses frequently have an abnormally low head carriage.
- A short-strided gait is common, although there is no ataxia or loss of proprioception.
- Many horses have a raised tail head, and excessive sweating is seen in >50% of cases.
- Ophthalmic examination reveals a mosaic pattern of dark brown to yellow-brown pigment in the tapetal zone and a horizontal band of pigment at the tapetal junction.

Diagnosis

Although the clinical course in severe cases is characteristic, important differentials include botulism, grass sickness, myositis, malabsorptive disorders, and neglect. Antemortem diagnosis can be difficult, since laboratory findings are nonspecific.

- Mean plasma CK and AST activities are usually elevated (>1200 and >1300 IU/L, respectively).
- Plasma vitamin E is significantly lower than on-farm controls.
- Needle electromyographic studies under general anesthesia are consistently abnormal in affected animals.

Histopathologic examination of a biopsy of dorsal coccygeal muscle can confirm the presence of neurogenic-type muscle atrophy. Biopsy of the ventral branch of the spinal accessory nerve is another valuable antemortem diagnostic tool.

Treatment and prognosis

There is currently no definitive treatment. Signs often stabilize or improve 1 to 2 months after onset, but progression after a period of stabilization is common. A few cases have improved with oral vitamin E supplementation (see the section on treatment and prevention of equine degenerative myeloencephalopathy). Athletic ability of surviving animals is permanently impaired.

Equine Degenerative Myeloencephalopathy

Equine degenerative myeloencephalopathy (EDM) is a diffuse degenerative disease of the spinal cord and brainstem.

- It is most common in the northeastern United States, but has been recognized all over the United States and northern Europe in most breeds of horse.
- The disease is hereditary in Appaloosas, Standardbreds, and Paso Finos, and a genetic basis is suspected in Norwegian fjord horses, Arabians, Welsh ponies, Haflingers, and Morgans.
- The exact pathogenesis is unknown; however, vitamin E deficiency is a causative factor.
- EDM usually occurs in foals but may affect horses up to 3 years of age.
- It may occur in a single animal or affect groups of young horses (especially if related).

Clinical signs

There is an insidious or abrupt onset of symmetric ataxia, paresis, and dysmetria. Typically, hind limb signs are worse than forelimb signs by at least one grade. Clinical signs may progress to the point of causing recumbency or may be stable for many months.

Diagnosis

Presumptive diagnosis usually can be made by careful evaluation of the history and clinical signs. Confirmation involves assessment of vitamin E status.

- Normal serum vitamin E is at least 1.5 μg/mL.
- Serum vitamin E levels <1 μg/ml κg/ml have been associated with EDM; however, values may be normal, depending on the stage of disease.
- Daily vitamin E intake should be estimated and compared with the recommended dietary level.
- The vitamin E status of any stablemates or pasturemates should also be determined.

- Cervical radiographs should be taken to rule out cervical vertebral malformation.

Treatment and prevention

If vitamin E intake is found to be suboptimal, all horses on the farm should receive vitamin E supplementation at 1.5 mg (2.25 IU)/kg/day.

- Affected horses should also receive vitamin E in oil at 1000 to 3000 IU/day IM for up to 1 week, followed by 6000 IU orally in feed for several months or even years.
- Response to therapy may be seen within a few weeks and continues for more than a year.
- Serum vitamin E should be measured periodically to assess treatment effectiveness.
- The presence of EDM within a family should be considered when selecting breeding stock.

Cervical Vertebral Malformation-Malarticulation

Cervical vertebral malformation (CVM) describes a group of malformation-malarticulation anomalies involving the cervical vertebrae of ataxic horses ("wobblers"). Affected horses have one or more focal compression-type lesions in the cervical spinal cord. Two subdivisions of CVM have been described.

- ***cervical vertebral instability:*** typically involves deformation of the vertebral bodies, with malarticulation and subluxation on flexion of the vertebrae
  - The size, shape, and integrity of the articular processes frequently are abnormal.
  - This type typically occurs in the midcervical vertebrae of weanlings and yearlings.
- ***cervical static stenosis:*** generally involves the caudal cervical vertebrae and results from degenerative joint disease of the articular processes, with bony and occasionally soft tissue protrusion into the vertebral canal
  - This type is most often seen in horses between 18 months and 3 years of age.

Contributing factors

The precise abnormalities of bone and joint development resulting in CVM are not completely known.

Many factors likely interact to alter development of the cervical vertebrae, including:

- nutrition, especially copper deficiency and high dietary protein and carbohydrates
- genetics, including the propensity for large body size for the horse's age
- biomechanical forces (possibly caused by conformation)
- exercise
- trauma

Cervical vertebral malformation is one of a group of developmental orthopedic diseases (see Chapter 15, Musculoskeletal System). Thoroughbred, Quarter Horse, and Warmblood breeds have a high incidence of CVM, although the condition occurs in all breeds. Both sexes can be affected, but males tend to be over-represented.

Clinical signs

The principal neurologic signs are ataxia, weakness, and spasticity.

- Ataxia and paresis usually begin acutely, progress, and then may stabilize or regress.
  - Complete recovery is uncommon, but cycles of improvement and deterioration often are seen.
- Generally, the hind limbs are most affected, with forelimb signs being less obvious (usually one grade less) and occasionally developing later in the course of the disease.
  - Some horses show an apparent single hind limb lameness.
  - Occasionally, severe forelimb signs can result from malformation at the C6-C7 or C7-T1 junctions.
- Slight asymmetry of signs is common and may be marked, depending on the degree of lateral compression.
- Palpable swellings of the cervical vertebrae occasionally are detectable, particularly if the midcervical vertebrae are involved.
  - Pain on palpation or lateral bending of the neck can sometimes be detected, and reduced range of lateral motion may result from degenerative joint disease of the facet joints.
- Discrete lameness without obvious neurologic deficits can also occur but is nearly always accompanied

by neck pain or stiffness and radiologic evidence of caudal cervical arthropathy.

Diagnosis

Differential diagnoses include protozoal myeloencephalitis, degenerative myeloencephalopathy, and vertebral trauma. A detailed analysis of the history and careful neurologic examination are helpful in establishing a tentative diagnosis, but radiography and myelography are most useful in confirming CVM.

◆ Many affected horses are well grown, and some have a history or signs of other developmental orthopedic diseases, such as osteochondritis dissecans or physitis.

  • There often is a history of a minor fall or training incident.

◆ Tentative diagnosis usually can be made with plain radiographs, based on narrowing of the vertebral canal, degenerative joint disease of the facet joints, and malalignment of vertebrae.

  • The midcervical area should be scrutinized carefully.

  • Measuring the vertebral canal diameter has been advocated as an objective index of vertebral canal stenosis and spinal cord compression.

  • Severe degenerative joint disease and lamina changes can be incidental findings and not sources of spinal cord compression.

◆ CSF collection and analysis is helpful in ruling out some of the differential diagnoses.

  • CSF from animals with CVM generally is normal; mild xanthochromia and a slightly elevated protein content (70 to 130 mg/dL) may be found.

Measurement of vertebral canal diameter and myelographic techniques are described in *Equine Medicine and Surgery V.*

Treatment

Medical treatment is aimed at reducing edema and inflammation within the spinal cord.

◆ Stall rest is recommended to minimize further spinal cord damage.

  • If signs stabilize during stall rest, the horse may eventually be turned out to a small pasture.

◆ In the acute stages, phenylbutazone, corticosteroids, and DMSO are the most frequently used antiinflammatory drugs.

  • The effects usually are positive, but signs frequently worsen on drug withdrawal.

  • Chronic spinal cord compression responds less definitively to medical management.

Surgical stabilization with interbody fusion or arthrodesis is indicated in horses with vertebral instability. Dorsal laminectomy had been recommended for decompression of static stenosis lesions, although interbody fusion is now used to provide slow decompression through remodeling of the bony malformations. These techniques are described in *Equine Medicine and Surgery V.*

Prognosis

Conservative therapy rarely returns a horse to useful purposes, even breeding. The prognosis is improved by surgical therapy, though surgery by no means returns all animals to their intended use. The severity and duration of clinical signs and the adequacy of the diagnostic workup and surgical decompression often dictate the eventual outcome.

IDIOPATHIC DISEASES

Arthrogryposis (Contracted Foal Syndrome)

Arthrogryposis describes a wide range of contractures and curvatures of the limbs and vertebral column in neonatal foals. The cause usually is not known, although ingestion of locoweed *(Astragalus mollismus),* Sudan grass, or other *Sorghum* spp. grasses by pregnant mares is implicated in some cases. The success or failure of treatment for limb contracture depends in a large part on the degree of involvement of the central and peripheral nervous systems. In some cases there is depletion of lower motor neurons in the spinal cord and lesions in the peripheral nerves and muscles. Symptomatic management will not cure such cases.

Postanesthetic Myelopathy

A syndrome of postanesthetic hemorrhagic myelopathy has been reported in horses. It involves hypoxic-ischemic neuronal damage, most likely caused by hypotension during halothane anesthesia and local venous congestion from compression of the caudal vena cava by abdominal viscera. The majority of affected animals are young (6 months to 2 years) and weigh >300 kg (660 lb).

Clinical signs

Neurologic abnormalities occur after periods of anesthesia in dorsal recumbency of >45 minutes.

- In most cases, anesthesia and the initial recovery period are uneventful, but weakness soon becomes evident.
- Initial signs range from difficulty standing to tetraplegia with flaccid paralysis and anesthesia of the hind limbs.
  - A characteristic sign is depression of sensation and spinal reflexes over several contiguous segments.
- Affected horses become recumbent or remain in lateral recumbency until euthanasia 1 to 8 days after surgery.

Treatment and prognosis

The prognosis is hopeless in severely affected horses. However, milder cases may benefit from supportive care and treatment with corticosteroids and DMSO. It is probably wise to position heavy horses slightly off true dorsal recumbency when this position is necessary during general anesthesia.

Diseases of the Cauda Equina *(pages 972-975)*

Caroline N. Hahn, I. G. (Joe) Mayhew, and Robert J. MacKay

DISEASES WITH PHYSICAL CAUSES

Sacral Fractures

The neurologic signs of sacral fracture result from damage to the sacral and caudal nerve roots of the cauda equina.

- Varying degrees of paralysis, hypalgesia, and hyporeflexia of the bladder, rectum, anus, vulva, tail, penis, and perineal skin as far ventrally as the udder or prepuce are found.

- Fecal obstipation, bladder distention, and urinary and fecal incontinence result.
- Signs may be evident immediately after injury or may occur days or weeks later; once present, signs usually do not worsen.
- Sacral fracture is suggested by a history of trauma.
  - Palpation of the sacrum per rectum can reveal a fracture and/or callus formation.
  - Radiographs of the area are difficult to take and interpret.
  - Nuclear scintigraphy may be helpful in making a diagnosis.
- Differential diagnoses include cauda equina neuritis, sorghum-Sudan grass toxicity, EHV-1 myeloencephalopathy, epidural empyema, cryptococcosis, listeriosis, and EPM.
- Conservative treatment usually is undertaken.
  - Particular attention must be given to evacuation of the rectum and bladder and promoting exercise.
  - Antiinflammatory treatment (corticosteroids, NSAIDs) can be given for the first 3 days.
- Without improvement in 6 to 12 weeks, the prognosis for long-term improvement is very poor.

INFLAMMATORY, INFECTIOUS, AND IMMUNE DISEASES

Neuritis of the Cauda Equina (Polyneuritis Equi)

Neuritis of the cauda equina is a condition that primarily involves the nerve roots of the cauda equina. Because cranial nerves or other peripheral nerves may be concurrently or exclusively affected, *polyneuritis equi* is a more accurate term. The cause is unknown but may involve an immune-mediated response to a virus (e.g., adenovirus, EHV-1). Affected animals are mature and aged.

Clinical signs

Presenting signs are quite variable, though usually referable to sacrococcygeal nerve root involvement.

- Onset usually is insidious and progression occurs over several weeks, though in most cases signs are noticed acutely.

- There may be a recent history of rubbing and abrasion of the tail head and perineum, colic caused by obstipation, or hypersensitivity to pressure over the gluteal area.
- There usually is a well-demarcated area of cutaneous analgesia and areflexia involving the tail, perineum, caudal gluteal area, and penis (but not the prepuce).
  - Often the area of analgesia is surrounded by a band of hyperesthesia.
- The tail hangs limply and the anal sphincter, rectum, bladder, urethral sphincter, and vulva or penis are paralyzed.
  - After 1 to 2 weeks there is marked coccygeal muscle atrophy, persistent bladder distention, and continual dribbling of urine from a gaping vulva or prolapsed penis.
- Appetite and vital signs usually are normal.
- Hind limb weakness may occur as the disease progresses.
  - Gait abnormalities often are subtle and asymmetric, at least initially.
  - There may also be atrophy of the gluteal, biceps femoris, or other muscles.
- Involvement of other nerve roots and peripheral nerves is common but may be less obvious.
  - Cranial nerve abnormalities can include masseter atrophy and weakness, facial paralysis, head tilt, nystagmus, tongue weakness, and difficult swallowing.

Diagnosis

Definitive diagnosis can be difficult.

- Differential diagnoses include sacral or coccygeal trauma, EHV-1 myeloencephalopathy, EPM, rabies, and equine motor neuron disease.
- CSF usually reveals moderate elevations in protein and numbers of leukocytes (mixed population).
- Use of an ELISA to detect serum anti-P2 antibodies might help differentiate this disease from other peripheral neuropathies.
  - Elevated anti-P2 antibodies have been noted in normal horses and some with sacral fractures, space-occupying vertebral lesions, and EHV-1 myeloencephalopathy.
- Electromyography may be useful.

Treatment and prognosis

Despite clinical fluctuations, cauda equina neuritis typically persists and is fatal. Regular manual evacuation of the rectum, catheterization of the bladder, and management of urinary tract infections may prolong the horse's life for many months. Corticosteroids may be beneficial in cases in which the cranial nerves are primarily affected.

TOXIC DISEASES
Sorghum Poisoning

A syndrome characterized by ataxia and cystitis occurs in horses grazing hybrid crosses of sorghum (*S. vulgare*) and Sudan grass (*S. vulgare* var *sudanense*); other species, including Johnson grass (*S. halepense*), have also been incriminated. Well-cured *Sorghum* hay apparently does not cause the disease. Symmetric ataxia and weakness of the hind limbs usually are the first signs noted.

- Flaccid paralysis of both hind limbs and the tail occasionally develop 24 hours later.
- Urinary incontinence develops soon after neurologic signs and is manifested as continual dribbling from a relaxed vulva or penis; cystitis is common and may be severe.
- Removal from sorghum-Sudan pasture usually effects improvement but not full recovery.

Diseases of the Peripheral (Spinal) Nerves *(pages 975-980)*

Caroline N. Hahn, I. G. (Joe) Mayhew, and Robert J. MacKay

PERIPHERAL NERVE TRAUMA
Suprascapular Nerve

Damage to the suprascapular nerve at the cranial border of the scapula results in atrophy of the supraspinatus and infraspinatus muscles (Sweeney) and laxity or instability of the shoulder joint, which allows the shoulder to subluxate laterally during weight-bearing. Causes include collision with a solid object or another horse, wounds to the front of the shoulder, and stretching of the nerve when the horse stumbles while the limb is retracted.

Treatment and prognosis

Initial treatment involves use of anti-inflammatory therapy.

* Dexamethasone (0.05 mg/kg IM q12h), flunixin meglumine (0.5 mg/kg IM q12h), or phenylbutazone (2.2 mg/kg PO q12h) may be given for 3 days.
* Stall confinement is recommended, and immediate application of icepacks should be considered.
* Function returns in days or weeks when loss of function is simply due to concussion (neurapraxia).
* When the nerve has been severed, surgical reconstruction may be attempted.
  * If reconstruction is not possible, proximal axons regrow at about 2.5 cm (1 inch) a month.
* Surgical decompression can improve return to normal function and probably should be performed within 8 to 12 weeks of injury (see *Equine Medicine and Surgery V*).
  * Treatment may be unnecessary if the horse is not used for performance.

Radial Nerve and Brachial Plexus

The radial nerve principally innervates the triceps brachii and digital extensor muscles. It can be damaged by direct trauma, prolonged lateral recumbency, and rib or humeral fractures. Inability to extend the limb and flex the shoulder joint and thus bear weight on the forelimb reflects total radial paralysis.

* The elbow, knee, fetlock, and interphalangeal joints are flexed, and the dorsum of the toe rests on the ground.
* The elbow is maintained in a "dropped" position during locomotion, and the limb is advanced only half a stride, usually with the toe dragging.
* Radial paralysis of >2 weeks' duration results in atrophy of the triceps, extensor carpi radialis, ulnaris lateralis, and digital extensor muscles.
* Radial nerve function should be evaluated before humeral fracture repair because of the poorer prognosis that accompanies radial nerve damage.

Treatment of uncomplicated radial nerve paralysis is as described for suprascapular nerve damage. In addition, the distal limb should be protected from abrasion and flexor contracture with a supportive bandage or light cast.

Musculocutaneous, Median, and Ulnar Nerves

These nerves innervate the flexors or the elbow, carpus, and digit. Paralysis rarely occurs as a singular event, and the resulting syndromes are not well documented. Brachial plexus injuries and spinal cord lesions involving gray matter of the brachial intumescence may cause signs related to involvement of some or all of these nerves. Elbow fractures potentially may affect the ulnar and median nerves. Following are some features of specific nerve injury.

* *musculocutaneous nerve:* Damage results in decreased elbow flexion and toe dragging.
  * Sensory loss is expected over the craniomedial aspect of the knee and metacarpal region.
* *median nerve:* Damage results in a stiff gait, with toe dragging as a result of decreased flexion of carpus and fetlock; hypalgesia is found on the medial aspect of the pastern.
* *ulnar nerve:* Damage results in a gait alteration that is similar to, though more pronounced than, that seen with median nerve damage.
  * There is decreased flexion of the carpus and fetlock, and the foot may be projected in a jerky fashion.
  * There is hypalgesia on the lateral metacarpus and caudal forearm.
  * Obvious atrophy of the digital flexor muscles becomes apparent.

Aggressive therapy may be unnecessary because of the remarkable improvement of these gait alterations with time (usually 2 to 3 months).

Femoral Nerve

The femoral nerve innervates the major extensor muscles of the stifle, so paralysis results in inability to extend the stifle.

- Because of the reciprocal arrangement between stifle and hock, femoral nerve damage results in extensor paralysis, with the affected limb resting in a flexed position and the ipsilateral hip lower than the other.
  - No weight is supported on the affected limb during locomotion.
- If the horse is recumbent, the patellar reflex is depressed or absent.
- There may be hypalgesia of the medial thigh (saphenous branch involvement), and eventually there is quadriceps atrophy.

Causes
The femoral nerve is well protected from external injury but may be damaged by penetrating wounds in the caudal flank. Other possible causes of femoral nerve paralysis include:
- abscesses and tumors in the region of the external iliac arteries
- fractures of the pelvis and femur
- postfoaling hemorrhage around the pelvic canal
- spinal cord lesions of the ventral gray matter or nerve roots at L4 and L5
  - EPM, helminths, and trauma can cause such lesions.

Exertional rhabdomyolysis and postanesthetic myopathy may cause unilateral or bilateral extensor weakness in the hind limbs that clinically resembles femoral nerve damage.

Treatment and prognosis
The principles of medical and surgical management of such nerve injuries are discussed in the section on the suprascapular nerve. The prognosis is guarded unless the nerve can be repaired.

Sciatic Nerve
The sciatic nerve supplies the main extensor muscles of the hip and flexor muscles of the stifle and divides into peroneal and tibial branches (see below). Total sciatic paralysis results in a profoundly abnormal gait and posture, mainly from flexor weakness.
- At rest, the limb hangs behind the horse, with the stifle and hock extended, the fetlock and interphalangeal joints partly flexed, and the dorsum of the hoof on the ground.

- During locomotion, the foot is dragged, or the distal limb is jerked up and forward.
- If the foot is manually advanced and placed on the ground, the horse can support weight with some flexion of the hock and take a stride.
- The muscles of the caudal thigh and limb distal to the stifle become atrophied.
- Hypalgesia over most of the limb, except for the medial thigh, is reported.

Causes
The sciatic nerve is well protected, but it may be damaged by pelvic fractures, especially of the ischium. In foals, deep injections caudal to the proximal femur and *Salmonella* osteomyelitis of the sacrum and pelvis have resulted in sciatic paralysis. Syndromes of sciatic palsy and flexor weakness can occur with spinal cord lesions, such as EPM affecting the L5-S3 ventral gray matter or nerve roots.

Treatment and prognosis
Treatment of the primary problem may resolve sciatic paralysis, but if the nerve is severed, the prognosis is unfavorable. Support and protection should be given to the distal limb.

Peroneal Nerve
This branch of the sciatic nerve supplies the flexor muscles of the hock and extensor muscles of the digits. Thus paralysis results in extension of the hock and flexion of the fetlock and interphalangeal joints.
- At rest, the horse holds the limb somewhat extended, with the dorsum of the hoof resting on the ground.
- During locomotion, the foot is dragged along the ground, then jerked back when an attempt is made to bear weight.
- If the limb is advanced manually and the toe extended, the horse can bear weight.
- Hypalgesia occurs on the craniolateral aspect of the hock and metatarsal regions.
- Atrophy of the craniolateral aspect of the gaskin can be expected.

The peroneal nerve is most vulnerable to external injury where it crosses the lateral condyle of the femur. Injury from a kick or from lateral recumbency usually does not sever the nerve, so many horses with traumatic peroneal nerve damage eventually improve. The limb should be supported and protected; other aspects of therapy are as described for suprascapular nerve injury.

Tibial Nerve

The tibial branch of the sciatic nerve innervates the gastrocnemius and digital flexor muscles.

- Paralysis causes the limb to be held with the hock flexed and the fetlock resting in a flexed or partly knuckled position; the hip is held lower on the affected side.
- The horse overflexes the limb when walking, and the foot is raised higher than normal, then abruptly dropped to the ground.
  - The overall stride is similar to that seen with stringhalt.
- Atrophy of the gastrocnemius muscle and anesthesia of the caudal metatarsal region and heel bulbs also occur.

  Tibial paralysis is very uncommon, partly because the nerve is well protected.

Obturator (Postfoaling) Paralysis

The obturator nerve innervates the adductors of the thigh and its paralysis is an infrequent sequel to foaling. Signs range from mild stiffness to paraplegia. In mild cases, unilateral involvement may be apparent as abduction and circumduction of the limb at the walk. The limb may slip laterally on slippery surfaces, especially when the mare attempts to rise. Antiinflammatory therapy (corticosteroids, phenylbutazone) is indicated, as well as basic nursing care in recumbent horses. Function generally returns over a period of weeks.

IDIOPATHIC DISEASES
Stringhalt, Shivering

Stringhalt is characterized by an abnormal gait, with involuntary and exaggerated hock flexion in one or both hind limbs during attempted movement. It occurs in both outbreak and sporadic forms.

- Outbreaks of stringhalt (Australian stringhalt) have been associated with grazing weed-infested pastures during periods of drought.
  - Plants incriminated include *Hypocoeris radicata* (dandelion, cat's ear, flatweed) *Taraxacum officinale* (European dandelion), and *Malva parviflora* (mallow plant).
  - Involvement of an environmental mycotoxin has also been suggested.
  - Ingestion of hay containing *Lathyrus hirsutus* (caley pea) results in a syndrome (neurolathyrism) of hind limb dysmetria that in its chronic form is similar to stringhalt.
- Sporadic cases have been linked to various musculoskeletal disorders of the hind limb, as well as to lumbosacral spinal cord disease.
- A related condition of draft breeds, known as "shivers," is characterized by hind limb muscle tremors and elevation of the tail.
  - Signs are most pronounced when the animal is forced to turn tightly or move backward.
  - Lifting the affected limb may be impossible or may induce considerable muscle trembling.
  - Bilateral "shivers" is thought to be hereditary in some draft breeds and usually is progressive.

Clinical signs

Signs of stringhalt often develop suddenly.

- In mild cases, exaggerated hock flexion is seen only during turning or backing and may disappear with exercise.
- In its most severe form, stringhalt is disabling; the affected limb(s) is flexed so violently that the fetlock slaps the abdomen or point of the elbow with each step.
- Inspiratory stridor as a result of left laryngeal hemiparesis also is seen in some cases of Australian stringhalt (and of lathyrism).

Treatment and prognosis

Horses with Australian stringhalt can recover, although recovery may take more than a year. Treatment in these cases is supportive.

- Horses should be removed from the offending pasture and given stall or paddock rest.
- Successful treatment with phenytoin at 15 to 25 mg/kg PO q24h has been reported.

Some cases of sporadic stringhalt also improve with rest, though this is not a consistent finding. Mildly to moderately affected horses may improve after tenectomy of the lateral digital extensor tendon see (*Equine Medicine and Surgery V*).

Diseases of the Neuromuscular Junction *(981-983)*

Caroline N. Hahn, I. G. (Joe) Mayhew, and Robert J. MacKay

INFLAMMATORY, INFECTIOUS, AND IMMUNE DISEASES

Botulism

Botulism results from absorption of a toxin produced by *Clostridium botulinum*, a Gram-positive anaerobic bacillus. Eight toxigenic types are recognized; types B, C, and D have been incriminated in cases of equine botulism. The prevalence of each serotype varies with geographic location. The most common cause of botulism is ingestion of preformed toxin in contaminated or spoiled feedstuffs, such as grain or hay containing small animal carcasses, and "big bale" silage. Toxin can also be elaborated in necrotic tissue (toxicoinfectious botulism), including gastric ulcers, foci of hepatic necrosis, umbilical or pulmonary abscesses, and wounds in skin and muscle. Toxicoinfectious botulism in foals is referred to as "shaker foal" syndrome.

Clinical signs

Regardless of the route of entry and type of toxin, the clinical picture is consistent.

- Locomotor abnormalities usually are noticed first.
  - Affected horses move with a shuffling, stilted gait, dragging their toes, and may stand with head and neck hanging below horizontal.
- Complete absence of facial expression creates a dull, sleepy appearance.
  - Mydriasis and sluggish pupillary reflexes usually appear early, as does flaccid paresis of the tongue and eyelids.
  - Awareness is normal, but facial weakness conveys an impression of stupor.
- Saliva frequently drools from the mouth; though appetite is unaffected, mastication and lingual movements may be so feeble that partly chewed food drops from the mouth.
  - Difficulty in swallowing often causes water and feed material to appear at the nostrils.
  - Inhalation pneumonia often complicates the clinical course.
- Skin sensation is normal, although spinal and cranial nerve reflexes generally are depressed.
- Some horses experience abdominal pain, with complete cessation of intestinal sounds; rectal examination may reveal dry, mucus-covered feces.
- The bladder often is distended, and there may be frequent passage of small amounts of urine, accompanied by penile protrusion and paralysis in males.
- Trembling and generalized sweating develop as weakness becomes more profound.
  - Breathing becomes labored, with prominent abdominal effort.
- Once adult horses with botulism become recumbent, they seldom rise again and soon become too weak to maintain a sternal position; they should be euthanized if antiserum is not given.

"SHAKER FOAL" SYNDROME. This form of botulism most often affects fast-growing foals 1 to 2 months (range, 2 weeks to 6 months) of age. It is endemic in central Kentucky. Signs are typical of botulism: stilted gait, muscle tremors, and inability to stand for more than a few minutes. Nasal reflux of milk is also a common sign in these foals. Without intensive nursing care and serotherapy (see

below), death occurs in 1 to 3 days in >50% of foals.

Diagnosis

Definitive diagnosis is seldom made antemortem, although clinical signs are highly suggestive.

- *Clostridium botulinum* toxin is rarely detectable in the serum, but serum samples from horses with early signs should be frozen and submitted for toxin detection.
- At necropsy, stomach and intestinal contents, feces, liver, suspect feed, and areas of tissue necrosis should be submitted for anaerobic culture and toxin assay.
  - *C. botulinum* organisms normally present in the intestine may elaborate toxin postmortem, so only fresh or frozen samples should be submitted for toxin detection.

Treatment

The University of Pennsylvania produces a homologous type B and type C and D antisera that may improve survival rates when given early (200 mL slowly IV in foals and 500 mL in adults). The sera are now available through the British Equine Veterinary Association. If toxicoinfectious botulism is suspected, high levels of crystalline penicillin (25,000 to 100,000 IU/kg IV q6h) may be given. Wounds should be debrided and irrigated and any abscesses cultured and drained.

Death from botulism usually is due to respiratory failure. In shaker foals, assisted ventilation and parenteral nutrition can improve survival. Less severely affected horses may need intensive support for several weeks during recovery.

- If gastric emptying and intestinal motility are adequate, placement of an indwelling nasoesophageal tube ensures adequate hydration and nutrition.
  - Mineral oil should be given as needed to avoid or treat constipation.
- Recumbent horses should be encouraged to remain sternal and, if possible, assisted to stand for short periods and to posture for urination.
- Recumbent horses may require catheterization to prevent bladder distention and necrosis.
- Urinary and respiratory tract infections must be treated vigorously.
  - Drugs that may potentiate neuromuscular blockage, such as aminoglycosides, tetracyclines, and procaine penicillin, must be avoided.

Prognosis

Without specific serotherapy, the mortality rate in naturally occurring cases ranges from 69% to >90%. Death may occur within several hours or may take up to a week. Recovery may take weeks or even months but is complete when it occurs.

Prevention

Type-B toxoid is commercially available in the United States and can be effective at preventing shaker foal syndrome. Pregnant mares initially are vaccinated with the toxoid in the eighth, ninth, and tenth month of gestation and thereafter in the tenth month of each pregnancy.

Postanesthetic Myasthenia

A botulism-like syndrome occurring immediately after general anesthesia has been reported. With supportive care, affected horses are able to walk within 5 to 7 days and totally recover within a month.

12

Reproductive System: The Stallion

Examination of the Stallion *(pages 998-1006)*

Dickson D. Varner
and James Schumacher

Examination of a breeding stallion (breeding soundness examination) is to:
* evaluate the quality and quantity of ejaculated spermatozoa
* assess the libido and mating ability of the stallion
* reveal congenital defects that may be transmissible to offspring and/or decrease the stallion's fertility
* identify infectious diseases that may be transmitted venereally
* find any other lesions that may reduce breeding longevity

HISTORY AND IDENTIFICATION

Pertinent historical information regarding the stallion includes:
* lineage
* present use
* previous breeding performance
* prior fertility evaluation results
* illnesses, injuries, medications, and vaccinations, with explicit information regarding previous and current reproductive management and veterinary medical programs

Positive stallion identification also is important.

GENERAL PHYSICAL EXAMINATION

General physical examination should comprise:
* assessment of general body condition
* appraisal of conformation, especially with respect to traits that potentially are heritable (e.g., cryptorchidism, parrot mouth) or that may affect mating ability (e.g., leg or back problems)
* methodical examination of the general body systems
* ophthalmic examination

EXAMINATION OF THE REPRODUCTIVE TRACT

External Genitalia

The penis and the scrotum and its contents should be thoroughly examined. Inspection of the penis is aided by first stimulating penile tumescence through exposure of the stallion to a mare in estrus. This procedure also permits assessment of sexual behavior, including erection capability. Tranquilization with promazine-derived drugs should be avoided because it can result in penile paralysis or priapism (see p. 305).

Penis and prepuce

Examination of the penis is limited to the body and glans:

- The fossa glandis and urethral process require careful examination.
- Common penile lesions include those of traumatic origin, vesicles/pustules of equine coital exanthema, cutaneous habronemiasis, squamous cell carcinomas, and papillomas.
- The prepuce should be examined for evidence of inflammatory or proliferative lesions.

Scrotum and testes

Both testes and attached epididymides should be freely movable within the scrotal pouch. Other evaluations include:

- size, texture, and position of each testis
  - Testicular size is highly correlated with daily sperm production, so this measurement helps predict a stallion's breeding potential (see *Equine Medicine and Surgery V*).
- palpation of the spermatic cord through the neck of the scrotum

Internal Genitalia

The internal genital organs can be examined by palpation per rectum.

- Adequate restraint is important to prevent rectal damage and injury to the operator.
- The two internal inguinal rings are palpable as small (2 to 3 cm [0.75 to 1.25 inch]), slitlike openings ventrolateral to the pelvic brim.
  - The deferent duct and pulse of the testicular artery usually can be detected at the opening.
- The paired ampullae and lobes of the prostate gland can be identified per rectum.
- The vesicular glands usually are palpable only when distended during sexual stimulation.
  - They sometimes become thickened (and hence palpable during sexual quiescence) following vesicular adenitis.
- The bulbourethral glands usually are not palpable.

Examination for Venereal Disease

Depending on the etiologic agent involved, venereal disease may cause overt clinical signs in the stallion, but, more commonly, infected stallions are asymptomatic carriers.

Bacterial genital infections

A variety of environmental bacteria can be isolated from the equine prepuce, penis, and distal urethra, many contributing to the normal non-pathogenic bacterial flora in healthy stallions. Documentation of a bacterial infection depends on serial isolation of a pathogen (e.g., *Klebsiella pneumoniae, Pseudomonas aeruginosa*), preferably in large numbers and in relatively pure culture. The exception is culture of *Taylorella equigenitalis* (the contagious equine metritis organism), for which a single isolation is considered diagnostic.

Following are some practical guidelines for sample collection:

- Swabs of the fossa glandis, free portion of the penile body, and folds of the external prepuce should be taken for bacteriologic culture before cleaning the penis.
- Briskly rubbing the glans penis during washing usually stimulates secretion of clear fluid from the urethral and/or bulbourethral glands.
  - Some of this fluid may be collected for bacterial culture and cytologic examination if infection of the urethra or bulbourethral glands is suspected.
  - A preejaculation urethral swab then is obtained for bacterial culture.
- Semen can be collected in an artificial vagina and a postejaculation urethral swab taken
  - The semen can be sampled for bacterial culture, if indicated.
- Passage of a small catheter or culture swab into the seminal vesicles allows culture for seminal vesiculitis (see p. 302).
- Secretions from the prostate gland, ampullae, and ductus deferens may be collected in the first jet of an ejaculate, using an open-ended artificial vagina.
- Infections of the epididymides or testes usually induce palpable changes, and the causative organism may be recoverable from the semen.

Viral genital infections

The two known viral venereal diseases in horses are:

- equine coital exanthema (equine herpesvirus 3)
  - Diagnosis is made by physical examination, which reveals characteristic blisters on the penile body and prepuce (see p. 307).
  - Similar lesions may be found on the external genitalia of exposed mares.
- equine viral arteritis (EVA)
  - Infected stallions can remain long-term asymptomatic carriers, with virus sequestration in the genital tract and shedding in the semen.
  - Diagnosis is based on virus isolation from ejaculated semen or on development of serum neutralization antibodies in seronegative mares that were bred to the suspect stallion.

OBSERVATION OF LIBIDO AND MATING ABILITY

The ability of a stallion to copulate normally should be assessed before the horse is considered a satisfactory breeding prospect. Sexual behavior can be analyzed by exposing the stallion to a mare in estrus. Typically, a stallion with good libido shows immediate and intense desire for the mare.

ANCILLARY AIDS TO EXAMINATION

Semen Collection

Accurate assessment of semen quality relies on proper semen collection techniques (discussed in *Equine Medicine and Surgery V*). Once semen is collected, it should be promptly taken to a laboratory, avoiding injury to spermatozoa induced by sunlight, temperature shock, agitation, and chemicals.

Semen Evaluation

No single semen characteristic has an absolute correlation to fertility. Routine tests are described below. More involved tests that may be indicated in selected cases include chemical analysis of semen plasma and electron microscopic study of spermatozoal ultrastructure (see *Equine Medicine and Surgery V*).

Gross evaluation

Volumes of gel and gel-free semen are measured, and the color and consistency are noted.

- The average volume of an ejaculate is 60 to 70 mL (range, 20 to 250 mL)
  - Ejaculate volume varies among stallions and is affected by frequency of ejaculation, intensity and length of precopulatory. sexual stimulation, and season.
  - The actual volume is not important to fertility, but is necessary to calculate the total sperm numbers in the ejaculate (see below).
- Gross evaluation provides a rough estimate of sperm concentration and permits detection of color changes that may be associated with blood, urine, or purulent material.

Sperm concentration

The total sperm number in an ejaculate is one of the more important measurements used in estimating a stallion's fertility.

- It is derived by multiplying sperm concentration and semen volume.
  - Sperm concentration of the gel-free semen can be determined using a hemacytometer, but use of a spectrophotometer or densimeter is faster.
- Sperm concentration in ejaculated semen averages 120 to 180 million sperm/mL (range, 20 to 600 million/mL); it is inversely proportional to ejaculate volume.
- Total sperm number is subject to seasonal variation and is affected by frequency of ejaculation, age, testicular size, and various reproductive diseases.

pH

The pH of gel-free semen should be determined using a properly calibrated pH meter, preferably within an hour after semen collection.

- The pH of normal semen ranges from 7.2 to 7.7, depending on the season, frequency of ejaculation, and spermatozoal concentration.
  - It increases with successive ejaculates and during the nonbreeding season.
- Abnormally high semen pH can be associated with contamination of the ejaculate by urine or soap or

with inflammatory lesions of the internal genital tract.

Spermatozoal motility

Spermatozoal motility reflects the viability of the sperm population. Subjective analysis can be made by visual evaluation, using a microscope with phase-contrast optics and a heated stage. Visual assessment of sperm motility should include:

- gross or total motility (percentage of progressively motile and nonprogressive motile sperm)
- progressive motility (percentage of progressively motile sperm)
- spermatozoal velocity (on an arbitrary scale of 0 to 4)

Both *initial* motility and *longevity* of motility should be assessed and recorded. It is best to estimate initial spermatozoal motility of raw (undiluted) semen samples as a control for testing possible ill effects of seminal extenders on sperm motility. Longevity of spermatozoal motility can be determined on raw semen samples stored at room temperature (20° to 25° C [68° to 77° F]) and on samples diluted in extender and stored at room temperature or refrigerated (4° to 5° C [39° to 41° F]). Assessment of longevity is important if the stallion owner anticipates breeding mares with cooled transported semen.

Spermatozoal morphology

Spermatozoa are less susceptible to artifactual changes in morphology than in motility, so assessment of spermatozoal morphology is an integral part of a fertility evaluation. Spermatozoal structure typically is examined using a light microscope at ×1000 magnification.

- Several staining techniques have been described.
  - Specific sperm stains include those developed by Williams and Casarett.
  - General-purpose cellular stains (e.g., Wright's, Giemsa, hematoxylin-eosin) are used to accent both germinal and somatic cells in semen smears.
  - Background stains (eosin-nigrosin, India ink) are widely used because of their ease of use.
- Structural detail of the sperm can be enhanced by fixing the cells in buffered formol-saline or buffered glutaraldehyde solution, then viewing the unstained cells as a wet mount.
  - Artifactual changes are minimized in comparison with those of stained smears.
- At least 200 spermatozoa should be evaluated, and the type and incidence of each defect recorded.
  - The current trend is to record the numbers of specific morphologic defects, such as knobbed acrosomes, proximal protoplasmic droplets, swollen midpieces, and coiled tails.

Because some stallions may have normal fertility despite sperm abnormalities, the total number of morphologically *normal* sperm in the ejaculate may provide more information regarding the stallion's fertility than does the percentage or absolute number of morphologically *abnormal* sperm.

Diagnostic Imaging

Various diagnostic imaging techniques may be used in selected cases.

- *Urethral endoscopy* generally is reserved for use in stallions with hemospermia or those with suspected urethral or bladder lesions.
- *Ultrasonography* allows precise testicular measurements, and assessment of testicular masses, scrotal fluid accumulation, the cavernous spaces of the penis, and the accessory genital glands; it also allows abdominal exploration for an intraabdominal testis.
- *Contrast radiography* can be used to evaluate the patency of the urethra and ductus deferens and to examine the corpus cavernosum penis (e.g., in stallions with chronic penile paralysis).

Other Diagnostic Tools

Karyotype studies permit detection of numeric and structural changes in chromosome composition that could affect reproductive performance. Hormone assays can be difficult to interpret in stallions, although cryptorchidism can be confirmed by measuring blood testosterone and estrogen concentrations (see p. 295).

Aspiration and Biopsy

Percutaneous aspiration of epididymal contents has been used to differentiate azoospermia resulting from aspermatogenesis from that associated with an ejaculatory disturbance. Likewise, testicular biopsy has been advocated by some clinicians for diagnosis of infertility in stallions. However, untoward sequelae of these procedures can include adhesions, sperm granulomas, and formation of antisperm antibodies.

Principles of Therapy

(pages 1006-1029)

Dickson D. Varner
and James Schumacher

MANAGEMENT OF THE BREEDING STALLION

Management of breeding stallions is discussed at length in *Equine Medicine and Surgery V*. Topics covered include feeding, exercise, immunization, and deworming programs, use of artificial lighting, estimating a stallion's book (determining the optimum number of mares to be bred to that stallion during the breeding season), natural service and artificial insemination programs, and semen collection, handling, and preservation. In addition, Table 12-1 provides recipes for various semen extenders.

Artificial Insemination

Following are some practical guidelines for maximizing stallion fertility when breeding mares by artificial insemination:

- The pregnancy rate of fertile stallions usually is maintained when mares are inseminated within 48 to 72 hours before ovulation.
  - Daily or twice-daily insemination until ovulation is detected may be required to enhance pregnancy rates of subfertile stallions.
  - Timing of ovulation and preparation of the mare are discussed in Chapter 13, Reproductive System: The Mare.
- The optimum number of sperm in a standard artificial insemination

dose is 500 million progressively motile sperm.
- In some stallions, this number can be reduced to 100 million without reducing fertility.
- The typical insemination volume of extended semen is 10 to 25 mL, although larger or smaller volumes can be used successfully.
- Cooled semen does not need to be warmed before insemination unless an extender is used that forms a gel when cooled (e.g., cream-gel extender).

CASTRATION TECHNIQUES

Surgical techniques for open, closed, and modified-closed castration are detailed in *Equine Medicine and Surgery V*. Following are some practical guidelines for preparation and aftercare:

- Before castration, the scrotal region should be closely inspected to document the presence of two normal scrotal testes and the absence of a scrotal or inguinal hernia.
- *Standing castration* should be reserved for well-mannered stallions with well-developed scrotal testes and no history of signs that suggest inguinal herniation.
  - If the testes cannot be easily and safely palpated within the scrotum, the horse should be anesthetized and castrated while in a recumbent position.
- The emasculator must be applied with the crushing portion toward the abdomen; that is, the wing nut of the emasculator is positioned toward the testis ("nut to nut").
  - The emasculator should be left in place for 30 to 60 seconds.
- Immediately before or after castration, both tetanus antitoxin and tetanus toxoid should be given to all horses not previously immunized with tetanus toxoid.
- A tetanus toxoid booster should be given to previously immunized horses if >1 year has passed since it was previously vaccinated.
- Prophylactic antibiotics generally are not required.
- The horse should be confined to a clean stall for the first 24 hours

after surgery; thereafter, it should be exercised twice daily for 2 weeks.

Postoperative Complications

Excessive hemorrhage

Hemorrhage is the most common immediate postoperative complication of castration and often is caused by an improperly applied or malfunctioning emasculator.

* If blood flow does not diminish within 20 to 30 minutes, the severed end of the cord can be grasped with the fingers and stretched, and a crushing forceps, ligature, or emasculator can be applied.
* If the end of the severed spermatic cord is inaccessible, sterile gauze rolls can be packed tightly through the scrotal incision into the inguinal and scrotal cavities.
  * The skin incision is closed with closely placed sutures or towel clamps.
  * The pack can be removed the following day; if hemorrhage continues, the horse must be anesthetized and the hemorrhaging vessel(s) ligated.
* 10 to 15 mL of 10% formalin in 1 L of 0.9% saline solution IV may promote hemostasis.

Preputial/scrotal swelling

Swelling of the prepuce and scrotum is expected following castration and, unless excessive, is no cause for alarm.

* Manual massage of the swollen tissue is beneficial, if the horse will tolerate it.
* If the castration wound seals prematurely, it should be opened by gentle massage or dilation with a gloved finger.
* Hydrotherapy may help prevent the wounds from resealing prematurely and may decrease edema in the scrotum and prepuce.
* Infection of the scrotal cavity usually can be resolved with local and systemic antibiotics, hydrotherapy, and establishment of proper scrotal drainage.

Clostridial infections of castration wounds are particularly catastrophic. Treatment consists of large doses of penicillin, NSAIDs, supportive therapy, and radical debridement of all necrotic tissue from the scrotal wound.

Septic funiculitis

Acute infection of the spermatic cord (funiculitis) can cause scrotal swelling, pain, and fever. Antimicrobial treatment, drainage, and hydrotherapy usually resolve the infection, but removal of the infected stump may be necessary.

Chronic infection of the spermatic cord ("scirrhous cord") often results in draining tracts from the cord to the scrotal skin. Palpation may cause only mild pain, and affected horses usually are afebrile. Surgical removal of the scirrhous cord usually results in uncomplicated recovery.

Septic peritonitis

Septic peritonitis is an uncommon complication of castration.

* Signs include fever, depression, weight loss, tachycardia, hemoconcentration, colic, and constipation or diarrhea.
* Development of any of these signs following castration may warrant collection of a peritoneal fluid sample.
  * Nucleated cell counts in peritoneal fluid >10,000/µL are common for at least 5 days after uncomplicated castration, and counts >100,000/µL occasionally are detected.
  * Thus, a diagnosis of septic peritonitis should not be based on a high cell count alone.
  * Degenerative neutrophils or intracellular bacteria in the peritoneal fluid are more indicative of peritoneal sepsis.

Management of septic peritonitis is discussed in Chapter 10, Alimentary System.

Hydrocele

A hydrocele (a slowly increasing collection of fluid within the vaginal cavity; may appear several months after castration as a circumscribed, fluid-filled, painless swelling in the scrotum. Hydroceles are uncommon after castration; the highest incidence is seen in mules. Surgical removal of the vaginal tunic is indicated.

Evisceration

Evisceration following castration of horses with normally descended testes is an uncommon but potentially fatal complication.

- It may occur up to 1 week after castration but usually happens within the first 4 hours.
- If intestine appears in the incision after castration, the horse should be anesthetized immediately.
  - IV fluids should be given in amounts adequate to combat hypotensive shock.
  - The horse should be positioned in dorsal recumbency and the intestine cleaned meticulously with copious amounts of sterile saline.
  - The prolapsed bowel must be reduced as soon as possible; it may be necessary to apply intraabdominal traction on the intestine through a paramedian or ventral midline celiotomy.
  - For castrations performed in the field, transport to a surgical facility is necessary if intestinal resection or peritoneal lavage seems indicated.
- Parenteral antimicrobial treatment should be initiated immediately.

OMENTAL PROLAPSE. Occasionally, a strand of omentum prolapses through the scrotal incision after castration. When this occurs, the vaginal ring should be palpated per rectum to determine whether there is any accompanying intestine protruding through the ring. Unless inguinal herniation is detected, the exposed omentum is removed with emasculators, usually with the horse standing, and the horse is confined for 48 hours.

Diseases Affecting Multiple Sites

(pages 1029-1034)

Dickson D. Varner
and James Schumacher

SEXUAL BEHAVIOR DYSFUNCTION
Lack of Libido

Reduced or absent libido in a mature stallion may be a response to a negative experience, such as a breeding accident, overuse, or punishment for sexual behavior. Review of the history should include evaluation of the stallion's social environ-ment, handling and training techniques, changes in environment, previous reproductive experiences, breeding procedures used, and time of onset and events surrounding the deviation in sexual behavior. Physical examination should include assessment of visual, olfactory, and auditory function and palpation of external genital organs.

Management

Patience, persistence, and positive reinforcement are indispensable elements of treatment for low libido in stallions. Specific recommendations are discussed in the text. Drug therapy is effective in some cases.

- Human chorionic gonadotropin and gonadotropin-releasing hormone have been used, but their long-term effects on spermatogenesis have not been firmly established.
  - Exogenous androgen administration is contraindicated.
- Slow IV infusion of diazepam (0.05 mg/kg, maximum dose of 20 mg) 10 minutes before breeding sometimes reverses sexual inhibition associated with a novel environment or a previous negative sexual experience.

Erection Failure

Inability to develop and maintain a normal penile erection may be a repercussion of suppressed libido, or it may result from an organic dysfunction, such as neuromuscular or vascular disease resulting from a breeding accident or other genital injury. Management must address these possibilities.

Mounting or Intromission Difficulty

Stallions with hind limb lameness, pelvic pain, or spinal lesions often are hesitant to mount, even though precopulatory behavior is quite intense. In others, penile injuries can lead to penile deviations during erection that impair intromission. Treatment should be directed at correction or attenuation of the underlying ailment, such as:

- administering NSAIDs
- reducing the number of mares the stallion is expected to breed during a season

♦ converting from natural service to
artificial insemination

Ejaculatory Dysfunction

Nonejaculatory coitus is relatively
common in breeding stallions and
often is manifested by normal or
heightened libido and normal copulatory behavior without corresponding ejaculation. Rhythmic
twitching of the tail or urethral pulsa-
tions may be observed despite lack of
ejaculation. Discharge of semen fluid
free of spermatozoa (azoospermia)
also may occur.

Causes and diagnosis

The cause often is difficult to establish. Diagnosis initially is directed at
differentiating psychogenic from organic causes.

♦ Psychogenic causes include abusive
handling, previous breeding accidents, an unfamiliar environment,
and sexual overuse.
♦ Organic causes include damage to
the dorsal nerve of the penis due to
penile trauma, and insufficient penile friction during mating (e.g., incomplete penile erection, inadequate copulatory thrusts,
pneumovagina).
♦ Occluded ejaculatory ducts or aspermatogenesis should be considered if normal copulatory efforts
end in sexual satiety.
  • These disorders often are associated with production of sperm-
  free ejaculates.

Managment

Management of suspected organic
ejaculatory dysfunction can take either physical or chemical forms, depending on the specific ailment.

♦ Azoospermia from occluded ejaculatory ducts sometimes can be corrected with repeated semen collection in conjunction with intermittent massage of the ampullae
per rectum.
  • Refractory cases have been corrected by deferent duct catheterization and flushing.
♦ Azoospermia resulting from aspermatogenesis may be temporary or
permanent.
  • Removal of inciting factors (e.g.,
  increased testicular temperature)

improves testicular function in
some cases.

♦ Pharmacologic manipulation of ejaculation has been attempted in horses
with disruption of the neural mechanisms that control semen emission.
  • L-Norepinephrine at 0.01 mg/kg
  IM 15 minutes before breeding induces contraction of musculature
  enveloping the deferent ducts and
  accessory genital glands.
  • This treatment can be combined
  with carazolol (a β-adrenergic
  blocker), at 0.015 mg/kg IM 10
  minutes before breeding, to improve the likelihood of semen
  emission.
  • This regimen is contraindicated
  in stallions with chronic obstructive pulmonary disease.
♦ Imipramine (a tricyclic antidepres-
sant) can also be effective in treating
ejaculatory failure in some stallions.

Aggressive Behavior

Excessive aggression in breeding stallions generally takes the form of
dominance/irritable aggression or
self-mutilation.

♦ Aggressiveness sometimes develops
in stallions experiencing ejaculatory
failure.
  • Treatment is directed at correcting the ejaculatory disturbance (discussed above).
♦ Stallions may exhibit similar behavioral patterns if they have
normal libido but cannot copulate
because of limb, pelvic, or spinal
cord problems.
♦ Short-term progestin therapy may
be indicated in the early retraining
period for stallions with aggressive
behavioral disorders.
♦ Daily exercise or full-time housing
in an outdoor paddock may eliminate or reduce self-mutilation, but
in some stallions physical restraint
is required.
  • Cross-ties, neck-cradles, side-poles,
  or muzzles may be necessary.
  • Progestins and diazepam may
  have some effect.
  • This neurosis often is a chronic
  problem, and, despite treatment
  efforts, few stallions revert to a
  normal tranquil state.

Diseases of the Scrotum

(pages 1034-1039)

Dickson D. Varner
and James Schumacher

CONGENITAL AND FAMILIAL DISEASES

Intersexuality

An intersex is an individual with disparities among genotype, phenotype, and gonadal sex caused by a defect in embryologic development. These horses can have a wide spectrum of physical appearance, behavior, and reproductive organ composition.

- **True hermaphrodites** have both ovarian and testicular tissue; the rest of the reproductive tract is intermediate between the two sexes.
  - This condition is uncommon in horses.
- **Male pseudohermaphrodites** have only male gonadal tissue; this is the most common form of intersexuality in horses.
  - Affected horses exhibit stallion-like behavior; phenotype is quite variable.
  - The testes usually are intraabdominal, inguinal, or subcutaneous, and the horse has no scrotal development.
  - There may be an underdeveloped penis that is directed caudally or a vulva containing an enlarged clitoris that resembles a glans penis.
  - Affected horses can have a 64,XX sex-chromosome complement, but mosaic karyotypes are more common.
- **Testicular feminization** is a specific type of male pseudo-hermaphroditism, characterized by an XY karyotype and female phenotype; these horses have abdominal testes, so psychosexual behavior is distinctly masculine.
- **Female pseudohermaphrodites** have only female gonadal tissue; this defect is rare in horses.
- **X-Y sex reversal** produces a phenotypic mare with female genitalia but a male (XY) karyotype; these horses have small, inactive ovaries and a hypoplastic tubular genital tract.

Tentative diagnosis of intersexuality is based on external and internal physical examination. Confirmation requires cytogenetic studies and documentation of gonadal sex.

DISEASES WITH PHYSICAL CAUSES

Scrotal Trauma

Scrotal trauma usually is associated with a breeding accident, such as a kick during mating. Resulting edema and inflammation, and subsequent fibrosis, can compromise spermatogenesis by altering testicular thermoregulation, so these injuries must receive prompt attention.

Diagnosis

Blunt scrotal injury usually can be diagnosed from the history and clinical findings, but the specific lesion often is difficult to identify.

- The scrotal surface should be thoroughly examined for injuries, including abrasions, lacerations, puncture wounds, and foreign bodies (e.g., thorns).
  - If the testes and epididymides are readily palpable, the scrotal swelling is not caused by edema and probably originates in the testis (i.e., orchitis).
- It sometimes is difficult to differentiate massive scrotal edema from hemorrhage of scrotal, spermatic cord, or testicular origin.
  - Needle aspiration of the affected scrotum helps make this distinction.
  - It is *essential* that the inguinal rings first be palpated to ensure that the scrotal swelling is not associated with a scrotal hernia.
  - Torsion of a spermatic cord should be included in the differential diagnosis of acute scrotal swelling.

Treatment

Treatment initially is aimed at controlling local inflammation, edema, and hematoma formation.

- Cryotherapy is the most important therapeutic method.
  - Cold, in the form of ice packs or immersion of the testicles in cold water, should be applied for up to 20 minutes, every 1 to 3 hours.

- Simultaneous gentle massage of the scrotum mechanically reduces edema.
- Cold water sprays are not recommended because they can cause further skin damage if the tissue has been compromised.
- Systemic antiinflammatory and diuretic medications are useful adjuncts to local therapy.
- Prophylactic antibiotic therapy should be instituted to control infection.
- A tetanus toxoid booster is recommended if the horse has not been vaccinated against tetanus within the past year.
- Emollients should be applied to the skin to protect against maceration.
- Management of scrotal lacerations should follow general principles of wound care (cleansing, debridement, irrigation, and primary closure if feasible).
  - Scrotal lacerations often fail to heal by first intention after surgical closure, but wound closure should be attempted if the testis is exposed.

Significant intrascrotal hemorrhage can result in fibrosis, which may permanently compromise testicular function. To save the compromised testis, surgical removal of the organized blood clot can be attempted 4 to 7 days after injury. If the hemorrhage was caused by a rent in the testicular capsule, unilateral castration is recommended to preserve normal thermoregulatory function in the other testis.

Prognosis
Unless fibrosis results in permanent impairment of testicular thermoregulation, semen quality generally is restored within 3 to 5 months of the injury.

Temperature-Induced Scrotal Edema
Some stallions develop scrotal edema during the hot summer months. Affected horses often respond to daily exercise and diuretic therapy. Hot weather also may induce a hydrocele (see p. 290).

Contact Dermatitis
Various chemicals, such as fly spray, disinfectants, and detergents, can cause scrotal inflammation and edema. Repeated scrotal contact with chemical irritants can produce chronic skin reactions, such as hyperkeratosis with fissure formation, that permanently interfere with testicular thermoregulation. Treatment involves preventing further contact with the irritant and suppressing local inflammation with cryotherapy and corticosteroids (systemic and/or topical). Systemic antibiotics are advised if secondary bacterial infection is present or imminent.

INFLAMMATORY, INFECTIOUS, AND IMMUNE DISEASES
Dourine
Dourine is a chronic systemic disease caused by the organism *Trypanosoma equiperdum*. The disease, presently eradicated from the United States, is transmitted venereally. Scrotal or preputial edema is a consistent manifestation in the early stages.

Scrotal Infection
Scrotal infections usually are a sequela to breaks in the protective scrotal skin (e.g., castration, scrotal lacerations, puncture wounds, blunt trauma).
- Aerobic and anaerobic bacterial cultures of these wounds are important for optimal care.
- General principles of wound care also should be followed, including removal of any foreign material, thorough debridement, irrigation, and establishment of drainage.
  - Puncture wounds should be examined meticulously for foreign bodies.
  - Ultrasonography can help identify foreign material.
- Systemic antibiotics should be initiated and continued for at least 5 days.
- Tetanus prophylaxis is essential.
- Extension of infection to a testis usually necessitates removal of that testis (see p. 289).

Other Causes of Scrotal Edema
Equine infectious anemia (EIA) and the acute phase of equine viral arteritis (EVA) can cause scrotal edema. These diseases are discussed in Chap-

ters 19, Hemolymphatic System. Scrotal edema may be seen with diseases that cause hypoproteinemia (and thus generalized edema), including protein-losing enteropathies, malnutrition, liver disease, and kidney disease. Local venous and/or lymphatic obstruction can also produce noninflammatory scrotal edema.

Diseases of the Testes
(pages 1039-1050)
Dickson D. Varner
and James Schumacher

CONGENITAL AND FAMILIAL DISEASES
Testicular Agenesis
Testicular agenesis, or anorchism, is rare in horses; to date only unilateral agenesis has been reported. Some horses with apparent testicular agenesis actually have a severely atretic testis (e.g., caused by spermatic cord torsion of an abdominal testis). Unilateral testicular agenesis may be associated with agenesis of ipsilateral structures, such as the ureter or kidney.

Cryptorchidism
Cryptorchidism is a condition in which one or both testes fail to descend into the scrotum. Retained testes are aspermic, but cryptorchid horses develop secondary sexual characteristics and male sexual behavior. Several reports suggest a genetic basis in horses. In descending order, the following breeds are most commonly affected: Percherons, Palominos, and Quarter Horses; cryptorchidism apparently is least prevalent in Thoroughbreds.
Location of the retained testis
Right and left testicular retention occurs with nearly equal frequency, but unilateral retention occurs about 9 times more often than bilateral retention. In horses, most retained left testes are located abdominally (75%) and most retained right testicles are located inguinally (60%). In ponies, a retained abdominal testis is equally likely to be found on the right side as on the left.

Diagnosis
Cryptorchidism is easily diagnosed if the horse's castration history is known. Horses purchased as geldings but displaying stallionlike behavior pose more of a diagnostic challenge.
- Examination of a suspect cryptorchid horse begins with palpation of the scrotal contents and superficial inguinal ring.
  - Sedation may relax the external cremaster muscles, making a subcutaneous or inguinal testis more accessible for palpation.
- The scrotum should be palpated and visually inspected for scar tissue that might indicate previous surgery.
  - However, a scrotal scar indicates only that an incision has been made, not that a testis has been removed.
- If external palpation fails to reveal both testes, palpation per rectum can be performed; it is difficult to locate an abdominal testis, but palpating the vaginal rings can be informative.
  - If the vaginal ring can be identified, the testis, or at least the epididymis, probably has descended.
  - In horses with complete abdominal testicular retention, the vaginal ring usually is difficult to identify.

HORMONE ASSAYS. When the castration history is incomplete and external and/or internal genital examinations are inconclusive, hormonal assays are of considerable diagnostic value.
- Comparison of plasma testosterone concentrations before and 30 to 120 minutes after IV injection of hCG (5000 to 12,000 IU) can distinguish cryptorchids from geldings.
  - Prestimulation (baseline) testosterone <40 pg/mL indicates the absence of testicular tissue, and values >100 pg/mL indicate its presence.
  - Paired samples (before and after stimulation) are necessary to distinguish geldings with relatively high basal testosterone from cryptorchids with relatively low concentrations.
- Single-sample assays for conjugated estrogen are accurate for diagnosis

of cryptorchidism, except in horses <3 years of age and in donkeys.

- In geldings, plasma conjugated estrogen is markedly lower (<400 pg/mL) than that of cryptorchids and normal stallions.
- The HCG-stimulation test should be used for diagnosis of cryptorchidism in donkeys and horses <3 years of age.

Treatment

In horses with unilateral cryptorchidism, a search for the cryptorchid testis should precede removal of the descended testis. The retained testis can be removed via an inguinal, flank, paramedian, or parainguinal approach. Surgical techniques are described in *Equine Medicine and Surgery V*. Although a theoretical argument can be made for the administration of testosterone or hCG to stimylate testicular descent, there are no controlled studies to substantiate their use.

DISEASES WITH PHYSICAL CAUSES

Testicular Lacerations

Testicular lacerations generally result from a severe blow to the scrotum or from extensive scrotal laceration. Testicular lacerations without associated scrotal lacerations are manifested clinically as acute and pronounced scrotal enlargement. Definitive diagnosis generally requires surgical exploration.

Treatment

Unilateral castration often is the treatment of choice; removal of extravasated blood and primary skin closure are indicated to minimize interference with thermoregulation of the contralateral testis. Aseptic surgical technique is critical to healing.

Testicular Hematoma

Testicular hematomas are caused by extravasation of blood into the testis, usually as a result of blunt trauma or as a sequela to locally invasive testicular tumors or testicular biopsies. Considerable hemorrhage can result from rupture of testicular vessels, and the testis eventually becomes small and atrophic.

Diagnosis

Diagnosis based solely on physical findings is difficult. High-resolution ultrasonography is the most reliable diagnostic method. Recent intratesticular hemorrhage produces focal hypoechoic areas, whereas regional scar formation associated with previous hemorrhage causes increased echogenicity.

Treatment

Surgical intervention is of questionable benefit. If massive hematomas are present, hemicastration often is performed to preserve function in the contralateral testis.

Traumatic Orchitis

Blunt scrotal trauma can produce acute noninfectious orchitis, characterized by hot, tense, painful testes. Swelling of the affected testes may not be perceptible because of the nonexpansive tunica albuginea, although testicular and scrotal edema invariably are present. In severe cases or untreated horses, irreversible atrophy and fibrosis of the seminiferous epithelium usually occurs.

Treatment

Treatment is directed at counteracting local inflammation, as described for scrotal trauma. Sexual rest is indicated. Serial (monthly) measurements of testicular size and texture, as well as evaluation of semen quantity and quality, help in assessing the prognosis.

INFLAMMATORY, INFECTIOUS, AND IMMUNE DISEASES

Bacterial Orchitis

Bacterial orchitis is rare in stallions. Possible routes of infection include hematogenous spread, invasion via the inguinal canal secondary to infectious peritonitis, and, most commonly, penetrating wounds of the scrotum. Bacterial orchitis may be unilateral or bilateral, depending on the route and extent of infection.

Clinical signs and diagnosis

Affected testes are hot, tense, slightly swollen, and acutely painful; testicular enlargement is limited by the inelastic tunica albuginea. The testes remain freely movable within the scrotum, unless periorchitis also is present. Fever and scrotal edema are common. Marked testicular degeneration is the usual sequela, manifested by oligospermia or azoospermia and an eventual decrease in testicular size.

Treatment

Medical management includes:

* systemic antibiotic therapy effective against the causative organisms(s)
* NSAIDs and local cryotherapy
* treatment of associated problems, such as scrotal infection or infectious peritonitis

Despite treatment, bacterial orchitis often necessitates orchiectomy. Prompt excision of a unilaterally affected testis can minimize damage to the contralateral gonad.

Viral Orchitis

Orchitis may result from equine infectious anemia, equine viral arteritis, or influenza. These diseases are discussed in other chapters.

Parasitic Orchitis

Migrating larvae of the nematode, *Strongylus edentatus,* can produce focal inflammatory lesions in the testes and occasionally in other parts of the external genitalia. Most of these lesions probably are subclinical. Ivermectin eliminates the larvae.

Autoimmune Orchitis

Escape of germinal cells from the lumen of the seminiferous tubules produces a local granulomatous reaction. Possible causes include testicular lacerations, biopsies, neoplasms, trauma, or degeneration. The immune response to displaced sperm potentially can induce antisperm antibodies and local or widespread testicular degeneration.

TOXIC DISEASES
Anabolic Steroids

Testicular degeneration, decreased sperm production and quality, diminished testicular size, and increased aggression are the most obvious sequelae to anabolic steroid use in stallions. These effects are temporary in adult stallions, but effects on the prepubertal testis are unknown.

NEOPLASIA

Testicular neoplasia is uncommon in stallions. Primary testicular neoplasms occur more frequently than do secondary neoplasms. Germinal tumors, such as seminomas, teratomas, and embryonal carcinomas, are more common than Leydig cell tumors, Sertoli cell tumors, lipomas, fibromas, and leiomyomas. Metastasis of germinal tumors has been documented. Many tumor types, including seminomas, teratomas, Leydig cell tumors, and Sertoli cell tumors, have been associated with cryptorchidism in stallions.

Clinical signs and diagnosis

Clinical findings often are nonspecific.

* Testicular tumors usually are unilateral.
* Small tumors are not likely to be detectable by palpation alone, but as the neoplasm expands, testicular enlargement occurs.
* Usually, the testis remains freely movable within the scrotum.

Differential diagnoses include orchitis, periorchitis, hydrocele, testicular scrotal hematoma, and scrotal hernia.

* Ultrasonography is an important diagnostic tool.
* Palpation per rectum should be performed, especially if tumor dissemination is suspected.

Treatment

Prompt orchiectomy is the primary treatment for testicular neoplasms, regardless of type.

* Unilateral orchiectomy is recommended when only one testis is involved.
* The proximal end of the spermatic cord should be ligated before removal of the testis, and the affected testis should be handled minimally during the surgical procedure.
  * Radical spermatic cord removal is advised.
* Radical scrotal ablation should accompany orchiectomy if the tumor has invaded peritesticular tissues.
* Excision of adjacent lymphatic chains is indicated if metastatic sites are suspected.

MULTIFACTORIAL DISEASES
Testicular Hypoplasia

Testicular hypoplasia is relatively common in horses. It is characterized by incomplete gonadal development and must be differentiated from testicular degeneration or atrophy.

Causes

Testicular hypoplasia is thought to be congenital; both genetic and teratogenic causes are suspected. It occurs in association with cryptorchidism but also can occur in scrotal testes. Infections, intoxications, malnutrition, endocrinologic disturbances, irradiation, and other factors may precipitate testicular hypoplasia. The testes of male equine hybrids (mules or hinnies) typically are hypoplastic.

Clinical findings

♦ Testicular hypoplasia can be mild or severe, and can involve one or both testes.
♦ The testes may be soft, but eventually they become firm as connective tissue replaces the parenchyma.
♦ Depending on the severity, affected stallions are oligospermic or azoospermic.
  • There usually is a high incidence of spermatozoal morphologic defects and poor motility.
♦ Libido often is unaffected, and semen volume may be normal.

Diagnosis and treatment

Diagnosis can be difficult in stallions <3 years of age. The condition is indistinguishable from testicular degeneration by physical examination or histologic evaluation; the history is critical to differentiation of these two conditions. There is no known therapy.

Testicular Degeneration

The susceptibility of the germinal epithelium to damage makes testicular degeneration a major cause of infertility/subfertility in stallions. Testicular degeneration can affect one or both testes, depending on whether the causative factor is localized (e.g., a locally aggressive tumor) or generalized (e.g., fever). It can be temporary or permanent, depending on severity and duration of the insult.

Causes

Testicular degeneration has a multitude of causes, including:

♦ thermal injury (e.g., high environmental temperature, fever, orchitis/periorchitis, hydrocele, scrotal hemorrhage, edema, or dermatitis, and incomplete testicular descent)

♦ systemic and/or local infections
♦ injury to essential vasculature (e.g., torsion of the spermatic cord, inflammation of the testicular artery, degenerative changes in testicular arterioles)
♦ uncontrolled intratesticular hemorrhage
♦ hormonal disturbances, ionizing radiation, malnutrition, toxic plants, testicular tumors, efferent/epididymal duct obstruction, and production of antisperm antibodies
♦ advanced age (possibly)

Diagnosis

Diagnosis involves:

♦ a good history, which is essential for differentiating testicular degeneration from hypoplasia
♦ general and genital physical examinations
♦ specific evaluations of testicular size and consistency
  • Testes with only mild degenerative changes tend to be slightly small, with normal turgid or abnormal soft consistency.
  • Acutely affected testes have a soft, flabby consistency, whereas chronically affected testes become abnormally firm.
  • Severe degeneration results in a marked reduction in testicular size; the tunica albuginea often becomes wrinkled and has a corrugated texture.
  • With advanced testicular degeneration, the epididymis may feel disproportionately large.
♦ semen evaluation
  • Oligospermia or azoospermia usually is noted on semen evaluation, but libido and semen volume often are normal.

Treatment and prognosis

Testicular degeneration can be reversible.

♦ Treatment is directed at removing the factor(s) responsible for the degenerative changes.
♦ Chronic GnRH administration has been used to improve semen quality in aged stallions with suspected testicular degeneration.
♦ Periodic measurements of testicular size and consistency, and serial (monthly) evaluations of semen

quality help evaluate testicular improvement or deterioration.

◆ Complete restoration of normal spermatogenic function takes several months after removal of the causative factor.

• In many instances, the preinjury level of spermatogenic activity is never fully recovered.

Diseases of the Epididymis *(pages 1050-1052)*

Dickson D. Varner and James Schumacher

CONGENITAL AND FAMILIAL DISEASES

Epididymal Aplasia and Cysts

Epididymal aplasia is rare and epididymal cysts are uncommon in stallions. Uncomplicated cystic dilations usually do not interfere with transit of spermatozoa. But large epididymal cysts, detectable as circumscribed, fluctuant masses at the craniodorsal aspect of the testis, can become impacted with spermatozoa, leading to a local sperm granuloma.

DISEASES WITH PHYSICAL CAUSES

Epididymal Lacerations

Although rare, epididymal lacerations can occur along with severe trauma to the scrotum, even if the insult is nonpenetrating. If the lacerated epididymis is not removed surgically, extravasated spermatozoa are likely to produce a granulomatous reaction. This becomes recognizable when scrotal swelling associated with the scrotal injury has subsided. The most plausible treatment is unilateral castration, including removal of the epididymis.

INFLAMMATORY, INFECTIOUS, AND IMMUNE DISEASES

Infectious Epididymitis

Infectious epididymitis rarely occurs as a primary entity in stallions. More commonly, it is secondary to orchitis. Acute epididymitis results in severe pain and local swelling, usually in conjunction with fever. Treatment is similar to that of infectious orchitis (see p. 296).

Sperm Granulomas

Spermatozoa are antigenic and elicit a granulomatous reaction when they escape the seminiferous tubules or excurrent duct lumina and come in contact with stromal tissue. Epididymal sperm granulomas occur infrequently in stallions.

◆ Possible causes are varied, and include the following:

• parasitic migration (*Strongylus edentatus*)

• bacterial or traumatic epididymitis

• epididymal adenomyosis (outgrowth of the epithelial lining into the epididymal musculature)

• impaction of blind efferent ductules, aberrant ductules, or the appendix of the epididymis with spermatozoa

◆ In the acute phase, sperm granulomas exist as locally painful swellings, but they become indurated, painless masses with time.

• Obliteration of the epididymal lumen can occur and usually is permanent.

◆ There is no effective treatment.

IDIOPATHIC DISEASE

Spermiostasis

Some stallions have an impaired ability to emit epididymal and deferent ductal spermatozoa during sexual quiescence, even though they may ejaculate normally. As a result, spermatozoa abnormally accumulate in the epididymis and deferent ducts during sexual rest.

◆ Retained spermatozoa undergo senile degenerative changes, including reduced motility and head-tail separations.

◆ Semen samples have an unusually high spermatozoal concentration (600 to 1800×10^6/mL), but normal semen volume.

◆ Spermatozoa occasionally become impacted within the epididymal/deferent duct lumina to the point that they are not released even during ejaculation

- Serial ejaculations (e.g., 10 to 20 ejaculates over a 1- to 2-week period) usually are required to restore normal semen quality in these stallions.
- Relapse is likely if an affected stallion does not ejaculate regularly (3 to 4 times per week).

Diseases of the Tunica Vaginalis *(pages 1052-1055)*

Dickson D. Varner
and James Schumacher

MULTIFACTORIAL DISEASES

Hydrocele

A hydrocele is an abnormal collection of clear, serous fluid between the visceral and parietal layers of the tunica vaginalis. Usually, both sides of the scrotum are affected. Hydroceles may accompany either inflammatory or noninflammatory scrotal edema, but also can arise without scrotal edema. They have been known to occur in hot weather, resolving in the fall when the ambient temperature drops. The condition may be temporary or permanent.

Diagnosis

A hydrocele feels like a large, compressible, fluid-filled bag. Generally it is not painful, although marked distention of the vaginal cavities can cause discomfort. The testis and epididymis often are not palpable. Definitive diagnosis is based on aseptic needle aspiration of fluid.

Treatment

Treatment is aimed at removing the underlying cause, if it can be identified. Aspiration of the hydrocele(s) occasionally is effective, but often the fluid reaccumulates. Persistent hydrocele results in temperature-induced testicular/epididymal dysfunction.

Inguinal Herniation

An inguinal, or scrotal, hernia is a protrusion of abdominal viscera, usually small intestine, through the inguinal ring. Inguinal/scrotal hernias

in horses occur almost exclusively in intact males. Most are present at birth or develop soon after as a result of congenitally large vaginal rings. Inguinal or scrotal hernias also may result from trauma, such as a fall, or develop following breeding or exercise. There is a higher incidence in Standardbreds.

Congenital hernias

Congenital hernias usually are of the scrotal type and appear soon after birth as a viscera-filled scrotum.

- The condition may be unilateral or bilateral.
- These hernias can easily be manually reduced into the abdomen, and most show no tendency to incarcerate; the hernia usually resolves spontaneously over 3 to 6 months.
- Typically, congenital inguinal hernias cause no problems; however, if long-standing, testicular hypoplasia/atrophy or adhesions between the testicle, viscera, and vaginal tunic may occur.
  - Occasionally, the intestine becomes strangulated, requiring surgical reduction.
  - Some congenital inguinal hernias become apparent only after castration, when the hernial contents eventrate through the scrotal incision.

  MANAGEMENT. Treatment in young foals generally is not required. In the absence of abdominal pain or gross enlargement of the scrotum, only close observation of the colt is necessary. Conservative therapy, when indicated, comprises:

- manual reduction of the herniated viscera several times daily
- application of a "foal diaper" to correct persistent hernias
  - The foal is sedated and placed in dorsal recumbency.
  - The hernia is completely reduced, and the external inguinal rings are packed with cotton pledgets, which are covered by an elastic bandage applied in a figure-8 fashion over both inguinal rings.
  - Care should be taken to prevent occlusion of the anus or

preputial orifice and compression of the penis.

- The bandage can be left in place for up to a week, although the superficial inguinal rings should be palpated under the bandage each day to ensure that herniation has not recurred.

♦ Surgical intervention is indicated only as a last resort, particularly if the foal has a potential career as a breeding stallion, although it is necessary if intestinal incarceration has occurred.

Acquired hernias

Acquired inguinal/scrotal hernias occur most commonly in adult horses and usually are accompanied by acute abdominal pain.

- The possibility of an inguinal or scrotal hernia should be considered in all stallions exhibiting abdominal pain.
- The scrotum on the affected side usually is enlarged.
- Examination per rectum reveals viscera entering the vaginal ring.

MANAGEMENT. Most acquired inguinal/scrotal hernias require immediate treatment to avoid irreversible vascular damage to the hernial contents.

- Reduction of the hernia by external massage may be successful, particularly if herniation is diagnosed soon after the onset of clinical signs.
- If external reduction fails, retraction of the entrapped viscera per rectum may be attempted.
  - Sedation and epidural anesthesia are required; an alternative is general anesthesia with the horse's hindquarters raised.
- Nonsurgical reduction does not permit assessment of the hernial contents, so the horse should be closely observed for several days after reduction for signs of intestinal infarction.
- Surgical reduction of the hernia is indicated if manual reduction fails, if there is evidence of enlarged or damaged vaginal rings, or if infarction of the entrapped viscera is suspected.
- Surgical techniques are discussed in *Equine Medicine and Surgery V.*

Diseases of the Spermatic Cord

(pages 1055-1057)

*Dickson D. Varner
and James Schumacher*

INFLAMMATORY, INFECTIOUS, AND IMMUNE DISEASES

Funiculitis

Funiculitis (inflammation of the spermatic cord) generally occurs following castration; trauma, parasite migration (*S. edentatus* larvae), and generalized infections are other possible causes. Management of funiculitis is discussed in the section on postoperative complications of castration.

IDIOPATHIC DISEASES

Torsion of the Spermatic Cord

Torsion of the spermatic cord (rotation or twisting of the cord about its long axis) is occasionally observed in stallions. Torsion may be unilateral or bilateral, and can be transient or permanent.

180-Degree torsion

With 180-degree torsions, the cauda epididymis and scrotal ligament are located cranially within the scrotum, rather than being in their normal caudal position.

- The scrotal ligament is readily palpable and serves as an excellent landmark for identification of the cauda epididymis.
- In most instances, 180-degree torsions are subclinical and found incidentally.
  - Infrequently, affected stallions display mild, intermittent scrotal pain that becomes most pronounced during athletic activity.
- The consensus is that spermatic cord torsions up to 180 degrees do not produce local circulatory disturbances and so are considered of minor consequence.
  - Treatment generally is unnecessary, although orchiopexy may be warranted in some cases (see *Equine Medicine and Surgery V*).

360-Degree torsion

With 360-degree torsion, the scrotal ligament and cauda epididymis are in their proper caudal positions, but occlusion of the arterial supply results in ischemic necrosis of the scrotal contents.

♦ Findings include acute, severe testicular pain and scrotal enlargement.
  • The spermatic cord is thickened and firm, and the attached testis may be enlarged; both structures may be pulled dorsally in the scrotum.
  • Palpation of scrotal contents becomes difficult as scrotal edema and swelling progress.
  • Unrelenting colic and a stilted gait may also be evident.
♦ A primary differential diagnosis is inguinal/scrotal herniation.
  • Examination of the suspect vaginal ring per rectum helps differentiate these conditions.
  • Other considerations are scrotal trauma, orchitis/periorchitis, testicular neoplasia, varicocele formation, and thrombosis of spermatic cord vasculature.
♦ Typically, this type of torsion is unilateral and permanent, although temporary torsions are possible and recurrent episodes may occur.

A 360-degree spermatic cord torsion is considered a surgical emergency. Unilateral castration generally is recommended because the affected testis rarely is salvageable and antibodies against sperm liberated from the ischemic testis may permanently damage the contralateral testis. Early diagnosis and treatment are imperative if the affected testis is to be saved.

Varicocele

The term *varicocele* describes abnormally distended and tortuous veins of the pampiniform plexus. Diagnosis is based on palpation of the characteristic "bag of worms" texture within the spermatic cord, created by the dilated, tortuous vessels. Varicoceles are uncommon findings, and their relationship to fertility has not been critically studied in stallions. It is speculated that varicoceles could compromise testicular thermoregulation, although unilateral varicosities have been re-

ported in stallions with normal spermatozoal quality and quantity.

Thrombosis of Spermatic Cord Vessels

Thrombosis of vessels within the spermatic cord is rare in stallions. Verminous migration and previous spermatic cord torsion are possible causes. Clinical signs resemble those of 360-degree spermatic cord torsion. Definitive diagnosis is made during exploratory surgery. Unilateral castration is the only viable treatment.

Diseases of the Accessory Genital Glands *(pages 1057-1059)*

Dickson D. Varner
and James Schumacher

INFLAMMATORY, INFECTIOUS, AND IMMUNE DISEASES

Bacterial Infections

Bacterial infections of the accessory genital glands are uncommon in stallions. Causative bacteria include *Pseudomonas aeruginosa, Klebsiella pneumoniae, Streptococcus* spp, *Staphylococcus* spp, and *Brucella abortus*. The vesicular glands are the most frequently involved sites.

Clinical findings

Clinical manifestations are varied.
♦ Acute infections may cause reluctance to breed or ejaculate or cause pain during ejaculation.
♦ More often, the stallions exhibit normal breeding behavior, and signs of accessory genital gland infection are not clinically evident.
♦ Examination of the accessory genital glands via rectal palpation is indicated.
  • Infected vesicular glands are enlarged and firm, occasionally with a lobulated texture and irregular borders.
  • In the acute stages, signs of pain are elicited by palpation.
  • Unilateral or bilateral involvement is possible.

Sample collection techniques

Localization of an infection to a specific accessory genital gland often is difficult. Culture and cytologic examination of accessory gland fluid aid diagnosis. Techniques for sample collection are outlined below (and discussed in more detail in *Equine Medicine and Surgery V*).

* **seminal vesicles**
  * The stallion is sexually stimulated, and the penis is washed with surgical scrub.
  * A sterile 100-cm rubber catheter with an inflatable cuff is passed into the urethra until the tip is adjacent to the orifices of the ejaculatory ducts (palpable per rectum).
  * The cuff is inflated and fluid in the suspect vesicular gland is expressed by manual compression of the gland per rectum.
  * Passage of a small catheter or culture swab into the seminal vesicles, by threading the device through the biopsy port of a pediatric endoscope, is a more current technique.
* **bulbourethral glands**
  * The glans penis is rubbed briskly while the stallion remains in close proximity to a mare exhibiting behavioral estrus.
  * This stimulates release of clear preejaculatory fluid from the bulbourethral glands because the fluid is contaminated by contents of the urethral lumen, bacterial urethritis is difficult to distinguish from infection of the bulbourethral glands.
* **prostate glands or ampullae**
  * Selective fluid collection from the prostate gland or ampullae alone is not possible.
  * Semen collection using an open-ended artificial vagina may allow detection of prostate gland, ampullae, and deferent duct infection (see *Equine Medicine and Surgery V*).

Ejaculates from stallions with accessory genital gland infections contain numerous neutrophils, bacteria, and red blood cells. Air-dried semen smears can be stained with Giemsa, Wright's, or hematoxylin-eosin stains to differentiate inflammatory cells from round primordial germ cells prematurely released from the seminiferous epithelium. Gram stain aids identification of the causative organism(s).

Treatment and prognosis

Bacterial infections of the accessory genital glands usually cause infertility, and transmission of the bacteria to the mare during natural mating is unavoidable. Treatment of bacterial infections involving accessory genital glands, although often unsuccessful, is described below.

* Trimethoprim-sulfamethoxazole may be the best antibacterial for systemic treatment if the causative organism is susceptible to it.
  * Most other antibacterial drugs do not achieve therapeutic concentrations in the accessory genital glands when given systemically.
* Other antibacterial drugs may be effective when instilled into the gland lumina using a small-diameter catheter passed through the urethral opening of each gland (see *Equine Medicine and Surgery V*).
* If treatment is unsuccessful but fertility has been maintained, venereal transmission of bacteria is avoided by using a minimum-contamination breeding technique.
  * Semen is collected using an artificial vagina, then placed in semen extender containing an appropriate antibacterial drug before artificial insemination.
  * If the stallion is to breed by natural service, 100 mL of semen extender containing appropriate antibacterial drugs are infused into the mare's uterus before natural service.
  * It may be advantageous to irrigate the mare's uterus with physiologic saline for 2 consecutive days after ovulation and instill antibacterial drugs after each irrigation.

Diseases of the Urethra
(pages 1059-1061)
Dickson D. Varner
and James Schumacher

DISEASES WITH PHYSICAL CAUSES
Urethral Trauma

Penetrating or blunt trauma to the penis can result in urethral laceration or rupture. Ischial injuries can produce similar urethral lesions. Other causes of urethral trauma include stallion rings, urethral calculi, and improper or repeated urethral catheterization or urethroscopy.

Diagnosis

Diagnosis of urethral trauma begins with close inspection of the penile/perineal integument; penetrating wounds should be thoroughly explored. Urethral endoscopy allows definitive diagnosis of urethral lesions. The patency of the penile urethra and integrity of the wall can also be assessed with retrograde urethrograms. Ultrasonography is useful for locating lodged urethral calculi.

Treatment

Therapeutic measures depend on the form of urethral injury.

- Sexual rest (at least 2 months) is indicated to allow urethral healing to be completed.
- Curettage, in conjunction with local urethral dilation, can be used to treat strictures, prolapsed urethral vessels, and proliferative granulation tissue.
- Iatrogenic injury to the urethral wall generally resolves without complications or special therapeutic measures.
- Calculi lodged within the urethral lumen can be removed via urethrotomy (see *Equine Medicine and Surgery V*).
- Rents or lacerations of the urethral wall that communicate with the adjacent corpus spongiosum penis often heal poorly.
- Ischial urethrotomy in conjunction with prolonged sexual rest facilitates healing in these cases (see *Equine Medicine and Surgery V*).

INFLAMMATORY, INFECTIOUS, AND IMMUNE DISEASES

Bacterial Urethritis

Bacterial urethritis is uncommon in horses. It occurs as a primary disease, or as a sequela to infectious cystitis, accessory genital gland infection, or local injury. Diagnosis is based on isolation of the causative organism from urethral swabs. Urethral endoscopy permits direct visual examination of the mucosal lining for evidence of inflammatory changes.

Treatment

Bacterial urethritis usually responds to systemic antibiotic therapy in conjunction with instillation of nonirritating antibiotics into the urethral lumen. Sexual rest (at least 2 weeks) is mandatory. Underlying conditions, such as cystitis or penetrating wounds, also must be managed properly. Posttreatment urethral cultures are required to ensure elimination of the infection.

Protozoal Urethritis

Dourine (see p. 294) may be manifested as urethritis, with a mucopurulent urethral discharge, early in the disease. Tentative diagnosis is based on clinical signs. Confirmation requires demonstration of the organism or serologic testing.

TOXIC DISEASE

Cantharidin Intoxication

Cystitis/urethritis are common manifestations of cantharidin ("blister beetle") toxicosis. Frequent urination, dysuria, and hematuria may be seen (see Chapter 10, Alimentary System).

Diseases of the Penis

(pages 1061-1075)

Dickson D. Varner
and James Schumacher

DIAGNOSTIC AND THERAPEUTIC CONSIDERATIONS

Phimosis

Phimosis is inability of the penis to protrude from the prepuce as a consequence of preputial injury or disease. It is discussed in the section on diseases of the prepuce.

Paraphimosis

Paraphimosis refers to inability to retract the penis into the prepuce. Paraphimosis often follows acute preputial trauma and resulting edema, but it can also develop as an aftermath of protracted penile prolapse, as with penile paralysis or priapism (see below). Regardless of the cause, inability to retract the penis causes impaired venous and lymphatic drainage and, within hours, edematous swelling of the penis and prepuce. Without proper treatment, the process becomes self-perpetuating, and gangrenous changes of the penile tissue can result.

Treatment

The first consideration is to support the penis and reduce gravitational edema.

* If possible, the penis should be replaced within the preputial cavity and retained there with towel clamps or a purse-string retention suture.
* The penis also can be kept within the preputial cavity with a retention device fabricated from a 500-mL narrow-neck plastic bottle and rubber tubing or gauze bandages (see *Equine Medicine and Surgery V*).
* The penis should be removed from the preputial cavity at least twice daily for examination and topical application of medication and emollients.
  * If the integument has been damaged, local and systemic antibacterial therapy is indicated, as well as judicious use of diuretics and NSAIDs.
* In acute cases, penile/preputial edema usually can be relieved by gentle massage with emollients, cold therapy (see p. 290), and the supportive measures described above.
  * Temporarily wrapping rubber or pneumatic bandages around the penis hastens reduction of edema in pronounced or refractory cases.
* If the penis cannot be placed or retained within the preputial cavity, it should be supported against the ventral abdominal wall with abdominal wraps.
* Once the penis is adequately supported, the horse should be exercised regularly to promote local venous and lymphatic drainage.

Extensive preputial fibrosis may necessitate resection of the scar tissue by elliptic incision or circumcision. If unresponsive penile paralysis or priapism is responsible for the paraphimosis, surgical retraction of the penis or amputation may be required (see below).

Penile Paralysis and Priapism

The terms *penile paralysis* and *priapism* often are used interchangeably to describe a pathologically prolonged erection not associated with sexual desire and caused by failure of the detumescence mechanism(s). Initially, penile paralysis/priapism is characterized by an erection of varying rigidity not associated with edema or other clinically detectable genital lesions. If the erection does not subside within a few hours, penile and preputial swelling ensue, and the penis undergoes progressive necrotic changes.

Causes

Penile paralysis/priapism is a relatively common disorder with a multitude of causes, including:

* phenothiazine tranquilizers—probably responsible for most cases
* viral diseases (e.g., rhinopneumonitis, rabies)
* other infectious diseases (e.g., strangles, dourine)
* debilitation, starvation, exhaustion
* spinal injuries and penile injuries

In many patients, the cause cannot be identified.

Medical treatment

Medical management consists of:

* penile massage
* application of slings to support the penis
* diuretic administration
* possibly ganglionic blockage (e.g., benztropine mesylate at 8 mg IV)

If medical management is unsuccessful within the first few hours after penile paralysis/priapism, the horse should be anesthetized and the corpus cavernosum penis flushed with heparinized saline to evacuate the sludged blood (see *Equine Medicine and Surgery V*). However, nonsurgical treatment generally is ineffective if the collecting veins are occluded.

Surgical treatment

Surgical management is indicated if conservative therapy does not restore venous outflow. Creation of a venous shunt is recommended in horses that fail to respond to medical therapy or to three sessions of irrigation of the corpus cavernosum. Refractory cases require phallopexy (permanent penile retraction) or partial phallectomy (penile amputation).

- Phallopexy (Bolz operation) is the more conservative of the two procedures, but surgical candidates must meet the following qualifications.
  - The penis must be capable of being fully retracted into the prepucial cavity.
  - Inflammation/infection of the penis and prepuce must be controlled before surgery.
  - Castration must be performed within a reasonable time after phallopexy; preferably, the horse should be castrated several weeks before surgery.
  - The horse should not be allowed exposure to mares after surgery for several weeks.
- Partial phallectomy is reserved for horses with intractable paraphimosis, extensive penile injury, or serious penile disease such as squamous cell carcinoma.
- Surgical techniques are described in *Equine Medicine and Surgery V.*

Prognosis

Following damage to the corporeal tissue, the prognosis for return to normal reproductive function is quite bleak. However, some stallions can impregnate mares successfully even though the penis does not become rigid when fully engorged. These stallions require assistance with intromission. Repeated breeding attempts may encourage recanalization of damaged cavernous tissue.

DISEASES WITH PHYSICAL CAUSES

Lacerations/Abrasions

Lacerations, contusions, and abrasions of the penis generally occur when the penis is erect. Kicks from a nonreceptive mare, and lacerations from the mare's tail hair or an improperly placed "breeding stitch" in the mare's vulva are common causes of penile injury during intromission.

Treatment

Prompt and appropriate therapy is the key to successful treatment of penile injuries. Initial treatment is directed at controlling acute inflammation and edema.

- As described for scrotal trauma, cold therapy, massage, antiinflammatory and diuretic medications, antibiotic therapy, and tetanus prophylaxis are important.

- Returning the prolapsed penis to its normal detumescent position within the preputial cavity is critical to prevention of penile paralysis and/or paraphimosis.

Superficial penile lacerations heal remarkably well as open wounds if local infection and edema are controlled and sexual rest is enforced until healing is complete. Debridement and suturing are recommended for deep lacerations, especially those that penetrate the urethral wall. Severe penile injury may necessitate amputation.

Stallion Ring–Induced Ischemic Necrosis

Stallion rings are nonexpansive bands that are placed immediately proximal to the glans penis to discourage masturbation in breeding stallions. Tightly fitting rings or prolonged applications compress the underlying penile and urethral tissue, leading to ischemic necrosis and constricting fibrosis. Such injury often results in urethral strictures or erection failure. In most instances, the regenerative capacity of the urethra is remarkably good; but repair of damaged erectile tissue is difficult. Corrective measures involve repeated sexual stimulation to encourage erection and reestablish patency of the constricted sinusoidal spaces.

Rupture of the Penile Suspensory Ligaments

The paired suspensory ligaments of the penis attach the proximal shaft to the ventral pelvis. Rupture of this suspensory apparatus is rare. The affected penis develops a characteristic ventral bow proximal to the prepuce. Surgical repair has not been reported.

Penile Hematoma

Penile hematomas usually result from blunt trauma to the erect penis during breeding. In many instances, the swelling becomes so pronounced that the penis can no longer be retracted; progressive preputial edema also develops. For this reason, paraphimosis is a common sequel to untreated penile hematomas.

Treatment

Treatment is directed at countering penile swelling and preventing paraphimosis.

◆ Efforts are made to reduce the swelling sufficiently so that the penis can be replaced within the preputial cavity.

- Initially, compression bandages are applied to the penis to reduce hemorrhage.
- Cold therapy and systemic anti-inflammatory and diuretic medications also are indicated.

◆ Once the acute phase of the injury has subsided and the penis can be retracted voluntarily, efforts should be made to minimize formation of fibrous tissue.

- Daily penile massage with emollients is recommended to maintain tissue pliability.

◆ 3 weeks after injury, the stallion should be exposed to an estrous mare to evaluate the integrity of the penis during erection.

- Penile deviations should be treated by daily manipulation of the erect penis, pulling the penis back into its normal position to override the restriction caused by scar tissue.

Smegma Accumulation

Secretions of the preputial sebaceous and sweat glands combine with dirt and desquamated epithelial cells to form a gray-black, caseous, foul-smelling, and often puttylike substance termed *smegma*. If penile hygiene is ignored, excessive amounts of smegma collect on the prepuce and penis, occasionally becoming impacted within the recesses of the fossa glandis and producing low-grade balanoposthitis. Abnormally large accumulations of smegma may cause discomfort during urination or, possibly, ejaculation. The penis and prepuce of geldings and stallions should be cleansed occasionally, using warm water. Use of soaps is discouraged.

INFLAMMATORY, INFECTIOUS, AND IMMUNE DISEASES

Coital Exanthema

Coital exanthema is a venereal disease of horses caused by equine herpesvirus 3 (EHV-3). Lesions generally are confined to the external genitalia of stallions and mares. The penis and prepuce are the most commonly affected areas in stallions.

◆ Lesions begin as small (5 to 15 mm), white-gray, discrete, circumscribed vesicles or pustules that often become confluent.

- Within a few days, the vesicles rupture to form superficial ulcers.
- Although an uncommon occurrence, infected horses can develop transient fever and lethargy.

◆ Clinical disease typically is self-limiting, with complete resolution occurring in 3 to 5 weeks.

- Focal areas of depigmentation may remain.

◆ Treatment consists of sexual rest and daily applications of protective emollients.

- Sexual rest should be enforced until genital lesions are completely healed.
- Secondary bacterial infection is a rare complicating factor.

Contagious Equine Metritis

Contagious equine metritis (CEM) is a highly contagious bacterial disease caused by *Taylorella equigenitalis* (see Chapter 13, Reproductive System: The Mare). Horizontal transmission primarily occurs via coitus. In marked contrast to mares, stallions never become clinically infected; rather, they serve as asymptomatic carriers of the organism. If untreated, *Taylorella equigenitalis* can persist on the surface of the penis and prepuce indefinitely.

Diagnosis

Diagnosis of CEM is especially difficult in stallions because clinical signs are absent and superficial contamination of the external genitalia does not stimulate a humoral response. Confirmation of the disease in stallions usually is based on bacterial isolation from the external genitalia.

◆ Culture swabs are obtained from the urethral sinus (within the fossa glandis), urethra, penile skin, and preputial folds.

◆ Preejaculatory fluid should be collected for bacteriologic culture, if possible.

◆ All swabs must be separately placed in Amies' transport medium, then shipped to an appropriate diagnostic laboratory within 24 hours.

- Samples should be cooled (4° C [39° F]), but not frozen, during shipment.

To overcome the problems of laboratory isolation of this fastidious organism, suspect stallions can be bred to test mares, or smegma from the urethral fossa can be inoculated into the uterus of selected mares, which are then evaluated for disease transmission. If CEM is suspected, federal veterinarians must be contacted immediately.

Treatment

Treatment of infected stallions has been quite successful.

* The extruded penis and prepuce are thoroughly washed for 5 minutes each day with 2% chlorhexidine solution (Nolvasan) for 5 consecutive days.
  * Particular attention is given to cleansing the recesses of the fossa glandis.
* Following each cleansing session, the penis and prepuce are dried and liberally coated with nitrofurazone ointment.

Bacterial Colonization

The normal microflora of the stallion's external genitalia rarely produce genital infection in immunologically competent mares. Occasionally, the normal flora is disrupted, and potentially pathogenic bacteria colonize the penis and prepuce. Although these organisms rarely produce clinical disease in stallions, they can be transmitted to the mare's genital tract at breeding, causing infectious endometritis and associated infertility. *Pseudomonas aeruginosa* and *Klebsiella pneumoniae* are the most common venereal pathogens.

Diagnosis

Pathogenic bacterial colonization of a stallion's external genitalia is suspected if postcoital endometritis and infertility are noted in a high percentage of mares bred. Bacteriologic culture of the fossa glandis, penile body, and external folds of the prepuce provides an overall perspective of the microbial population. However, interpretation of the findings can be difficult. When this problem is suspected, the most reliable approach is to test breed the stallion to suitable maiden mares.

Treatment

Once a stallion's penis becomes colonized with pathogenic bacteria, it is very difficult to reestablish the normal bacterial microflora. If the stallion is to remain in the breeding program, minimum-contamination breeding strategies must be used, as described for bacterial infections of the accessory genital glands (see p. 302).

Balanitis

Balanitis (inflammation of the penis) often is accompanied by posthitis (inflammation of the prepuce). It most frequently occurs following penile paralysis, paraphimosis, or injury at the time of breeding. Primary venereal disease (coital exanthema or dourine) also can produce balanoposthitis, as can smegma irritation. Treatment, consisting of thoroughly rinsing the area, daily applications of antibacterial ointment, and sexual rest, results in uneventful recovery in about 2 weeks.

Cutaneous Habronemiasis (Summer Sores)

Cutaneous habronemiasis is a mildly pruritic, granulomatous skin condition caused by the infective larvae of *Draschia megastoma, Habronema musca,* and *Habronema microstoma.*

* Cutaneous habronemiasis primarily occurs in the spring and summer, when flies are prevalent.
* The nematode larvae are deposited by houseflies and stable flies onto moist skin surfaces or wounds, where they stimulate rapid production of granulation tissue.
  * The external genitalia (scrotum, prepuce, glans penis, and urethral process) are common sites of infestation.
* Small, yellow, caseous masses are found throughout the granulation tissue.
  * Finding these masses helps differentiate this disease from squamous cell carcinomas, sarcoids, and exuberant granulomas.
  * In the Gulf states, pythiosis is another differential diagnosis.

Treatment

Treatment is directed at reducing the hypersensitivity reaction and eradicating the larvae from the wound.

* Organophosphates administered intralesionally, PO, IV, or topically kill the parasitic larvae.

♦ Ivermectin also prevents and cures cutaneous habronemiasis.

♦ Antiinflammatory drugs, such as diethylcarbamazine and corticosteroids, alleviate the foreign body reaction against the larvae.

Chronic infestation of the urethral process causes marked periurethral fibrosis, necessitating amputation of that structure. Cutaneous habronemiasis is discussed further in Chapter 17, Integumentary System.

NEOPLASIA

Squamous cell carcinoma is a common neoplasm of the equine penis. It is locally invasive and capable of metastasis. Squamous papillomas may occur on the prepuce and penis of horses, although the incidence is very low. Genital papillomas generally are quite refractory to treatment.

Diseases of the Prepuce

(pages 1075-1077)

Dickson D. Varner
and James Schumacher

DIAGNOSTIC AND THERAPEUTIC CONSIDERATIONS

Phimosis

Phimosis refers to inability to exteriorize the penis. It is a result of congenital or acquired constriction of the preputial orifice (exterior) or preputial ring (interior) or other local lesion that causes compression/fixation of the penis within the preputial cavity.

♦ The free portion of the penis in a newborn colt *normally* is adhered to the internal lamina of the prepuce during the first few weeks of life.

♦ Acquired phimosis usually is secondary to acute or chronic posthitis (preputial inflammation) or space-occupying preputial lesions (abscesses, neoplasia, granulomas).

• Excessive preputial edema can induce prolapse of the external prepuce while trapping the penis in the swollen internal prepuce.

• Preputial edema can be relieved by diuretics, vigorous exercise,

cold therapy, and local massage with demulcents.

♦ The preputial skin can become sclerotic and nonpliable following chronic posthitis, sometimes to the extent that the normal telescoping ability of the prepuce is impaired.

• Affected horses urinate within the preputial cavity, heightening inflammation.

• Cicatricial constriction of the preputial orifice and phimosis eventually occur, requiring surgical intervention (preputiotomy; see *Equine Medicine and Surgery V*).

♦ Large neoplastic or granulomatous lesions of the prepuce may require surgical correction.

• Preputial resection (reefing operation, circumcision, posthioplasty) is indicated when diseased preputial skin must be removed *en bloc* to restore normal preputial function.

INFLAMMATORY, INFECTIOUS, AND IMMUNE DISEASES

Posthitis/Balanoposthitis

Acute posthitis

Acute inflammation of the prepuce usually occurs with penile inflammation; this condition is called *balanoposthitis*. Infectious causes include coital exanthema, dourine, microfilariasis (*Onchocerca* and *Setaria* organisms), and possibly treponemiasis. More often, balanoposthitis occurs secondary to trauma, paraphimosis, or penile paralysis.

Chronic posthitis

Smegma accumulation may irritate the genital skin, causing a chronic inflammatory response (posthitis or balanoposthitis). Thickening and induration of the preputial lamina can develop if the inflammation does not subside. Treatment consists of thoroughly cleansing the prepuce and penis to remove smegma from these areas. Frequent application of lotions or ointments containing a corticosteroid may help control persistent or recurrent posthitis. Some refractory cases require preputial resection.

Preputial Abscesses

Abscess formation in the prepuce is uncommon but may be a complication of penetrating injuries or a sequela to a systemic infection, especially with *Streptococcus equi* or *Corynebacterium pseudotuberculosis*.

Diseases Affecting Semen *(pages 1078-1081)*

OLIGOSPERMIA/AZOOSPERMIA

Oligospermia is to a deficiency of spermatozoa in ejaculated semen, whereas azoospermia is an absence of spermatozoa in an ejaculate. The causes of these disorders are similar, the only difference being the magnitude of the problem. Causes include reduced spermatogenesis (e.g., testicular hypoplasia or degeneration), obstruction of the extragonadal duct lumina, and sexual overuse. However, with overuse, libido usually decreases and the stallion fails to copulate before ejaculatory sperm numbers drop to a level insufficient for impregnation.

IATROGENIC REDUCTION OF SEMEN QUALITY

Improper handling of collected semen, whether for evaluation or insemination, can adversely affect sperm motility and morphology, and thus stallion fertility.

♦ Physical causes include temperature extremes, agitation, and exposure to light.
  • Artificial vagina temperatures should not exceed 45° to 48° C (113° to 118° F).
  • Semen should not be kept at body temperature (37° to 38° C [98.6° to 100.4° F]) in vitro.
  • Refrigeration (4° to 6° C [39° to 43° F]) is well tolerated once the semen is placed in a semen extender and slowly cooled.
♦ Toxic causes include improperly selected or maintained artificial vagina liners and semen collection receptacles or storage containers, and improper semen extender composition.

CONTAMINATION WITH BODY FLUIDS

Hemospermia

Hemospermia is contamination of the ejaculate with blood, either in minute or large quantities.

♦ Specific causes include penile lacerations, cutaneous habronemiasis of the urethral process or glans penis, urethritis, urethral rents into the corpus spongiosum penis, and infection or inflammation of the accessory genital glands.
  • A disproportionately elevated number of leukocytes (especially neutrophils) to erythrocytes in ejaculated semen suggests internal genital infection as the cause.
♦ Stallions with overt hemospermia are considered highly subfertile.
  • A certain amount of blood contamination of an ejaculate is compatible with fertility, especially if the semen is properly diluted with semen extender before insemination.

Successful management relies on the cause being identified and addressed.

Urination During Ejaculation (Urospermia)

Urospermia, or contamination of the ejaculate with urine, is uncommon in stallions.

♦ The problem may be incessant or intermittent and unpredictable.
♦ Affected stallions generally exhibit normal libido and mating ability.
♦ The etiology likely involves a disturbance in the nervous pathway controlling ejaculation.
  • Neuropathies causing bladder paralysis, such as cauda equina neuritis, EHV-I infection, and sorghum/Sudan grass poisoning, could create urinary incontinence during ejaculation.
  • However, most stallions with urospermia do not exhibit signs of a neurologic deficit other than urinary incontinence at the time of breeding.
♦ Generally, effects on spermatozoal motility and fertilizing capacity are dose dependent.
  • Minute amounts of urine are tolerable in ejaculated semen, but the critical depressive concentra-

tion of urine contamination probably is very low.

- ◆ Gross contamination of semen with urine is easily detected by the sample's color and odor.
  - Elevated semen concentrations of urea nitrogen (>25 mg/dL) or creatinine (>2 mg/dL) are required to document scant urine contamination.

Management

Urospermia can be a frustrating problem; management should involve:

- ◆ Delaying semen collection (or breeding) until immediately after the stallion has urinated.
  - Urination can be stimulated by administration of a diuretic, such as furosemide
- ◆ Fractionating ejaculates (using an open-ended artificial vagina) to obtain urine-free semen samples.
- ◆ Diluting the semen in an appropriate extender to help protect the spermatozoa from urine-related damage.

13

Reproductive System: The Mare

Examination of the Mare *(pages 1088-1094)*
Atwood C. Asbury

BREEDING HISTORY

An in-depth history is essential because improper management often is the principal cause of infertility. Details should include:

* a complete account of the mare's entire career, including the years before she was first bred
* known or suspected abortions, early embryonic deaths, twinning, and neonatal deaths
* a complete list of live foals, their sires, and foaling dates
* teasing and breeding data for the most recent seasons when foals were produced
* treatment history, including culture results, treatment schedules, and routine prophylactic measures
* a list of all stallions to which the mare was bred
* assessment of the level of management on the breeding farm

GENERAL PHYSICAL APPRAISAL

A brief physical assessment of the mare should be a routine part of every reproductive examination. Details to note include:

* extremes in body condition, from debilitation to obesity
* painful injuries (acute or chronic)
* behavioral quirks and disposition

Diseases causing poor body condition must be evaluated and treated. Painful injuries may also require treatment.

EXAMINATION OF THE REPRODUCTIVE TRACT
Restraint

Acceptable methods of restraint for reproductive examination include:

* placing the mare's hindquarters in the corner of the stall near the door and if necessary applying a twitch or lip chain
* examination stocks (evaluate for safety before use)
* a front leg strap
* chemical restraint, which can be unpredictable; when sedation is necessary, a combination of detomidine and butorphanol or a moderate dose of chloral hydrate is recommended

Examination of the External Genitalia

The vulva is best evaluated during estrus. The following features should be noted:

* The dorsal commissure of the vulva should be no more than 4 cm dorsal to the pelvic floor.
* A defective vulvovaginal sphincter, which allows aspiration of air and feces into the vagina, can be identified by parting the labia and listening for the characteristic "windsucking" sound.
* Color and moistness of the vaginal mucosa should be glistening pink

to red in estrus, pale and dry in anestrus, and dark red or muddy colored when inflamed.

Rectal Palpation

Ovarian palpation

Ovarian size may vary from 3 × 3 cm during deep winter anestrus to 10 × 5 cm during peak sexual activity. The entire surface of each ovary must be palpated. Following are the typical features palpable during the estrous cycle:

- Follicles are fluid-filled, symmetric structures that, as they mature, enlarge, project above the ovarian surface, and progress from firm and thick-walled to very fluctuant and thin-walled.
  - Occasionally a follicle that is still firm and tense ovulates with no change in turgidity.
- Collapse of the follicle occurs with ovulation. A crater or pit is felt where the follicle was located. During palpation, the mare responds by tensing the flank muscles on that side or raising the hind leg.
- The mushy consistency of the cavity becomes progressively more firm until 24 hours after ovulation, when the clot and serum that fill the crater may feel like another follicle (although this corpus hemorrhagicum is smaller than the original follicle).
- A mature (5 days postovulation) corpus luteum is seldom detectable by rectal palpation.

These changes are best evaluated by repeated examination and by combining rectal palpation with ultrasonography. Consideration of estrual signs is also helpful.

Uterine palpation

Palpation of the nonpregnant uterus should define the size, tone, consistency, and general conformation, followed by a detailed examination for abnormalities. Normal findings are as follows:

diestrus: The uterus has a tubular, compact feeling.

proestrus and estrus: Characterized by progressive relaxation and soft thickening, the uterine wall is easily compressed. Endometrial folds (small ridges) are prominent if deep digital pressure is applied. NOTE: *Deep dig-*

ital pressure should never be used if there is any possibility of pregnancy.

anestrus: The uterus is flaccid, thin-walled, and often quite indistinct.

Abnormalities that may be either palpated or detected with deep digital pressure include:

- ventral enlargements at the junction of the horn and body, which may indicate myometrial and endometrial atrophy or diffuse lymphatic stasis or lacunae
- abnormal fluid accumulation in the uterine lumen
- absence of endometrial folds, which is suggestive of fibrotic lesions or denuded endometrium at that site
- endometrial cysts; cysts as small as 2 to 3 mm often can be detected with deep digital pressure

Areas with notable differences in consistency, either firmer or softer than the rest of the uterus, should be evaluated further (e.g., with endometrial biopsy).

Cervical palpation

Cyclic changes in cervical size and consistency are similar to those of the uterus.

diestrus: The cervix is long, tubular, and readily palpable.

proestrus and estrus: Progressive softening, shortening, and edema occur. During estrus the cervix flattens readily when digital pressure is applied.

anestrus: The cervix is soft and indistinct.

Vaginoscopic Examination

Visual inspection of the vaginal lumen and external cervical os is important for:

- determining the stage of the estrous cycle (see below)
- determining the character of uterine, cervical, and vaginal secretions
- identifying anatomic abnormalities or traumatic lesions

Practical considerations

- The metal trivalve (Caslick's) speculum or one of the tubular types is satisfactory. A separate sterile instrument should be used for each examination.
- Artifactual reddening develops quickly when air contacts the tissues, so evaluation of color must

be made shortly after dilation of the vagina.

+ Repeated exposure of the vagina, cervix, and uterus to air and accompanying contaminants causes irritation and inflammation. After every speculum examination the air should be expressed by compression per rectum.

Determining the stage of the cycle

In conjunction with teasing and rectal palpation, the following vaginoscopic changes help determine the stage of the estrous cycle:

diestrus: The cervical and vaginal mucosae are pale (grayish-yellow) and dry, and a heavy, sticky mucus often is present. The external cervical os is high on the vaginal wall and tightly contracted.

estrus: The cervix progressively relaxes and softens, droping toward the floor of the distended vagina. Mucosal edema, mucus secretion, and hyperemia increase (cervix and vagina). The external cervical os has edematous mucosal folds that resolve as ovulation approaches.

anestrus: The cervical and vaginal mucosae are blanched, almost white. The cervix becomes atonic and flaccid and may gape open to reveal the uterine lumen. Blood vessels are scarce on the vaginal wall, and little hyperemia occurs after exposure to air.

Manual Examination of the Vagina

Digital palpation is useful for identifying:

+ minute rectovaginal defects (sometimes more easily felt than seen)
+ lacerations and adhesions in the cervical canal
+ lesions in the uterine lumen, detected during rectal examination (e.g., adhesions, endometrial cysts, neoplasms)

For intraluminal palpation of the uterus, the cervix must be dilated either manually or with estradiol cypionate (given 12 to 24 hours before examination). Aseptic technique is essential. This procedure may not be feasible in maiden or primiparous animals; it should be reserved for mares with reproductive problems.

Ancillary Diagnostic Aids *(pages 1094-1117)*

Atwood C. Asbury, Angus O. McKinnon, and Edward L. Squires

ENDOMETRIAL CYTOLOGIC EXAMINATION

Atwood C. Asbury

Because uterine culture is prone to contamination from nonuterine sources, cytologic examination is a more reliable method of diagnosing endometritis. Samples of endometrium and luminal fluid are obtained with a disposable guarded uterine culture instrument. Material from the swab tip or plastic cap can be smeared on a microscope slide, air-dried, and stained with Diff-Quik.

Interpretation

Two questions are pertinent when interpreting the smears:

Are there endometrial epithelial cells in the sample? If not, another specimen should be obtained. (See *Equine Medicine and Surgery V*, Figure 13-7, p. 1095.)

Are there significant numbers of neutrophils in the sample? If so, inflammation is present. In samples with only a few neutrophils, the ratio of neutrophils to epithelial cells should be calculated; >1 neutrophil per 10 epithelial cells indicates significant inflammation.

Other cell types are occasionally seen but are unimportant.

CULTURE OF THE REPRODUCTIVE TRACT

Atwood C. Asbury

The best time to recover uterine organisms is the first day of standing estrus. Results from samples obtained at other times of the estrous cycle may be misleading.

Sample handling

Refrigeration or addition of sterile saline extends bacterial viability in samples, but ideally, immediately after collection uterine swabs are placed directly onto the final medium for culture. This allows positive correlation between numbers of organisms on the swab and numbers of colonies on the plate. Transporting or storing swabs in nutrient broth promotes proliferation of some contaminants, and stabbing swabs into semisolid holding medium may reduce the numbers of some organisms.

Following are some practical guidelines for in-house bacterial culture:

- Plate swabs onto blood agar and one selective gram-negative medium.
- Incubate plates at 37° C (98.6° F), preferably in a candle jar to provide microaerophilic conditions.
- Inspect the plates at 24 and 48 hours.

Interpretation

In most cases therapeutic decisions can be made after inspecting the colonies on the plates and making Gram's stains. The following organisms, in significant numbers and in fairly pure cultures, are considered pathogenic:

- β-hemolytic streptococci
- *Pseudomonas* spp.
- hemolytic *Escherichia coli*
- *Klebsiella* spp.
- *Monilia* (*Candida*) spp.

Other organisms, when isolated repeatedly, may be suspect in the presence of inflammation. However, α-hemolytic streptococci, staphylococci, and enteric organisms other than those listed above generally should be viewed as contaminants. Culture results must be compared with cytologic findings to be most useful.

- Any organism is considered a pathogen when it is recovered in pure culture in large numbers from mares with demonstrable inflammation.
- When cultures are positive and cytologic findings repeatedly are negative, contamination is likely.

Culture of caudal areas

With contagious equine metritis and some cases of *Klebsiella* infection, bacteria are concentrated in the caudal vagina, urethral opening, clitoral fossa, and clitoral sinuses. Sampling of these areas is warranted when either condition is suspected.

ENDOMETRIAL BIOPSY

Atwood C. Asbury

Endometrial biopsy is indicated in the following situations:

- in barren mares with a clinically evident reproductive tract abnormality and a history of early embryonic death or cyclic failure during the breeding season that fail to conceive after repeated breedings to a stallion of known fertility
- as part of a fertility evaluation before purchase
- to help determine the presence or absence of endometritis when clinical findings and culture results are inconclusive

Practical considerations

- *It is essential to establish that the mare is not pregnant before performing endometrial biopsy.*
- Deep palpation of the uterus to detect physical abnormalities enhances the value of endometrial biopsy.
- When focal lesions are palpated, multiple biopsies are indicated and should include the area(s) in question as well as a portion of endometrium that feels normal.
- In the absence of clinically detectable pathologic changes, a single endometrial sample taken from the base of either horn is considered representative of the entire endometrium.
- The safest method of biopsy is to turn the instrument on its side and press a portion of endometrium between the side walls of the punch with the index finger of the hand in the rectum.
- The sample should be immediately placed in fixative, preferably Bouin's solution, for 12 to 24 hours, followed by transfer into 80% ethanol.

Histologic changes

The characteristic histologic changes at various stages of the estrous cycle are given in *Equine Medicine and Surgery V*. Significant pathologic changes in endometrial biopsies are:

- *inflammation:* Increased numbers of inflammatory cells are seen in the lamina propria, either focally or diffusely. Neutrophils predominate in acute inflammation, whereas infiltration with lymphocytes and a few plasma cells and macrophages is typical of chronic endometritis.
- *fibrosis:* This condition most commonly occurs around the glands in response to inflammation or glan-

dular damage. Severe periglandular fibrosis is well correlated with failure to sustain pregnancy beyond 70 to 80 days.

* *lymphatic stasis:* This appears as large, fluid-filled spaces lined with endothelial cells. When widespread and accompanied by a jellylike consistency of the uterus on rectal palpation, this lesion is correlated with reduced fertility.

Interpretation

Mares can be divided into three diagnostic and prognostic groups.

* *Category I:* The endometrium is compatible with conception and capable of supporting a foal to term.
  * Any pathologic changes are slight and widely scattered.
  * No endometrial atrophy or hypoplasia is seen (during the breeding season).

  These mares have ≥70% chance of producing a live foal.

* *Category II:* Mares in this category have endometrial changes that reduce the chance of conception and pregnancy maintenance but that are reversible or only moderately severe. This may include combinations of any of the following:
  * slight to moderate, diffuse cellular infiltration of superficial layers
  * scattered but frequent inflammatory or fibrotic foci in the lamina propria
  * scattered but frequent periglandular fibrosis of individual gland branches
  * ≤3 nests of gland branches per low-power field in 5 fields
  * widespread lymphatic stasis without palpable changes in the uterus

  These mares have a 50% to 70% chance of producing a live foal with proper management.

* *Category III:* Mares in this category have endometrial changes that reduce the chances of conception and pregnancy maintenance and that are essentially irreversible. This may include any of the following:
  * widespread periglandular fibrosis with ≥5 gland nests per low-power field
  * widespread, severe cellular infiltration of superficial layers

* lymphatic stasis accompanied by palpable changes in the uterus
* endometrial atrophy or hypoplasia with gonadal dysgenesis
* pyometra accompanied by palpable endometrial atrophy or widespread, severe inflammatory cell infiltration

These mares have <10% chance for fertility.

ULTRASONOGRAPHIC EVALUATION OF THE REPRODUCTIVE TRACT

Angus O. McKinnon and Edward L. Squires

Examination of the Ovaries

Ultrasonography is useful for monitoring dynamic follicular and luteal changes. However, it does not replace essential management techniques, such as regular teasing and rectal palpation and is not the sole diagnostic criterion for determining the stage of the estrous cycle. A 5-MHz transducer is more suitable than a 3- or 3.5-MHz transducer.

Determining the stage of the cycle

Follicles are nonechogenic and appear as black, roughly circumscribed structures. Compression by adjacent follicles, luteal structures, or ovarian stroma often causes irregularly shaped follicles. Following are some other sonographic features:

* *anestrus:* Small (2 to 5 mm) follicles occasionally are present, but anestrus is suggested by the absence of a corpus luteum.
* *transitional mares:* Multiple large follicles are characteristic before the first ovulation of the year. Observation of a corpus luteum may confirm that the mare has entered the ovulatory season.
* *proestrus and estrus:* Selective, accelerated growth of an ovulatory follicle beginning 6 days before ovulation and regression of large nonovulatory follicles a few days before ovulation characterize this phase.
* *diestrus:* Multiple 2- to 5-mm follicles are seen during early diestrus and growth of larger follicles beginning midcycle. With a 5-MHz

transducer, the corpus luteum should be visible for 16 to 17 days.

Predicting ovulation

Various characteristics can be used to predict the time of ovulation:

- Softening of a large follicle occurs 24 hours before ovulation in 70% of mares and is a particularly useful sign when associated with pain on rectal palpation.
- The follicular shape can change from spherical to irregular.
- The follicle wall can thicken, but generally this occurs too early to be useful.
- The follicular fluid can have increased echogenicity, but this can be inconsistent.

Ultrasonography is not a substitute for rectal palpation. However, some ovulations are detected ultrasonographically and not by rectal palpation. They often are associated with well-circumscribed corpora lutea that, though smaller in size, feel similar to fluid-filled follicles.

Identifying a corpus luteum

Following are the sonographic features of a corpus luteum (CL):

- The CL is first visible on the day of ovulation (day 0) as a strongly echogenic, circumscribed mass. Echogenicity gradually decreases throughout diestrus, although it increases just before CL regression.
- About 50% of CLs are "uniformly echogenic." Echogenicity remains constant throughout diestrus.
- "Centrally nonechogenic" CLs (or corpus hemorrhagicum), in which a nonechogenic center develops on day 0 or 1, are less common.

Ovarian irregularities and lesions

- **Anovulatory hemorrhagic follicles:** These are preovulatory follicles that grow to an unusually large size (70 to 100 mm), fail to ovulate, but fill with blood and then gradually recede.
  - The blood in these follicles is distinctly echogenic, unlike the central clot of a corpus hemorrhagicum, which generally is anechoic and discrete (15 to 35 mm).
  - Scattered, free-floating echogenic spots within the follicle swirl during ballottement of the ovary. Over time the contents organize into fibrous bands.

- There may be an echogenic rim (4 to 7 mm) of luteal tissue.
- Maturation and ovulation of another follicle during the same cycle may cause an unusually long period of behavioral estrus (about 12 days, or 5 days after demonstration of the anovulatory follicle).
- The subsequent luteal phase is either normal or prolonged.
- Anovulatory hemorrhagic follicles occur toward the end of the breeding season; they are rare during the ovulatory season.
- There is currently no treatment; hCG does not appear to be beneficial.

- **luteinized unruptured follicles:** These may be quite common in pregnant mares, in association with secondary CL formation.

- **prolonged maintenance of the corpus luteum:** This can be differentiated from anovulatory or anestrous conditions by identifying a mature CL.

- **granulosa–theca cell tumors:** These tumors may be solid or cystic on palpation and feel smooth, knobby, hard, or soft (with obvious follicular development).
  - The unaffected ovary usually is small and inactive.
  - Ultrasonographic examination helps differentiate tumors from other large nonneoplastic structures, but in general, definitive diagnosis requires histologic or gross examination.

- **Embryonic vestiges and cystic accessory structures:** Quite common in mares, these cysts, though often small, may be confused with an ovarian follicle. Rectal palpation generally is more accurate in determining whether the structure is part of the ovary.
  - Small fimbrial cysts (<10 mm) probably do not cause infertility.
  - Hydrosalpinx is uncommon in mares but can be identified ultrasonographically.

Examination of the Uterus

Pregnancy detection

The developing blastocyst can first be recognized 9 to 10 days postovulation using a 5-MHz transducer and at 13 to 15 days using a 3-MHz transducer. But because considerable embryonic loss occurs in early pregnancy, it may be best to postpone the first scan until days 18 to 20, except in mares with a history of twinning or double ovulations. Pregnancy should not be confirmed until day 50. Following is a timeline of events that can be documented using ultrasonography:

- Day 15: Mobility of the conceptus begins to decrease. The yolk sac vesicle is spherical.
- Days 16 to 17: Fixation occurs, usually at the base of the uterine horn. The yolk sac vesicle may become irregular in shape.
- Days 20 to 25: The embryo is first detected, located ventrally within the vesicle.
- Day 22: A heartbeat is often detectable.
- Day 24: Growth of the allantois begins, concurrent with contraction of the yolk sac.
- Days 24 to 40: The embryo moves from the ventral to the dorsal aspect of the vesicle.
- Days 40 to 50: The umbilical cord elongates from the dorsal pole, al-

lowing the fetus to gravitate back to the ventral floor, where it is seen in dorsal recumbency from day 50.

Size of the chorionic vesicle and fetus at various stages of pregnancy is presented in Table 13-1.

Apposition of the yolk sac and allantois creates a sonographically visible line, normally oriented horizontally. Occasionally this junction has a vertical configuration similar in appearance to twin vesicles. Knowing the approximate gestational age helps differentiate an abnormally oriented singleton from twins.

Manual reduction of twins

In almost all instances (96%), single embryonic reduction can be achieved by manually crushing one of two twin vesicles between 12 and 30 days of pregnancy.

- *before day 16:* The smaller vesicle should be manipulated into the tip of one uterine horn and squeezed. A distinct popping sensation may be noticed when the vesicle ruptures.
- *after day 16:* The vesicles are likely to be fixed, making manual reduction more difficult, particularly if

Table 13-1
Size of the chorionic vesicle and fetus at various stages of pregnancy

Days of gestation	Size and shape of chorionic vesicle	Crown-rump length of fetus
16	2-4 cm, bantam's egg (round)	0.32 cm
20	2.5-4.5 cm, small hen's egg (slightly oval)	0.66 cm
25	2.5-4.5 cm, small hen's egg (slightly oval)	0.6-0.85 cm
30	2.5-5.0 cm, hen's egg (oval)	0.9-1.0 cm
35	3.5-6.5 cm, goose's egg (oval)	1.5-2.0 cm
40	4.5-7.5 cm, small orange (oval)	2.5-4.0 cm
45	6-10 cm, large orange (oval)	2.6-4.5 cm
50	12 × 7.5 cm, small melon (oval)	3.0-6.0 cm
60	13.3 × 8.9 cm, melon (oval)	4-7.5 cm
90	14 × 23 cm, football (oval)	10-14 cm
120		10-14 cm
150		25-37 cm
180		35-60 cm
210		55-70 cm
240		60-80 cm
270		80-90 cm
300		70-130 cm
330		100-150 cm

From Roberts SJ: *Veterinary obstetrics and genital diseases (theriogenology)*, ed 3, North Pomfret, Vt, 1986, David & Charles.

both are fixed on the same side.
One vesicle must be crushed in situ.
Management of twin pregnancy is discussed further on p. 331.

Predicting early embryonic death

Early embryonic death is diagnosed when an embryonic vesicle is not observed on two consecutive sonograms or when only remnants of a vesicle are seen. It should be *suspected,* particularly after day 30, when:

- No fetal heartbeat is observed.
- Definition of fetal structure is poor.
- The largest diameter of the vesicle is significantly less than average for that specific day of gestation (see Table 13-1).
- Vesicle growth is slow or undetectable.

Criteria for *impending* early embryonic death include:

- an irregular and indented vesicle
- an echogenic ring within the vesicle
- vesicular fluid that contains echogenic spots
- prominent endometrial folds
- fluid in the uterine lumen
- a mass floating in a collection of fluid
- fixation failure
- a gradual decrease in volume of placental fluid with disorganization of placental membranes

Uterine size and endometrial folds

- Ultrasonographic evaluation of postpartum mares before breeding helps identify mares with poor uterine involution and excessive uterine fluid. These mares are unlikely to conceive.
- Prominent endometrial folds during estrus should not be considered pathologic, but impending abortion is suggested during routine scanning for pregnancy when the embryonic vesicle is located in a uterus with prominent endometrial folds.
- Uterine edema and endometrial folds can also be used to determine whether large follicles in transitional mares are producing estrogen.

Uterine fluid accumulation

Ultrasonography is valuable for estimating the quantity and quality of fluid in the uterine lumen. It is as accurate as uterine cytology and endometrial biopsy and more accurate than uterine culture in diagnosing en-

dometritis. The degree of echogenicity is correlated with the amount of debris and white blood cells in the fluid. Grade I fluid has large numbers of neutrophils, while grade IV fluid has very few neutrophils. Following are some guidelines for interpretation of uterine fluid at various stages of the estrous cycle:

- *diestrus:* Fluid accumulation results in lower pregnancy rates at both days 11 and 20 and is correlated with a worsening biopsy score (indicative of inflammation).
- *estrus:* Fluid accumulation does not affect pregnancy rates at either day 11 or 50, but fluid accumulation 1 or 2 days *after ovulation* is associated with a significant increase in early embryonic death and reduced day-50 pregnancy rates.
- *postpartum:* Uterine fluid accumulation is associated with significantly decreased pregnancy rates when found in the first postpartum ovulatory period; however, delay of the first ovulation to day 15 postpartum or later, by administering progestin, improves pregnancy rates (see p. 328)

Uterine cysts and other lesions

Endometrial cysts usually are ≤10 mm; their incidence and significance are largely undetermined. Uterine cysts of *lymphatic origin* generally are larger than endometrial cysts. They are common in older mares and sometimes are associated with abnormal uterine biopsy findings, including chronic lymphocytic endometritis and senility. Following are some guidelines for differentiating uterine cysts from embryonic vesicles:

- It is uncommon for cysts to enlarge at a rate similar to early embryonic vesicles.
- Cysts commonly are rounded but with irregular borders; occasionally they are multiple or compartmentalized.
- The early equine conceptus (days 10 to 16) is mobile.

Intrauterine air:

- This is a less common lesion, recognized as multiple hyperechoic reflections (occasionally with ventral reverberation artifact) slightly cranial to the cervix

- It is considered normal within 24 hours of artificial insemination, but it is not to be expected in normal mares >48 hours after breeding.
- When found in mares that have not been recently bred, it reflects impaired competency of the labia, vestibulovaginal sphincter, and/or cervix. It often is associated with uterine fluid accumulation.

ENDOSCOPIC EXAMINATION OF THE UTERUS

Atwood C. Asbury

Endoscopic examination should be considered when palpable changes in the uterus require further evaluation or when other diagnostic procedures fail to identify a cause of infertility.

Practical considerations

- A flexible endoscope used for examination of the equine upper respiratory tract is adequate, although the accompanying biopsy instruments do not provide an endometrial sample large enough for meaningful evaluation.
- Examination of the uterus is best performed during diestrus, since distention is more easily maintained with a tight cervix.
- Distention of the uterus with fluid, such as saline or water, allows complete examination of the body and both horns and causes markedly less straining than does air inflation. In older mares, 1 to 2 L of fluid can be instilled into the uterus without causing discomfort.

Interpretation

The uterine bifurcation appears as a vertical pillar that should not be confused with an intraluminal adhesion. Typical lesions found with endoscopy are lymphatic cysts, polyps, and other nodules (35%); adhesions (20%); and changes in texture and color (15%).

INDIRECT PREGNANCY TESTS

Angus O. McKinnon and Ed L. Squires

Reasons to use a blood or urine sample to diagnose pregnancy include:

- inconclusive findings on rectal palpation
- inadequate examination facilities

- evaluation of vicious or wild equidae, Miniature Horses, small ponies, or mares with previous rectal tears
- confirmation of early embryonic death

Progesterone

Serum progesterone concentrations between 4 and 9 ng/mL are found 5 to 10 days after ovulation. If pregnancy ensues, higher concentrations are observed by days 16 to 20 in pregnant mares than in mares returning to estrus: >6.3 ng/mL in pregnant mares and <1.0 ng/mL in nonpregnant mares.

Limitations

Regardless of the method of progesterone measurement, some pregnant mares have low serum progesterone concentrations and some diestrous mares (with retained CLs) have values in the range found in pregnant mares. Thus measurement of serum progesterone is not recommended for pregnancy diagnosis.

Equine Chorionic Gonadotropin

Serum concentrations of equine chorionic gonadotropin (eCG) parallel the growth and regression of endometrial cups. This hormone is first detectable on days 35 to 40, peaks at days 60 to 65, and decreases to low or undetectable levels by 120 to 150 days of gestation. Serum assays should be performed between days 40 and 120.

Limitations

When abortion occurs after day 35, endometrial cups may persist, resulting in a false-positive pregnancy diagnosis. In mares carrying a mule fetus, levels of eCG are extremely low or undetectable, despite the persistence of pregnancy.

Immunologic tests

Tests available include the hemagglutination inhibition or mare immunologic pregnancy (MIP) test (e.g., MIP-Test), radioimmunoassay, direct latex agglutination (DLA; e.g., Rapitex), and enzyme-linked immunosorbent assay (e.g., D-TEC-MP ELISA). The MIP test, DLA assay, and ELISA are all 90% to 100% accurate after 50 days' gestation, but none are reliable before 40 days.

Estrogen

A major increase in serum estrogen concentration occurs after day 60 and peaks on about day 210 of gestation.

Limitations

Estrogen detection in serum or urine has only limited value for pregnancy diagnosis because it becomes reliable only relatively late in pregnancy. Testing is not recommended before day 150. Also the presence of estrogen in the urine is not specific for pregnancy. Mares with ovarian cysts, nymphomania, and chronic genital disease may have urinary estrogen excretion similar to that in pregnant mares.

Specific tests

- Direct measurement of conjugated estrogen in serum or milk allows differentiation between pregnancy and estrus after about 50 days.
- Enzymatic determination of unconjugated estrogen in feces has also been used for pregnancy diagnosis. With this test it is possible to confirm pregnancy after 120 days of gestation.
- Measurement of conjugated estrone sulfate in serum, milk, or urine can be used to provide evidence of a viable conceptus after about 60 days of pregnancy. Rapid drops in estrone sulfate before 250 days indicate fetal loss; this may be useful in mares that begin to lactate in the second or third trimester. Changes in urinary concentrations are more significant than changes in serum concentrations.

Pathophysiology and Principles of Therapy

(pages 1117-1148)

Michelle M. LeBlanc

NORMAL PREGNANCY

Diagnosing Pregnancy by Rectal Palpation

Following are some guidelines for pregnancy diagnosis:

- As early as 17 or 18 days postovulation, the uterine wall increases in thickness and tone.

- To confirm pregnancy, the conceptus in its chorionic vesicle must be identified. At day 17 or 18 the vesicle, which is only about 2.5 cm diameter, appears as a distinct, fluid-filled, spherical structure on the ventral aspect of the uterus, usually at the base of either horn.
- Some "curling" of the base of the uterine horn normally occurs during pregnancy and should not be mistaken for a chorionic vesicle.
- The vesicle reaches 3 cm in diameter by 25 days and 4 to 4.5 cm by 30 days. The approximate size through 90 days is presented in Table 13-1.
- The vesicle can be mistaken for the urinary bladder if a thorough evaluation is not made.
- It is important to diagnose pregnancy by 35 to 38 days postovulation because if therapeutic abortion is necessary (e.g., for twinning), it must be performed before the endometrial cups form. Mares aborted after day 38 have a poor chance of conceiving until the endometrial cups regress (day 120).
- From 50 to 90 days of gestation, the uterus extends cranially over the pelvic brim and becomes too large and heavy to retract and delineate completely. This makes positive pregnancy diagnosis more difficult until the fetus can be palpated (120 to 150 days).
- If the uterus is not retractable, its fluid contents are confirmed by ballottement. If the uterine wall feels thin and pliable, and if the fluid is not viscous, a positive diagnosis of pregnancy can be made.
- Pyometra can be mistakenly diagnosed as pregnancy, although the uterine wall is thick and doughy and the fluid contents are much more viscous.
- From about 150 days until birth, the fetus is readily palpable.

Other palpable changes

- An elongated, tubular, and very firm cervix (greater than that expected during diestrus) is supportive evidence of early (17 to 20 days) pregnancy; however, persistence of the CL without pregnancy causes similar findings.

- Ovarian activity is of no help in pregnancy diagnosis.

Vaginoscopic changes

Speculum examination of the cervix and vagina helps confirm pregnancy.

- During pregnancy, a thick, dry, tenacious, white secretion usually is present on the vaginal wall.
- The cervix is tightly closed and is centrally located. There should be no cervical discharge.

NORMAL PARTURITION
Physical Signs

Gestational length is extremely variable, with a mean length for light breeds of 335 to 342 days and a range of 305 to 365 days. Foals born before day 300 rarely survive without intensive care and are considered premature if born before day 320. Donkeys and mares carrying mule foals have slightly longer gestational periods.

Signs of impending parturition

Signs often are subtle and vary from mare to mare. They include:

- slight relaxation of the sacrosciatic ligaments in late pregnancy (may not be obvious in heavily muscled mares)
- slight swelling (edema) of the vulva and lengthening of the vulvar cleft during the last few weeks of pregnancy
- udder development, beginning about 4 weeks before parturition, with "waxing" usually occurring 6 to 48 hours before foaling

Some mares leak milk for several days before foaling; others, notably maiden mares, foal with no external signs of impending parturition.

Normal parturition

Parturition in mares is divided into three stages:

Stage 1: lasts 15 to 90 minutes

- The mare is restless, walks around with a raised tail, and urinates small amounts frequently.
  - The mare shows signs of colic, alternately lying down and standing up.
  - Slight sweating becomes noticeable on the flanks and behind the elbows.

- The foal rotates into a dorsosacral position.
- Uterine contractions cause rupture of the allantochorionic membrane, allowing escape of the allantoic fluid.

Stage 2: averages 12 to 15 minutes and commences with the release of allantoic fluid

- The foal's forelimbs, still encased in the amniotic membrane, appear at the vulva within 5 minutes of rupture of the chorioallantois.
- Strong contractions progressively move the foal through the birth canal.
  - Delivery is accomplished very quickly once the foal's hips clear the maternal pelvis.
- It is typical for the entire foal to be delivered before the amniotic membrane ruptures; in most cases movement of the foal's forefeet and head tears the amnion.
- The umbilical cord ruptures spontaneously about 50 mm from the foal's body. The cord may be manually separated within seconds of birth with no harmful effects.
- Most mares foal in lateral recumbency; unless disturbed, the mare tends to remain recumbent for a few minutes after delivery.

Stage 3: fetal membranes are expelled within 3 hours of delivery

- The membranes may be expelled while the mare is still in lateral recumbency. It is not unusual for the entire placenta to be passed within 10 minutes of delivery.
  - Retention of the membranes for up to 3 hours is normal.
  - Continued uterine contractions cause abdominal discomfort until the placenta is passed.

Management of Foaling

Following are some guidelines for foaling management:

- Where climatic situations allow, mares can foal outdoors (and still be supervised).
- Foaling stalls should be roomy, well ventilated, easily cleaned, and used only for foaling.
- Straw bedding is preferred over wood chips.

EQUINE MED.

SF 951, E57

= =

m36

c932

Status Title
Overdue Ancient Egypt : anatomy of a civ
        Kemp.
Overdue The Oxford history of ancient Eg
        Shaw.
Overdue The twilight of ancient Egypt :
        / by Karol My{226}sliwiec

• If foaling proceeds without complication, the mare and foal should be left alone to bond in the immediate postpartum period.

Intervention during parturition

Identifying a mare that is having difficulty foaling and deciding when to intervene take experience. Following are some guidelines:

• Minimal intervention is indicated during stage 1 because mares can arrest the foaling process if disturbed; rather, the mare should be quietly observed under minimal lighting conditions.

• If the amnion or foal's forefeet do not appear at the vulva within 5 to 10 minutes of chorioallantoic rupture, manual vaginal examination is indicated.

• If both forefeet and the tip of the muzzle can be detected in the birth canal, the mare should be allowed to continue attempts to deliver the foal.

• If strenuous abdominal contractions fail to deliver the foal within the next 10 minutes, assistance in delivery is indicated (see the section on dystocia).

• If the fetal membranes are not passed within 6 hours of foaling, systemic treatment should be instituted (see the section on retained placenta).

Induction of Parturition

Indications

Cases should be selected carefully, since it is difficult to ensure maturity of the foal when inducing parturition. Induction is indicated in mares that previously have had:

• premature placental separation
• a rectovaginal fistula
• a foal with neonatal isoerythrolysis

and in those with:

• preparturient colic
• uterine atony
• impending rupture of the prepubic tendon

Criteria

Criteria to aid the decision to induce parturition include:

• gestation of not less than 330 days (calculated from a known breeding date)

• relaxation of the pelvic ligaments and cervix

• colostrum in the udder (the most important criterion)

• concentrations of calcium, sodium, and potassium in mammary secretions

If the mare has a history of 350- to 365-day gestations, induction should be delayed, since chances for survival are best when parturition is induced within 5 to 7 days of term.

COLOSTRAL ELECTROLYTES. Unless the mare is dripping milk or has placentitis (indicated by abnormal vaginal discharge), the concentration of electrolytes in the colostrum is a reliable indicator of impending parturition. A scoring system that evaluates prepartum colostral electrolyte concentrations has been developed (Table 13-2). A score of ≥35 points suggests that the mare is within 24 hours of foaling and that induction would likely result in a mature foal. Mares with electrolyte scores between 20 and 30 points are more likely to deliver premature, weak foals if induced at that time.

Preparation

• Irrespective of induction technique, it is advisable to place an indwelling jugular catheter so that the mare can be anesthetized quickly if dystocia occurs.

• If the mare had Caslick's operation, the labia should be reopened under local anesthesia.

• Resuscitation equipment and a small surgical pack should be available in case complications occur.

Table 13-2

Scoring system for prepartum colostral electrolyte concentrations

Calcium (mg/dL)	Sodium (mEq/L)	Potassium (mEq/L)	Points for each electrolyte
≥40	≥30	≥35	15
≥28	≥50	≥30	10
≥20	≥80	≥20	5

Total score ≥35 suggests safe induction.
From Dusey JC et al: *Equine Vet J* 16:259-263, 1984.

- Parturition should be induced in a quiet, clean, dry area, preferably removed from other farm activities.

Induction with oxytocin

Oxytocin is the drug of choice for induction of parturition in mares. It usually results in delivery within 15 to 90 minutes of administration. Various methods of oxytocin induction have been described:

- bolus injection of 60 to 120 IU oxytocin IM or IV
- IM or SC injection of 2.5 to 20 IU oxytocin at 15-minute intervals
- IV administration of 60 to 120 IU oxytocin in 1 L of physiologic saline, delivered at a rate of 1 U/min

There are apparently no differences in time to foaling or neonatal health among these methods. Following are some guidelines for safe induction with oxytocin:

- Most mares foal within 60 minutes of administration of oxytocin. Mares that have cervical dilation at the time of induction tend to foal more quickly.
- After oxytocin administration, mares become restless and colicky, swish their tails, and frequently get up and down and stretch. Sweat appears over their shoulders and neck, behind the elbows, and on the flanks within 20 minutes.
- Chorioallantoic membrane rupture and strong abdominal contractions usually occur within 40 minutes of administration. If strong abdominal contractions are present but the chorioallantoic membrane does not rupture, the vagina should be examined manually.
- Premature separation of the placental membranes can occur with this procedure. When this happens the chorioallantois should be incised with scissors and the foal delivered with assistance.
- If the placenta is not passed within 3 hours of delivery, treatment for retained placenta must be instituted.

Induction with prostaglandins

Both natural ($PGF_{2\alpha}$) and synthetic (fluprostenol, fenprostalene, prostalene, cloprostenol) prostaglandins may be used to induce parturition in mares. However, neonatal adaptation abnormalities, weakness, and fractured ribs can result when prostaglandin is administered before clinical signs of impending foaling. In addition, the induction-parturition interval with fluprostenol, fenprostalene, and prostalene is more variable (1 to 6 hours) and may take longer than spontaneous foaling or induction with oxytocin. Dexamethasone does not induce parturition in mares.

TREATMENT AND MANAGEMENT TECHNIQUES

Hormonal Therapy

Inducing ovulation in transitional mares

Increasing the photoperiod stimulates reproductive activity in mares. *Artificial lighting*, added in the evening to provide a total of 16 hours of light per day, is used to advance the breeding season. However, too much light (>16 hours per day) may actually delay the onset of cyclic activity. Sufficient light can be provided with:

- a 100-watt incandescent bulb placed in a 12 x 12-ft box stall
- eight 1000-watt metal halide flood lights, at a height of 20 ft, for a paddock 84 x 66 ft

An interrupted photoperiod of 10 hours of light, 8 hours of dark, 2 hours of light, and 4 hours of dark, initiated early in December, also is effective. Adding 1 to 2 hours of light after about 10 hours of dark may be an economical means of inducing cyclicity.

HORMONE THERAPY. Progestin or progesterone used in combination with human chorionic gonadotropin (hCG) and artificial lighting is most effective. The efficacy of progesterone or progestin treatment depends on the stage of the transitional period; several 25- to 35-mm follicles should be present on the ovaries before treatment. The following regimen is recommended:

- Mares should be exposed to artificial lighting for 60 days before administration of progesterone.
- Progesterone in oil (150 to 200 mg IM) or altrenogest (0.044 mg/kg PO) is given daily for 12 to 15 days.

This usually stops prolonged estrous activity within 2 days.

- After the last treatment mares usually exhibit estrus within 3 days, with ovulation occurring in 7 to 10 days; hCG given on day 2 of estrus assists ovulation.

Another effective regimen combines an increased photoperiod with injections of progesterone (150 mg IM) and estradiol-17β (10 mg IM) daily for 10 days, followed by an injection of prostaglandin $F_{2\alpha}$ on the last day of treatment. In 90% of mares, ovulation occurs 10 to 12 days after the last day of treatment.

Inducing ovulation in cycling mares

hCG is the hormone most commonly used to induce ovulation in cycling mares. Ovulation occurs 36 to 48 hours after IV or IM injection of 2000 IU of hCG, provided the follicle is sufficiently developed (it must be >35 mm in diameter and be a developing or dominant follicle). Repeated use results in development of antibodies against this hormone, although there is no cross-reactivity with endogenous equine luteinizing hormone, so mares continue to ovulate. *Gonadotropin-releasing hormone* (GnRH) or its analogs have also been tried for induction of ovulation, with inconsistent results. A new slow-release GnRH analog, deslorelin, is a small implant that is placed SC in estrual mares when the dominant follicle is ≥30 mm in diameter. It causes ovulation within 48 hours in 88% of mares.

Prostaglandins

Prostaglandin F_{2a} and synthetic analogs are effective luteolytic agents in mares. Indications include:

- termination of diestrus, either normal or prolonged: e.g., when breeding is passed or missed because of twin ovulations or foal heat, and when diestrual ovulation prevents normal return to estrus; the best response is seen when prostaglandins are administered between days 6 and 9 of the estrous cycle
- termination of pregnancy
- hastening or synchouronization of ovulation: e.g., fenprostalene (250 mg) given 60 hours after the onset of estrus causes ovulation within 48 hours in >80% of mares

- cervical relaxation for diagnostic or therapeutic procedures
- treatment of mares with pyometra accompanied by a persistent CL
- treatment of mares with persistent, postmating uterine fluid and endometritis

TERMINATION OF PREGNANCY. Pregnancy can be terminated at up to 38 days of gestation with a single injection and after 38 days with multiple injections (daily for 3 to 5 days). Mares at >80 days of pregnancy can be safely aborted with cloprostenol (250 µg IM once daily for up to 5 days; abortion occurs within 3 to 5 days of the first injection). Incidence of dystocia and retained placenta are not increased.

ENHANCED UTERINE CLEARANCE. Prostaglandins may be used to clear the uterine lumen of fluid after breeding and to enhance uterine lymphatic drainage in mares with persistent mating-induced endometritis. Not all prostaglandins effectively induce uterine clearance; cloprostenol is the most reliable. Following is a recommended protocol:

- Four to 8 hours after breeding, lavage the uterus with saline and give 10 to 20 U of oxytocin IV or IM.
- Give 250 to 500 µg of cloprostenol IM 12 hours after breeding.
- Perform an ultrasound examination of the uterus (using a 5- or 7.5-MHz probe) 24 hours after breeding. If there is intraluminal or intramural fluid, repeat the procedure.

Cloprostenol should not be given any later than 48 hours after ovulation.

DOSAGE AND ADVERSE EFFECTS. The usual luteolytic doses in light breeds of horses (400 to 500 kg) are 5 to 10 mg IM of prostaglandin $F_{2\alpha}$ and 2 mg SC of prostalene. Transient sweating, increased gastrointestinal (GI) motility, and slight caudal ataxia are the main adverse reactions seen when natural prostaglandin is used.

Estrogens

Clinical uses of estrogens include:

- induction of estrus in anestrous or ovariectomized mares used for semen collection: 2 to 4 mg of estradiol cypionate or 10 mg of estradiol may induce signs of estrus within 6 to 10 hours.

- demonstration of estrus behavior in mares with "silent heats," such as in maiden mares or mares with foals at foot: Provided a large follicle is present, 1 mg of estradiol may induce signs of estrus, thus allowing natural mating with safety.
- synchronization of estrus (when combined with progesterone therapy)
- delay of the first postpartum ovulation (when combined with progesterone therapy)
- management of endometritis, either alone or in combination with antibiotics: A suggested regimen is 1 to 2 mg of estradiol IM daily for 3 to 5 days during estrus.

A combination of progesterone (150 mg) and estradiol-17β (10 mg) daily for 10 days induces estrus within 3 to 4 days of the last injection. The first postpartum ovulation can be delayed with this combination if treatment is begun within 12 hours of parturition and continued once daily for 5 days.

Progesterone

Progesterone therapy is used to:

- treat transitional-phase ovaries (see the section on inducing ovulation in transitional mares)
- delay first postpartum estrus
- suppress signs of estrus in performance horses
- synchronize estrus (discussed later)
- supplement endogenous progesterone for maintenance of pregnancy

SUPPRESSION OF ESTROUS BEHAVIOR. In most mares, signs of estrus can be suppressed with daily administration of progesterone in oil (100 to 300 mg IM) or altrenogest (30 mg PO). Mares usually cease estrous behavior after 2 to 3 days of treatment, although estrus persists for 6 days or more in some mares.

MAINTENANCE OF PREGNANCY. Mares that habitually abort may be given exogenous progesterone until days 120 to 150 of gestation. Typically, treatment is started at the time of pregnancy diagnosis (15 to 20 days), although it can be commenced shortly after breeding in mares thought to have luteal insufficiency. Following are some points for consideration:

- Many pregnant mares are treated with progesterone unnecessarily.

- A diagnosis of progesterone insufficiency should not be based on a single blood sample, but rather on 2 or 3 samples collected over a week. Mares with serum progesterone >4 ng/mL are less likely to abort than mares with concentrations <4 ng/mL.
- Progesterone treatment can be detrimental in mares with chronic endometritis. Before using progesterone in a problem mare, prebreeding uterine biopsy, cytologic examination, and culture should be performed.
- In ovariectomized mares, the following dosages are necessary to maintain pregnancy: 200 to 300 mg of progesterone in oil daily; 1000 mg of repository progesterone every 4 to 7 days; 0.044 mg/kg altrenogest daily.
- Progesterone (300 mg IM daily) and altrenogest (44 mg PO daily) can prevent abortion in mares in which pregnancy is at risk because of diseases associated with excess prostaglandin $F_{2\alpha}$ secretion (such as endotoxemia).

Synchronizing estrus

Methods of estrus synchronization include administration of:

- *prostaglandin alone:* Two injections are given 14 to 18 days apart in cycling mares. Sixty percent of mares show estrus 4 days after the second injection, and 75% to 90% show estrus by 6 days. Ovulation can be hastened by giving hCG on the second day of estrus.
- *progesterone plus prostaglandin:* Progesterone in oil (150 to 200 mg IM) or altrenogest (27 to 44 mg PO) is given daily for 8 to 10 days, with an injection of prostaglandin given on the last day. Most mares show estrus 2 to 5 days after the last injection and ovulate 8 to 15 days after treatment ends.
- *progesterone and estradiol-17β plus prostaglandin:* Progesterone (150 mg) and estradiol-17β (10 mg) are given IM daily for 10 days, and an injection of prostaglandin is given on the last day. Most mares ovulate 10 to 12 days after treatment ends. This regimen provides the best synchronization of estrus and ovulation.

Oxytocin

Clinical uses of oxytocin in mares include:

+ clearance of intrauterine fluids during estrus and after foaling (see p. 325)
+ induction of parturition (see p. 324)
+ treatment of retained placenta (see p. 354)
+ enhancement of milk letdown: Milk ejection often can be stimulated with 10 to 15 IU of oxytocin IV.
+ postbreeding management (see p. 332)

Oxytocin therapy is *contraindicated* in mares with dystocia or uterine torsion. However, it may be used to stimulate uterine involution after dystocia, cesarean section, or uterine prolapse. Oxytocin is ineffective in mares with agalactia caused by fescue toxicity.

Intrauterine Therapy

General guidelines

Antimicrobial concentrations typically are higher in the endometrial layers and last longer after intrauterine treatment than with systemic treatment. But if metritis is present, systemic antimicrobials are indicated.

ADVERSE EFFECTS

+ endometrial irritation
+ treatment failure and refractory secondary bacterial or fungal infections caused by random selection of antimicrobials (e.g., *Pseudomonas* or yeast infection after penicillin administration)

Antimicrobial selection should be based on culture and sensitivity results. Mares with endometritis are especially susceptible to recurrent infection.

PRACTICAL CONSIDERATIONS

+ Intrauterine infusions should be administered with sterile equipment after aseptic preparation of the mare.
+ Uterine size, determined by palpation, can be used to estimate the volume to be instilled. Total infusion volumes of 50 to 200 mL are usually recommended.
+ Exudate in the uterine lumen reduces the efficacy of antimicrobial therapy. When exudate is present, lavage should be performed before infusing antibiotics.
+ Aminoglycosides must be buffered before infusion; e.g., 1 mL of 7.5% sodium bicarbonate solution

should be used to buffer 50 mg of gentamicin or amikacin.

+ Chlorhexidine is highly irritating even in diluted (1:10,000) solutions and can cause endometrial, cervical, and vaginal adhesions.
+ Povidone-iodine preparations may irritate the endometrium unless diluted at least 1:10.

Antimicrobials and detergents

Guidelines for intrauterine use of various drugs are listed in Table 13-3.

Uterine lavage

Irrigation with large volumes of saline is useful when treating endometritis and acute postpartum metritis.

TECHNIQUE

+ 24- to 30-Fr Foley catheter with an 80-cm autoclavable flushing catheter (Bivona EUF-80) is preferred.
+ Sterile physiologic saline solution is infused by gravity flow, 1 L at a time, and is then recovered in a container.
+ Lavage is repeated until the recovered fluid is clear.
+ Measurement of the recovered fluid or ultrasonographic examination of the uterus ensures that all fluid has been recovered.
+ If fluid remains, oxytocin (10 to 20 IU IV or IM) or cloprostenol (250 to 500 µg IM) is given.

Plasma infusion

Intrauterine plasma infusion may be beneficial in mares with chronic and chronic-active endometritis. In lactating and barren mares pregnancy rates are improved when mares are treated with intrauterine plasma and antibiotics 12 to 36 hours after breeding.

PRACTICAL CONSIDERATIONS

+ Blood should be collected aseptically and heparin (5 to 10 U/mL of blood) added.
+ Prompt separation and infusion are recommended. Gravity sedimentation is acceptable, particularly if the blood is refrigerated during sedimentation.
+ Plasma can be stored frozen (−20° C [−4° F]) for 100 days without losing its potency, but overheating by using hot water to thaw plasma inactivates the proteins.

Minimum-contamination technique

With this technique, 100 to 300 mL of semen extender containing antimicrobials is infused into the uterus immediately before natural breeding. It is most effective when breeding susceptible mares to stallions infected with *Pseudomonas aeruginosa* or *Klebsiella pneumoniae*. Selection of drugs and their concentrations in the semen extender is critical (see Chapter 12, Reproductive System: The Stallion).

Applications of therapy

ACUTE ENDOMETRITIS

- When a causative agent is identified, a combination of uterine lavage and specific antimicrobial therapy is more effective than either treatment alone.

- Use of uterine lavage on alternate days during estrus plus daily infusions of the appropriate antimicrobial works well.

CHRONIC INFECTIOUS ENDOMETRITIS

- Chronic infection often results from contamination of the uterus by fecal and genital flora.
- The first step should be to correct any predisposing causes, such as by performing Caslick's vulvoplasty, urethoural extension, or cervical repair as needed.
- Local and/or systemic antibiotics should be administered based on culture and sensitivity results.

Table 13-3
Guidelines for administration of intrauterine drugs

Drug	Dose per infusion	Comments
ANTIBACTERIALS		
Amikacin	2 g	Use for *Pseudomonas, Klebsiella,* and persistent gram-negative organisms
Ampicillin	3 g	Use only the soluble product
Amphotericin B	200 mg	For fungi, dilute in 100-250 mL sterile water
Carbenicillin	6 g	Broad spectrum
Gentamicin sulfate	2 g	Excellent gram-negative spectrum, buffer with bicarbonate or large volume of saline (200 mL)
Ticarcillin	6 g	Effective against streptococci, *E.coli, Pseudomonas;* not effective against *Klebsiella*
PENETRATING AGENTS		
EDTA-TRIS (1.2 g Na EDTA with 6.05 g TRIS/L H_2O titrated to pH 8.0 with glacial acetic acid)	250 mL, then 3 hours later infuse antibacterial	EDTA binds Ca in bacterial cell walls, making cell wall permeable to antibacterials
Dimethylsulfoxide (5% stock solution)	50-100 mL	Does not appear to be effective as a carrying agent
ANTISEPTICS		
Povidone iodine (1%-2% stock solution)	250 mL	Good irrigation for nonspecific inflammation and for fungal infections; concentrations >10% cause irritation
ANTIMYCOTICS		
Nystatin	5×10^6 U	Dissolve in 30 mL 0.9% saline solution; daily for 7-10 days
Clotrimazole	500 mg	Suspension or cream; daily for 1 week
Vinegar	2%	20 mL wine vinegar to 1 L of 0.9% saline solution; use as uterine lavage
Amphotericin B	200-250 mg	Daily for 1 wk

From Asbury AC: *Compend Cont Educ Pract Vet* 9:585-592, 1987.

- If free fluid and inflammatory debris are present in the uterine lumen, the uterus should be lavaged before intrauterine treatment. A 3- or 5-day regimen of once-daily intrauterine therapy is most common.
- Rest from breeding for 45 to 60 days may aid recovery from chronic inflammation.
- After the infection is cleared, breeding should be limited to once per estrus.

YEAST OR FUNGAL INFECTIONS

- Yeast or fungal infections often are the result of extensive use of intrauterine antibiotics.
- These infections are difficult to treat and tend to recur.
- Antimycotic drugs used include nystatin and clotrimazole.
- Uterine irrigations with diluted povidone-iodine solution, vinegar, or diluted acetic acid have been used with varying results.
- For treatment to be successful, several weeks of daily treatment may be needed.

PERSISTENT MATING-INDUCED ENDOMETRITIS

- Mares with persistent mating-induced endometritis usually are free of bacteria before breeding but have delayed uterine clearance.
- Treatment is directed at rapid removal of intrauterine fluids after breeding. A combination of uterine lavage and oxytocin (alone or with antibiotics) improves pregnancy rates.
- Prostaglandin $F_{2\alpha}$ also enhances uterine clearance and induces more prolonged uterine contractions than oxytocin (5 hours for cloprostenol versus 40 minutes for oxytocin).
- To be effective, treatment must be performed after each mating.

Systemic Antimicrobial Therapy

Though intrauterine therapy is the preferred treatment for endometritis, systemic antibiotic administration has some advantages:

- Higher antimicrobial concentrations are achieved throughout the genital tract with systemic administration.
- Drugs administered locally may be degraded by conditions in the uterine lumen.
- Systemic therapy eliminates the need to invade the vestibule, vaginal canal, and cervix, thus minimizing contamination of the reproductive tract.

Antimicrobials considered effective by the systemic route are listed in Table 13-4.

Reproductive Management of Mares

It is standard management practice to recommend breeding 1 to 2 days before ovulation. If a stallion is known to have spermatozoa that survive for only a short period, breeding within

Table 13-4
Antimicrobials suitable for systemic treatment of endometritis

Drug	Dose	Times daily
Amikacin sulfate	7 mg/kg	2
Ampicillin trihydrate	10-15 mg/kg	2
Enrofloxacin	6-7 mg/kg	1
Gentamicin sulfate	2 mg/kg	3
	or 6 mg/kg	1
Procaine penicillin G	20,000 U/kg	2
Trimethoprim and sulfamethoxazole	3 mg/kg (trimethoprim) 15 mg/kg (Sulfamethoxazole)	2

Note: These dosages are based on anecdotal reports and may not conform with FDA regulatory approval.
From Bennett DG et al: *Equine Pract* 3:37-44, 1981.

6 hours of predicted or controlled ovulation may be required.

Management of maiden mares

A complete reproductive examination of all maiden mares is advisable before breeding, including:

- evaluation of the size and function of the ovaries and uterus
- palpation of the pelvic canal, noting the size and any impingements from old traumatic episodes
- routine vaginal examination and inspection for remnants of the hymen (treated by stretching or incision); if pneumovagina and concurrent vaginitis and cervicitis are found, Caslick's operation is indicated.
- uterine culture, if required by the breeding farm; maiden mares rarely have endometritis, so in the absence of clinical signs of inflammation, a positive culture should be viewed skeptically.

Management of foaling mares

The first postpartum estrus ("foal heat") occurs quickly, and the mare can conceive within 9 to 15 days of parturition.

- The mean interval from foaling to first ovulation is 10.2 days; 43% of mares ovulate by 9 days postpartum, 97% by day 20.
- Mares foaling later in the year have a shorter interval between foaling and first ovulation, so use of artificial lighting for pregnant mares during the winter may be worthwhile.

ENHANCING UTERINE CLEARANCE.

Pregnancy rates at foal heat and at the 30-day postfoaling estrus can be increased by administration of prostalene (1 mg SC) twice a day for 10 days, starting the day of foaling. Pregnancy rates at the 30-day heat are 67%, compared with 29% in untreated mares.

DELAYING FOAL HEAT.

Conception rates are higher in mares bred after postpartum day 10 than in those bred on or before day 10. Thus delaying foal heat can improve fertility rates. One protocol, which begins the day after foaling, involves:

- daily administration of progesterone (150 mg) and estradiol-17β (10 mg) for 6 to 10 days or altrenogest (0.044 mg/kg) for 8 days
- injection of prostaglandin (10 mg) on day 9

In one study, more mares (82%) became pregnant when ovulation occurred after day 15 postpartum than when it occurred before day 15 (50%).

ESTRUS DETECTION.

Mares nursing foals often do not exhibit estrous behavior, particularly if it is the mare's first foal. Failure to detect estrus by the expected time is an indication for ultrasonographic examination.

PREBREEDING EVALUATION.

A complete genital examination is indicated for all foaling mares before the first postpartum breeding. This is best performed on the first day on which signs of estrus are strong, and should include:

- vaginoscopy and direct palpation of the vagina and cervix for uterine discharge and damage caused by delivery
  - A mucoid, chocolate-brown discharge (blood) seldom warrants treatment.
  - Purulent discharges accompanied by inflammation should be cultured; however, results from samples obtained during foal heat should be interpreted cautiously because invariably there are some residual organisms.
- ultrasonographic examination for intrauterine fluid
  - Mares with intrauterine fluid at foal heat should be treated appropriately before breeding or should not be bred.
  - Mares that are not bred can be given prostaglandin $F_{2\alpha}$ 5 days after the first postpartum ovulation.

Dystocia, retained placenta, persistent purulent exudate, and physical damage to the reproductive tract are valid reasons for not breeding during foal heat. Therapeutic or corrective measures should be initiated as soon as possible.

BREEDING STRATEGIES.

The number of natural services should be kept to a minimum in postpartum mares. Artificial insemination, when permitted, increases conception rates.

Management of barren mares

MANAGING MARES WITH ENDOMETRITIS

- Natural service should be kept to a minimum. Artificial insemination, postbreeding treatment, or minimal contamination techniques (see the section on intrauterine therapy) should be used when possible.

♦ Treatment includes intrauterine therapy, uterine lavage, and systemic antimicrobials administered before breeding or after ovulation.

♦ Oxytocin or cloprostenol after breeding is very beneficial in mares with persistent mating-induced endometritis.

Artificial lighting is especially useful in barren mares. The more ovulatory cycles available during the breeding season, the greater the chance of returning the mare to production.

Management of twinning

Twinning is a common cause of abortion in mares. To maximize a mare's reproductive potential, twins must be identified early in gestation and one conceptus reduced before formation of the endometrial cups (day 35 to 38). Following are some practical guidelines:

♦ It is not necessary to delay breeding until the next cycle in mares with more than one preovulatory follicle.

♦ Mares should be checked for twins 13 to 16 days after ovulation, regardless of the number of detected ovulations.

♦ Two vesicles fixed in the same horn may be pressed together and irregular in shape, causing the thin apposing walls to be undetectable. Reexamination of the vesicle at 20 to 23 days aids correct diagnosis.

♦ Vesicles must be differentiated from uterine cysts. Recording the location and size of cysts found during routine examinations helps differentiate them from a small vesicle (see the section on ultrasonographic evaluation of the reproductive tract).

♦ If unilaterally fixed embryos are present after day 17, the best approach is to wait a few days and evaluate the success of natural reduction.

MANUAL REDUCTION. Manual reduction of one embryo is most successful when performed before day 25. The vesicles are easier to rupture when large (12 to 18 mm, days 13 to 15) than when small (6 to 9 mm, days 11 to 12). Administering antiinflammatory drugs during manual reduction does not appear to improve the success of this technique. Manual reduction is also discussed on p. 318.

REDUCTION AFTER 30 DAYS' GESTATION. A number of reduction techniques have been attempted in mares at >30 days of gestation:

♦ Surgical removal of one fetus at 41 to 65 days has been successful when the twins were in separate horns.

♦ Allantoic aspiration of one vesicle using a transvaginal ultrasound–guided technique has been performed.

• When the vesicles are not in intimate contact, twin pregnancy can be reduced to a viable singleton in about 30% of cases.

• The technique is most applicable for bilateral twins but has shown promise for unilateral twins at <40 days' gestation.

♦ Intracardiac injection of potassium chloride in one fetus can successfully reduce twin pregnancies to singletons in 56% of cases when performed after 115 days of gestation.

• If performed before 112 days, only 12% of mares subsequently deliver a live foal.

When twins are diagnosed late in pregnancy, progesterone supplementation at 150 to 200 mg/day IM may be helpful. Mares may give birth to a full-term foal and a mummified fetus.

THERAPEUTIC ABORTION. Sometimes it is better to induce abortion rather than attempt to reduce the pregnancy to a singleton or manage a twin pregnancy. The preferred method depends on the stage of gestation.

♦ Before 38 days a single injection of prostaglandin is effective. This is the most satisfactory approach because mares return to estrus and may be bred again that season.

♦ Between 38 and 100 days, multiple injections of prostaglandin are effective. However, once the endometrial cups have formed, mares do not return to estrus for some time.

♦ After 100 days, manual dilation of the cervix and irrigation of the uterus with large volumes of warm (38° C [100.4° F]), sterile saline, using strict asepsis, induces abortion.

• Cloprostenol (250 µg IM once daily) has been used successfully to induce abortion between 80 and 150 days.

After 100 days' gestation, the risks of uterine damage, dystocia, retained placenta, and other complications increase. Though abortion may be induced midterm by cervical dilation or later in gestation by oxytocin injection, it often is best for future fertility to allow the mare to foal naturally.

Management of mares to be bred with shipped, cooled semen

Before ordering the semen, the veterinarian managing the mare should clarify several points with the stallion manager:

- days of the week the stallion's semen is collected
- times during the breeding season when the stallion will not be available
- longevity of the stallion's semen
- first-cycle conception rate of the stallion
- method of air transport used (same-day air or overnight)

GUIDELINES FOR MAXIMIZING CONCEPTION

- Knowing the idiosyncrasies of a mare's estrous cycle, especially the number of days she is in estrus and on what day and what size follicle she typically ovulates, is important.
- The stallion manager should be notified on the first day of estrus.
- Estrus can be determined by teasing the mare daily or by daily ultrasound examinations, complemented by vaginoscopy to determine the degree of cervical relaxation.
- Beginning on day 2 of estrus, the mare should be palpated and examined with ultrasound daily.
- When the dominant follicle reaches 35 mm in diameter, the semen should be ordered and hCG or deslorelin administered (see the section on inducing ovulation in cycling mares).
- When managing unfamiliar mares or mares that typically ovulate small follicles, it may be prudent to order the semen on day 3 of estrus; hCG or deslorelin is then given when the mare is inseminated. Use of a stallion to identify estrus is critical for success in these cases.

PREDICTING OVULATION. Ultrasonography is extremely helpful in timing ovulation.

- Beginning 24 to 48 hours before ovulation, the endometrial folds recede and the uterus develops a more homogeneous appearance.
- At least 6 to 12 hours before ovulation, the dominant follicle changes from spherical to pear shaped.

SEMEN HANDLING AND INSEMINATION

- It is important to identify that the semen sent is from the correct stallion.
- The semen does not need to be warmed before insemination, unless it has been extended in a cream gel extender.
- All but 1 to 2 mL of semen is drawn up into a syringe and the mare is bred.
- Sperm motility is determined from the remaining sample after it has been warmed at 37° C (98.6° F) for 2 to 5 minutes. Progressive motility of the warmed sample should be >30%.
- Ultrasonography is used to confirm ovulation and to check for intrauterine fluid accumulation 24 hours after insemination. If fluid is present, postbreeding treatment is indicated (see p. 319).
- If the mare does not ovulate within 36 hours, she should be rebred.

Management of mares to be bred with frozen semen

First-cycle pregnancy rates with frozen semen are 31% to 64%. To maximize conception rates, mares should be:

- examined every 6 hours during late estrus
- given hCG
  - If hCG is given when the follicle is 35 mm, most mares ovulate 36 to 48 hours later.
  - The mare should be palpated at 24, 30, and 36 hours after hCG administration.
  - If at any of these times the mare has ovulated, she should be inseminated immediately.
  - If the follicle is still present 36 hours after hCG administration, the mare should be inseminated.
- examined by ultrasound 12 hours after insemination
- If the mare has not ovulated, she should be reinseminated.

  Alternative I:

- The mare is examined every 6 hours once the follicle reaches 35 mm.

- Insemination is performed once (immediately after ovulation) or twice (before and after ovulation) when the follicle develops a teardrop shape and the endometrial folds diminish.

Alternative II:

- If monitoring every 6 hours is impractical, the mare must be examined at least every 24 hours, preferably every 12 hours.
- Insemination should be delayed as long as possible.
- Once the mare has been inseminated, she should be checked at intervals of 12 hours and reinseminated at each inspection until ovulation occurs.

Postbreeding treatment:

- In some mares insemination of thawed semen induces a severe inflammatory reaction and intrauterine fluid accumulation.
- If fluid is found on ultrasonography, uterine lavage should be performed and oxytocin administered (see p. 328).

Diseases Affecting Multiple Sites

(pages 1148–1157)

Michelle M. LeBlanc

Abdominal pain is the most common clinical sign in periparturient mares experiencing difficulty. Causes include:

- normal contractions as the uterus involutes and expels the placenta
- internal hemorrhage from rupture of the uterine artery or uterus
- rupture of the cecum or right ventral colon
- ischemic necrosis of the small colon
- colonic torsion
- uterine torsion
- retained placenta
- rupture of the urinary bladder or diaphragm

DISEASES WITH PHYSICAL CAUSES

Postpartum Hemorrhage

Hemorrhage from a uterine artery is common in older mares (>11 years of age), although it can occur in young mares. Hemorrhage from the artery is not always fatal; it may slowly dissect into the broad ligament and form a hematoma. But if the broad ligament ruptures or the serosal surface of the uterus tears, the mare bleeds to death quickly.

Diagnosis and treatment

- Colic is the predominant sign of postpartum hemorrhage, although many mares are not discovered until they are weak or dead.
- Diagnosis is made by rectal palpation, which causes extreme discomfort. The degree of enlargement of the uterus indicates the extent of hemorrhage.
- Treatment consists of confining the mare to a dark, quiet stall and using mild sedation if necessary.
- Blood transfusions, plasma volume expanders, and fluid therapy do not alter the course of the illness and may even be contraindicated if the mare becomes excited by treatment procedures.
- Naloxone, formaldehyde, hypertonic saline, and Chinese herbs have also been used.

Gastrointestinal Complications

GI complications in postpartum mares include:

- rupture of the cecum or right ventral colon
  - Affected mares appear normal at the beginning of parturition, but subsequent abdominal straining is either weak or absent, and the foal must be manually delivered.
  - The mare does not recover from foaling as expected, and shock develops quickly (within 4 to 6 hours of delivery).
  - The mare should be euthanized if abdominocentesis reveals ingesta in the peritoneal cavity.
  - When the large bowel is damaged but not ruptured, necrosis results in slowly developing peritonitis.
  - Feeding less hay to mares a few days before parturition helps prevent large bowel damage.
- colonic torsion (see Chapter 10, Alimentary System)
- ischemic necrosis of the small colon
  - Contusions of the small intestine, small colon, or mesentery during parturition produce mild, transitory signs of colic.

- More severe trauma may result in mesenteric rupture, possibly leading to intestinal incarceration or vascular occlusion and ischemic necrosis.
- Abdominal pain may be seen at any time from foaling to 24 hours after parturition.
- Rectal palpation reveals inconsistent and varied findings, from no palpable abnormalities to an impacted small colon.
- Results of peritoneal fluid analysis are consistently abnormal (see Chapter 10, Alimentary System).
- Exploratory celiotomy is recommended. Survival rates after ischemic necrosis of the small colon are poor.

INFLAMMATORY, INFECTIOUS, AND IMMUNE DISEASES

Metritis-Laminitis-Septicemia Complex

Acute metritis with concurrent laminitis and/or septicemia is a serious sequel to retained placenta or any gross contamination of the uterus during foaling. This syndrome must be managed rapidly and vigorously. It often is fatal in mares that do not receive adequate care.

Signs and diagnosis

- Signs may begin as early as 12 to 24 hours after foaling.
- The mare becomes severely depressed, anorectic, and painful.
- Fever, elevated pulse and respiratory rates, and congested mucous membranes are noted.
- The digital pulse may increase 12 hours to 5 days later, indicating the beginning of laminitis.
- The uterus usually contains several liters of chocolate-colored, fetid fluid.
- A small piece of placenta frequently is retained in one horn.

Treatment

- uterine lavage
  - Large volumes of warm, diluted povidone-iodine solution or saline are infused into the uterus by gravity flow, using a large-bore nasogastric tube.
  - The uterine contents are then siphoned off, and lavage is repeated until the fluid drained out is similar to that being infused.

- The procedure is repeated 2 to 3 times daily.
- Before each treatment, the uterus should be palpated per rectum to evaluate the amount of fluid accumulating between treatments.
- Mares responding with uterine involution have a thickened corrugated uterine wall, whereas mares not responding have a thin, flaccid uterine wall.
- Treatment is discontinued when the intrauterine fluid is clear or only slightly cloudy.
- systemic broad-spectrum antimicrobials, IV fluids, and nonsteroidal antiinflammatory drugs (NSAIDs)
  - *Bacteroides fragilis* is commonly involved. It frequently is resistant to penicillins and aminoglycosides but is susceptible to metronidazole.
- monitoring with a complete blood count (CBC) every 48 to 72 hours
  - Extremely low white blood cell (WBC) counts (<2000 cells/μL) with left shift and toxic neutrophils are common. The WBC count should return toward normal as the mare responds to treatment.
  - Fibrinogen, which may be >500 mg/dL, returns to normal 2 to 3 days after the rise in WBC count.
- antiinflammatory drugs and supportive therapy (laminitis; see Chapter 15, Musculoskeletal System)
  - It is uncommon if acute metritis is treated vigorously from the outset.
  - It develops quickly, often necessitating euthanasia.

MULTIFACTORIAL DISEASES

Dystocia

Dystocia is uncommon in mares, but when it occurs, it generally is severe. The life of the foal usually is in serious jeopardy, and the health and future reproductive capacity of the mare also is at risk.

Fetal causes of dystocia

Most cases of dystocia are due to postural abnormalities of the fetus, such as:

- simple retention of a forelimb at the fetlock or carpus and deviation of the head

- Lateral or ventral deviation of the head usually is due to the foal's being weak or dead.
- It must be differentiated from congenital curvature of the cervical vertebrae ("wry neck"), which cannot be corrected manually.
- Correction of a laterally deviated head requires repulsion of the foal. An obstetric chain placed over the poll and through the mouth may also be necessary; blunt eye hooks are helpful in some cases.
- Retention of a forelimb must be differentiated from flexor contracture. It is sometimes impossible to vaginally deliver a foal with contracted tendons.
- ◆ "dog sitting," in which the hind limbs are flexed at the hips and folded under the foal's body
  - Attempts to deliver a foal with this malpresentation uncorrected are unsuccessful. The foal quickly dies because the umbilical cord is occluded by the pelvic brim.
  - Delivery of a dead foal is effected by partial fetotomy (transverse division of the trunk, caudal to the last rib).

Posterior presentations are relatively uncommon. Amputation of the affected limb(s) may be necessary if the foal is dead. Transverse presentation is extremely rare and is an indication for cesarean section.

Twins may cause dystocia, as can disparity of fetal size and maternal pelvic diameter (unusual if the maternal pelvis is of normal dimensions). Dystocia as a result of fetal monsters is uncommon. Hydrocephalus is encountered occasionally; most affected fetuses can be delivered after collapsing the skull.

Maternal causes of dystocia

Maternal causes of dystocia include:

- ◆ pelvic abnormality, such as ileal or acetabular fractures and other pelvic injuries that may result in stenosis of the birth canal
  - Examination before breeding identifies mares with these problems.
  - Elective cesarean should be considered.
- ◆ abdominal hernia or rupture of the prepubic tendon

- Sudden ventral displacement of the caudal abdomen with accompanying edema suggests prepubic tendon rupture.
- Mechanical support of the abdomen is needed until parturition.
- Restrictions of exercise and diet are important until after foaling.
- Elective cesarean or induction of parturition should be considered.
- ◆ vaginal cystocele
  - Eversion of the bladder through the urethra or prolapse through a tear in the vaginal wall may impede delivery.
  - The bladder must be drained and replaced, after first abolishing abdominal straining and repelling the fetus. The vaginal wound is then sutured and the foal delivered.
- ◆ uterine inertia
  - This condition is uncommon. It is seen more often in older mares and in debilitated, weak, metabolically imbalanced, or systemically ill mares.
  - Affected mares begin labor but cannot deliver the foal; assistance is needed.
- ◆ uterine torsion (see p. 344)
- ◆ immaturity (inadequate pelvic size)
- ◆ premature separation of the chorioallantois
  - Premature separation has been associated with placentitis, induction of parturition before fetal maturity, systemic illness, and fetal death.
  - A large, red, glistening "bag" is seen protruding through the labia.
  - *This complication must be handled as an emergency;* the placenta should be incised and the foal delivered immediately.
  - Oxygen supplementation of the foal via nasal intubation may aid survival.

Treatment guidelines

Some restraint is advisable in all cases. A twitch or lip chain often suffices; sidelines may also be used.

SEDATION AND ANESTHESIA

- ◆ Sedation may be indicated, but drugs that might depress the fetus (e.g., tranquilizers, narcotics, and inhalant and intravenous anesthetics) must be used with discretion.

- The respiratory depression caused by narcotics can be reversed with levallorphan or naloxone.
- Small doses of thiobarbiturates are tolerated, and inhalation anesthetics are readily eliminated via the lungs if the foal breathes adequately after delivery.
- Sedation of the mare with acepromazine (5 to 6 mg/100 kg IV) has a minimal effect on the foal.
- Xylazine or detomidine alone is a poor choice. Good sedation and analgesia can be achieved with xylazine (0.5 mg/kg IV) plus butorphanol (0.025 to 0.05 mg/kg IV).
- Xylazine (0.5 mg/kg IV) followed by morphine (0.1 to 0.2 mg/kg) provides excellent sedation for fetotomy, although GI stasis for up to 4 hours is a frequent complication. Mares should receive 4 L of mineral oil via stomach tube after the dystocia is corrected.

♦ Epidural anesthesia is of questionable value in delivering a live foal (time factor), and it has no effect on abdominal contractions.
  - An epidural may be indicated if the mare needs to be shipped to a referral institution for fetotomy or cesarean section.
  - A combination of xylazine (100 mg) and lidocaine (5 mL of 2% lidocaine) in the epidural space (S1-S2) is preferred over lidocaine alone.

♦ Short-term general anesthesia may be indicated for correction of minor postural abnormalities.
  - Xylazine (0.5 mg/kg IV) plus ketamine (2 mg/kg IV) provides 10 to 15 minutes of good relaxation, with some degree of anesthesia.
  - Addition of guaifenesin IV (1 L of 5% guaifenesin in 5% dextrose) gives an additional 10 to 20 minutes of anesthesia.
  - None of these drugs significantly depress neonatal respiration.

♦ General anesthesia may be necessary for apparently serious dystocias requiring a major obstetric procedure.
  - If the foal is alive, premedication with xylazine (0.5 mg/kg IM) and induction with ketamine (2.2 mg/kg IV) and guaifenesin (100 mg/kg IV) is preferred.

- If the foal is dead, thiobarbiturate (1 to 2 g of thiamylal sodium) added to guaifenesin may be used as the induction agent.
- Anesthesia should be maintained using minimal concentrations of halothane, with the mare in lateral recumbency or with her hindquarters raised by ropes attached to the rear limbs.
- Until the foal is delivered, many mares have great difficulty breathing adequately and spontaneously without mechanical assistance.

MANAGEMENT PRINCIPLES

♦ During any obstetric procedure, the emphasis should be on asepsis, adequate lubrication, rapid assessment of the problem, and minimal use of traumatic instruments.

♦ Presentation, position, and posture of the fetus must be determined quickly.

♦ The size and viability of the fetus, the condition of the tissues of the mare's reproductive tract, and the adequacy of pelvic size also need to be assessed.

♦ The possibility of twin fetuses should be explored in every case.

♦ Hip lock may be overcome by placing a halter on the foal and applying traction along the foal's spinal column instead of along the forelimbs. Rotation of the foal does not help.

♦ The vaginal and cervical mucosae are highly sensitive to prolonged or traumatic procedures and often respond with multiple and irreversible adhesions.
  - *Fetal extractors are contraindicated in equine obstetrics.*
  - Fetotomy must be undertaken carefully and quickly and should be limited to 1 or 2 cuts. *Total fetotomy is contraindicated in equine obstetrics.*
  - Epidural anesthesia is helpful when partial fetotomy must be performed.

CESAREAN SECTION

♦ Timing of an *elective* cesarean is important. The same criteria used for induction of parturition should be applied (see the section on induction of parturition).

- Maturity of the foal is a prime consideration. The safest approach is to wait for the mare to actually begin labor.
- With *emergency* cesareans (dystocias), an early decision to perform surgery is critical for a successful outcome.
- The surgical approaches are the low flank (Marcenac, which offers the best exposure to the uterus), paracostal, and ventral midline. Techniques are detailed in *Equine Medicine and Surgery V.*
- Systemic antimicrobials are given before, during, and after surgery.
- Tetanus prophylaxis should also be given; fluids or plasma are administered as needed.
- To stimulate placental expulsion, 100 IU of oxytocin in 3 L of sterile saline is given IV over 1 hour.
  - The incidence of retained placenta is high (80%), but attempts to remove the placenta during surgery can cause extensive uterine damage.
  - It is vital that the placenta not be included in any of the uterine suture lines.
- Systemic treatment for laminitis should be initiated, and the mare should be given light daily exercise.
- Postoperative adhesions between the uterus and adjacent abdominal structures can be prevented or minimized by daily palpation of the uterus per rectum, beginning day 2 or 3 postsurgery.
  - Uterine involution is evaluated, and the uterus is cleared from adjacent structures.
- Survival rates in mares range from 61% to 100% (average 81%). The survival rate in foals is 30%.
- Subsequent conception rates in mares are only about 50%, and of those that conceive, about 25% abort. Fertility rates also are reduced after fetotomy (38% overall).

Disseminated Intravascular Coagulopathy

Disseminated intravascular coagulopathy (DIC) is a possible sequel to severe dystocia or cesarean section.

Signs and diagnosis

- Mares with DIC bleed from the uterus for prolonged periods (2 to 5 days).

- Large volumes of bright red, unclotted blood are seen dripping from the labia.
- The mare appears depressed, toxic, weak, and anorectic.
- The PCV may drop as low as 10%.

Treatment and prognosis

- Treatment consists of whole blood transfusions, IV fluids, and supportive nursing care in a quiet environment.
- Systemic antimicrobials and antiinflammatories are indicated. The use of heparin is controversial (see Chapter 19, Hemolymphatic System).
- The mortality is high in mares whose condition does not stabilize within 48 hours.

Diseases of the Ovary

(pages 1157-1154)
Michelle M. LeBlanc

DIAGNOSTIC AND THERAPEUTIC CONSIDERATIONS

An accurate breeding history should be obtained and ovarian structures and uterine/cervical status thoroughly evaluated in mares presented because of cyclic irregularities or lack of estrous behavior (see the section on examination of the mare). Table 13-5 offers guidelines for diagnosis.

Ovarian Enlargement

A history of overt masculine behavior, in conjunction with a crested neck and enlarged clitoris, strongly suggests a testosterone-secreting ovarian neoplasm. If the opposite ovary is active and the mare is cycling, the enlarged ovary is more likely caused by a hematoma, mature teratoma, or cystadenoma.

Guidelines for diagnosis

- A presumptive diagnosis of ovarian tumor or hematoma is based on palpation and ultrasonographic detection of a persistently large (6 to 40 cm), firm or lobulated, unilateral mass.
- Repeated rectal examinations should be performed before making a final diagnosis.

Table 13-5
Findings and differential diagnoses in nonpregnant, noncycling mares

Ovaries	Season	Tubular tract	Behavior	Other findings	Probable cause
Normal size, active, may have follicles	Summer	Excellent tone	Rejects stallion	None	Spontaneous prolonged CL
Normal size, active	Spring	Poor tone	Passive or irregular estrus	Pale, dry cervical and vaginal mucosa	Transition from anestrus to ovulatory stage
Small, inactive	Winter	Flaccid	Passive or irregular estrus	Pale, dry cervical and vaginal mucosa	Winter anestrus
Very small, inactive	Any	Infantile	Passive	Small body size	Gonadal dysgenesis
Very small, inactive	Any	Infantile	Passive irregular estrus stallion-like behavior	Large, athletic	Testicular feminization
One ovary enlarged, other ovary smaller than normal	Any	Variable (flaccid)	Masculine (aggressive) or constant estrus	No ovulation fossa on large ovary	Secreting ovarian tumor

CL, Corpus luteum.

* Endometrial biopsy is indicted to determine the breeding prognosis before surgery is considered.

Ovariectomy

In *normal* mares, removal of both ovaries can be performed with the mare standing, via either colpotomy or a flank approach, using tranquilization and epidural anesthesia, and a chain ecraseur (colpotomy) or an emasculator (flank approach). Techniques and aftercare are discussed in *Equine Medicine and Surgery V*.

REMOVAL OF OVARIAN TUMORS

* Unilateral ovariectomy for removal of tumors can sometimes be performed under local anesthesia via colpotomy or flank approach.
* Hemostasis is very important—the increased vascularity of tumescent ovaries requires complete ligation of the ovarian vessels (extremely difficult or impossible in a standing animal).
* Excessive traction on the ovary causes intense pain and may cause the mare to rear or fall.
* For these reasons, general anesthesia is usually recommended.
  * The approach is dictated by tumor size and width of the paralumbar fossa.
  * Large tumors are more readily removed via a ventral midline or paramedian approach.
  * Colpotomy may be used if the ovary is <10 cm, and the flank approach can be used for ovaries up to 15 cm in diameter.

CONGENITAL AND FAMILIAL DISEASES

Gonadal Dysgenesis

Gonadal dysgenesis is occasionally seen in infertile phenotypic females. Findings include:

* persistent anestrus or irregular periods of behavioral estrus
* extremely small ovaries (usually <1 cm)
* an infantile uterus, often no more than a thin band of tissue
* a flaccid, pale, dilated cervix
* normal external genitalia
* small stature in some affected mares

The main karyotypic abnormality is 63, XO. Other abnormal karyotypes reported to cause gonadal dysgenesis include 63, XO/64, XX or XY; 65, XXY/64, XX; and autosomal deletion 64, XX del2q-.

Testicular Feminization

Testicular feminization is a type of male pseudohermaphroditism. The chromosomal complement invariably is 64, XY. This is an inherited defect. Affected mares have the following features:

* Larger than average for their breed, they are athletic, and some have the appearance of a stallion.
* They have small, firm, inactive ovaries.
* The cervix is pale and dilated, and the uterus and cervix are small or nonexistent.
* Affected mares display erratic stallionlike behavior.

Karyotyping is essential to confirm the diagnosis because not all mares with hypoplastic ovaries have abnormal chromosomes or are infertile.

DISEASES WITH PHYSICAL CAUSES

Hematoma

Ovarian hematomas are relatively common and can vary in size from 50 mm to 50 cm. Hemorrhage typically occurs into the follicular cavity after ovulation. Normal cyclic ovarian activity continues, though the hematoma may persist for 2 weeks to 6 months.

Differentiating hematoma from neoplasia

Hematomas are differentiated from ovarian neoplasia by:

* the timing of their formation (after estrus)
* the presence of a palpable ovulation fossa
* their progressive shrinkage, usually over 2 weeks
* continued normal cyclic activity
* ultrasonographic appearance

Management

Ovarian hematomas usually resolve without treatment. Rarely a hematoma becomes large enough to persist for several months, eventually destroying germinal tissue and leaving a firm, mineralized ovary that is devoid of follicular activity.

Abscesses

Ovarian abscesses are rare, generally resulting from aspiration of an ovarian "cyst" or retrieval of an egg for in vitro fertilization. Affected mares continue to cycle normally. Ultrasonography is useful for differentiating an abscess from other ovarian conditions. Abscesses are treated by surgical drainage and appropriate antimicrobial therapy or by ovariectomy.

Ovarian Cysts

Follicular and luteal cysts do not occur in mares. A misdiagnosis of "cystic ovaries" may be made in mares with any of the following:
- large or multiple follicles
- ovarian hematoma
- prolonged estrus
  - During the cyclic season prolonged estrus (8 to 12 days) may occur, with multiple follicles that ovulate synchronously or asynchronously.
  - Daily rectal palpation, in conjunction with ultrasonography, can be used to determine when to breed mares with twin follicles (best bred 12 to 24 hours before ovulation of the second follicle).

Germinal inclusion cysts are small (1 to 2 mm), fibrous, encapsulated cysts that occur at the ovulation fossa, potentially obstructing ovulation. They are more common in aged mares with hard, multifollicular ovaries that do not change palpably during the estrous cycle. Ovariectomy may be warranted in these mares. Parovarian cysts commonly occur in tissues surrounding the ovary but are not clinically significant.

Hemorrhagic Follicles

Although rare, the dominant preovulatory follicle may not ovulate during the cyclic season, but instead may fill with blood (see the section on ovarian irregularities and lesions). Mares that experience this problem may do so over a number of estrous cycles and are presented for infertility. Anovulatory hemorrhagic follicles are identified by repeated ultrasonographic examinations of the ovaries during estrus.

NEOPLASIA
Granulosa–Theca Cell Tumor

Granulosa–theca cell tumors are the most commonly reported ovarian neoplasm. They generally are benign, steroid-producing neoplasms. Affected mares display the following signs and symptoms:
- Anestrus or continuous or intermittent estrus is exhibited.
- Masculine behavior, including mounting mares in estrus, aggressiveness, squealing, and striking, may be shown.
- Plasma testosterone concentrations may be elevated
  - Aggressive or masculine demeanor occurs with plasma testosterone concentrations >100 pg/mL.
  - Serum testosterone >40 to 100 pg/mL (depending on the assay method) is diagnostic for granulosa–theca cell tumors.
  - Only arrhenoblastomas (see below) cause similarly elevated serum testosterone levels.
  - Testosterone concentrations may not be elevated in mares in anestrus or in persistent estrus.
- Elevated concentrations of inhibin are common.
  - Only 54% of mares with granulosa cell tumors have elevated testosterone concentrations, whereas 87% have elevated inhibin concentrations (>1 pg/mL).
  - Plasma progesterone levels usually remain <100 pg/mL.
  - Abnormally high serum estrogen concentrations are associated with persistent signs of estrus or nymphomania.

Diagnosis

Granulosa–theca cell tumors are suspected based on:
- the history, especially abnormal behavior
- rectal palpation: an enlarged, abnormally–firm ovary or a multicystic ovary, usually without apalpable ovulation fossa
  - The unaffected ovary is small and inactive.
  - If the contralateral ovary is producing follicles that ovulate, the enlarged ovary is more likely caused by an ovarian hematoma, mature teratoma, or cystadenoma.

- During the transitional period (early spring and late fall), an ovary containing numerous anovulatory follicles may be confused with an ovarian neoplasm.
- ultrasonography: a solid ovarian mass or a single, large, fluid-filled cyst
  - The mass varies from multilocular and honeycombed to dense, knobby, or smooth.
  - The opposite ovary usually shows little or no follicular activity.
- Gross appearance of the excised ovary: multiple cystic structures separated by yellowish stroma
  - Cysts may contain blood, blood-tinged fluid, or, most often, straw-colored serumlike fluid.

Definitive diagnosis is by histologic examination after excision.

Treatment and prognosis

Treatment is ovariectomy of the affected ovary. The prognosis for fertility after surgery is favorable. Most mares begin to cycle within 2 to 16 months after surgery (mean, 8.5 months), depending on the time of year.

Teratoma

Teratomas are the second most common ovarian tumor. They are benign, nonsecretory tumors that contain misplaced embryonic structures, such as bone, skin, teeth, cartilage, nerves, blood vessels, and hair. They are either solid or contain large cystic spaces.

Diagnosis and management

- During rectal examination the ovary feels firm and enlarged, with rough, irregular surfaces.
- Differentiation from other nonsecretory ovarian tumors is difficult without excision or biopsy. Ultrasonography may aid diagnosis.
- Affected mares continue to cycle and ovulate from the unaffected ovary, but surgical removal is indicated if the tumor grows large enough to drop within the abdomen.

Adenoma and Adenocarcinoma

Other nonsecretory ovarian tumors are extremely rare.

- Ovarian adenomas usually are formed from the surface of the ovulatory fossa or oviductal fimbriae. They typically are unilateral and may be unilobular or multilobular.
- If cystic, these tumors are referred to as cystadenomas.
- Rarely adenomas metastasize (then classified as adenocarcinomas), causing weight loss, ascites, and/or recurring abdominal pain.
- Excision is indicated for adenomas and for localized adenocarcinomas.

Dysgerminoma and Ovarian Lymphosarcoma

Though rare, dysgerminomas and ovarian lymphosarcomas are highly malignant.

- If dysgerminomas can be detected before metastasis, the affected ovary should be removed. This tumor has been associated with hypertrophic osteopathy (see Chapter 9, Respiratory System).
- Ovarian lymphosarcoma causes debilitation.
  - Visceral abdominal metastases are common. Abdominocentesis may reveal exfoliated tumor cells.
  - There is no satisfactory treatment. Euthanasia is recommended.

Arrhenoblastoma

Arrhenoblastomas are rare, masculinizing ovarian tumors. Affected mares may.

- have an elevated serum testosterone concentration
- exhibit masculine behavior
- have a small, inactive contralateral ovary

It can be difficult to differentiate an arrhenoblastoma from a granulosa–theca cell tumor except by histologic examination of the excised ovary.

IDIOPATHIC DISEASES

Prolonged Diestrus

Mares may fail to return to estrus after a normal ovulatory cycle for a number of reasons:

- pregnancy
- conception with early embryonic death: may not show signs of estrus for 7 to 12 days
- abnormal uterine contents, such as pyometra or mucometra
- estrous signs not displayed or detected, despite normal cyclic ovarian activity
- persistence of the CL (35 to 95 days)
  - Rectal findings are typical of diestrus: a firm, elongated, pale

cervix, excellent uterine tone, and active ovaries.

- On ultrasonography a CL usually is evident and there is no embryonic vesicle in the uterus.
- Treatment is directed at luteolysis: administration of prostaglandin or an analog (see section on hormonal therapy) or indirect stimulation of natural luteolysis by uterine infusion.

Anestrus During the Ovulatory Season
Idiopathic

◆ Mares occasionally develop ovarian atrophy and loss of uterine tone during the breeding season, similar to changes seen in winter anestrus.

◆ The cause is not known but may involve constant exposure to prolonged daylight (>16 hours/day) or poor nutrition.

◆ Diagnosis is based on physical findings (see the section on rectal palpation) plus periodic assays for circulating progesterone.

◆ There is no treatment. It is necessary to simply wait until the mare begins cycling again.

Lactational anestrus

Anestrus after foaling is seen occasionally.

◆ Affected mares have a normal postpartum estrus 8 to 15 days after foaling but do not show signs of estrus again for 60 to 120 days.

◆ Repeated rectal examinations reveal small, firm, inactive ovaries, a soft, flaccid uterus, and an open cervix.

◆ Periodic serum progesterone assays show levels <1 ng/mL.

◆ There is no consistently effective treatment.

This condition must not be confused with a mare that is overly protective of her foal and does not show signs of estrus (behavioral anestrus). Such mares, when palpated, have ovarian follicular activity, and they ovulate and form CLs.

Diestrual Ovulation

Ovulation without signs of estrus is relatively common in cycling mares and may be regarded as normal. However, diestrual ovulation can prolong diestrus. When it occurs 1 to 4 days before days 15 or 16 of the cycle (when luteolysis normally occurs), the mare does not show signs of estrus. The same situation can result in failure of exogenous prostaglandin therapy.

Ovulatory Failure

Persistent follicles are large, tense, fluid-filled structures, usually observed during the spring transitional period. They remain static and enlarged for up to 60 days. Once ovulation occurs at the end of the transitional period, mares with persistent follicles cycle normally. *Autumn follicles* are follicular structures that persist without ovulation throughout autumn. Anovulatory hemorrhagic follicles are a cause of ovulatory failure during the breeding season (see p. 340).

Diseases of the Oviduct
(page 1164)
Michelle M. LeBlanc

Lesions of the oviduct in mares are rare. The incidence of infundibulitis and endometritis, as well as gross infundibular adhesions, increases with age. However, the effect on fertility of such lesions is unknown. With chronic uterine infections, sperm transport through the oviducts may be delayed.

Diseases of the Uterus
(pages 1165-1173)
Michelle M. LeBlanc

DIAGNOSTIC AND THERAPEUTIC CONSIDERATIONS

Endometritis is a major cause of reduced fertility in mares. Some inflammation follows each episode of uterine contamination, so fertility depends on the efficacy of uterine defenses. Impaired physical clearance is the main factor involved in susceptibility to persistent endometritis. Perineal conformation is an important contributing factor in many mares.

Because treatment for endometritis is time-consuming and expensive, it is important to be certain of the diagnosis before proceeding with therapy. A summary of the criteria for diagnosis is presented in Table 13-6.

Table 13-6
Diagnostic criteria for endometritis

Physical examination	Uterine culture	Endometrial biopsy	Endometrial smear	Ultrasonography findings (uterus)	Diagnosis, comments
Gross inflammation and/or discharge	Pathogen isolated repeatedly	Significant inflammation	Many neutrophils	Intraluminal fluid	Endometritis
Inconclusive physical findings	Pathogen isolated	Significant inflammation, probably chronic	Many neutrophils	Intraluminal fluid	Endometritis, probable chronic
	No growth	Significant inflammation	Many neutrophils	+/− fluid	Persistent mating-induced endometritis
	Pathogen or non-pathogen isolated repeatedly	Insignificant or no inflammation	No or few neutrophils	No fluid	Normal endometrium, culture results reflect contamination
No signs of inflammation	No growth	No growth	No or few neutrophils	No fluid	Normal endometrium

Management

Successful management of endo-metritis must:

1. Correct any contributing causes (e.g., by performing Caslick's operation or vaginoplasty).
2. Reverse the inflammatory process by eliminating causal organisms and excess fluid after mating.
3. Avoid recurrent infection by using proper breeding and management practices:
   - limit breeding to once per estrous cycle
   - determine the optimal breeding time with teasing and ultrasonography
   - time ovulation with hCG or deslorelin (see p. 326)
   - lavage the uterus and administer oxytocin ± intrauterine antibiotics after breeding (see p. 327)

CONGENITAL AND FAMILIAL DISEASES

Endometrial Hypoplasia

Underdevelopment or delayed development of the endometrium frequently is associated with gonadal dysgenesis, ovarian neoplasia, or immaturity. It may be suspected after rectal palpation of the uterus and confirmed by endometrial biopsy. Immature mares have:

- relatively small (<3 cm) ovaries with little evidence of follicular development
- a small uterus
- persistent anestrus or weak behavioral estrus

Mating is unproductive and is often followed by persistent acute endometritis. Unless endometrial hypoplasia is associated with gonadal dysgenesis or ovarian neoplasia, most affected mares improve with time.

DISEASES WITH PHYSICAL CAUSES

Uterine Torsion

Torsion of the gravid uterus is uncommon in mares, but it should be a consideration in mares showing signs of abdominal discomfort late in pregnancy. Colic signs may be mild to severe; secondary GI disturbances can result from the altered position of the uterus. Necrosis of the uterus, with subsequent rupture, occasionally occurs.

Diagnosis

Rectal findings with the typical clockwise torsion are as follows:

- The left broad ligament is stretched across the dorsal aspect of the uterus from left to right, and the right broad ligament disappears ventrally down the right body wall toward the right ovary.
- Occasionally, twisting can be palpated just cranial to the cervix.
- The fetus usually is displaced cranially.

Vaginal signs of uterine torsion are inconclusive.

Treatment and prognosis

Though uterine torsion can be corrected by rolling the mare, the basic approach to correction is surgical. In simple uterine torsions, the objective is to return the uterus to its normal position and allow the pregnancy to continue to term.

- When possible, a standing flank laparotomy is the best approach. Simple 180-degree torsions often can be corrected by rolling the twisted uterus back into normal position by elevating the uterus from beneath and repelling the fetus.
- Correction in mares at term often results in immediate delivery of a normal foal.
- More complex cases, particularly those with secondary bowel involvement, may require paramedian or midline approaches.

When uterine torsion results in uterine rupture, the prognosis is grave. Formation of adhesions or other damage to the abdominal viscera typically results in loss of the mare.

Uterine Rupture

Uterine rupture in mares can occur before or during parturition.

- Prepartum uterine rupture has been associated with uterine torsion.
- Rupture during parturition has been associated with dystocia and manipulative procedures. It can also occur during second-stage labor in an apparently normal delivery.

Full-thickness injuries result in peritoneal contamination, but red blood cell (RBC) leakage and peritoneal contamination may also occur with partial-thickness tears.

Signs and diagnosis

Clinical signs depend on the extent of uterine rupture.

+ If the rupture is large, the mare rapidly shows signs of hemorrhagic shock and may die.
+ If the serosa remains intact, the mare may not show any signs until significant peritonitis has developed.

Diagnosis is confirmed by rectal palpation, uterine palpation (via the cervix), and abdominocentesis. Inability to identify a tear by palpation does not preclude its presence because many are difficult to find. Uterine rupture usually occurs at the dorsal aspect of the uterus.

Treatment

Supportive therapy includes:

+ appropriate systemic antimicrobials
+ NSAIDs
+ IV fluids
+ peritoneal lavage using large volumes of warm, sterile fluid containing antimicrobials, followed by ventral drainage

Attempts should be made to repair the wound as soon as possible. A ventral midline approach under general anesthesia is recommended.

Uterine Prolapse

Prolapse of the uterus may follow dystocia, retained placenta, or normal delivery, particularly in multiparous mares. It should be treated as an emergency because these mares are particularly predisposed to shock and hemorrhage (from stretching of the broad ligaments and rupture of the uterine artery). *Treatment of shock is as essential as replacing the prolapse.*

Treatment guidelines

+ Cleansing and replacement of the prolapsed uterus should be attempted as soon as possible.
+ Additional trauma to the exposed endometrium increases straining.
+ Epidural anesthesia reduces straining, greatly facilitating replacement; however, general anes-

thesia may be needed in fractious mares.

+ Administration of oxytocin after replacement speeds uterine involution.

The combination of shock, hemorrhage, contamination, and/or uterine trauma warrants a poor prognosis in most cases. (Uterine artery rupture is discussed earlier in the section on postpartum hemorrhage.)

INFLAMMATORY, INFECTIOUS, AND IMMUNE DISEASES

Endometritis is categorized into four groups:

1. persistent mating-induced endometritis
2. chronic infectious endometritis
3. sexually transmitted diseases
4. chronic degenerative endometritis (periglandular fibrosis)

The distinctions between categories are not always clear, and a mare can switch from one category to another or have pathologic changes that place her in more than one category. It is important to continually reevaluate each case of endometritis.

Persistent Mating-Induced Endometritis

Intrauterine deposition of semen causes a transient physiologic endometritis. Normal mares are able to clear this uterine contamination within 24 hours of breeding, but mares susceptible to endometritis cannot and accumulate fluid within the uterine lumen. Older, infertile, multiparous mares are most susceptible.

Diagnosis

Clinical findings vary widely.

+ Early in the season, before breeding, there may be no significant abnormalities on rectal examination, vaginal speculum examination, or ultrasonography.
  + No bacteria may be isolated, and cytology frequently is negative.
  + Biopsy scores may be Kenney II(a) or II(b), with only mild inflammatory or fibrotic changes noted.
+ Later in the season, after being bred once or twice, signs of inflammation are frequently present.

- The vagina may be hyperemic, and the uterus may have a doughy texture.
- There may be intrauterine fluid on ultrasonographic evaluation, and if the mare has conceived, the embryo may appear abnormally shaped and be lying in fluid.
- Cytologic specimens may have >5 neutrophils per high-power field.
- Bacteria may be cultured.
- Biopsies taken at this time frequently reveal a mild to moderate, diffuse, subacute endometritis with moderate lymphangectasia and endometrial edema.

Treatment

The aim of treatment is to rapidly remove intraluminal fluids and administer drugs that increase uterine contractions (see the section on hormone therapy). Rest from breeding may also be indicated. If the uterus is not treated quickly after breeding and given time to heal between insults, or if the insult is severe, uterine inflammation persists.

Chronic Infectious Endometritis

Any compromise to the vulva, vestibule, vagina, or cervix predisposes the mare to a chronic uterine infection. The major pathogens involved in endometritis are:

- *Streptococcus equi-zooepidemicus:* >66% of infections
- *Escherichia coli:* almost always associated with anatomic defects that predispose mares to pneumovagina and fecal contamination
- *Pseudomonas aeroginosa* or *Klebsiella pneumoniae:* may be transmitted by coitus; common in mares repeatedly treated with intrauterine antibiotics or with marginal resistance to contamination
  - Once established, infection with either organism is difficult to treat.
  - Resistance to antimicrobial therapy is common.
- yeasts: commonly recovered in mares repeatedly treated with intrauterine antibiotics or with marginal resistance to contamination

Other bacterial species occasionally are incriminated, including *Staphylococcus, Corynebacterium, Enterobacter, Proteus,* and *Pasteurella* spp. If clinical signs of infection accompany the recovery of these bacteria, they must be regarded as significant.

Diagnosis

Findings include:

- hyperemic vaginal and cervical mucosae and vaginal discharge
- fluid accumulation within the uterus
- neutrophils in cytologic specimens
- positive bacterial culture
- Kenney II or III biopsy scores, depending on the severity of the insult and duration of the uterine infection

Treatment

- Goals of treatment are to promote clearance of fluid from the uterus and to inhibit bacterial infection with appropriate antibiotics.
- Anaerobes may be recovered in mares with acute endometritis, especially after parturition.
  - *Bacteroides fragilis* is the predominant anaerobe cultured in these mares. It is resistant to gentamicin and penicillin, which contributes to treatment failure in cases of retained placenta or postpartum metritis.
  - Treatment with metronidazole is necessary.

Contagious Equine Metritis

Contagious equine metritis (CEM) is a venereal disease caused by a gram-negative, nonmotile coccobacillus tentatively named *Taylorella equigenitalis.*

- It causes a mucopurulent vulvar discharge and reduced fertility in mares but no clinical signs in stallions.
- The organism can survive for long periods on the external genitalia of stallions and in the caudal vagina and clitoral area of mares.
- It may be transmitted directly from mare to mare by contaminated instruments, materials, or personnel. There is no evidence the infection spreads directly from mare to mare.
- The endometritis of CEM is of fairly short duration, but after the acute signs resolve, the mare is an asymptomatic carrier for long periods.

Clinical signs

Clinical signs in mares are those of acute endometritis:

- Profuse, gray-white, mucoid vulvar discharge may be seen 2 to 3 days postinsemination or may not be evident until a premature return to estrus 8 to 10 days later.

- Some mares are infected without any clinical signs and may conceive and foal; however, conception and pregnancy rates may be markedly reduced.

Clinical signs in stallions are absent; they act as asymptomatic carriers. The organism resides on the penis, in the urethoural diverticulum, and in and around the prepuce, where it can persist for many months.

Diagnosis

CEM is diagnosed by identification of *T. equigenitalis* on culture. However, culture is complicated by the organism's fastidious nature and propensity to reside in areas with many contaminants.

PRACTICAL CONSIDERATIONS

- Sterile swabs should be used to obtain samples from the cervix, clitoral fossa, clitoral sinuses, and uterus early in estrus and at weekly intervals for at least 3 weeks.
- Swabs should be smeared on a sterile glass slide, placed in Amies medium with charcoal or in Stewart's medium, refrigerated at 4° to 6° C (39° to 43° F), and transported within 24 to 48 hours to an approved laboratory for special culture.
- The presence of neutrophils containing many ingested organisms in swab samples is helpful in screening mares.
- A transient rise in humoral antibody levels occurs from 7 or 8 days to about 45 days after infection. Antibodies can be detected by agglutination, complement fixation, and ELISA.

Treatment and control

- Treatment is ineffective. The acute endometritis resolves on its own, with or without antimicrobial therapy.
- About 20% of infected mares remain asymptomatic carriers regardless of treatment.
- Mares with continually positive cultures should not be considered for further breeding until cultures are negative (which may take >1 year).
- Control is directed at preventing spread of the disease.

- Quarantine measures and breeding restrictions have successfully confined outbreaks.
- In the United States, the disease is reportable.

Fungal Endometritis

Candida spp., especially *Candida albicans,* can cause endometritis. There almost always is a history of repeated antimicrobial therapy for bacterial endometritis. *Candida* grows readily on media used for routine microbiologic culture; identification is aided by examining wet mounts or stained smears for budding yeasts. Recovery of fungi from clinically normal mares can be disregarded.

Pyometra

Pyometra (accumulation of pus in the uterus) is an occasional sequel to metritis and sometimes cervicitis. It often causes pronounced pathologic changes in the uterus, especially in older, "infection-prone" mares with defective uterine defense mechanisms.

Signs and diagnosis

- The uterus may be palpably enlarged.
- Pyometra sometimes results in prolonged diestrus; other mares with pyometra cycle regularly.
- Culture of uterine fluids may yield any of the common bacterial or fungal agents responsible for endometritis; occasionally the fluid is sterile.
- Systemic signs of disease are not evident, although mild neutropenia or anemia is noted in a few mares.

Treatment and prognosis

Once established, pyometra is a difficult problem to manage.

- Severe inflammatory changes and endometrial atrophy are common, so endometrial biopsy is indicated as a prognostic step before attempting treatment.
- Treatment includes mechanical evacuation of the retained pus (repeated lavage) and appropriate intrauterine antimicrobials.
- Recurrence is common, and even with diligent treatment the prognosis for fertility is poor.
- Mares that expel pus during estrus have a somewhat better prognosis.

- If severe cervical or intrauterine adhesions are present, the prognosis is hopeless.

NEOPLASIA

Leiomyoma

Endometrial tumors are rare in mares. Leiomyomas or fibroleiomyomas are the most common, usually occurring in older mares as firm, small (2.5 to 5 cm) nodules. Often they are diagnosed by rectal palpation as a firm, nodular enlargement that sometimes extends into the cervix. Frequently they are pedunculated, extending into the uterine lumen, and thus can be easily removed with a surgical snare.

Other Uterine Tumors

Other tumors are fibromas, fibroadenomas, adenosarcomas, lymphosarcomas, rhabdomyosarcomas, and leiomyosarcomas. Ultrasonography, uterine biopsy, and fiberoptic examination are useful diagnostic aids.

MULTIFACTORIAL DISEASES

Endometrial Fibrosis

Endometrial fibrosis occurs in response to inflammation, glandular damage, increasing age, and other undefined causes. Periglandular fibrosis affects glandular support of the 35- to 90-day-old conceptus, leading to embryonic death. If the embryo survives, periglandular fibrosis causes delayed microcotyledon development between 80 and 120 days of gestation, leading to placental insufficiency and retarded fetal growth.

Endometrial Cysts

Endometrial cysts are fluid-filled structures that arise from the endometrium, most often in mares >10 years of age. If found in large numbers or if a single cyst is >10 mm, pregnancy may be adversely affected. However, in one large study, there was no effect of the presence, number, diameter, or volume of endometrial cysts on the establishment or maintenance of pregnancy.

Large cysts may be drained by needle aspiration, ruptured with an endoscopic instrument, or removed by mechanical curettage, laser, or electrocoagulation.

IDIOPATHIC DISEASES

Shortened Diestrus

Shortened intervals between periods of estrus may be:

- normal: Premature return to estrus or "split heat" is relatively common. It can be missed if mares are not teased systematically throughout the cycle. Mares should be rebred on the split heat.
- associated with a uterine abnormality, such as endometritis: It is a good indicator of endometritis and is more common with acute infections than with chronic ones.

Diseases of the Cervix

(pages 1173-1175)
Michelle M. LeBlanc

DIAGNOSTIC AND THERAPEUTIC CONSIDERATIONS

Cervical lesions usually are caused by foaling trauma, although adhesions may also result from chronic endometritis or pyometra. Congenital abnormalities and neoplasia are uncommon.

Diagnosis

Vaginoscopy and digital palpation are essential for accurate detection and definition of cervical abnormalities.

- Examination during estrus aids detection of cervical canal lesions.
- Cervical tone and competence are best assessed during diestrus.

Treatment and prognosis

- Adhesions involving the intravaginal cervix and vaginal fornix can be ignored, circumvented by artificial insemination, or surgically corrected, depending on their severity.
- Surgery often is unsuccessful in all but the simplest cases, so prognosis for fertility is guarded.
- In the absence of obvious structural damage, progesterone supplementation has been used.

DISEASES WITH PHYSICAL CAUSES

Cervical Trauma

After any prolonged spontaneous or assisted foaling, a detailed vaginoscopic examination and digital palpation should be performed to detect mucosal defects or lacerations in the cervix or vagina.

Treatment guidelines

- Areas of roughened mucosa or exposed submucosa should be cleansed daily with warm saline solution, followed by ample application of antimicrobial ointment. Most lesions epithelialize by the first postpartum estrus.
- Newly formed adhesions should be manually debrided and antimicrobial ointment applied twice daily for 7 to 10 days.
  - Adhesions have a tendency to recur, especially if there is concurrent pyometra or endometritis, so treatment for any uterine problems must be instituted.
  - Mature adhesions are best treated surgically.
- Lacerations caused by excessive stretching during parturition must be surgically repaired; however, the long-term breeding prognosis is guarded because the cervix invariably tears again at foaling.

Cervicitis from Irritating Solutions

Irritating solutions, including certain unbuffered antibiotics and undiluted antiseptics, must be avoided for treatment of endometritis. Though endometrial damage may not occur from use of such compounds, they may adversely affect the vagina and/or cervix, rendering the mare infertile.

IDIOPATHIC DISEASES

Failure of Cervical Dilation

Occasionally in maiden mares (especially those >12 years of age) the cervix fails to dilate during estrus.

- Examination reveals a tightly closed cervix without adhesions or uterine lesions.
- Usually these mares fail to conceive by natural breeding but do conceive when artificially inseminated.

Manual dilation of the cervix before natural breeding is unreliable.

- These mares experience a delay in uterine clearance, so it is frequently beneficial to perform uterine lavage and administer either oxytocin or cloprostenol after breeding.
- No problem with cervical dilation occurs at foaling.

Diseases of the Vagina, Vestibule, and Vulva

(pages 1175-1193)
Michelle M. LeBlanc

CONGENITAL AND FAMILIAL DISEASES

Persistent Hymen

A common cause of minor, transient postbreeding hemorrhage in maiden mares is rupture of hymenal tissue.

- Most maiden mares have some semblance of a hymen forming a low ridge across the floor of the vagina.
- Less commonly, the hymen is more complete. Incision of the membrane is necessary in these mares.

Cystic Gartner's Ducts

- Cystic or infected Gartner's (mesonephric-Wolffian) ducts are found on the floor of the vagina, opening lateral and slightly caudal to the urethral orifice. Infection may occur subsequent to perineal or vaginal abscesses.

Varicose Veins

Varicose veins in the region of the perforated hymen are relatively common and may cause intermittent vulvar bleeding.

- When observed at breeding, the bleeding must be differentiated from vaginal rupture (see p. 350).
- Varicose veins may also cause bleeding during gestation.
- The veins are detected by speculum examination of the hymen (1 to 2 cm diameter, bluish vessels).
- They are not detrimental to life or fertility, so treatment is not necessary. Surgical attempts at ligation,

cryotherapy, or thermocautery can be tried.

Pseudohermaphroditism

Intersexes are rare congenital malformations. Part or all of the genital organs of both sexes are present. The gonads are of one sex and accessory reproductive organs are predominantly of the opposite sex. The external genitalia may consist of an enlarged clitoris or a hypospadia-like vestigial penis.

DISEASES WITH PHYSICAL CAUSES

Vulvar Laceration/Vulvar Insufficiency

Vulvar lacerations are a common aftermath of foaling.

- Failure to adequately open the previous year's Caslick's operation is a frequent cause.
- If the laceration is severe, the inflammation must be resolved before repair is attempted. Immediate care should include cleansing of the laceration and administration of systemic antimicrobials and tetanus toxoid.
- In the worst cases, it is prudent to delay repair until after the mare is mated.

Small tears in a previously sutured dorsal vulvar commissure occurring at the time of breeding usually are of no consequence, although repair of the Caslick's vulvoplasty may be necessary.

Caslick's operation

- Caslick's operation is the most important procedure in the treatment of pneumovagina and infertility caused by genital tract infection. Endometritis may resolve spontaneously after the procedure.
- The mare must remain sutured for the remainder of her reproductive life, although incision and resuturing for breeding and foaling are necessary. A delay in resuturing of only a few days may allow reinfection.
- Caslick's operation is necessary when the dorsal vulvar commissure is located more than 4 cm dorsal to the pelvic floor.

Techniques and aftercare are discussed in *Equine Medicine and Surgery V*.

Vestibulovaginal Sphincter Insufficiency

If labial vestibular sphincter function is not reestablished by Caslick's procedure, surgical reconstruction of the perineal body is indicated. Techniques and aftercare are discussed in *Equine Medicine and Surgery V*.

Vaginal Laceration/Rupture

Minor lacerations

- Vaginal lacerations incurred during breeding most commonly involve the cranial dorsolateral vaginal wall, close to the cervix.
- They generally are <5 cm long and accompanied by minor transient hemorrhage.
- Such lesions have minimal clinical significance, although mixing of blood with semen could reduce fertility.
- Spontaneous healing is rapid and complete.
- A breeding roll sometimes is used to prevent this injury.

Vaginal rupture during breeding

Severe lacerations to the vagina after breeding can result in rupture of the vaginal wall with eventration of bowel or the urinary bladder. Management guidelines are as follows:

- Preventive antimicrobial therapy should be started immediately. Acute, severe peritonitis can develop in 2 to 3 days if a vaginal rupture is overlooked.
- The mare should be cross-tied for at least 48 hours to prevent eventration of abdominal viscera when she lies down. Medication should be administered to prevent straining.
- If a portion of bowel eventrates through the rent, it should be washed with normal saline containing antimicrobials before replacement in the abdominal cavity.
- The vagina should be flushed with 500 mL of saline containing a nonirritating antimicrobial solution.
- Unless surgical repair of vaginal damage can be achieved easily and quickly, it is counterproductive.

Rupture during foaling

Vaginal rupture may be caused by the foal's foot or by obstetric manipulation.

- The vagina may rupture at any point, but the dorsal wall is the most susceptible to perforation by the foal's feet.
- Cranial vaginal ruptures communicate directly with the peritoneal cavity; however, bowel seldom eventrates through a laceration in this location.
- The edges of the laceration should be apposed with absorbable sutures after epidural anesthesia in the standing mare. Caslick's procedure reduces the possibility of air aspiration into the peritoneal cavity.
- When the ventral wall of the vagina is lacerated, herniation of abdominal viscera is a frequent sequela.
  - This complicates delivery of the foal, and vigorous attempts to deliver the foal vaginally lead to serious trauma and contamination of the bowel.
  - Immediate cesarean section is indicated.

Urine Pooling

Pooling of urine in the cranial vaginal vault (vesicovaginal reflux) and uterine lumen is a well-recognized cause of infertility. Vaginitis, cervicitis, and endometritis are common sequelae. Contributing factors include abnormal perineal conformation, increased age in multiparous mares, weight loss, relaxation of the reproductive tract during estrus, and slow postpartum uterine involution in large, pluriparous mares.

Diagnosis

- Vesicovaginal reflux should be suspected in mares that repeatedly fail to conceive, particularly old, thin, infertile mares, those with poor external conformation, and mares with uterine fluid accumulation before and after ovulation.
- Diagnosis is made by vaginal speculum examination (best performed during estrus; urine does not pool during diestrus).
- Fluid in the vaginal fornix may be confirmed as urine by visual inspection or biochemically (osmolality, urea content)

Treatment

- When first diagnosed, sexual rest, improved nutrition, and if necessary, external conformation modification (e.g., perineal body reconstruction)

alleviates vesicovaginal reflux. Resolution occurs in most postpartum mares after uterine involution.
- If the condition recurs, surgical correction is indicated (urethral extension; see *Equine Medicine and Surgery V*).

Rectovestibular and Perineal Injuries

Primiparous mares are particularly susceptible to reproductive tract injury during parturition. Remnants of the hymen are responsible for most of these injuries. Astute observation and prompt intervention by attendants at foaling may prevent serious vaginal and perineal injuries.

Classifications

Perineal lacerations are classified by the extent and severity of tissue damage:

- *First-degree lacerations* involve the mucosa of the vestibule and skin of the dorsal commissure of the vulva. They are readily repaired by a routine Caslick's procedure.
- *Second-degree lacerations* involve the vestibular mucosa and submucosa, skin of the dorsal commissure of the vulva, and perineal body musculature.
  - In most cases, healing does not result in complete return of the vulva's constrictor function. Air and feces can be aspirated into the vagina, causing chronic irritation, inflammation, and infertility.
  - Caslick's procedure may not completely prevent contamination. Surgical reconstruction of the perineal body is necessary.
- *Third-degree perineal lacerations* involve the floor of the rectum and ceiling of the vestibule, musculature of the perineal body, perineal septum, and anal sphincter.
- *Rectovestibular fistulas* involve the ceiling of the vestibule, floor of the rectum, and a variable amount of the perineal septum and musculature.

Principles of treatment

- A 3- to 6-week interval should pass before repair of perineal and rectovestibular lacerations is attempted. If there is a live foal, it is advisable to delay repair until weaning.
- Immediate care consists of administration of tetanus toxoid, systemic antimicrobials, and NSAIDs.

- Daily cleansing of the wound during the first week is beneficial.
- Before surgery the mare should be placed on a diet that softens and reduces the volume of her stools. Feeding lush green pasture, pelleted rations, or wet bran mashes and administering danthron or laxatives (e.g., mineral oil and magnesium sulfate) are recommended.
- The prognosis for fertility after successful surgical repair is good.
  Surgical techniques and aftercare are detailed in *Equine Medicine and Surgery V.*

INFLAMMATORY, INFECTIOUS, AND IMMUNE DISEASES
Bacterial Vaginitis
Inflammation of the vagina may be caused by a variety of insults:

- pneumovagina: When pneumovagina alone is responsible for vaginitis, a rapid return to normal should follow correction of the predisposing anatomic defect.
- endometritis: In many cases endometritis is a *result* of vaginal or cervical infection.
- intravaginal use of irritant chemicals, such as diluted iodine (2% solution) and chlorhexidine: These chemicals can cause vaginal mucosal ulceration and necrosis.
- delivery of a dead, necrotic fetus: Severe vaginitis occurs if hair and necrotic tissue become imbedded in the wall because of improper lubrication.

Treatment
Treatment of severe necrotic vaginitis consists of:

- lavage with warm saline and a nonirritating antimicrobial to loosen necrotic vaginal tissue; proper aseptic technique and ample sterile lubrication minimize further vaginal irritation
- broad-spectrum antibiotics and metronidazole (these mares often are systemically ill)

Coital Exanthema
Coital exanthema is a disease of the external genitalia caused by a herpesvirus. Though it is primarily a venereal disease, coital exanthema may be transmitted by grooming, veterinary instruments, and possibly insects.

Signs and diagnosis
- Lesions appear on the vulva of mares and on the penis and prepuce of stallions.
- Initially, vesicles rapidly progress to pustules and then to shallow, necrotic ulcers; lesions may spread to the surrounding perineal skin.
- Edema, tenderness, and painful urination are seen in the acute stages.
- Intranuclear inclusion bodies can be demonstrated histologically in affected tissues.

Treatment and prognosis
- Treatment usually is unnecessary. Healing occurs in 7 to 10 days (in the absence of secondary bacterial infection), and mares can be bred at the next estrus.
- When signs develop spontaneously after minor vulvar abrasions, stretching, or episiotomy, mating should be postponed until healing is complete.
- Antiseptic creams may prevent secondary bacterial infections.
- The effect on fertility is negligible. Permanent loss of pigmentation may occur at the site of healed lesions.

Diseases Involving the Placenta *(pages 1193-1199)*
Michelle M. LeBlanc

DIAGNOSTIC AND THERAPEUTIC CONSIDERATIONS

Often the best information on the cause of abortion or on management of a compromised neonate may be obtained by careful examination of the fetal membranes:

- Both surfaces of the allantochorion should be visually examined. The placenta is laid out and both horns and the body are thoroughly evaluated.
- The placenta's weight is estimated.
- If abnormalities are evident, samples are taken for bacterial culture and histologic examination, including an area adjacent to the cervical star.

* The inner surface of the amnion has small (1 to 2 mm) yellow nodules of hyperkeratosis near the cord and overlying major vessels. These nodules should not be mistaken for fungal plaques.

Identification and Treatment of the High-Risk Fetus

Antepartum evaluation may identify high-risk candidates, such as mares that:
* had problems in previous pregnancies
* develop vaginal discharge
* exhibit premature mammary development and lactation
* develop serious medical or surgical problems in late pregnancy

Evaluation

Evaluation may include:
* palpation per rectum
* vaginal examination
* collection of blood for hormonal analysis
* amniocentesis
* fetal electrocardiography
* fetal and placental ultrasonography (transabdominal or rectal): fetal heart rates >120/min indicate fetal stress; repeated observation of fetal heart rates <65/min usually indicates impending fetal death

EQUINE BIOPHYSICAL PROFILE. This set of data can be used to assess fetal well-being from 298 days gestational age to term. It includes assessment of:
* fetal heart rate
* fetal aortic diameter
* maximal fetal fluid depths
* uteroplacental contact
* uteroplacental thickness
* fetal activity

A low score indicates an impending negative outcome; however, a high score is not assurance of a positive outcome.

Placental abnormalities

Fetoplacental infections cause nearly one third of all abortions or fetal mortality; 90% of these infections are due to an ascending placentitis. Early signs of placental abnormalities or detachment associated with placentitis usually occur in the area of the cervical star. These changes are best evaluated by transrectal ultrasonography.
* At this site, uteroplacental thickness that is >8.5 mm in the eleventh month (301 to 330 days) or >11.8 mm in the twelfth month (331 to 360 days) may indicate placentitis.
* Detachment of the placenta or increased echogenicity of the allantoic or amniotic fluids may indicate placental failure or fetal hypoxia.

CONDITIONS WITH PHYSICAL CAUSES

Hypoplastic Villi of the Allantochorion

In older mares and those with a history of degenerative endometritis, placental insufficiency (as a result of areas of chorion with absence, atrophy, or hypoplasia of villi) may cause fetal growth retardation.
* These abnormalities have been associated with endometrial fibrosis and extensive cystic lymphatic disorders.
* Affected foals are carried for more than 365 days and are small and sometimes weak.
* Endometrial fibrosis is essentially irreversible, so it is prudent to cull the mare.

INFLAMMATORY, INFECTIOUS, AND IMMUNE DISEASES

Bacterial Placentitis

Streptococcus spp. are the bacteria most frequently isolated from aborted fetuses and from placentae with gross lesions. Other commonly encountered organisms are *Escherichia coli, Pseudomonas* spp., *Klebsiella* spp., and *Staphylococcus* spp.

Signs and diagnosis

* Often mares with bacterial or fungal placentitis have a vaginal discharge, and they prematurely lactate.
* Vaginal speculum examination should be performed to determine the source of the discharge and the extent of cervical relaxation.
* Ultrasonography can provide evidence of fetal viability and the degree of placental separation.
* After delivery or abortion, the placenta may be edematous and heavy, with local areas of marked thickening. The infected chorionic surface is brown, with varying amounts of fibrinonecrotic exudate.

- Culture and examination of stained smears are necessary for diagnosis.
- Gross fetal lesions are nonspecific and may be no more than an enlarged liver and increased fluid in body cavities.
- Organisms can be recovered from many fetal organs, most consistently from the stomach.

Leptospirosis

Leptospiral abortion is difficult to diagnose because mares rarely exhibit clinical signs of disease. Preliminary diagnosis is based on postmortem findings in aborted fetuses and placentae and is confirmed by demonstration of spirochetes in fetal tissues and placentae by immunofluorescent techniques or with Warthin-Starry stain.

Fetal and placental abnormalities

- An aborted fetus may have no gross lesions, or it may exhibit icterus and a swollen, yellow liver.
- Placental lesions are common and vary from thickening to exudate.
- Histologically, nephritis and placentitis are commonly observed, and spirochetes are found in the kidney, liver, and placenta.

Treatment and prevention

- Prolonged treatment with either procaine penicillin G (20,000 IU/kg IM bid) or oxytetracycline (5 mg/kg IV bid) may decrease shedding.
- Antibiotics may also be useful in preventing fetal infections in mares with high titers during late pregnancy.
- Currently there are no approved vaccines for use in horses.
- Sanitation and hygiene are essential for control.
  - Transmission is by contact with environmental sources such as wildlife, low-lying or swampy areas, stagnant water, and runoff water.
  - Exposure to contaminated feed and water and infective urine and abortuses must be eliminated.

Fungal Placentitis

Aspergillus is the most common fungal cause of placentitis. The placental exudate tends to be mucoid, but otherwise fungal placentitis is grossly indistinguishable from bacterial placentitis.

Diagnosis

- The chorioallantois is the specimen of choice for diagnosing mycotic abortion.
  - The placenta is diffusely yellowish, thickened, and leathery; affected areas are clearly demarcated from normal areas.
  - The chorionic surface is necrotic and usually covered with thick, adherent, mucoid exudate.
  - Impression smears reveal fungal hyphae.
- The amnion may have irregular necrotic plaques (in about 10% of *Mucor* spp. infections).
- The fungal organism may be isolated from a bacterial culture of the mare's uterus after parturition.

Premature Placental Separation

Premature placental separation has been associated with placentitis, induction of parturition before fetal maturity, systemic illness, and fetal death in utero. When this condition is recognized at term, the foal must be delivered immediately.

MULTIFACTORIAL DISEASES

Retained Placenta

Retention of fetal membranes is a common postpartum disorder. It is often associated with abnormalities of parturition, such as dystocia, twin delivery, abortion, and cesarean section. The membranes are more frequently retained in the nongravid horn.

Treatment

Retention of fetal membranes should be managed as an emergency. Acute metritis can develop and rapidly lead to toxemia, septicemia, and laminitis, so appropriate treatment must be initiated within 6 hours of parturition. Objectives are the atraumatic expulsion of the entire placenta and control of bacterial growth in the uterus.

- Oxytocin is the drug of choice.
  - A single injection of 40 to 80 units IM or 10 to 20 units IV can be given.
  - The dose is repeated twice at 2-hour intervals if the placenta has not been expelled.
  - Uterine contractions occur within minutes of injection and cause abdominal discomfort and sweating.

Giving 80 to 100 units of oxytocin in 1 L of saline IV over 30 to 40 minutes minimizes discomfort.

- Most mares respond to one or two injections, and if these are successful before 6 hours postpartum, no further treatment is required.

♦ Alternatively, redistension of the allantois with 10 to 12 L of diluted (0.01%) warm povidone-iodine solution or saline, infused via stomach tube, can be used to stimulate uterine contractions. Usually the membranes are passed within 30 minutes.

♦ If fetal membranes are retained for >6 hours, broad-spectrum systemic and intrauterine antimicrobials and systemic antiinflammatory drugs (e.g., flunixin meglumine, phenylbutazone) are indicated.

♦ Careful aseptic examination of the uterus should be performed in mares that fail to deliver the placenta within 8 hours and in mares requiring several injections of oxytocin.

- Membranes lying free in the uterine lumen should be brought to the outside to add traction to the retained portions.
- Forcibly stripping the chorion from the endometrium is hazardous and may lead to permanent endometrial damage and hemorrhage.

♦ All membranes should be examined carefully after expulsion. If large defects indicate that portions are still retained, treatment should be continued to manage bacterial growth.

♦ If acute metritis develops, uterine lavage with large volumes of saline is indicated.

IDIOPATHIC CONDITIONS
Hydroallantois

Hydroallantois is rare in mares.

♦ Affected mares are usually multiparous.

♦ The condition generally becomes apparent at 7 to 10.5 months of gestation, developing over 10 to 14 days.

♦ Dramatic accumulation of uterine fluid prevents ballottement of the fetus and results in reluctance to move, an altered gait, and dyspnea on recumbency.

♦ Affected mares should be watched closely; during parturition, the abdominal contractions are weak and assistance with delivery often is necessary.

♦ Induction of parturition using oxytocin should be considered.

♦ After delivery, affected mares may go into hypovolemic shock and must be treated accordingly.

Disease of the Embryo
(pages 1199-1202)
Michelle M. LeBlanc

EARLY EMBRYONIC LOSS

Early embryonic death loss (loss of the conceptus between fertilization and day 40 of gestation) is an important cause of reduced fertility of aged subfertile mares.

- Studies using pregnancy detection with ultrasonography before day 20 postovulation reported higher losses than those conducted after day 20.

♦ The highest losses occurred between days 11 and 15 postovulation.

Diagnosis

The ultrasonographic morphology of both spontaneous and induced embryonic losses have been described. Indications of death of the embryo are:

♦ the presence of intraluminal uterine fluid, especially 3 to 10 days after ovulation

♦ prolonged mobility of the vesicle in the uterus

♦ an undersized vesicle

♦ and an irregularly shaped vesicle

Many spontaneous embryonic losses at days 11 to 20 postovulation are not preceded by a detectable ultrasonographic changes in the embryo or uterus.

Prevention

Many practitioners supplement mares with exogenous progesterone if serum progesterone levels are low on day 12, if the mare has previously lost a conceptus, or if owners believe it is beneficial. Progesterone supplementation is contraindicated in mares that chronically lose their fetus because of endometritis. Treatment protocols are discussed in the section on patho-physiology and principles of therapy earlier in chapter 13 of *Equine Medicine and Surgery V*.

CONGENITAL AND FAMILIAL CONDITIONS
Loss from Chromosomal Defects
Investigators have proposed that chromosomal defects may cause embryonic losses in mares, because karyotypic abnormalities have been described in mares and stallions. Aged gametes have been proposed as a factor in chromosomal anomalies in equine embryos because of the relatively long estrus in mares and the prolonged survival of spermatozoa in the mare's reproductive tract.

DISEASES WITH PHYSICAL CAUSES
Loss from Delayed Oviductal Transport
Oviductal function may affect embryonic loss by delaying transport of the embryo from the oviduct to the uterus or by interfering with the ability of sperm to attach to the oviductal epithelium.

Loss in Postpartum and Lactation Mares
Mares bred on foal heat may have higher embryonic and early fetal losses than foaling mares bred at later estrous periods. Delaying the breeding of mares until 15 days after foaling improves pregnancy rates.

Restriction of Conceptus Mobility
Unrestricted conceptus mobility is essential to maintaining pregnancy and preventing luteolysis. If uterine contractions are not sufficient to move the embryo throughout the uterus and inhibit luteolysis, the embryo may die. Uterine pathology such as transluminal adhesions or endometrial cysts restrict conceptus mobility.

INFLAMMATORY, INFECTIOUS, AND IMMUNE DISEASES
Endometritis
Endometritis is an important factor in embryonic and early fetal loss in mares at days 14 to 48 postovulation. These losses may be related to uterine inflammation and the subsequent decline in progesterone concentration resulting from luteolysis.

Salpingitis
Salpingitis does not appear to occur frequently in mares.

MULTIFACTORIAL DISEASES
Periglandular Fibrosis
Periglandular fibrosis and endometritis detected on histopathologic examination of endometrial biopsies are associated with embryonic and early fetal loss in mare between 40 and 90 days of gestation. Mares with more than five fibrotic nests per low-power field of endometrial tissue examined have less than a 10% chance of sustaining pregnancy to term.

IDIOPATHIC CONDITIONS
Loss from Embryonic Factors
Embryos collected from the uterus or the oviduct of subfertile mares do not appear to be as viable as those collected from reproductively normal mares.

TOXIC AND METABOLIC CONDITIONS
Loss from High Environmental Temperature
Heat stress may be important in embryonic loss in mares in certain climates.

Loss from Maternal Stress
When *Salmonella typhimurium* endotoxin was administered as a single intravenous infusion (0.33 µg/kg) to mares during various stages of pregnancy, mares less than 55 days pregnant lost their fetuses.

NUTRITIONAL CONDITIONS
Low protein or energy intake may adversely affect pregnancy. Mares that lost body condition during the first 90 days after parturition have lower 30-day pregnancy rates and more pregnancy losses between gestational days 30 and 90 than mares that retained body condition.

Abortion *(pages 1202-1207)*

Michelle M. LeBlanc

DIAGNOSTIC AND THERAPEUTIC CONSIDERATIONS

Twinning is the most common overall cause of abortion, and equine herpesvirus (EHV-1) infection is the single most important infectious cause. Abortion is more common in older mares.

Indicators

- Signs of impending abortion vary; frequently no premonitory signs are observed.
- In protracted abortions involving placental separation, there often is premature mammary development. Some mares "run milk" for weeks before aborting.
- Signs of impending parturition are common, but dystocia is uncommon.
- Complications are infrequent, although retained placenta and its sequelae (laminitis and metritis) are possible.

Examination of the Fetus and Placenta

The cause can be definitively diagnosed in 50% to 60% of cases if the fetus and placenta are methodically examined, appropriate samples are submitted, and a thorough history is obtained.

- *history:* Should include gestational age of the fetus, vaccination history of the mare, any record of illness in the mare or other horses on the farm, and past reproductive performance.
- *placenta:* The placenta should be weighed and the texture, color, thickness (normal, increased, decreased), and consistency (edematous, fibrotic, leathery) noted.
  - Any necrosis, ulceration, denuded areas, and adherent exudate should be recorded.
  - Duplicate specimens of any lesions should be submitted fresh and in 10% buffered neutral formalin.
- *specimens:* The best specimens to submit are the fetus and an intact placenta, chilled but not frozen. The samples must be properly handled, preserved, and submitted to the laboratory without delay.
- *field necropsy:* If a field necropsy is performed on the fetus, specimens must be taken at the appropriate stage during the procedure to avoid contamination.
  - The crown-to-rump length is measured to assess fetal age and the possibility of retarded fetal growth.
  - The abdomen is opened and two pieces of liver are collected, one for bacteriologic examination and one for virus isolation.
  - The stomach is tied off at the esophagus and pylorus and submitted for bacterial culture.
  - Small pieces ($1 \times 2 \times 2$ cm) of liver, lymph node, kidney, adrenal gland, and spleen are placed in 10% buffered neutral formalin for histologic examination.
  - The amount of fluid in the thorax is noted, and samples of lung are immediately and aseptically collected for bacteriologic and virologic study. A sample of thymus is also taken for virology.
  - Samples of lung and thymus are taken for histologic examination.
  - Swabs of abdominal and thoracic fluid and cardiac blood from the fetus and a uterine swab from the mare are taken for microbiologic examination.
- *serology:* Immunoglobulin concentrations in umbilical cord blood may be useful in diagnosing fetal infection. In mares, high or rising serum titers may indicate viral arteritis and leptospirosis.

Treatment and Prevention

Following are some general guidelines:

- Use of ultrasonography to detect early pregnancy allows identification and correction of twin pregnancy (see the section on ultrasonographic evaluation of the reproductive tract).
- Results of uterine biopsy can be used to select against mares that are likely to abort (those with extensive and severe endometrial fibrosis).
- EHV-1 infection can be prevented by routine vaccination, avoidance of stress, and maintenance of closed herds.

- Equine viral arteritis can be controlled with routine vaccination of stallions, by only breeding stallions shedding the virus to vaccinated or seropositive mares, and by providing an appropriate period of isolation from other nonvaccinated horses.
- Bacterial abortion is prevented by managing endometritis in barren mares (see p. 345).

PHYSICAL CAUSES OF ABORTION

Torsion of the Umbilical Cord

Fetal death may occur as a result of twisting of the umbilical cord and obstruction of the umbilical vessels. In these cases the umbilical cord is long (>90 cm), is twisted excessively, and is edematous and hemorrhagic.

INFLAMMATORY, INFECTIOUS, AND IMMUNE CAUSES OF ABORTION

Equine Herpesvirus 1 Infection

The most frequent infectious cause of abortion is EHV-1 infection.

- The virus is transmitted via the respiratory tract by ingestion of contaminated feedstuffs or by fomites.
- Its prevalence varies from year to year, and abortions tend to occur in outbreaks ("abortion storms"), especially when pregnant mares are crowded and there are additions during the final months of the foaling season.
- Immunity after abortion is of short duration (4 to 6 months).
- Pregnant mares abort without warning, and the fetus usually is encased in the amnion. Abortion can occur after 5 months of gestation but more commonly between 9 months of gestation and term.
- Sometimes the foal is born alive but dies in a few hours to a few days.

Diagnosis

Diagnosis of EHV-1 abortion is based on gross and microscopic changes in the aborted fetus, immunofluorescence, and virus isolation.

- Aborted fetuses are fresh and free from postmortem autolysis at delivery.
- The most consistent gross lesion is severe edema of the lungs, which

are heavy and rubbery and remain pitted on digital pressure.
- Other findings include excessive cellular fluid in the pleural cavity, edema of the pharyngeal tissues and subcutis, and slight jaundice of the mucous membranes.
- Hepatic lesions consist of small, grayish-white foci of subcapsular necrosis from pinpoint size to 5 mm in diameter.
- Pericardial effusion is occasionally seen, with numerous petechiae on the pericardium.
- The placenta sometimes is edematous but has no characteristic lesions.
- Fluorescent antibody staining of fetal tissues is the best method of diagnosis, followed closely by virus isolation and then by observation of viral inclusion bodies in the liver, lung, and thymus. Inclusion bodies seldom are found in affected late-term foals or those born alive.
- Serologic changes in the mare are not helpful, although fetal and neonatal serology may be useful (serum from aborted fetuses, stillborn foals, and weak foals before colostrum ingestion may have significant virus-neutralizing antibody titers).

Prevention

- *vaccination:* The decision on which vaccination regimen, if any, to use depends on the exposure potential and general farm management.
  - Typically mares are vaccinated with a killed product at 5, 7, and 9 months of gestation.
  - An additional dose can also be administered during the third month of gestation.
  - The efficacy of vaccines for prevention of EHV-1 infection is variable.
- *management strategies:* Regardless of the vaccination program used, pregnant mares should not be stressed or allowed prolonged contact with younger horses. Introduction of new animals to the herd should be minimized.
- *prevention during an outbreak:* Mares that have aborted should be isolated until the diagnosis is confirmed.

- Any bedding used by the mare should be burned. If the abortion occurred in a paddock, it should be cleared of all horses for 4 weeks.
- Staff attending the mare should wear plastic gloves and rubber boots, and these items must be disinfected thoroughly before other mares are attended.
- The aborted fetus and placenta should be placed in a plastic bag and taken directly to a diagnostic laboratory.

Viral Arteritis

Equine viral arteritis (EVA) is a severe systemic and respiratory infection of low incidence. The virus is transmitted venereally and as an aerosol, and the incubation period is 7 to 10 days.

Signs of EVA infection

- moderate to severe depression
- fever (40.6° to 41.1° C [105.1° to 105.9° F])
- keratoconjunctivitis
- generalized edema, particularly of the extremities
- fetal death after acute signs of infection, with abortion occurring 7 to 10 days later

Diagnosis of EVA abortion

- There may be no gross lesions in the aborted fetus, although fetal autolysis is common.
- When present, gross lesions can include petechial hemorrhages on the pleural surface, with slight edema of the lungs and clear fluid within the pleural cavity.
- Diagnosis is made by virus isolation and immunofluorescent staining.

- Serum neutralization tests on serum samples from acutely infected and convalescent mares that have aborted can also confirm the diagnosis.

Control

Recommendations for control include:

- immunizing stallions with a modified-live vaccine
- restricting the breeding of stallions
- shedding the virus to vaccinated or seropositive mares
- isolation from other unvaccinated horses

MULTIFACTORIAL CAUSES OF ABORTION

Fetal Mummification

Mummified fetuses are aborted when one of twin fetuses dies in utero and the pregnancy continues, or in cases of bacterial or mycotic placentitis in which the mare is treated with systemic antimicrobials and progesterone. Thus practitioners must be cautious in administering antimicrobials and progesterone to pregnant mares with vulvar discharge.

TOXIC AND NUTRITIONAL CAUSES OF ABORTION

Fescue grasses, Sudan grasses, and sorghum are toxic to the fetus. Phenothiazine derivatives and organophosphates are the anthelmintics most commonly associated with abortion. Selenium and iodine deficiencies can also cause abortion.

14

Ocular System

Examination of the Eye

(pages 1218-1221)
William C. Rebhun

ROUTINE EXAMINATION OF THE EYE

Initial Examination

A history, including information on prior ocular and systemic disease, should be obtained. The necessary ophthalmic instruments include:

- focal light source (e.g., pen light, transilluminator, or flashlight)
  - A source of magnification, such as a loupe, also is helpful.
- direct ophthalmoscope
- blue cobalt filter light or ultraviolet light source (e.g., Wood's lamp)

In a well-lit area, the skull, orbits, palpebral fissures, and eyes are inspected for asymmetry and obvious abnormalities, and the menace response is assessed in each eye. The rest of the ocular examination should be performed in a darkened room or box stall. Using a focal light source, the eyelid margins, conjunctiva, nictitans, cornea, anterior chamber, iris, and lens are examined and the pupillary light responses assessed.

Ophthalmoscopic Examination

Following is a recommended routine for examination using a direct ophthalmoscope:

- Begin with the scope set at 0 diopters and held 45 to 60 cm (18 to 24 inch) from the horse's eye.
  - This highlights opacities in the cornea, anterior chamber, lens, or vitreous.

- Assess direct and consensual pupillary light responses by quickly swinging the beam from one eye to the other.
- Move the scope to within 2.5 to 5 cm (1 to 2 inches) of the cornea and examine the fundus.
  - Adjust the setting to keep the fundus in focus (-3 to -5 diopters for most humans).

Mydriasis usually is not necessary; however, if the examination cannot be completed in a very dark area, mydriasis can be achieved with topical 1% tropicamide.

Fluorescein Dye Test

Disposable fluorescein-impregnated strips can be moistened with topical anesthetic to facilitate examination. Excess dye should be flushed off the eye with physiologic saline or an ocular irrigating solution. A blue light source (e.g., Wood's lamp) highlights staining of small corneal abrasions and fine linear injuries.

Digital Tonometry

Intraocular pressure can be compared by exerting gentle finger pressure through the upper eyelids against the globes. This test is fairly accurate for assessing gross differences in intraocular pressure between the two eyes.

OPHTHALMIC EVALUATION OF FOALS

Ophthalmic examination in neonatal foals (>2 weeks of age) is identical to that in adult horses, except for restraint considerations. Following are some normal ophthalmic differences between foals and adult horses:

♦ Foals tend to have rounder pupils and lighter colored irises than adult horses.
  • The corpora nigra in foals tend to be smaller and less obvious, and corpora may be observed at both the dorsal and ventral pupillary borders of the iris.
♦ There is less pigmentation of limbal conjunctiva in neonates.
♦ The menace response is less obvious in young foals.
♦ The pupillary light responses must be evaluated with very bright light because neonatal foals are easily excited (resulting in dilated pupils that appear to respond poorly to light).
♦ It is common to find "suture lines" (a gray or whitish Y-shaped opacity) on the lens.
  • They are most common in neonatal foals but may persist through the yearling period.
♦ Persistent remnants of the hyaloid artery may be found in newborn foals, especially premature foals.
  • The vessel is seen as a dark or refractile, waving, linear opacity traversing the vitreous from posterior lens capsule to optic disc.
  • Such remnants generally are bilateral and disappear by 2 to 3 months of age.

The normal fundus color of neonatal foals is no different than that of adult horses.

Common Ophthalmic Problems in Foals

Corneal lesions

Corneal lesions in neonatal foals generally suggest exposure- or trauma-induced injuries or lid abnormalities (e.g., entropion in sick foals and trichiasis in pony and Miniature Horse foals).

Uveal problems

Septic or endotoxin-induced uveitis is most common in neonatal foals suffering from gram-negative septicemia; in fact, uveitis in a neonatal foal is certain evidence of septicemia. Signs may be obvious (e.g., conjunctival and ciliary injection, miosis, and fibrin, hypopyon, or hyphema in the anterior chamber) or very subtle (e.g.,

greenish discoloration of the iris). In addition to treatment for septicemia, the eyes should be treated for septic uveitis (see p. 378).

Vision problems

If a foal has reduced vision or apparent blindness, yet no ocular abnormalities are found and pupillary light responses are intact, a visual cortex lesion must be considered. Most such foals have mild or focal hypoxicischemic cerebrocortical lesions (a manifestation of neonatal maladjustment syndrome; see Chapter 6, Neonatal Evaluation and Management). Other possibilities are hydrocephalus or another developmental condition of the central nervous system (CNS).

Ancillary Diagnostic Aids *(pages 1221-1223)*

William C. Rebhun

REGIONAL ANESTHESIA

Auriculopalpebral Nerve Block

The auriculopalpebral nerve block provides eyelid akinesia, which allows easy manipulation of the upper eyelid without pressure on the painful eye.

♦ 5 mL of 2% lidocaine is injected SC over the nerve as it courses over the highest point of the zygomatic arch (the nerve is palpable at this site).
♦ In an extremely painful eye or an exceptionally dangerous horse, sedation (e.g., routine doses of an α_2-agonist) or use of a twitch may be necessary.

Topical Anesthesia

Proparacaine (0.5% to 1% solution) is the topical anesthetic of choice. For best results, several drops are instilled onto the painful eye at 30-second intervals for 2 minutes. When indicated, samples for bacterial culture should be obtained before topical anesthesia is applied.

CORNEAL CULTURES AND SCRAPINGS

These procedures are important in the diagnosing and managing of corneal infections.

• Corneal cultures should be collected from the necrotic edges of ulcers or after removal of necrotic epithelium in cases of stromal infection.
  • A moistened swab or sterile scalpel blade is used to collect samples. The instrument and sample are then placed in enrichment broth or agar.
• For corneal scrapings, infected corneal lesions are gently scraped with a no. 15 Bard Parker or no. 64 Beaver blade, and the tissue is placed on a clean microscopic slide.
  • Gram's staining allows identification of bacterial and most fungal pathogens.
  • Wright's-Giemsa, new methylene blue, or Grocott's methenamine silver stains are helpful for identifying fungi and characterizing inflammatory infiltrates.

OTHER DIAGNOSTIC TOOLS AND TECHNIQUES

Following is a list of diagnostic aids that may be used in selected cases or at specialist centers:
• *Anterior chamber paracentesis* is reserved for drastic infections that extend into the anterior chamber and are not accessible by routine corneal scrapings.
  • The risks are obvious, so this procedure should be reserved for use in eyes that have a very guarded prognosis for vision.
• *Electroretinography* may be indicated to assess retinal function when visual impairment exists but funduscopic lesions are absent or the fundus cannot be visualized.
  • Its major use in horses is to confirm a diagnosis of night blindness.
• *Ultrasonography* may be helpful when ophthalmoscopic examination is limited by an anterior segment lesion.
  • Orbital trauma or suspected orbital masses, foreign bodies, and posterior segment lesions masked by corneal changes are indications for its use.
• *Tonometry* is indicated when intraocular pressure must be assessed

more accurately than is possible with digital tonometry (e.g., for glaucoma).
• *Slit lamp*, with its exceptional clarity and magnification, is helpful in characterizing anterior segment lesions and for identifying very small conjunctival or corneal foreign bodies.

Principles of Ocular Therapy *(pages 1223-1229)*
William C. Rebhun

ANTIMICROBIAL THERAPY
Topical Therapy
Topical medications are the mainstay of therapy for diseases of the conjunctiva, cornea, and anterior uveal tract. Frequent topical application of antimicrobial drugs (Table 14-1) remains the best treatment for conjunctival or corneal infection.
• Uninfected injuries may be treated prophylactically q8h.
• Infected corneal ulcers may require treatment q1-2h (drops) or q2-4h (ointments).

In horses with severe infections or other painful ocular conditions requiring frequent topical application of drugs, use of a subpalpebral or nasolacrimal lavage system should be considered.

Subconjunctival Therapy
Subconjunctival injection is a means of briefly attaining high therapeutic levels of antimicrobial agents in the cornea, anterior segment, and to some degree the vitreous. This technique is a useful adjunct to (but not a substitute for) frequent topical therapy in horses with severe corneal infections. Following are some commonly used drugs:
• *ampicillin (50 mg):* used to treat streptococcal infections
• *cefamandole or cephalothin (100 mg):* for gram-positive infections
• *gentamicin or tobramycin (20 mg):* for gram-negative infections
• *ticarcillin with clavulanic acid (100 mg):* for either gram-positive or gram-negative infections

Table 14-1
Commonly used topical ophthalmic antibiotics

Antibiotic	Available preparations	Organisms most likely to be effective against	Recommended frequency
Chloramphenicol 1%	Commercial drops or ointment	Gram-positive organisms, some gram-negative organisms	3-12 times daily, depending on severity
Cefamandole (50 mg/mL) Cefazolin (50 mg/mL)	Need to make solution	Gram-positive organisms, severe *Staphylococcus* or *Streptococcus* infections	12-24 times daily in severe lesions
Bacitracin, polymixin B, neomycin combinations	Commercial drops or ointment	Mild gram-negative or gram-positive infections, prophylaxis for uninfected injuries	3-6 times daily
Sulfacetamide	Commercial drops or ointment	Gram-positive conjunctivitis, prophylaxis	3-6 times daily
Gentamicin	Commercial 0.3% drops or ointments	Gram-negative infections, *Pseudomonas*	3-12 times daily
	Fortified homemade 1%-2% solutions	*Pseudomonas*	12-24 times daily
			12-24 times daily
Tobramycin	Commercial 0.3% drops or ointments	*Pseudomonas*	12-24 times daily
Chlortetracycline, polymixin B	Commercial ointment	Conjunctivitis, prophylaxis	3-6 times daily
Ciprofloxacin	Commercial drops	Gram-negative and *Staphylococcus* infections	6-12 times daily
Ofloxacin	Commercial drops	Gram-negative and *Staphylococcus* infections	6-12 times daily

Subconjunctival agents are effective only when injected under the bulbar conjunctiva, not when injected into the eyelid or palpebral conjunctiva.

Systemic Therapy

Systemic antimicrobial therapy generally is of value only when the blood-aqueous barrier has been compromised by inflammation involving the anterior segment and uveal tract (e.g., deep corneal stromal abscess, septic uveitis). Systemic antimicrobial drugs never attain corneal concentrations as high as those attained by frequent topical application or subconjunctival injection. Systemic therapy is, however, indicated before and after intraocular surgery.

CORTICOSTEROID THERAPY

Topical Therapy

Uveitis is the primary ocular disease requiring corticosteroid therapy in horses.

- Chronic nonulcerative keratitis, nonspecific or allergic conjunctivitis, and corneoconjunctival granulomatous lesions also may require corticosteroid therapy.
- Topical 1% prednisolone acetate drops penetrate the eye better than other topical corticosteroid preparations, although frequent application may be necessary.
  - Dexamethasone phosphate ointment (0.1%) often is preferred because of its longer contact time.

Subconjunctival Therapy

Subconjunctival injection of corticosteroids may be used as an adjunct to topical therapy in patients with uveitis. Generally, 20 mg of methylprednisolone (0.5 mL of 40 mg/mL) or betamethasone is injected. Unless corneal injury or ulceration has been absolutely ruled out and uveitis definitively diagnosed, injection of a repository corticosteroid is contraindicated.

NONSTEROIDAL ANTIINFLAMMATORY DRUGS (NSAIDS)

Systemic administration of phenylbutazone (2.2 to 4.4 mg/kg q12h) or flu-nixin meglumine (0.55 to 1.1 mg/kg q12h) frequently is used for managing painful ocular conditions in horses. At least one ophthalmic NSAID preparation is currently available (flurbiprofen [Ocufen]). These products may be useful in reducing intraocular inflammation and for preoperative treatment.

ATROPINE

Atropine may be the single most important topical drug used to treat uveal diseases.

- Topical atropine induces cycloplegia and pupillary dilation, thereby reducing ocular pain, patient resistance, and the potential for synechia formation.
- Side effects can usually be prevented by limiting the dose to either one drop of a 1% solution or a 1.25 cm ($^1/_2$ inch) ribbon of 1% atropine ointment per application.
  - Initially, topical atropine is applied q6-8h until cycloplegia occurs; it is then used as necessary to maintain mydriasis.
  - Gastrointestinal stasis (ileus) may result from overzealous use.
- Once dilated, the pupil may remain dilated for 2 to 6 weeks in some horses.

ANTIFUNGAL THERAPY

Antifungal medications should only be used when fungal infection is confirmed by corneal scrapings or culture. Most topical antifungal agents do not penetrate the intact corneal epithelium very well, so primary treatment of fungal keratitis usually includes superficial keratectomy. Following are some antifungal regimens that have been used to treat keratomycosis in horses:

- Natamycin 5% solution, given topically q1-2h, is the best available preparation against *Aspergillus* spp.
- Miconazole, an intravenous (IV) preparation (Monistat I.V.), is used either undiluted (as drops) or as part of an "ulcer mix" and is given q1-2h.
- Ketoconazole (2% solution given topically q1-2h) is an excellent choice for yeast infections.

- It may also be given by mouth (PO) at 4.4 mg/kg q12h for deep fungal or yeast infections of the eye.
- Silver sulfadiazine cream can be a useful drug for treatment of fungal keratitis.
- Itraconazole 1%, suspended in 30% DMSO and applied topically q6h, achieves excellent corneal tissue levels and has given encouraging clinical results.
  - The product must be formulated by hand.
- Clotrimazole and thiabendazole (as liquid, paste, or cream) can be effective, although their antifungal spectrum is narrower than that of natamycin or miconazole.
- Amphotericin B has been used topically after dilution of 50 mg of amphotericin B powder in 33.3 mL of diluent; drops are instilled into the eye q1-2h.
  - Most ophthalmologists no longer use it because amphotericin B is extremely irritating to ocular tissues.

NURSING CARE

Various nursing procedures help reduce ocular pain and make the horse more comfortable.

- Warm compresses relieve inflammatory edema in the eyelids and also soften discharge or debris around the eyelid margins.
- All discharges and remnants of medications should be gently washed away with warm water before application of more medication.
- Keeping the environment as dark as possible decreases photophobia, blepharospasm, and lacrimation.

Diseases of the Orbit and Globe *(pages 1229-1232)*
William C. Rebhun

CONGENITAL AND FAMILIAL DISEASES
Microphthalmia
Microphthalmia occurs as a sporadic congenital malformation in all breeds of horses. It may be unilateral or bilateral, and the degree varies from subtle to severe. In mild cases, pupillary light response, funduscopic examination, and menace response may be normal, but vision is poor. There is no treatment.

Congenital Buphthalmos
Congenital buphthalmos, or enlarged globe, is rare and generally associated with multiple ocular anomalies that result in chronic glaucoma. If the other eye is normal, enucleation of the buphthalmic globe is recommended to avoid injury and exposure keratopathy.

DISEASES WITH PHYSICAL CAUSES
Trauma
Traumatic damage to the orbit is very common in horses.

- Minor injuries may simply cause eyelid edema or lacerations.
- More serious injuries may result in orbital fractures, orbital edema, chemosis, neuroparalytic keratitis, blindness (traumatic optic neuropathy), sinus or skull fractures, and concussion.
- Complete examination of the orbit, ocular adnexal tissue, and eye is indicated.
  - Unless there are neurologic signs, the horse should be sedated for careful palpation of the orbit and examination of the eye.
  - Skull radiographs should be obtained if orbital fractures are suspected.
  - Warm compresses and antiinflammatory medications may be required to relieve orbital edema before thorough examination of the eye is possible.

Treatment
Treatment varies with the location and severity of the damage.

- If the eye has vision and the pupillary light response is normal, only supportive therapy is necessary.
- If the eye is blind, the pupillary light response is reduced or absent, or optic disc abnormalities are found, antiinflammatory therapy must be intensive.

- DMSO is used at 1 g/kg diluted to a 10% solution in 5% dextrose and given slowly IV.
- Dexamethasone is given at 0.044 to 0.22 mg/kg IV once, then 0.044 mg/kg/day for 3 days.
- Phenylbutazone (4.4 mg/kg PO q12h) or flunixin meglumine (1.1 mg/kg q12h) also is indicated.
- The prognosis for return of vision in such cases is guarded.
- Orbital fractures should be repaired once the horse's condition is stable.
- If the globe has sustained expulsive trauma, proptosis, rupture, or corneal laceration, surgery is necessary to enucleate the globe or repair the corneal laceration.
  - If the ocular damage is irreparable, surgery may be delayed 24 to 72 hours while warm compresses and antimicrobial and antiinflammatory drugs reduce the inflammation.
  - Surgery to repair corneal lacerations should be performed as soon as possible.

Traumatic optic neuropathy

Traumatic optic neuropathy is a common cause of blindness resulting from orbital trauma. Obvious hemorrhage or peripapillary edema may be seen in the optic disc region, but the disc may appear totally normal, because the actual damage is retrobulbar or even intracranial. In horses that do not respond to intensive antiinflammatory therapy, blindness persists and obvious optic nerve atrophy is apparent within a few weeks or months of injury.

Acquired Buphthalmos

Most buphthalmic globes are associated with glaucoma secondary to intraocular inflammation (e.g., uveitis, physical damage resulting in lens luxation); rarely, intraocular neoplasia causes buphthalmos. Enlargement of the globe caused by glaucoma results in blindness. If exposure keratopathy occurs, the eye should be enucleated or an ocular silicone ball implant considered.

Phthisis Bulbi

Phthisis bulbi is atrophy or shrinkage of the globe secondary to chronic uveitis or ocular perforating wounds. The small globe predisposes to chronic conjunctivitis and ocular discharge, with subsequent irritation by flies. If ocular irritation becomes chronic or unmanageable, enucleation should be performed.

INFLAMMATORY, INFECTIOUS, AND IMMUNE DISEASES

Periorbital Cellulitis

Periorbital cellulitis most often results from a minor and usually inapparent injury (e.g., puncture by a nail or wire) to the eyelid skin or palpebral conjunctival surface.

- Periorbital trauma to the eyelids or facial area is a more obvious but less common cause.
- Signs are unilateral and include diffuse, painful periorbital soft tissue swelling, chemosis, mucopurulent ocular discharge, and possibly fever.
- Therapy consists of systemic antimicrobial drugs, analgesics, and warm compresses.
  - The cornea should be protected with frequent application of a broad-spectrum antibacterial ointment.
  - If a puncture wound can be found, it should be debrided to facilitate drainage.

Retrobulbar Abscess

Retrobulbar abscessation may develop from periorbital puncture wounds or trauma, migration of bacteria or foreign material from the oral cavity, or from *Streptococcus equi* infection.

- Signs include progressive exophthalmos, conjunctivitis, a swollen nictitating membrane, and eyelid edema.
  - Eating is painful, so the horse may be inappetent; fever is noted in some cases.
- Differential diagnoses include periorbital cellulitis and retrobulbar neoplasia.
- CBC, measurement of serum albumin and globulins, skull radiographs, ultrasound evaluation of the orbit, and aspiration from the retrobulbar area are indicated.

✦ Treatment requires drainage of the abscess before initiation of antibacterial therapy.
  • Drainage usually must be established ventral or lateral to the globe, which carries a significant risk of injury to the optic nerve and other vital structures.
  • Use of ultrasound to guide drainage is recommended.
  • Once drainage is established, appropriate antibacterial drugs (based on Gram's stain and/or culture results) are indicated, as are analgesics and warm compresses.

NEOPLASIA

The two more common neoplasms involving the orbit and globe are squamous cell carcinoma and lymphosarcoma. These tumors may involve the conjunctiva, cornea, eyelids, or nictitating membrane. Rarely, multicentric lymphosarcoma can cause a large retrobulbar mass with resulting proptosis of the globe. These tumors are discussed in specific sections later in this chapter.

IDIOPATHIC DISEASES
Adipose Tissue Prolapse

Occasionally, periorbital fat prolapses and appears as soft, conjunctival-covered masses protruding from under the eyelids or nictitating membrane. This benign condition may be unilateral or bilateral and is easily confused with neoplasia.

Diseases of the Eyelids
(pages 1232-1259)
William C. Rebhun

CONGENITAL AND FAMILIAL DISEASES
Entropion

Entropion, or inversion of the eyelid, is the most common congenital eyelid defect in foals. It may be present at birth or acquired within the first few days of life.
✦ Usually the lower eyelid is affected in one or both eyes.

✦ Signs include blepharospasm, lacrimation, and photophobia in the affected eye.
  • Secondary corneal abrasions or ulcerations may occur. *Pseudomonas* spp. and *Streptococcus* spp. are commonly isolated from these lesions.
✦ Focal light examination highlights the inverted lower eyelid margins, and tear-soaked eyelid hair can be found contacting the corneal surface.
  • Fluorescein staining is recommended to highlight corneal abrasions or ulcers.

Treatment
Treatment involves eversion of the affected eyelid(s) and therapy for corneal injury.
✦ In early cases with no corneal damage, frequent manual eversion of the eyelid (e.g., q4-8h) and topical application of a broad-spectrum antibacterial ointment q8h is all that is required.
  • In many cases the problem resolves as the foal gains weight.
✦ In unresponsive cases and in those with corneal damage, other measures are necessary.
  • The lid margin is everted either with subcutaneous injection of lidocaine, saline, or penicillin into the eyelid or with mattress sutures.
  • Topical antibiotic and 1% atropine ointments are applied several times daily.
✦ In cases with severe corneal damage and when entropion recurs after simple techniques, surgical correction is required.
  • Culture and sensitivity tests and cytologic evaluation of corneal scrapings should direct the choice of antibacterial therapy, which should be intensive.
  • Topical atropine ointment is used as necessary.

DISEASES WITH PHYSICAL CAUSES
Eyelid Lacerations
To ensure good functional and cosmetic results, an attempt should be made to repair eyelid lacerations as perfectly as possible. With lacerations older than about 12 hours, eyelid

edema or infection can be managed medically with antibiotics and warm compresses for 1 to 4 days before surgical repair. Lacerations sustained more recently than that should be repaired immediately.

Treatment
Two-layer closure is recommended.
* In the first layer, absorbable suture material (e.g., 3-0 or 4-0 chromic catgut) is placed in an interrupted mattress pattern in the lid stroma between the conjunctiva and the skin.
  * The conjunctiva need not be sutured unless it is extensively displaced from the lid stroma.
* In the second layer, the skin is apposed using nonabsorbable suture material in a simple-interrupted pattern.
* In each layer, the first suture should be placed as close to the lid margin as possible, taking care that the suture, once placed, will not rub against the cornea.

Topical broad-spectrum antibacterial drugs are applied to the eye for 7 days, and systemic antibiotics and NSAIDs are given for 3 to 5 days. Tetanus prophylaxis is confirmed. The sutures should be left in place for 14 days.

Distichiasis
Distichiasis, the presence of abnormal hairs, is uncommon but should be ruled out in all cases of minor ocular irritation or recurrent conjunctivitis or corneal ulceration.
* Distichiae may be present in either or both eyelid margins as they exit the meibomian glands.
* Initial therapy simply involves plucking the distichias after administration of topical anesthesia.
  * The horse should become comfortable within a few days.
  * Concurrent corneal injury should be treated with topical broad-spectrum antibacterial drugs and atropine. Corneal injury should resolve within a week.
* In horses with only a few distichia, periodic plucking of the lashes or permanent electroepilation may be performed for long-term prevention of ocular irritation.
  * If many distichias are present, electroepilation or cryosurgical

destruction of the hair follicles is recommended.

Ectopic Cilia
Ectopic cilia are stiff hairs that originate at the base of a meibomian gland, penetrate the palpebral conjunctiva, and lie perpendicular to the corneal surface.
* These hairs, which are singular in most cases, cause persistent or recurrent corneal ulceration.
* Diagnosis is difficult because the cilia are small and difficult to see without magnification, and they are surrounded by reactive or hyperplastic palpebral conjunctiva.
* Treatment consists of en-bloc excision of the cilia and surrounding palpebral conjunctiva, including the base of the meibomian gland.
  * Cryosurgical or electrocautery destruction of the cilia is another option.
  * The corneal ulcer is treated in a routine fashion and should heal within 7 to 14 days.

Trichiasis
Trichiasis describes abnormally directed normal lashes.
* The most common cause is upper eyelid laxity.
  * The condition is more common in neonatal pony and Miniature Horse foals.
  * Trichiasis also occurs subsequent to eyelid injury in older horses and ponies.
* Signs include persistent or recurrent corneal ulceration that is refractory to standard therapy.
* In cases caused by eyelid laxity, treatment involves trimming the eyelashes and symptomatic therapy for corneal ulceration
* In horses with prior eyelid injuries, blepharoplastic procedures may be necessary to evert the eyelid and abnormally directed hairs or to close lid marginal defects.

INFLAMMATORY, INFECTIOUS, AND IMMUNE DISEASES
Habronemiasis
Habronema spp. can cause ulcerative granulomatous lesions ("summer sores") in the eyelids or conjunctiva.

- The medial canthus and naso-lacrimal duct region are typical locations.
- Firm, calcareous, yellowish-white concretions can be observed within the ulcerative granulomas and are virtually pathognomonic for habronemiasis.
- Diagnosis is relatively easy if multiple summer sores exist in various locations.
  - Biopsy is indicated if the diagnosis is in doubt.

Treatment

Treatment is instituted that kills existing larvae and reduces the body's reaction to dying larvae.

- Ivermectin at 200 µg/kg PO can be effective.

Alternatively, larvicidal ointment may be formulated from a mixture of 220 g nitrofurazone ointment, 30 mL of 90% DMSO, 30 mL dexamethasone, and 30 mL trichlorfon.

  - This product should be used only on skin lesions, not on conjunctival lesions.
- Echothiophate (phospholine iodide) drops (0.03%), at 1 drop q12h, also are larvicidal.
- Topical corticosteroids are indicated for conjunctival lesions.
  - If the cornea has been ulcerated, corticosteroids should not be used until the ulcer heals.
- Calcareous nodules should be debrided from the eyelid or conjunctival surface.

Onchocerciasis

The skin of the eyelids, temporal bulbar conjunctiva, temporal cornea, and uveal system all may show evidence of *Onchocerca* microfilariae infection.

- On the eyelids, bilateral alopecia or mild, pruritic, exudative dermatitis may be seen.
- Biopsy may be necessary for diagnosis.
- Systemic and topical corticosteroids should be administered before larvicidal therapy begins to control the host reaction to dying microfilariae.
  - Ivermectin (200 µg/kg PO) and diethylcarbamazine (4.4 to 6.6 mg/kg PO daily for 3 to 4 weeks) are effective larvicidal drugs.

- Levamisole (6 mg/kg PO once) also may be effective.

NEOPLASIA

Squamous Cell Carcinoma

Squamous cell carcinoma is a common lid neoplasm in middle-age and older horses.

- Lightly pigmented horses and ponies are affected most often.
- The lesions are pink, with a raised "cobblestone" ulcerative surface. They often have a white crust covering the pink surface.
  - This neoplasm often invades adjacent tissues.
- The gross appearance and origin in nonpigmented tissue suggest squamous cell carcinoma. If there is doubt as to the diagnosis, a biopsy should be performed.
- Cryosurgery, radiofrequency hyperthermia, irradiation, immunotherapy with *Bacillus* Calmette-Guerin (BCG) injections, and surgical resection are options, depending on tumor location and size.
  - Enucleation may be necessary for tumors with extensive eyelid involvement.
  - Tumors on the third eyelid should be treated by removal of the third eyelid.

Sarcoid

The second most common eyelid tumor is the sarcoid. The appearance of these tumors varies widely, from flat areas of alopecia and thickened skin to wartlike growths (verrucous form) to firm, round nodules that may be singular or clustered. The lesions may become ulcerated.

Treatment

The three most widely used treatments for sarcoids are:

- immunotherapy with intralesional BCG
  - The recommended dosage is 1 mL of BCG solution per 1 to 2 cm^3 of tumor, up to a maximum of 5 to 6 mL/tumor.
  - A total of 2 to 5 injections at 2-week intervals usually is needed for tumor regression.
- cryosurgery
  - The tumor is debulked and two freeze-thaw cycles are used.

♦ chemotherapy with intralesional cisplatin (in a sesame oil base)
  • The usual dosage is 1 mg cisplatin/cm³ of tumor.
  • Injections may be repeated at 2-week intervals.

Diseases of the Conjunctiva and Nasolacrimal System

(pages 1239–1243)
William C. Rebhun

CONGENITAL AND FAMILIAL DISEASES

Conjunctival Dermoid

Dermoids are rare, congenital, skin-like masses that appear as fleshy, hairy growths on the bulbar or palpebral conjunctiva. Equine dermoids tend to have short, stiff hairs that are very irritating. Treatment involves removal by wedge resection of the eyelid or by conjunctival resection.

Absence of Distal Nasolacrimal Duct Punctum

In some foals, one or both distal nasolacrimal duct puncta are absent.

♦ This condition causes persistent epiphora, conjunctivitis, and mucopurulent ocular discharge without ocular pain.
  • Affected foals may not have detectable epiphora or conjunctivitis until 2 to 6 months of age.
♦ The nostril should be examined for the presence of a distal punctum at the mucocutaneous junction; finding no punctum confirms the diagnosis.
  • Fluorescein applied to the eye fails to appear in the nostril within the usual 1 to 5 minutes.
♦ Treatment involves establishing a distal opening in the nasolacrimal duct.
  • Under either general anesthesia or sedation and topical anesthesia, stiff polyethylene tubing is passed rostrally from the proximal punctum in the upper or lower lid.

• Usually the tubing can be palpated beneath the mucosal surface in the floor of the nostril.
• An incision is made through the mucosa to retrieve the tubing, which is drawn through the newly created opening and sutured in place for 3 weeks.
• Antibacterial ointment is applied to the eye several times daily until the tubing is removed.

DISEASES WITH PHYSICAL CAUSES

Lacerations

Lacerations of the conjunctiva, unless extensive, seldom require surgical repair.

Obstruction of the Nasolacrimal Duct

Blockage of the nasolacrimal duct is common and usually is secondary to ocular or conjunctival diseases that produce excessive tear production or discharge.

♦ Failure of fluorescein dye to pass from the eye to the nostril is diagnostic.
♦ Flushing the duct with saline is curative.
  True obstructions of the nasolacrimal duct occur secondary to tooth root problems, sinus infections, tumors, and trauma; management must address the underlying condition.

Foreign Bodies

Foreign material may become entrapped in the palpebral conjunctiva, fornices, or bulbar side of the third eyelid.

♦ Most of these foreign bodies are plant material, such as seed awns, pieces of hay or straw, thorns, and burdock pappus bristles.
♦ Magnification may be necessary to identify some foreign bodies.
♦ Removal of the foreign material constitutes the primary treatment.
  • When the material is imbedded in the conjunctiva, it may be necessary to excise some attached conjunctiva to facilitate removal.
  • Corneal injuries are treated in a routine fashion.
♦ The eye should be comfortable within a few days or as soon as the corneal injury resolves.

INFLAMMATORY, INFECTIOUS, AND IMMUNE DISEASES

Bacterial Conjunctivitis

Primary bacterial conjunctivitis results in a mucopurulent ocular discharge, with no associated corneal lesions or pain.

* The conjunctiva is injected and the entire membrane may be edematous and swollen.
* Predisposing factors include irritation from dust, wind, dirt (during racing), flies, and viral upper respiratory infections (e.g., equine viral arteries, influenza, rhinopneumonitis, adenovirus infection).

Diagnosis

Diagnosis is based on:

* presence of mucopurulent ocular discharge in the absence of ocular pain
* negative fluorescein staining of the cornea
* absence of corneal or anterior segment inflammation
* conjunctival scrapings that demonstrate abundant neutrophils and bacteria
  * The predominant bacteria in normal equine conjunctival flora are gram-positive cocci.

Culture and sensitivity testing are indicated in patients resistant to standard therapy or with enzootic conjunctivitis in an equine facility.

Treatment

Treatment includes:

* topical broad-spectrum antibacterial agents, such as 1% chloramphenicol or neomycin-polymyxin-bacitracin ointment, applied q6-8h
  * The conjunctival sac should be cleansed and any facial discharge removed with warm water and cotton before each ointment application.
* checking the patency of the nasolacrimal duct with fluorescein dye and lavaging the duct as necessary

Most cases resolve in 4 to 7 days of therapy. If the problem has not resolved in a week, therapy should be stopped for 48 hours and swab samples obtained for culture and sensitivity testing. Also, nasolacrimal duct patency should be reassessed.

Parasitic Conjunctivitis

Habronemiasis

Habronemiasis lesions on the conjunctiva are similar to those involving the eyelids (see p. 368). Treatment is as described for eyelid lesions.

Onchocerciasis

Onchocerca microfilariae can cause pink or red raised lesions on the bulbar conjunctiva, especially in the temporal region. Lesions may progress into the cornea as a pannus-like growth. Diagnosis is based on routine biopsies or wet preparations of small conjunctival samples. Treatment is as described for onchocerciasis of the eyelids (see page 369).

Thelaziasis

Thelazia spp. can be found as free-moving worms in the conjunctival fornices, under the membrana nictitans, or in the nasolacrimal ducts. They cause minor irritation and occasional ocular discharge. Treatment consists of removal of visible worms and topical application of 0.03% echothiophate drops to kill the remaining parasites.

Dacryocystitis

Infections of the nasolacrimal duct (dacryocystitis) occasionally occur in horses

* Foreign bodies, chronic obstruction of the nasolacrimal duct, and infection by opportunistic microorganisms are possible causes.
* Signs are typical of nasolacrimal obstruction, and pus may exit the proximal punctum.
* Treatment should follow culture and sensitivity testing of the discharge and involve daily lavage of the duct and appropriate topical antibacterial drugs.
  * Contrast radiography is indicated if a foreign body or chronic obstruction is suspected.

Urticaria and Anaphylaxis

Chemosis (conjunctival edema) is often seen in cases of urticaria or anaphylaxis. Systemic treatment for anaphylaxis and removal of the offending antigen are of primary importance. Warm compresses and frequent application of hyperosmotic agents (e.g., 40% dextrose solution or 5% sodium chloride (NaCl) ophthalmic ointment) quickly reduces the chemosis in most cases.

NEOPLASIA

The most common tumor of the equine conjunctiva is squamous cell carcinoma (see p. 369). An important differential diagnosis is *angiosarcoma,* a slow-growing but malignant neoplasm that often metastasizes or invades deeper ocular tissues despite surgical excision and radiation therapy. These tumors tend to be redder in color than the classic pink squamous cell carcinoma. Particularly red, easily hemorrhaging ocular or periocular masses should be biopsied early to best identify vascular origin tumors.

Lymphosarcoma

Conjunctival tumors have been reported in some horses with lymphosarcoma. The conjunctiva may be very thickened and red or may merely appear chemotic and mildly inflamed. Diagnosis requires conjunctival biopsy and a complete physical examination to detect lymphadenopathy or other organ involvement. Treatment with topical and systemic corticosteroids may be palliative.

IDIOPATHIC DISEASES

Conjunctival Hypertrophy

Chronic unilateral or bilateral conjunctival hypertrophy occasionally is observed in ponies. It does not cause discomfort or ocular discharge, although the palpebral conjunctiva appears swollen, protruding from the fornix or lid margin. No treatment is necessary, but biopsy may be indicated to differentiate this condition from conjunctival lymphosarcoma.

Diseases of the Cornea

(pages 1243-1253)
William C. Rebhun

CONGENITAL AND FAMILIAL DISEASES

Corneal Dermoid

Corneal dermoids are uncommon, congenital, skinlike growths that at-

tach to the cornea, limbal area, or conjunctiva (see p. 370). Keratectomy of sufficient depth to remove the dermoid may result in significant corneal scarring. Topical antibacterial drugs and atropine are used postoperatively q6-8h until corneal healing is complete.

DISEASES WITH PHYSICAL CAUSES

Exposure Keratitis

Exposure keratitis most commonly results from facial nerve dysfunction (e.g., auriculopalpebral nerve injury from skull trauma or surgery, otitis media/interna and temporohyoid osteoarthropathy, and protozoal myeloencephalitis).

◆ Signs include lacrimation, photophobia, central corneal opacities that may progress to ulcerations, and signs of ipsilateral facial nerve dysfunction.
  • Signs of vestibular disease may accompany facial nerve dysfunction (see Chapter 11, Nervous System).
◆ Examination reveals a central horizontal area of corneal edema caused by desiccation; erosion or ulceration may develop in severe cases.
  • Blepharospasm is not present, because the eyelids cannot close effectively. For the same reason, the palpebral reflex is reduced or absent.
◆ Chronic exposure keratitis results in further corneal edema, vascularization, deeper ulceration, and a dried crust of necrotic corneal tissue at the site of ulceration.

Treatment and prognosis

Treatment consists of:

◆ gently irrigating any dried material off the cornea after application of topical anesthesia
◆ frequent application of topical broad-spectrum antibacterial drugs
  • Lubricating ointments may be all that is required in early cases.
◆ topical atropine as necessary (usually 1 to 3 times daily) to maintain cycloplegia
  • Atropine is not necessary in early cases without ulceration.
◆ temporary partial tarsorrhaphy

In very severe cases, complete tarsorrhaphy or a conjunctival flap may be necessary. A full-cup blinker can also be used to retain corneal moisture. The prognosis depends on the likelihood of resolution of the primary neurologic deficit.

Corneal Abrasion

Corneal abrasions are very common and usually are caused by trauma from feedstuffs, tail swishing, and dirt and stones in racing animals. Evidence of a painful eye (photophobia, blepharospasm, lacrimation) and fluorescein retention over the damaged area are found. Treatment consists of topical antibacterial drugs and atropine (if pain is severe). Small superficial abrasions (≤1 cm in diameter) should heal within 7 days.

Corneal Epithelial Erosion

Acute corneal erosions are merely large abrasions and should be managed as such. *Chronic* corneal erosions are nonhealing lesions that show loose-edged epithelial defects with poor healing tendencies over a period of weeks.

- Edema and vascularization are minimal, although pain is severe and fluorescein dye is retained in the damaged area.
  - Ectopic cilia, other lid abnormalities, and conjunctival foreign bodies must be ruled out.
- Treatment involves cautery with 2% tincture of iodine applied to the edges, followed by removal of the unattached epithelium.
  - Cautery may need to be repeated at 3- to 5-day intervals in refractory cases.
  - Punctate keratotomy is another option.
- Topical broad-spectrum antibacterial drugs and atropine are indicated q6-12h.
  - Drops are preferable to ointments in these cases.
- If treatment fails, topical hyperosmotic agents (e.g., 5% NaCl ointment), should be applied q6-8h to discourage stromal edema.
  - Application of soft contact lenses and surgical keratectomy are other options.

Stromal Ulcers

Ulcers that invade the corneal stroma induce more extensive inflammation involving corneal edema and vascularization.

- These ulcers cause lacrimation, photophobia, and blepharospasm; they retain fluorescein dye and have a concave or craterlike appearance.
- Topical broad-spectrum antibacterial drugs and atropine are necessary to aid healing and should be applied several times daily.
  - Antibacterial drugs should be continued until epithelialization is complete, which usually takes about 2 weeks for an uncomplicated ulcer 1 cm wide.
- *Corticosteroids must not be used in these cases.*

Corneal Lacerations
Partial-thickness lacerations

Nonperforating corneal lacerations usually are linear or triangular corneal wounds, possibly with an associated flap of cornea, that retain fluorescein dye. Treatment consists of topical antibacterial drugs applied several times daily, topical atropine to effect (cycloplegia), and systemic NSAIDs. Occasional cases require surgical debridement or suturing of large flaps of corneal tissue; deeper wounds may require bulbar conjunctival flaps for protection.

Full-thickness lacerations

Full-thickness corneal lacerations usually are severe and result in iris prolapse and a thick fibrin seal over the exposed iris and corneal defect.

- If the intraocular contents have not been expelled and the sclera is not badly torn, surgical repair is possible, although very difficult.
- In many cases, the complete extent of the injury cannot be determined until the horse is placed under general anesthesia.
  - Preoperative systemic bacteriocidal antibiotics and NSAIDs should be administered.

If proper instrumentation, including ophthalmic sutures swaged on fine needles, is not available, repair should not be attempted and the horse should be referred to an appropriate specialist.

If the intraocular contents have been expelled or if the corneal laceration extends far into the sclera, the eye probably should be enucleated.

Similarly, if the wound and anterior chamber are obviously infected, the eye should be enucleated.

Puncture wounds
Small corneal punctures caused by wire or a thorn may result in a leaking wound with an intact anterior chamber. If the wound is small enough, it may be sealed with 2% tincture of iodine or phenol cautery; cyanoacrylate also may be used to seal small punctures. If this does not work, corneal sutures are necessary. Topical and systemic antibacterial drugs and topical atropine should be administered.

Corneal Foreign Bodies
Foreign bodies imbedded in the cornea cause photophobia, blepharospasm, and lacrimation. If the foreign body has been present for several days, corneal vascularization and edema also are present. The foreign body should be removed as gently as possible.

- Most superficial foreign bodies can be flushed off the cornea with a stream of ocular irrigating solution or saline.
- If this does not work, the foreign body should be gently removed with a needle, foreign body spud, or fine forceps.
- Topical antibacterial drugs and atropine should be used until epithelialization is complete.

INFLAMMATORY, INFECTIOUS, AND IMMUNE DISEASES
Bacterial Corneal Ulceration
Infected corneal stromal ulcers are craterlike and have necrotic yellow or white edges.

- The affected eye is extremely painful, and corneal edema and vascularization are severe.
  - Necrosis may be evident at the base and periphery of the ulcer.
- Miosis is present, and inflammatory cells or fibrin may accumulate in the anterior chamber.

- Corneal scrapings should be performed and smears stained with Gram's, Wright's-Giemsa or other stains to demonstrate bacterial and fungal agents.
  - Samples for bacterial and fungal cultures should be obtained from the ulcer.

Treatment
Treatment comprises antibacterial medications, topical atropine, and, if necessary, collagenase inhibitors.

- A broad-spectrum antibacterial drug (see Table 14-1) should be applied as often as possible for the first several days.
  - Chloramphenicol, cefazolin, and cefamandole are good gram-positive choices.
  - Gentamicin, tobramycin, neomycin-polymyxin-bacitracin, or ciprofloxacin is indicated for gram-negative organisms.
- Rapid progression of the ulcer or evidence of extensive collagenase activity suggests *Pseudomonas* infection.
  - These ulcers should be treated with gentamicin, tobramycin, or ciprofloxacin.
- Systemic antibacterial drugs are indicated if endophthalmitis is suspected or if corneal lesions obscure intraocular structures.
  - Bulbar subconjunctival injections (e.g., 20 mg of gentamicin) also can be beneficial.
- Topical 1% atropine is applied q6-8h until pupillary dilation occurs or the eye appears more comfortable. Frequency of application then is tailored to the individual case.
- When collagenase activity is obvious or suspected, topical therapy with collagenase inhibitors is indicated.
  - To reduce irritation, 10% acetylcysteine drops can be used undiluted or diluted to a 1% to 2% solution with artificial tears.
  - Initial dosage is one drop per hour, decreasing the frequency only when ulceration stabilizes (reduced stromal necrosis, better-defined ulcer edges, and decreased corneal edema).
  - Collagenase inhibitors generally can be discontinued after 3 to 7 days.

- Systemic NSAIDs help control soft tissue pain and inflammation.
- *Corticosteroids are specifically contraindicated in corneal ulcerative disease.*
  Conjunctival or third eyelid flaps seldom are indicated unless corneal perforation is imminent. If a conjunctival flap is used, it should be narrow enough to allow observation of part of the cornea, anterior chamber, and pupil.

Mycotic Keratitis and Ulceration

Mycotic keratitis (keratomycosis) generally is manifested as chronic keratitis that does not respond to routine topical therapy.

- The history usually includes use of topical corticosteroids.
- Mild-to-severe lacrimation, photophobia, and blepharospasm are present.
- Typically the corneal lesion consists of multifocal stromal opacities that appear as white or yellowish 1- to 3-mm-wide densities; fluorescein uptake is variable.
  - Often the epithelium "lifts off," leaving a defect that retains stain.
  - Epithelial necrosis, corneal edema, and superficial vessels are variable findings.
- Less frequently, mycotic keratitis appears as a deep, craterlike ulcer or a stromal abscess.
  - Hypopyon, corneal neovascularization, corneal edema, and secondary iritis are common in these cases.
- Diagnosis requires stromal scrapings for staining to demonstrate fungal hyphae. This may necessitate removal of intact epithelium overlying fungal colonies.
  - Most fungi are easily demonstrated by Gram's stain.
  - The common organisms identified are *Aspergillus, Alternaria, Fusarium* spp., and yeasts.
- Superficial keratectomy should be performed before starting antifungal medication.
- *Corticosteroids are contraindicated.*
  The prognosis is guarded because of the unpredictable course and variable pathogenicity of fungal species. Healing is slow and usually requires weeks, even in apparently simple cases.

Stromal Abscesses

Corneal stromal abscesses result from small corneal puncture wounds and abrasions that become infected.

- Findings include severe ocular pain (lacrimation, photophobia, blepharospasm) and a yellow or white stromal or endothelial opacity with surrounding corneal edema and vascularization.
  - The severity of these changes is directly proportional to the duration of infection.
- An epithelial defect may or may not overlie the abscess. Often the corneal epithelium is intact and does not retain fluorescein dye.
- If the anterior chamber can be seen through the corneal lesion, fibrin clots or inflammatory cells (hypopyon) usually are present and the pupil is miotic.
  - If the cornea is too opaque to allow examination of the anterior chamber, endophthalmitis should be considered and the prognosis should be more guarded.
- Scrapings should be done to obtain samples for bacterial and fungal culture.
  - It may be necessary to remove a small area of epithelium over the abscess.
  - If the abscess involves the endothelium, anterior chamber paracentesis may be indicated (see p. 362).
- Sometimes fungi and other unusual organisms are identified. These infections result from inappropriate use of topical corticosteroids and have an extremely poor prognosis.

Treatment

Treatment should be started immediately.

- The choice of antimicrobial drug depends on the type of organisms found in the corneal scrapings.
  - Common isolates include *Streptococcus* spp., *Staphylococcus* spp., and *E. coli.*
  - In addition to topical therapy, antibacterial drugs should be injected subconjunctivally once daily for the first few days.

- Systemic antibacterial drugs also are indicated if endophthalmitis is present or suspected.
- The following medications may be effective against gram-positive organisms:
  - topical and systemic chloramphenicol (at 22 to 44 mg/kg PO q6h)
  - topical tobramycin
  - subconjunctival ticarcillin-clavulanic acid
  - systemic ceftiofur or ampicillin
- For gram-negative organisms, gentamicin, tobramycin, or ciprofloxacin should be selected for topical use, and ceftiofur or trimethoprim-sulfa for systemic administration.
- Removal of some epithelium over the abscess may facilitate absorption of water-soluble antibacterial drugs and is a good practice.
- Topical atropine is applied as necessary to maintain mydriasis.
- *Corticosteroids are contraindicated,* even when healing results in corneal vascularization and granulation tissue replaces the area of abscessation.

The healing lesion should change from red to pink to a white scar before medications are discontinued. Most of the corneal vascularization disappears without treatment within 2 to 4 weeks of healing. Because of the severity of the lesion, most healed eyes are left with some degree of corneal opacity, although the horse should have good vision.

Stromal Keratitis

Stromal keratitis is a category of corneal disease rather than a specific diagnosis. Infectious, immune-mediated, and degenerative conditions each might lead to the loose array of signs.

- Stromal infiltrates may appear as focal, multifocal, or diffuse gray-white opacities interspersed within surrounding zones of corneal edema.
  - Generally, such infiltrates attract corneal neovascularization and edema but do not cause necrosis or sloughing of the overlying corneal epithelium.

- The fluorescein dye test is negative.
- Topical corticosteroids may seem indicated and in fact are effective in some patients.
- In other cases corticosteroids cause a transient response followed by recurrence or worsening of the condition. This signals an infectious etiology.
  - Treatment may involve frequent topical application of ciprofloxacin, tobramycin, or amikacin for 1 to 3 months.
  - Oral rifampin (5 mg/kg q12h) also may be necessary.

Eosinophilic Keratitis

This rare condition is characterized by corneal opacities, neovascularization, leading-edge ulceration, and a white "cake frosting" exudate over the lesion.

- It has been reported in the mid-Atlantic states, Pennsylvania, and some other locations.
- Lesions are seasonal, occurring in mid- to late summer and frequently persisting until the fall.
- Affected eyes are painful, may be quite inflamed, and do not respond to antibiotic therapy.
- Abundant eosinophils are found in scrapings and biopsies. The conjunctiva also may have distinct eosinophilic infiltration.
- At this time, no uniformly successful therapy is available.
  - These lesions do not respond to topical or systemic larvicidal therapy.
  - Topical corticosteroids sometimes are necessary, but many cases fail to respond until the onset of cooler weather.
  - Using corticosteroids in the face of obvious corneal ulceration is contraindicated.

TOXIC DISEASES
Chemical Keratitis

Treatment of chemical keratitis consists of corneal lavage with sterile water or saline, followed by topical antibacterial and atropine therapy. Thermal injuries and exposure to smoke can cause corneal epithelial and stromal necrosis. Topical antibacterial drugs, collagenase inhibitors, and atropine are indicated, along with systemic analgesic therapy. Corneal scarring often is severe.

NEOPLASIA
Squamous Cell Carcinoma
Squamous cell carcinoma is the most common corneal tumor in horses.
* Middle-age and older horses without limbal pigmentation are at greatest risk.
* The tumor most often arises at the temporal limbal area and involves both bulbar conjunctiva and cornea.
* Small tumors (<1 cm diameter) may be treated with cryosurgery, radiofrequency hyperthermia, or keratectomy-conjunctivectomy with or without irradiation.
* Tumors >1 cm in diameter are best treated with keratectomy-conjunctivectomy followed by beta-irradiation or cryosurgery.
* Large tumors that involve the cornea, bulbar or palpebral conjunctiva, or eyelid have a poor prognosis. Enucleation may be required to preserve the horse's life.

Lymphosarcoma
Lymphosarcomata infiltrate from the limbus, appear pink, brown, or yellow, and tend to occur bilaterally. Corneal invasion is progressive and affected horses may have other evidence of lymphosarcoma, such as lymphadenopathy or visceral masses. Treatment is ineffective.

IDIOPATHIC DISEASES
Corneal Dystrophy
Endothelial dystrophies (irregularities in the corneal endothelium) may occur in otherwise normal eyes or may result from endothelial injury.
* Findings include nonpainful focal or diffuse corneal edema with an intact corneal epithelium.
* The affected area of cornea frequently is "coned" outward because of stromal swelling.
* Diagnosis is based on the signs and by ruling out other corneal lesions and glaucoma.

* Treatment consists of topical hyperosmotic agents (e.g., 5% NaCl ointment or 40% glucose ointment q4-8h) and topical corticosteroids q6-8h.
  * Primary problems, such as uveitis or corneal trauma, may necessitate other therapy.
* The prognosis is guarded. Many endothelial dystrophies respond poorly, if at all.
  * Response to therapy may not be obvious for several weeks.
* Endothelial dystrophies tend to persist, and owners should be prepared for long-term maintenance or intermittent therapy.

Calcific keratopathy
Superficial stromal and basement membrane dystrophic accumulations of calcium salts (calcific keratopathy) may be observed in some horses that have had multiple episodes of uveitis.
* The dystrophic accumulations may become so dense as to lift off the overlying epithelium, resulting in painful chronic corneal ulceration.
* Surgical removal of the lesion via keratectomy is indicated.
* The prognosis varies after keratectomy.
  * Some horses remain free of future dystrophic changes.
  * Others are doomed to reaccumulations because of multiple recurrences of uveitis.

Corneal Striae
Linear horizontal or vertical lesions that resemble railroad tracks and represent folds in Descemet's membrane are fairly common in horses, particularly in Warmbloods. The cause is unknown and most eyes are asymptomatic.

Diseases of the Uvea
(pages 1253-1260)
William C. Rebhun

CONGENITAL AND FAMILIAL DISEASES
Congenital abnormalities involving the uveal tract (iris, ciliary body, and

choroid) are uncommon. Reported iris anomalies include:

- *aniridia (absence of an iris):* reported in Belgian and Quarter Horse foals as a singular congenital defect and as part of multiple congenital anomalies
- *iris colobomas:* congenital, notch-like defects in the iris; may occur alone or as part of multiple congenital anomalies
- *heterochromia:* congenital mixture of color within the iris of one or both eyes; not an ocular abnormality

DISEASES WITH PHYSICAL CAUSES
Traumatic Uveitis

Traumatic uveitis usually is unilateral and results from direct injury to the globe or indirect injury via orbital trauma.

- Signs include blepharospasm, lacrimation, photophobia, miosis, aqueous protein and cellular deposits, hypotony, and ciliary and conjunctival injection.
  - Iris rents or detached corpora also may be observed.
  - Corneal edema may be present, but unless injured by trauma, the corneal epithelium does not retain fluorescein dye.
- Corneal disease must be ruled out, as must the possibility of embolic or septic uveitis.

Treatment and prognosis
Treatment consists of:

- topical atropine as necessary to induce cycloplegia
- topical corticosteroids, such as 0.1% dexamethasone ointment or 1% prednisolone acetate drops, q4-8h
  - Corticosteroids should not be used if the corneal epithelium has been compromised.
- systemic NSAIDs, such as phenylbutazone or flunixin meglumine, in standard doses
  - Topical NSAIDs, such as flurbinofen, may be used in the presence of corneal pathology.

The prognosis is good unless significant uveal hemorrhage, lens luxation, or retinal destruction has occurred. Uveitis should resolve over 4 to 14 days.

Iris Prolapse

Iris prolapse can result from penetrating corneal lacerations or punctures and perforating corneal ulcers that allow aqueous leakage.

- This is a very serious condition that requires immediate surgical repair of the corneal injury for best results.
- Many eyes with iris prolapse are irreparable because of expulsive loss of lens and vitreous; enucleation is indicated in these cases.
- If economics preclude corneal repair or enucleation, treatment should entail topical and systemic antibiotics and systemic NSAIDs for 2 to 4 weeks.
  - A blind, phthisical eye is the likely outcome, but the patient may be comfortable.

INFLAMMATORY, INFECTIOUS, AND IMMUNE DISEASES
Septic Uveitis

Septic uveitis occurs most commonly in neonatal foals with gram-negative bacteremia.

- It has also been reported in older Arabian foals with severe combined immunodeficiency (CID) and in adult horses with bacteremia secondary to endocarditis.
- In neonatal foals, gram-negative organisms such as *E. coli, Klebsiella* spp., *Actinobacillus equuli,* and *Salmonella* spp. are most commonly isolated.
- The earliest sign may be green discoloration of the irises.
- As the uveitis progresses, miosis, hypotony, ciliary and conjunctival injection, fibrinous and cellular anterior chamber accumulations (fibrin, hypopyon, hyphema, aqueous flare), and peripheral corneal vascularization develop.

Treatment
Treatment includes:

- intensive systemic antibiotic therapy
- topical antibiotic medications and atropine
  - Topical chloramphenicol, when appropriate, is an excellent choice as it penetrates the intact cornea well.

- Gentamicin (15 to 20 mg) or ticarcillin-clavulanic acid (50 mg) may also be injected subconjunctivally.
- systemic NSAIDs (used judiciously in young foals)

Prognosis

If the foal survives, the prognosis for vision usually is good. Large fibrinous clots in the anterior chamber generally are associated with more advanced septicemia and have a poorer prognosis. Septic uveitis in adult horses and older foals (e.g., those with CID) has a very guarded prognosis.

Immune-Mediated Uveitis

Immune-mediated uveitis ("periodic ophthalmia," "moon-blindness," "recurrent uveitis") is the most common cause of blindness in horses.

- It is characterized by persistent or recurrent uveitis in one or both eyes, the inflammation ranging from mild to severe.
- Possible inciting causes of this immune-mediated condition include infection with *Onchocerca* microfilariae, *Leptospira interrogans* serovar *pomona, Rhodococcus equi, Streptococcus equi,* and certain viruses (including equine herpesvirus [EHV-1])
- Genetic factors also may play a role; uveitis is more common in Appaloosas.

Clinical findings

The chief complaint generally includes a cloudy, painful, partially closed, discharging or blind eye. Other findings are numerous and variable:

- Blepharospasm, lacrimation, and photophobia may be extreme in acute uveitis but may be hardly recognizable in low-grade chronic uveitis.
- Miosis is consistently found.
- Usually there is conjunctival and ciliary injection with corneal edema and vascularization, which appear circumferentially as an infiltrate from the limbus.
- Aqueous flare, hypopyon, or hyphema may be present.
- The iris may appear edematous, dull, and darkened, and the normal concentric iris folds may not be discernible.

- In chronic or severe acute cases, neovascularization of the iris may be present.
- Adhesions, or synechiae, may have formed between the iris and the anterior lens capsule (posterior synechiae) or cornea (anterior synechiae).
  - The pupillary border of the iris may be distorted.
- A hypotensive globe is a result of severe, permanent damage to the ciliary processes, which eventually leads to phthisis bulbi.
- Cataracts may develop, and lens luxations can occur in chronic cases.
  - Angle-closure glaucoma can result from lens luxation (see p. 381).
- Vitreal opacities or "floaters" may be present.
  - Vitreal floaters can be found in many normal middle-age and older horses, but the debris and opacities associated with uveitis generally are more dense and extensive.
- Vitreoretinal traction bands (linear gray or white streaks extending from the optic disc through the vitreous) can occur and may detach the retinas over time.
  - As a result of slow contracture and traction of these adhesions, retinal detachment can occur weeks or months after apparent successful treatment of uveitis.
- Chorioretinal inflammation in the peripapillary area sometimes is present and consists of edema and exudate associated with the retinal vasculature (see p. 383).
  - As this lesion resolves, the classic "butterfly lesion" (a depigmented area containing many small hyperpigmented areas) forms on one or both sides of the optic disc.

Treatment

Topical corticosteroids are the mainstay of therapy for immune-mediated uveitis.

- Prednisolone acetate or dexamethasone is applied at least q4h for drops and q6h for ointments.
  - In acute cases, hourly application is optimal.
- Subconjunctival injection of a long-acting corticosteroid (e.g., 0.5

mL of methylprednisolone acetate or betamethasone valerate) should be included as part of the initial therapy.

* NSAIDs, such as phenylbutazone or flunixin meglumine in standard doses, also are helpful.
* Topical atropine (1% to 4%) is applied as often as necessary to induce and maintain cycloplegia.

Corticosteroid therapy should be continued for at least 4 weeks after clinical improvement. Atropine may be discontinued when signs of ocular pain have been controlled adequately for several days. Recurrence is always a possibility, so owners should keep atropine on hand and begin therapy when signs recur. Corticosteroids probably should not be given by the owner until the veterinarian has examined the eye and ruled out any corneal pathology.

Glaucoma

Glaucoma in horses usually is a sequela or complication of uveitis. But given the frequency of uveitis in horses, glaucoma is relatively uncommon.

* Glaucoma causes buphthalmos to varying degrees.
* *Acute* glaucoma is painful and is characterized by blepharospasm, lacrimation, photophobia, diffuse corneal edema, episcleral and conjunctival injection, and a partially to fully dilated pupil.
  * The lens may be normal or abnormal. The possibility of lens luxation should be considered.
* *Chronic* glaucoma is not painful unless the eye becomes so large as to suffer corneal exposure damage and subsequent corneal ulceration.

Treatment and prognosis

Treatment options are limited as a result of the already existing pathology.

* For eyes that do not have lens luxation to impede outflow, topical timolol (0.5%) drops q12h and oral acetazolamide (2.2 mg/kg PO q12h) are indicated.
* If active uveitis is present, atropine and topical corticosteroids also are indicated.
* If the pupil is fully dilated, miotics might be considered.

* If the lens has luxated into the anterior chamber, surgical removal of the lens, insertion of an ocular implant, or enucleation may be indicated.
* If corneal edema is severe, 5% NaCl ophthalmic ointment may be used several times daily.

Treatment success is rare, and the prognosis is poor for return of vision.

Endophthalmitis

Endophthalmitis is infection within the ocular media.

* Signs include intense blepharospasm, lacrimation, photophobia, and severe clouding of the ocular media.
* Intensive systemic, topical, and subconjunctival antimicrobial therapy is required to save the eye; nevertheless, most affected eyes require enucleation.
  * Culture of the aqueous humor via paracentesis is essential to identify the causative organism if treatment is elected.

Panophthalmitis

Panophthalmitis implies inflammation or infection throughout the ocular layers and fluid chambers. All parts of the eye are involved in this serious condition. Enucleation is the only treatment.

IDIOPATHIC DISEASES

Iris Cysts

Iris cysts appear sporadically in middle-age or older horses as unilateral or bilateral pigmented masses that arise from the iris epithelium.

* The cysts often originate from the posterior iris epithelium and appear in the anterior chamber as they move forward through the pupillary space.
* Transillumination or retroillumination allows differentiation of cystic structures from solid masses, such as melanomas, and from the normal corpora nigra.
  * Ocular ultrasonography also may be useful for diagnosis.
* Treatment usually is not necessary unless the cysts impair vision or worry the horse.

- Treatment involves aspiration of the cyst via limbal puncture under general anesthesia.

Diseases of the Lens and Vitreous *(pages 1260-1262)*
William C. Rebhun

CONGENITAL AND FAMILIAL DISEASES
Congenital Cataracts
Congenital cataracts occur sporadically in all breeds of horses and may be inherited in some breeds, such as Quarter Horses, Standardbreds, and paints.

- Congenital cataracts may be focal or diffuse and unilateral or bilateral.
  - When focal, they may be progressive or static.
  - When diffuse, they cause blindness in the affected eye.
- Surgical removal is the only effective treatment. The ideal age at surgery is 2 to 4 months.
  - Success rates approaching 75% are reported.

Inherited nuclear cataracts have been described in Morgan horses. These bilateral cataracts are subtle refractive opacities in the posterior central region of the lens nucleus. They usually cause no vision problems, and treatment is not indicated.

Congenital Lens Luxation
Congenital lens luxation or subluxation occurs in foals as a singular lesion or as part of multiple congenital ocular anomalies. Glaucoma is a common finding when the lens is fully luxated. Surgical removal of the luxated lens is the only treatment option.

DISEASES WITH PHYSICAL CAUSES
Traumatic Lens Luxation
Traumatic lens luxations may follow direct ocular trauma or skull trauma. Unless intraocular pressure increases, treatment is not necessary. With luxations that result in increased intraocular pressure, surgical removal of the lens is indicated.

Traumatic Cataracts
Traumatic cataracts occasionally develop after traumatic uveitis or ocular trauma with lens subluxation. These cataracts may be partial or complete. Treatment usually is not necessary unless the opposite eye also has visual impairment, in which case cataract surgery may be considered.

INFLAMMATORY, INFECTIOUS, AND IMMUNE DISEASES
Cataracts Associated with Uveitis
Cataracts associated with uveitis represent one of the most common reasons for blindness in patients with uveitis (see p. 379). Treatment seldom is possible because extensive posterior synechiae preclude lensectomy. In addition, attempts at surgical removal predispose to hemorrhage and induce a recurrence of severe uveitis.

IDIOPATHIC CONDITIONS
Vitreal Floaters, Asteroid Hyalosis, and Synchysis Scintillans
Various vitreal changes may be found in middle-age or older horses. In general, these changes are incidental findings, do not affect vision, and require no treatment. They include:

- *vitreal floaters:* refractile, thin, floating coils, ribbons, or veils in the vitreous
  - These are normal findings in older horses.
  - Rarely, horses with excessive accumulations of floaters or horses that find them distracting and frightening become "fly-eyed" (agitated).
- *steroid hyalosis:* a diffuse constellation of particulate "stars" (calcium salts) embedded in the vitreous gel
  - These opacities do not move about.
- *synchysis scintillans:* appear as falling snowflakes when the horse's head or eye is moved.
  - These white bodies swirl throughout the vitreous and then settle to the ventral aspect.
  - This condition is also known as cholesterolosis bulbi.

Acquired Cataracts

Acquired cataracts occur in horses of all breeds. If prior uveitis, trauma, and congenital lesions are ruled out, cataract formation is considered idiopathic. When only one eye is affected, surgical treatment seldom is necessary. When both eyes are diffusely affected, surgical treatment may be indicated; however, the prognosis for cataract extraction is guarded at best. Many horses with acquired focal cataracts continue to perform well without treatment.

Diseases of the Choroid and Retina *(pages 1263-1266)*
William C. Rebhun

DIAGNOSTIC CONSIDERATIONS
Normal Fundic Variations

Most fundic lesions occur in the nontapetal zone and optic disc. It is extremely rare to find lesions in the tapetal zone in horses. Following are common variations in the appearance of the normal equine fundus:

- The color of the tapetum varies somewhat with the coat color of the horse.
  - Black or dark bay horses have blue or blue-green tapetal coloration.
  - Bay or chestnut horses have green tapetal coloration.
  - Palomino horses may have yellow tapetal coloration.
- The nontapetal zone generally is black or dark brown in darkly pigmented horses but light brown to orange in lightly pigmented horses.
- Paint, pinto, and lightly pigmented horses and ponies of various colors often have partially albinotic or subalbinotic fundi.
  - This leads to zones in which the large choroidal vessel layer is visible in the fundus, usually most obvious in the nontapetal zone.
- The optic disc is extremely variable in terms of its borders, amount of pigmentation at the border, and degree of "scalloping" at the edges.
  - Variable degrees of myelination are possible, especially in older horses.

Benign Lesions in Older Horses

Proliferative optic neuropathy is a benign, raised-disc lesion occasionally observed as an incidental finding in older horses. Usually it is unilateral and does not appear to affect vision. Excessive myelinization of the optic disc also is an incidental finding that is most common in aged horses. Its importance lies in the fact that it can be mistaken for optic nerve edema or inflammation.

CONGENITAL AND FAMILIAL DISEASES
Coloboma

Atypical colobomas appear as blue or blue-gray, somewhat circular lesions near the tapetal-nontapetal junction. They represent defective choroidal and/or retinal development. Colobomas may be singular or multiple and found in one or both eyes. They are incidental findings.

Retinal Detachment

Congenital retinal detachment is most common in Standardbred and Thoroughbred foals. The condition often is bilateral, and affected foals are apprehensive, may collide with objects, and have dilated, unresponsive pupils. The detached retina appears as a thin, gray veil projecting from the optic disc. There is no effective treatment.

Night Blindness (Nyctalopia)

Night blindness has been observed in several breeds, but most cases occur in Appaloosas, suggesting a genetic mode of transmission in this breed. Night blindness is not a progressive disease. Visual disturbance is as serious at birth as in subsequent years, although the degree of visual disturbance among affected Appaloosas varies considerably.

- Mildly affected horses show vision problems only in reduced lighting or at night.
- More severely affected horses are apprehensive during daylight hours and appear totally blind in a darkened environment.
- The condition may be suspected from the history, ophthalmic examination, and observation of the

horse in a dark environment and is confirmed by performing an electroretinogram
- Ophthalmoscopic findings usually are normal and the eyes are free of lesions.
◆ There is no treatment.

DISEASES WITH PHYSICAL CAUSES
Traumatic Retinal Detachment
Retinal detachment secondary to skull or ocular trauma is rare in horses, occurring much less frequently than optic nerve damage. Traumatic retinal detachment usually is unilateral. If the detachment is acute and serous or serosanguinous, diuretic and antiinflammatory therapy may be attempted. Laser therapy is an option for partial retinal detachments. However, the prognosis is guarded.

INFLAMMATORY, INFECTIOUS, AND IMMUNE DISEASES
Chorioretinitis
Inflammation of the retina often originates in the vascular system (the choroid), a condition termed *chorioretinitis*.
◆ Small areas of active retinitis appear as gray-white circular lesions in the nontapetal area.
◆ These have been reported in horses and especially foals with active respiratory disease.
◆ In foals with large numbers of focal lesions, vision may be impaired and pupillary responses diminished until the lesions resolve over 1 to 2 weeks.
◆ Healed lesions leave "bullet-hole" scars in the nontapetal area.
  • Unless the scars are numerous or the horse appears to have visual problems, they are insignificant.
  • Horses with numerous (>20) scars should be carefully assessed during soundness examinations.
◆ Lesions occurring ventral to the optic disc can result in severe visual loss.
  • This zone seems to be critical for vision, so it should be carefully assessed.
◆ Large areas of chorioretinitis appear as comma-shaped, bar-shaped, or

vermiform zones within the nontapetal area.
  • In severe cases, the tapetal zone may also be involved.
  • During active inflammation, lesions are dull gray and serous retinal elevation may be seen.
  • As nontapetal lesions become inactive, they become depigmented, often with a central area of hyperpigmentation.
  • As tapetal lesions become inactive, they become hyperreflective and pigmented.
  • Optic nerve atrophy may occur in severe cases.

Peripapillary chorioretinitis
Peripapillary chorioretinitis is common in horses with immune-mediated uveitis.
◆ When active, these lesions may appear as zones of retinal edema and vasculitis around the optic disc.
◆ In the quiescent or healed phase, these lesions, described as "butterfly lesions," have an obvious depigmented zone interspersed with hyperpigmented spots.
  • Lesions can occur on one or both sides of the optic disc or circumferentially around it.
◆ Discovery of such lesions at prepurchase examination should prompt consideration of prior uveitis, and the lesions should be noted on the examination report.
  • The lesions may not necessarily result in poor vision, because they can be incidental findings in apparently normal horses with no history of uveitis.

Retinopathy Associated with Equine Motor Neuron Disease
A retinopathy has been identified in many horses affected with equine motor neuron disease. Ophthalmoscopic findings variably consist of excessive pigment that may appear as a horizontal linear band just dorsal to the optic disc, gridlike bars or reticulated pattern in the tapetal area and dorsal nontapetal zone, pigment clumps on the tapetum, tapetal dulling, and in the most severe cases, yellow-green-brown splotchy tapetal regions interspersed with hyperreflective zones of retinal degeneration.

Diseases of the Optic Nerve *(page 1267)*

William C. Rebhun

DISEASES WITH PHYSICAL CAUSES

Traumatic Optic Neuropathy

Traumatic optic neuropathy is common in horses. Hemorrhage or transudative edema may be apparent on ophthalmoscopic examination in cases of head trauma. Optic nerve atrophy and blindness may be sequelae in such cases.

INFLAMMATORY, INFECTIOUS, AND IMMUNE DISEASES

Optic Neuritis

Optic nerve inflammation may occur in conjunction with uveitis and peripapillary chorioretinitis or as a singular entity in uveitis.

- Exudative optic neuritis is characterized by sudden blindness with severe optic nerve inflammation (raised, nodular lesions that project into the vitreous).
- Optic nerve atrophy may result from optic neuritis or from optic nerve trauma or extensive chorioretinitis.
  - It appears as a chalk-white optic disc with loss of retinal vessels.
  - Blindness and a dilated, unresponsive pupil are other findings.

15

Musculoskeletal System

Examination of the Musculoskeletal System

(pages 1273-1292)

William A. Moyer, Leo B. Jeffcott, and David R. Hodgson

PHYSICAL EXAMINATION

Most horses have more than one problem, so it is advisable to examine the entire horse. After collecting the history, the examination should begin with observation of the horse from a short distance, noting any asymmetry (e.g., swelling, muscle atrophy) and the horse's general conformation. Each limb should then be thoroughly examined, while bearing weight and while lifted, and the neck and back carefully palpated. Important observations include swelling, pain, and altered range of motion. Detailed examination of the musculoskeletal system is described in *Equine Medicine and Surgery V*.

GAIT EVALUATION

Gait evaluation should be performed on a firm, flat surface. Assessment of the horse's gait is made at the walk and trot; while the horse is moving toward, away from, and past the examiner; and while the horse is worked in a circle. Observations include gross and fine limb movements, foot strike and balance, length and height of foot flight, and abnormal head movements (e.g., head bob) or excursions of pelvic prominences. If necessary, the gait also may be evaluated while the horse is walked or trotted up and down a hill, worked on different surfaces, and ridden or driven.

Manipulative Tests

Manipulative tests involve flexing a joint or applying pressure to a particular area (e.g., hoof, suspensory apparatus) for about 1 minute before releasing the limb and trotting the horse for 20 to 30 yards. For accurate interpretation, all four limbs should be evaluated, beginning with the least affected or apparently normal limb(s).

SERUM BIOCHEMISTRY

Muscle Enzymes

Assessment of muscle disorders often involves measurement of serum activities of muscle-specific enzymes:

* *creatine kinase (CK):* a sensitive indicator of myonecrosis
  * Serum CK peaks within about 6 hours of muscle insult; its serum half-life is 1 to 2 days.
  * Limited elevations may accompany training, transport, and strenuous exercise.
  * Moderate to extreme elevations (sometimes >100,000 IU/L) can occur with exertional rhabdomyolysis or nutritional muscular dystrophy.
  * If a delay of >12 hours is anticipated before analysis, the serum sample should be frozen.
* *aspartate aminotransferase (AST):* not specific for myonecrosis because AST is found in several types of tissue, including liver and RBCs, as well as in skeletal and cardiac muscle

- Serum AST rises more slowly than CK in response to myonecrosis, often peaking 12 to 24 hours after cell damage; its serum half-life is long (about 7 days).
- *lactate dehydrogenase (LDH):* electrophoretic separation of LDH into its isoenzyme forms is necessary to definitively diagnose myodegeneration
  - The isoenzymes that predominate in skeletal muscle are LDH_4 and LDH_5.

Serum Myoglobin

Measurement of serum myoglobin is useful for determining exercise-associated muscle damage because peak concentrations are reached shortly after exercise. Normal concentrations in resting horses are ≤ 9 µg/L. Concentrations after rhabdomyolysis may exceed 500,000 µg/L.

Ancillary Diagnostic Aids *(pages 1292-1344)*

P.O. Eric Mueller, William P. Hay, Dan L. Hawkins, Dean W. Richardson, Charles S. Farrow, Russell L. Tucker, Norman W. Rantanen, Clifford R. Berry, Douglas H. Leach, and Eleanor M. Green

REGIONAL ANESTHESIA

Regional anesthesia is used in conjunction with a thorough physical examination. Perineural anesthesia (nerve blocks) should be performed in a consistent manner, progressing from the distal aspect of the limb proximally. Intrasynovial anesthesia may be performed in the order of clinical suspicion. NOTE: *If a fracture (whether displaced or nondisplaced) is suspected, diagnostic regional anesthesia should not be performed.*

Perineural Anesthesia of the Distal Forelimb

Unless stated, local anesthetic is injected SC over the nerve to be desensitized.

Palmar digital nerve block

This block desensitizes structures in the palmar half to one third of the foot.

- An injection of 2 to 3 mL of anesthetic is administered over the medial and lateral palmar digital nerves as they run down the sides of the pastern immediately dorsal to the deep digital flexor tendon.
- The nerves are anesthetized as far distally as possible, usually just proximal to the lateral collateral cartilage.

Abaxial (basilar sesamoid) nerve block

This block desensitizes the foot, pastern and coffin joints, and proximal pastern. Sometimes lameness associated with the palmar aspect of the fetlock joint partially improves with this block.

- An injection of 2 to 3 mL of anesthetic is administered over the medial and lateral palmar nerves as they run along the abaxial surfaces of the sesamoid bones.
- Injection is performed near the base of the sesamoids, just palmar to the digital artery.
- Cutaneous sensation in the dorsal aspect of the fetlock and proximal pastern often persists.

Low palmar and palmar metacarpal nerve block (low four point)

This block desensitizes the fetlock joint and all structures distal to it. The block involves injection at four sites.

- The medial and lateral palmar nerves are blocked by injecting 3 to 4 mL of anesthetic SC between the suspensory ligament and deep flexor tendon, just proximal to the tendon sheath.
- The medial and lateral palmar metacarpal nerves are blocked by injecting 2 to 3 mL of anesthetic SC just distal to the ends ("buttons") of the splint bones.

High palmar and palmar metacarpal nerve block (high four point)

This block desensitizes the limb distal to the block, except for the proximal metacarpus and suspensory origin.

- The standard high four-point block involves four injections.
  - The medial and lateral palmar nerves are blocked just below the carpus by SC injection of 3 to 5 mL of anesthetic between the suspensory ligament and deep flexor tendon.

- The medial and lateral palmar metacarpal nerves are blocked at the same level by deeper injection of 2 to 3 mL of anesthetic axial to the splint bones.
- Anesthetizing the lateral palmar nerve at the base of the accessory carpal bone and the medial palmar nerve as described above desensitizes the proximal metacarpus, suspensory origin, and all distal structures.
  - An injection of 5 to 6 mL of anesthetic is administered SC beneath the carpal flexor retinaculum between the base of the accessory carpal bone and the head of the lateral splint bone.
  - The carpal canal may be inadvertently desensitized with this block.
- The proximal metacarpus and suspensory origin also can be blocked by direct infiltration.
  - An injection of 5 to 6 mL of anesthetic is administered between the suspensory origin and inferior check ligament just distal to the carpus, with the needle directed slightly proximal and axial.
  - The medial and lateral sides are infiltrated separately.

NOTE: *Regional anesthesia in the proximal palmar metacarpal region may result in inadvertent desensitization of the middle carpal and carpometacarpal joints.*

Perineural Anesthesia of the Distal Hind Limb

The palmar digital and abaxial nerve blocks in the hind limb are performed identical to those in the forelimb. Low and high plantar nerve blocks are performed in a similar manner to low and high palmar nerve blocks. Anesthesia of the proximal metatarsus and suspensory origin is achieved by direct infiltration of the suspensory origin, as described for the forelimb.

Dorsal metatarsal nerve block

To desensitize the dorsal metatarsus (excluding the skin), the medial and lateral dorsal metatarsal nerves must be blocked. The lateral nerve is closely associated with the metatarsal artery, and the medial nerve courses along the medial aspect of the long

digital extensor tendon; 2 to 3 mL of anesthetic is injected over each nerve.

Perineural Anesthesia Proximal to the Carpus or Tarsus

Diagnostic anesthesia proximal to the carpus or tarsus generally involves intrasynovial anesthesia; nerve blocks are not often used. Median, ulnar, medial cutaneous antebrachial, tibial, and peroneal nerve blocks are described in *Equine Medicine and Surgery V.*

Intrasynovial Anesthesia of the Forelimb

Distal interphalangeal (coffin) joint

The most common approach to the coffin joint is on the dorsal aspect of the coronet.

- The injection site is 1 to 2 cm (0.50 to 0.75 inch) proximal to the hoof wall, either on the dorsal midline or at the edge of the common digital extensor tendon.
- The needle is inserted at a 90-degree angle to the weight-bearing surface of the foot (vertically if the horse is weight bearing). The depth of penetration is ≤3.8 cm (1.5 inch).
  - Synovial fluid may or may not be retrieved; 8 to 10 mL of anesthetic is injected.
- The lateral approach (just proximal to the collateral cartilage on the lateral aspect of the pastern, with the needle directed toward the center of the frog) reportedly is less painful.

NOTE: *Diffusion of anesthetic from the joint pouch may desensitize the navicular structures and palmar digital nerves.*

Navicular bursa

The navicular bursa may be injected through a palmar or lateral approach.

- For the palmar approach, an 18-gauge, 3.5-inch spinal needle is inserted horizontally, midway between the heel bulbs, just above the hairline.
  - The needle is advanced until the navicular bone is encountered. The needle then is withdrawn 0.5 cm and the anesthetic injected.
- For the lateral approach, a 20-gauge, 1.5-inch needle is inserted just proximal to the lateral collat-

eral cartilage, between P2 and the deep digital flexor tendon.
  - The needle is advanced distally toward the opposite heel.
- With either technique fluid rarely is aspirated, but 2 to 3 mL of anesthetic should be easily injected without resistance.

Proximal interphalangeal (pastern) joint

The pastern joint may be injected from a dorsal or palmar approach.
- For the dorsal approach, the needle is inserted horizontally under the edge of the common digital extensor tendon, just distal to the distal eminence of P1, and directed axially.
- With the palmar approach, the needle is inserted in the groove formed by P1 dorsally, the branch of the superficial flexor tendon palmarly, and the distal eminence of P1 distally.
- Aspiration usually does not yield synovial fluid; 6 to 8 mL of anesthetic is injected.

Metacarpophalangeal (fetlock) joint

A lateral-palmar approach through the lateral collateral sesamoidean ligament causes less synovial hemorrhage than an approach through the palmar pouch or dorsal joint capsule. The fetlock is flexed 45 degrees and the needle is inserted perpendicular to the skin, in the depression between the cannon bone and the dorsal articular surface of the sesamoid bone.

Aspiration usually yields synovial fluid; 10 to 12 mL of anesthetic is injected.

Deep digital flexor tendon sheath

The flexor tendon sheath may be entered proximal to the sesamoids or at the palmar aspect of the pastern. With existing distension, fluid is easily aspirated and 10 to 15 mL of anesthetic injected.

Carpus

The radiocarpal and middle carpal joints both must be injected to desensitize the carpus.
- For each block, the capus is flexed 90 degrees and the needle is inserted on the dorsal aspect, medial or lateral to the extensor carpi radialis tendon, midway between the joint surfaces

- With the middle carpal joint, directing the needle 90 degrees to the long axis of the cannon bone prevents iatrogenic cartilage damage.
- Anesthesia of the middle carpal joint also desensitizes the carpometacarpal joint.
- Aspiration usually yields synovial fluid; 10 to 15 mL of anesthetic is injected into each joint.

NOTE: *Nerve fibers associated with the proximal palmar metacarpus (including the suspensory origin) may be anesthetized when the middle carpal joint is blocked.*

Humeroradial (elbow) joint

The elbow can be injected through a craniolateral or caudolateral approach (cranial and caudal to the lateral collateral ligament, respectively). The caudolateral approach is easiest with the elbow flexed. Landmarks for identifying the level of the humeroradial joint space are the lateral humeral epicondyle and the lateral radial tuberosity. The joint is penetrated at a depth of 5 to 6 cm (2 to 2.25 inches), and 10 to 20 mL of anesthetic is injected.

Scapulohumeral (shoulder) joint

To block the shoulder joint, an 18-gauge, 3.5-inch spinal needle is inserted in the depression between the cranial and caudal prominences of the lateral humeral tuberosity and advanced toward the opposite elbow. The joint is penetrated at a depth of 6 to 8 cm (2.25 to 3.25 inches), and aspiration usually yields synovial fluid; 20 to 40 mL of anesthetic is injected.

Bicipital bursa

An 18-gauge, 3.5-inch spinal needle is introduced 4 cm (1.5 inch) proximal to the deltoid tuberosity and directed toward the opposite ear. The depth of penetration is 5 to 7.5 cm (2 to 3 inches), and aspiration usually yields synovial fluid; 10 to 15 mL of anesthetic is injected into the bursa.

Intraarticular Anesthesia of the Hind Limb

Intraarticular injection techniques for the coffin, pastern, and fetlock joints are identical to those performed in the forelimb. Injection techniques for the hip joint and trochanteric bursa are described in *Equine Medicine and Surgery V.*

Tarsus

Complete desensitization of the tarsus requires injection into the tibiotarsal, distal intertarsal, and tarsometatarsal joints.

- ◆ The tibiotarsal joint is approached dorsally, either medial or lateral to the saphenous vein, and 2.5 to 3.8 cm (1 to 1.5 inch) distal to the medial malleolus.
  - Aspiration usually yields synovial fluid; 10 to 20 mL of anesthetic is injected.
- ◆ The distal intertarsal joint is approached medially, just distal to the cuncan tendon, in the depression between the central, third, and fused first and second tarsal bones.
  - The needle is directed 90 degrees to the skin surface.
  - Aspiration usually does not yield synovial fluid; 4 to 6 mL of anesthetic is injected.
  - The ease of injection and the amount of anesthetic that may be injected depend on the amount of existing degenerative joint disease.
- ◆ The tarsometatarsal joint is approached on the plantar-lateral aspect, just proximal to the head of the lateral splint bone and lateral to the superficial digital flexor tendon.
  - The needle is advanced distally and medially at a 45-degree angle. The depth of penetration is 2 to 3 cm.
  - Aspiration usually yields synovial fluid; 4 to 6 mL of anesthetic may be injected.

Femorotibial and femoropatellar (stifle) joints

Because of the variation in communication between joint compartments, each compartment should be injected separately to completely block the stifle.

- ◆ For a cranial approach to the femoropatellar joint, an 18-gauge, 3.5-inch spinal needle is inserted 2.5 to 3.5 cm (1 to 1.25 inch) proximal to the tibial crest, just medial or lateral to the middle patellar ligament, and directed dorsocaudally, beneath the patella.
  - The depth of penetration of the joint capsule is 6 to 8 cm (2.25 to 3.25 inches).

- Aspiration may yield synovial fluid; 40 to 60 mL of anesthetic is injected.
- ◆ For a lateral approach to the femoropatellar joint, a needle is inserted just caudal to the lateral patellar ligament, 5 cm (2 inches) proximal to the lateral tibial condyle.
  - This approach causes less cartilage damage and allows aspiration of more synovial fluid.
- ◆ The medial femorotibial joint is approached between the medial patellar and medial collateral ligaments, just proximal to the medial tibial condyle.
  - The needle is directed 90 degrees to the skin surface and advanced axially.
  - Aspiration usually yields synovial fluid; 20 to 30 mL of anesthetic may be injected.
- ◆ The lateral femorotibial joint can be approached either between the lateral patellar and lateral collateral ligaments or more caudally between the lateral collateral ligament and the origin of the long digital extensor tendon.
  - The needle is directed 90 degrees to the skin surface and advanced medially.
  - Aspiration usually yields synovial fluid; 20 to 30 mL of anesthetic may be injected.

SYNOVIAL FLUID ANALYSIS

The overall assessment of any joint should be based on clinical and radiographic evaluation, as well as results obtained from synovial fluid analysis.

Viscosity

Viscosity is a subjective assessment of joint fluid quality and the degree of synovial inflammation. It can be assessed by observing the fluid as it drips from the needle hub during collection: normal synovial fluid is viscous and strings out for several centimeters, whereas synovial fluid from a severely inflamed joint has a viscosity similar to water.

Protein Concentration

The protein concentration in synovial fluid normally is low (>2 g/dL) and increases with inflammation. In severe inflammatory processes, the synovial fluid albumin:globulin ratio changes as more globulins enter the fluid.

White Blood Cells

The total nucleated cell count normally is >300 cells/µL. Mononuclear cells comprise 70% to 95%, and the remainder primarily are nondegenerative neutrophils. The total WBC count is related to the degree of synovitis, although there is no definite upper limit for a nonseptic joint. Total nucleated cell counts >50,000/µL strongly suggest sepsis. A uniform population of degenerate neutrophils is stronger evidence for sepsis.

Red Blood Cells

Red blood cells normally are present in small numbers in synovial fluid, but even minor contamination during sampling markedly increases the numbers above normal. It is important to observe if there is streaking of a clear sample during collection or if the sample is uniformly discolored. Normally, the fluid is pale yellow, but mild xanthochromia (darker yellow) is normal in strenuously exercised horses.

Microbiologic Examination

A careful search for bacteria always should be performed if sepsis is suspected. Preliminary identification of an organism by Gram's stain can assist in antibiotic therapy.

RADIOGRAPHY

Radiography often is the most important single factor used in determining the probable cause of lameness and as such must be thorough and of excellent quality. Equipment, radiographic technique, common sources of error, and special procedures such as contrast studies are discussed in *Equine Medicine and Surgery V*.

Radiographic Protocols

Following are recommendations for routine equine radiographic examination; additional views may be indicated for specific conditions:

* *foot:* The five routine views are lateromedial, 30-degree dorsoproximal-palmarodistal oblique (ex-

posed for the navicular bone), two 50-degree dorsoproximal-palmarodistal obliques (one exposed for the navicular bone, the other for the distal phalanx), and a 45-degree palmar proximal-distal oblique (flexor skyline).
* *fetlock:* The four routine views are a 30-degree dorsoproximal-palmarodistal oblique, two 45-degree obliques (dorsolateral-palmaromedial and dorsomedial-palmarolateral), and a lateromedial (standing or flexed for both).
* *carpus:* The four routine views are two lateromedials (standing and flexed) and two 55-degree obliques (dorsolateral-palmaromedial and dorsomedial-palmarolateral).
  * Dorsopalmar and dorsal proximal-distal skyline projections frequently are indicated for specific conditions.
* *tarsus:* The four routine views are 10-degree dorsoproximal-plantarodistal oblique, 45-degree dorsolateral-plantaromedial oblique, 30-degree dorsomedial-plantarolateral oblique, and lateromedial.

ULTRASONOGRAPHY

Ultrasonography is important in the diagnosis and management of soft tissue injuries of the distal limb. Clinical ultrasonography is discussed in *Equine Medicine and Surgery V*, including basic theory, instrumentation, scanning techniques, and the appearance of some common lesions.

ALTERNATIVE IMAGING TECHNIQUES

Nuclear imaging ("bone scan"), computerized tomography (CT), and magnetic resonance imaging (MRI) are sophisticated imaging techniques that can provide information extra to that obtained with physical examination, regional anesthesia, and routine imaging procedures. Principles and indications are discussed in *Equine Medicine and Surgery V*.

THERMOGRAPHY

Thermography is a noninvasive diagnostic technique that can quantitate heat emitted from the body surface. Changes in surface temperature of as little as 0.5° C (33° F) can be identified. In many cases, thermography can detect the presence of inflammation well before abnormalities are found on physical examination or using routine imaging modalities. Techniques, indications, and interpretation are discussed in *Equine Medicine and Surgery V.*

Gait Analysis

The use of video analysis to examine the locomotion of lame horses is discussed in *Equine Medicine and Surgery V.*

Principles of Therapy

(pages 1344-1446)

Joerg A. Auer, Roger K.W. Smith, Peter M. Webbon, Dan L. Hawkins, Dean W. Richardson, Lawrence R. Bramlage, John P. Caron, Mimi Porter, Michael J. Wildenstein, and Anne E. Kraus-Hansen

EMERGENCY CARE AND TRANSPORTATION OF THE FRACTURE PATIENT

In patients with unstable fractures causing non–weight-bearing lameness, such as long-bone fractures, the fracture *must be stabilized* before the horse is transported to a surgical facility.

Emergency Care

The patient's physical status should be addressed first. After localization and assessment of the fracture, treatment options, prognosis, and costs should be discussed with the owner. Once the decision is made to treat the horse, the fracture is stabilized for transport. If sedation is required, the drug of choice is xylazine, either alone or in combination with morphine or butorphanol. Phenothiazine derivatives such as acepromazine should be avoided.

Splinting Techniques

A properly applied splint minimizes further soft tissue and bone damage, allows the horse to place some weight on the fractured limb, and reduces swelling and pain. Splinting techniques for unstable fractures vary with the location of the fracture. A useful approach is to view the limb as being divided into four anatomic areas.

Division 1 fractures

Division 1 includes fractures between the distal phalanx and the distal quarter of the cannon bone. For these fractures, it is important to splint the distal limb with the phalanges in the same frontal plane as the cannon bone.

- Suitable splint materials include 5- × 10-cm (2 × 4 inches) board or PVC pipe cut to specifications or a farrier's rasp.
- A thin layer of padding (<5 mm thick) is applied from the foot to the carpus/tarsus.
- In the forelimb the splint is taped to the padding over the dorsal aspect from toe to carpus.
- Nonelastic tape (e.g., duct tape or even fiberglass casting material) should be used.
- In the hind limb the splint is applied to the plantar aspect from toe to tarsus.
- Taping a wedge-shaped block of wood to the sole allows weight bearing and renders the patient more comfortable on the limb.
- Special splints, such as the Kimzey Leg Saver, can be used for first-aid treatment.
  - This splint also can be used for breakdown injuries involving the suspensory apparatus.

Division 2 fractures in the forelimb

Division 2 includes fractures between the distal quarter of the cannon bone and the distal radius.

- The best splinting technique uses a thick, firmly applied Robert-Jones bandage extending from the foot to the elbow.
- Likewise, the splint material (wood, PVC pipe, or any other rigid object) should extend from the foot to the point of the elbow.
- The limb should be splinted on *two surfaces* (e.g., lateral and caudal).
- The Robert-Jones bandage and splints must be applied as tightly as possible.

Division 2 fractures in the hind limb

Division 2 includes fractures from the distal quarter of the cannon bone to the base of the hock.

- The padding should extend above the hock, but excessive thickness should be avoided.
- Splints are applied to both the plantar and lateral aspect of the limb, extending to the proximal end of the tuber calcis.
- As for division 1 fractures, the phalanges should be extended and aligned in the same plane as the cannon bone.
  - Placement of a wooden wedge underneath the foot facilitates weight bearing.

Division 3 fractures

Division 3 includes fractures of the radius and ulna from distal radius to elbow joint or of the tarsus and tibia up to the level of the stifle joint.

- Forelimb fractures are bandaged as for division 2 fractures, except that the lateral splint should extend to the withers.
  - This splint should be well padded and in snug contact with the triceps muscle.
- Hind limb fractures in this region are difficult to stabilize with splints.
  - The limb should be bandaged with a thick, firmly applied Robert-Jones bandage from foot to stifle.
- A splint is firmly fixed to the lateral aspect of the limb from the foot to above the stifle.

Division 4 fractures

Division 4 includes fractures proximal to the elbow joint, including the olecranon, or proximal to the stifle joint.

- Olecranon fractures render the horse unable to bear weight on the limb.
  - It is important to support the carpus in an extended position to allow weight-bearing as described for division 2 fractures, although the bandage does not need to be bulky.
- With humeral or scapular fractures, bandaging is less important, although some lateral support, as described for proximal radial fractures, might be advisable.
- Because the femur is well protected by muscle, the hind limb generally does not require splinting, although it might be advisable to support the opposite hind limb.

PRINCIPLES OF FRACTURE REPAIR

The following techniques for fracture repair are discussed in *Equine Medicine and Surgery V*:

- external coaptation (fiberglass casts, transfixation casting, external fixation devices)
- internal fixation (bone screws, plates, pins, intramedullary nails)
- bone grafting (harvest sites, surgical technique, bone banking)

OTHER ORTHOPEDIC PROCEDURES

The following topics also are discussed in *Equine Medicine and Surgery V*:

- corrective osteotomies
- amputation and prosthetic devices
- arthrodesis
- surgical treatment of joint disease

MEDICAL TREATMENT OF DEGENERATIVE JOINT DISEASE

Rest and the relative merits of nonsteroidal antiinflammatory drugs (NSAIDs), corticosteroids, hyaluronan, polysulfated glycosaminoglycans, and oral supplements are discussed in this section of *Equine Medicine and Surgery V*. Specific recommendations for managing the condition in particular joints are given in later sections of this chapter.

MANAGEMENT OF TENDON INJURIES

Management of Subcutaneous (Strain) Tendon Injuries

The following recommendations primarily relate to management of superficial digital flexor tendonitis, although the same principles apply to strain injuries of other tendons.

Acute stage

In the acute stage (the first 2 to 4 weeks after injury), the aim is to minimize inflammation.

- Initial treatment includes cold hosing and/or use of ice packs for 10 to 15 minutes as often as possible and application of a firm but well-padded bandage.
- Therapeutic ultrasound can be used from 3 to 4 days after injury.

* NSAIDs can be given systemically but are not required long-term therapy.
  * Short-acting steroids can be beneficial when administered immediately after injury.
* Polysulphated glycosaminoglycans can relieve inflammation and are best administered intralesionally to horses with obvious core lesions on ultrasound.
  * They should not be injected intralesionally within 3 days of injury.
* Tendon splitting during this phase promotes more rapid resolution of core lesions.
  * It should be performed as soon as possible after the initial hemorrhage has subsided (any time beyond 4 days after injury).

Subacute stage

During the subacute stage (from 1 to 3 months after injury), the aim is to maximize the rate of repair and the quality of repair tissue.

* Light walking should begin immediately after the inflammation has resolved.
  * The amount of exercise is increased in line with the tendon's sonographic appearance.
* β-Aminoproprionitrile (BAPN, Bapten) administered during this phase prevents formation of crosslinks that limit remodeling of collagen into longitudinally arranged fibers.
  * It is administered intratendinously on alternate days for five treatments.
  * The exercise program must be carefully controlled with ultrasound monitoring.

Chronic stage

From 3 months after injury the aims are to maximize the remodeling of scar tissue into longitudinally arranged collagen fibers and to prevent reinjury.

* Remodeling is encouraged by a controlled ascending exercise regimen monitored by regular ultrasound examinations.
* Superior check desmotomy may help prevent recurrence of injury.

* Surgery usually is performed soon after injury, often in conjunction with tendon splitting, but its action is aimed at this later stage of tendon healing.
* Damage to tendon takes between 9 and 15 months to heal, inevitably leaving a residual scar. The ultrasonographic criteria indicating that the tendon has healed sufficiently for the horse to return to full exercise include:
  * normal echogenicity
  * no core lesion
  * good striated pattern in longitudinal images
  * no adhesions

Management of Percutaneous Tendon Injuries

Percutaneous injury to a tendon requires surgical intervention for evaluation and debridement and, if necessary, tenorrhaphy (see *Equine Medicine and Surgery V*). Application of a cast may be necessary.

HORSESHOEING

The corresponding section in *Equine Medicine and Surgery V* contains a discussion on shoeing for specific conditions. Recommendations for particular problems also are given in later sections of this chapter.

POSTOPERATIVE MANAGEMENT AND PHYSICAL THERAPY

In many cases, postoperative management is as critical to a successful outcome as the surgical procedure. Whether an injury is managed surgically or medically, physical therapy can aid recovery by restoring normal muscle strength and flexibility, preventing adhesion formation, and promoting tissue healing. Therapies discussed in *Equine Medicine and Surgery V* include:

* active and passive manipulation (controlled mobilization)
* therapeutic exercise
* hydrotherapy
* transcutaneous electrical nerve stimulation (TENS)
* therapeutic ultrasound

Diseases of Multiple Bones and Joints

(pages 1446-1483)

Brent A. Hague, G. Kent Carter, Joerg A. Auer, William P. Hay, P.O. Eric Mueller, J. Lane Easter, and Jeffrey P. Watkins, Gary D. Potter, and A.N. Baird

INFLAMMATORY, INFECTIOUS, AND IMMUNE DISEASES

Septic Arthritis

Infectious agents most commonly causing septic arthritis and/or osteomyelitis in foals are those associated with neonatal septicemia.

- gram-negative bacteria, particularly *Entamoeba coli, Actinobacillus equuli,* and *Salmonella* spp.
- gram-positive bacteria, such as *Staphylococcus* spp., *Streptococcus* spp., *Rhodococcus equi,* and *Corynebacterium* spp.

When septic arthritis is caused by a wound or iatrogenic contamination, causative bacteria tend to be skin and environmental pathogens.

- Gram-positive bacteria, particularly staphylococci and streptococci, are more common.
- *Staphylococcus aureus* is most often isolated after injection.
- *E. coli, Pseudomonas* spp., and *Proteus* spp. commonly infect joints secondary to wounds.

Diagnosis

Presumptive diagnosis is based on clinical findings.

- Signs can be variable, although lameness and joint swelling are consistent findings.
  - Often the lameness rapidly progresses to a complete inability to bear weight.
  - Joint swelling may be confined to synovial effusion or may include periarticular edema and cellulitis (acute) or fibrosis (chronic).
  - Infection of multiple joints is common in young foals; the physes also may be infected.
- The patient may be febrile, and other signs of systemic illness may be seen in affected foals.
- Radiography should be used to rule out bone trauma or osteomyelitis.

- Radiographic evidence of joint damage may not be seen until 2 to 3 weeks after infection.

Definitive diagnosis requires arthrocentesis and synovial fluid analysis.

- Initially, changes may be minimal, but typical findings include the following:
  - increased volume of turbid, yellow or serosanguineous fluid of low viscosity
  - elevated protein content ≥4 g/dL)
  - elevated WBC count (>30,000/µL and often >100,000/µL), with ≥90% being neutrophils
- *Culture and sensitivity testing always should be performed* if joint infection is suspected. However, results often are negative, despite joint infection.
- Gram's stain also should be performed; often bacteria are found despite negative culture.
- *If the possibility of infectious arthritis exists, it usually is best to treat the joint as if it were infected.*

Treatment

Optimal therapy includes:

- early initiation of systemic antibiotic therapy
  - Ideally, therapy is guided by culture and sensitivity or Gram's stain results.
  - Amikacin and cephalothin is a good combination for initial therapy.
  - Penicillin and gentamicin (once-daily dosing; see Chapter 4, Principles of Therapy) also is a good choice.
  - Enrofloxacin (5.5 mg/kg intravenously [IV] q24h or 7.5 mg/kg orally [PO] q24h) is another option in adults.
  - Intraarticular antibiotic therapy also should be considered.
  - Antibiotics should be continued for at least 2 weeks after resolution of clinical signs.
- removal of debris and harmful inflammatory products from the joint
  - Options include aspiration, synovial distention and irrigation, through-and-through lavage (using either needles/catheters or arthroscopy), and arthrotomy.

- Antibiotics and/or 100 mL of 99% DMSO can be added to the final liter of lavage fluid.
- Arthroscopic lavage and/or synovectomy may be considered for patients with chronically infected joints.

♦ supportive care
  - Stall rest and maintenance of a modified Robert-Jones bandage are recommended
  - Hand walking and passive joint flexion may improve joint function.
  - NSAIDs are indicated to relieve pain and inflammation.
  - Administration of hyaluronan or polysulfated glycosaminoglycans may be worthwhile once acute inflammation is controlled.

Prognosis

Early recognition and initiation of aggressive therapy may effect a cure, but the prognosis never is good. In general, foals respond to therapy better than do adult horses. But even in foals, the prognosis is guarded. Involvement of multiple joints and concurrent systemic illness worsens the prognosis, and osteomyelitis in conjunction with infectious arthritis carries a poor prognosis.

Osteomyelitis

Hematogenous osteomyelitis in young foals usually is caused by the same organisms responsible for infectious arthritis. In addition to the bacteria listed on p. 394, *Klebsiella* spp. and *Bacteroides* spp. also may be involved. Osteomyelitis in adult horses usually results from damage and inoculation at the time of trauma or surgery. *Staphylococcus* spp. are most often isolated; other common organisms are *Streptococcus* spp., *Proteus* spp., *Pseudomonas* spp., *E. coli*, and *Corynebacterium* spp. Anaerobic bacteria also may be involved.

Diagnosis

Diagnosis is based on the history, clinical findings, radiography, and culture and sensitivity.

♦ Clinical signs vary, depending on the duration and severity of infection.
  - Lameness may be the only apparent abnormality.

- In acute cases, fever may accompany local swelling and pain.
- Affected foals usually have concurrent septicemia, but systemic signs may not be apparent.
- In some cases, particularly when traumatically induced, draining tracts are present.

♦ Radiographic changes include irregular periosteal reactions and increased medullary density, possibly with sequestrum and involucrum formation.
  - In fracture cases, loosening of metal implants may be apparent.

♦ Culture and sensitivity testing should be performed when osteomyelitis is suspected.
  - Recovery of the causative organism is improved when cultures of infected bone or soft tissues are obtained.
  - Samples should be submitted for both aerobic and anaerobic culture.

Treatment

Acute osteomyelitis, particularly hematogenous, may respond to specific antimicrobial therapy if treatment is begun before significant bone necrosis has occurred.

♦ The same systemic antibiotics used for septic arthritis are used to treat osteomyelitis.
  - The combination of an aminoglycoside with a cephalosporin is the best initial choice.
  - Metronidazole, chloramphenicol, or clindamycin may be needed for the *Bacteroides* species and *Staphylococcus aureus* that are resistant to penicillin and cephalosporins.
  - Trimethoprim-sulfonamides are effective against many anaerobes, but they should not be used until culture and sensitivity results confirm susceptibility.
  - Enrofloxacin is useful for treatment of aminoglycoside-resistant gram-negative bacteria.

♦ Antimicrobial drugs also can be delivered directly to the site via regional limb perfusion, antibiotic-impregnated polymers, or subcutaneous infusion pumps (see *Equine Medicine and Surgery V*).

- Systemic antimicrobials should be continued for 4 to 6 weeks after clinical resolution.
- With superficial osteomyelitis resulting from a wound, sequestrum removal and debridement of the diseased bone may be all that is required for healing.

Once there is evidence of significant bone necrosis, surgical debridement is indicated. When infections are associated with implant failures, the implant should be removed and replaced with a more stable fixation device, and the infected sites should be drained.

Prognosis

Despite aggressive therapy, there is a substantial failure rate with bone infections. Severe osteomyelitis with significant loss of bone and/or involvement of multiple limbs (in foals) warrants a poor prognosis.

Lyme Disease (Borreliosis)

Lyme disease is a multisystemic illness caused by the spirochete *Borrelia burgdorferi.*

- The disease is principally transmitted by ticks.
- Clinical signs include lethargy, low-grade fever, and single or multiple painful and mildly swollen joints, resulting in stiffness and reluctance to move.
- Diagnosis usually is made by serology.
  - Initially, serum antibodies may be undetectable, and healthy horses in enzootic areas may have positive titers, so other causes of joint distention should be ruled out.
- Treatment consists of oxytetracycline, ampicillin, or procaine penicillin and NSAIDs.
- Signs should resolve after 1 week of therapy.

MULTIFACTORIAL DISEASES

Angular Limb Deformities

The term *angular limb deformity* describes a deviation from the normal axis of a limb in the frontal plane. Two types of angular limb deformity are described.

- *valgus:* The limb distal to the deformity deviates laterally (e.g., knock-kneed foal).
- *varus:* The limb distal to the deformity deviates medially (e.g., bow-legged foal).

In most cases, there also is a rotational component. Most foals are born with a slight angular limb deformity that spontaneously corrects during the first few weeks of life. In other foals the deformity becomes more pronounced during this period. In still others it develops later, during the first 6 months of life.

Diagnosis

Diagnosis is obvious, although the underlying defect should be investigated through physical examination and radiography.

- In newborn foals, an attempt should be made to manually straighten the limb.
  - Temporary correction of the deformity by manual pressure suggests incomplete cuboidal bone ossification or laxity of periarticular supporting structures as the cause.
  - If the deformity cannot be manually corrected, asynchronous growth likely is the cause.
- Radiographs allow localization of the deformity.
  - The dorsopalmar view is indicated for the carpal and fetlock regions; the lateromedial view is most diagnostic for the tarsal region.

Treatment

Depending on physical and radiographic findings, treatment may include:

- *exercise:* Foals with normal ossification but lax periarticular structures may respond to limited exercise (e.g., turn out in a small pasture for 2 to 3 hours per day).
- *stall rest:* This may be all that is required for foals with a mild degree of incomplete ossification but straight limbs and those with asynchronous bone growth at birth.
- *corrective trimming:* This can be effective in conjunction with stall rest or surgery; glue-on shoes with side extensions also may be beneficial.
- *external support:* PVC splints, commercial splints (e.g., Farley brace),

or tube casts should be applied as soon as possible after birth in foals with incomplete ossification.
- Foals with asynchronous bone growth should not be treated with external support.
- *surgery:* This is the preferred treatment for asynchronous bone growth.
  - Growth acceleration on the "concave" or "short" side by periosteal stripping is the most commonly used technique.
  - Growth retardation on the "convex" or "long" side using staples, screws and wires, or bone plates also is performed in foals with severe deformities and in older foals.
  - Surgery can be performed any time after 2 weeks of age but should be undertaken as soon as possible.

Surgical techniques are described in *Equine Medicine and Surgery V.* Specific recommendations for particular angular limb deformities are given in later sections of this chapter.

Flexural Deformities

Flexural deformities (flexor contractures) are discussed in specific sections later in the chapter. The pathogenesis is described in *Equine Medicine and Surgery V.*

Osteochondrosis/Physitis

Osteochondrosis is a multifactorial abnormality of bone development. Important contributors include genetic predisposition for rapid growth and large body size, nutritional imbalances, and trauma. Developmental orthopedic diseases attributed to osteochondrosis include osteochondritis dissecans, subchondral bone cysts, and physitis.

Osteochondritis dissecans

Osteochondritis dissecans (OCD) results when chondral and osteochondral fractures in the epiphyseal cartilage dissect to the articular surface.
- The most frequently affected sites are the lateral trochlear ridge of the femur, the intermediate ridge of the tibia, and the caudal aspect of the humeral head.
- Depending on the joint affected and use of the horse, the presenting complaint is joint distention, lameness, or both.
  - Lameness is variable in degree and may temporarily resolve when the horse is rested.
  - When present, the lameness usually is reduced or alleviated with intraarticular anesthesia.
- Radiographic lesions vary markedly and in some cases may be absent.
  - Osteochondral fragments are the classic manifestation of OCD.
  - Because osteochondrosis frequently occurs bilaterally, radiographic examination of the contralateral joint is recommended.
  - There is poor correlation between the severity of lesions identified radiographically and those found at surgery.
- Treatment may be conservative (rest, controlled exercise, intraarticular hyaluronan or polysulfated glycosaminoglycans) or surgical.
  - Arthroscopic removal of cartilage flaps and osteochondral fragments combined with curettage of the underlying defect is the standard approach for most OCD lesions.

Management of osteochondrosis at specific sites is discussed in later sections of this chapter.

Subchondral bone cysts

Subchondral bone cysts may be a manifestation of osteochondrosis.
- They are most common in the medial femoral condyle of the femorotibial joint.
- The presenting complaint most often is intermittent lameness of varying severity.
  - Lameness usually decreases in severity or resolves with rest; in some cases, it is not evident until the horse begins training.
  - Synovial effusion is not as obvious with subchondral bone cysts as with OCD.
- Intraarticular anesthesia is useful in localizing the lameness.
- Radiographs reveal lesions varying from mild flattening of the articular surface to large cystic areas, with an obvious channel communicating with the joint space.

- The contralateral joint also should be evaluated.
- Treatment options are much the same as for OCD.

Management of subchondral bone cysts at specific sites is discussed in later sections.

Physitis

Physitis is most common in the distal physes of the cannon bone, radius, and tibia.

- Affected horses typically are 4 to 8 months of age.
- Findings include metaphyseal flaring, pain on palpation, and stiffness or overt lameness.
  - Partial collapse of the defective physis may result in an angular limb deformity.
  - The pain may result in development of flexural deformities in the distal limb.
- Treatment is directed toward correcting underlying nutritional imbalances (see *Equine Medicine and Surgery V*), managing pain, and preventing further physeal damage.
  - NSAIDs may be used for pain relief.
  - If significant lameness exists, exercise restriction is indicated.
  - In patients with only mild or moderate lameness, controlled exercise is encouraged to maintain normal tendon and joint function.

IDIOPATHIC DISEASES

Hypertrophic Osteopathy

Hypertrophic osteopathy causes bilateral periosteal new bone growth in the distal limbs. Causes and management are discussed in *Equine Medicine and Surgery V*.

Diseases of Muscle

(pages 1483-1496)

David R. Hodgson

CONGENITAL AND FAMILIAL DISEASES

Myotonia

Myotonia is a congenital condition characterized by sustained muscle contraction after stimulation. Tentative diagnosis can be made on the basis of age (<1 year old), a stiff gait, muscle bulging, and prolonged, localized contraction after muscle percussion. Definitive diagnosis requires electromyographic examination (see *Equine Medicine and Surgery V*).

Hyperkalemic Periodic Paresis

Hyperkalemic periodic paresis is a disorder that affects Quarter Horses, American Paint Horses, and Appaloosas related to the Quarter Horse sire Impressive. It is characterized by episodes of muscle fasciculations and weakness and is transmitted as an autosomal dominant trait.

Clinical signs

Signs are highly variable, with some affected horses never showing clinical manifestations.

- A variety of stimuli may precipitate an episode, which begins with a brief period of myotonia. Some horses have prolapse of the third eyelid.
  - Sweating and muscle fasciculations are common.
  - Stimulation and attempts to move may exacerbate muscle fasciculations.
  - Some horses develop severe muscle cramping.
- Muscular weakness during episodes is characteristic.
  - Signs may progress to dog sitting or recumbency within a few minutes.
  - Respiratory distress occurs in some recumbent animals.
- Affected horses may appear stressed or anxious yet remain relatively bright and alert.
- Episodes usually last 15 to 60 minutes, with no apparent abnormalities between times.

Diagnosis

Episodic muscle tremors and weakness in a descendant of Impressive is strongly suggestive of this condition. Definitive diagnosis is made by submission of whole blood in ethylenediaminetetraacetic acid (EDTA) to an appropriate genetic laboratory.

Treatment

In acute cases, IV dextrose (6 mL/kg of a 5% solution) combined with bicarbonate (1 to 2 mEq/kg), or calcium gluconate (0.2 to 0.4 mL/kg of a

23% solution slowly IV) can be used to enhance intracellular movement of potassium. Strategies for reducing the incidence and severity of these episodes are discussed in *Equine Medicine and Surgery V*.

DISEASES WITH PHYSICAL CAUSES
Postanesthetic Myoneuropathy
This condition occurs as either a localized myopathy or generalized myopathy with neuropathy.

- Typically, affected horses are relatively large, well muscled, and subjected to prolonged and deep anesthesia on a hard surface.
- Signs include heat and pain in the muscles that were dependent during surgery, weakness, and reluctance or inability to bear weight on the affected limb(s) after anesthesia.
  - Local myopathy usually involves only a few muscles.
  - Generalized myopathy with neuropathy may prevent the horse from rising, and frequent violent attempts to stand may exacerbate the condition.
- Additional findings may include anxiety, tachycardia, tachypnea, profuse sweating, and myoglobinuria.

Many of the horses with localized myopathy recover within hours or days, with little or no treatment. In severely affected horses the same principles described for treatment of exertional rhabdomyolysis can be applied. Prophylaxis is discussed in *Equine Medicine and Surgery V*.

Exertional Rhabdomyolysis
Exertional rhabdomyolysis is a common and complex syndrome with numerous contributing factors, including diet, environment, and inherent muscle function.

- Classically, horses develop a stiff, stilted gait, with excessive sweating and a high respiratory rate during or after exercise.
  - The horse may stretch out as if to urinate, become extremely reluctant to move, and in severe cases become recumbent.
  - Affected muscles are painful when palpated; the back, hind

limb, and shoulder muscles are most often involved.
  - Myoglobinuria is a classic feature in more severely affected cases.
- Elevations in serum CK, AST, and LDH are common, with the degree reflecting the extent of myonecrosis (see p. 385).
- On occasion, examination of muscle biopsies helps establish the etiology, particularly in Quarter Horses and related breeds.
  - Defective glycolysis may be manifested by abnormal accumulations of carbohydrates.

Treatment
The aims of treatment for severely affected animals include limiting further muscle damage, reducing pain, and restoring fluid and electrolyte balance, thereby reducing the chances of renal impairment in animals with myoglobinuria.

- Further exercise is contraindicated in most cases of overt rhabdomyolysis.
  - Horses with simple muscle spasms and cramps may markedly improve with light exercise.
- If the circulatory system is not compromised, low doses of tranquilizers (e.g., acepromazine) relieve anxiety and may improve peripheral blood flow.
- NSAIDs are indicated, although they should be used judiciously when there is pigmenturia.
  - Corticosteroids may help by stabilizing cell membranes.
  - Anecdotally, DMSO (0.9 g/kg in a 20% solution IV) can be beneficial.
- Dantrolene sodium (2 mg/kg via nasogastric [NG] tube) sometimes is recommended.
- Balanced electrolyte solutions given IV and via NG tube are recommended for horses with myoglobinuria.
  - Fluid therapy should be maintained at a rate of 2 to 3 L/h until the urine is clear.
  - Diuretics usually are contraindicated.
  - Bicarbonate therapy is inappropriate if the myopathy occurred during an endurance ride.

- Recumbent horses require comfortable bedding and adequate nursing care.
  - It is ill advised to force these horses into frequent attempts to stand.

Prophylaxis

Reduction in dietary carbohydrate and provision of high-quality grass hay and a balanced vitamin and mineral supplement form the basis of prophylaxis for exertional rhabdomyolysis, regardless of etiology. Specific recommendations are discussed in *Equine Medicine and Surgery V*.

Fibrotic and Ossifying Myopathy

These conditions reflect a mechanical hind limb lameness that restricts normal function of the semitendinosus and sometimes the semimembranosus, biceps femoris, and gracilis muscles.

- In most cases this is an acquired disorder resulting from muscle trauma.
- Lameness usually is most apparent during walking and is characterized by an abrupt cessation of the anterior phase of the stride, causing the leg to be suddenly jerked to the ground.
- Firm, fibrous areas may be detectable on palpation of the affected muscle.
- Pain is not a feature of the lameness, and manipulative tests and antiinflammatory therapy have little if any effect on the degree of dysfunction.
- Surgical correction involves either excision or transection of the fibrotic portion of the muscle or tenotomy of the tibial insertion of the semimembranosus tendon (see *Equine Medicine and Surgery V*).

INFLAMMATORY, INFECTIOUS, AND IMMUNE DISEASES

Clostridial Myonecrosis

Clostridial myonecrosis can rapidly become a severe, life-threatening condition.

- Because most cases are sequelae to IM injections, common sites are the cervical, pectoral, and caudal hind limb muscles.

- Initially, affected muscles are warm and may have palpable crepitation (gas accumulation).
  - The horse may be lame, stiff, and reluctant to move.
- Clinical signs can rapidly progress to systemic illness (fever, depression, dehydration, tachycardia, tachypnea, and poor capillary perfusion) over a matter of hours.
- Ultrasonography often reveals fluid and gas accumulation SC and between tissue planes.
- Gram's stain of smears from affected muscle tissue frequently reveals clostridial organisms.
  - Definitive diagnosis requires anaerobic culture.

Treatment and prognosis

Treatment involves immediate institution of aggressive antimicrobial and supportive therapy.

- Initial treatment with crystalline penicillin G (30,000 to 50,000 IU/kg IV q2-8h) and possibly procaine penicillin G (25,000 to 30,000 IU/kg IM q6-12h) is appropriate.
  - Continual IV infusion of crystalline penicillin G (200 to 250 IU/kg/h) might be best until the animal's condition stabilizes.
- Radical debridement of affected tissues is important, as are fluid therapy, analgesics, NG feeding, and postoperative wound care.

Regardless of the intensity of therapy, horses with myonecrosis caused by *C. septicum* or *C. chauvoei* often die; those infected with *C. perfringens* (type A) may have a better survival rate.

Corynebacterium Pseudotuberculosis Abscesses

Large, deep, thick-walled abscesses in the pectoral muscles, and less commonly in the axillary region, ventral abdomen, and limbs, are features of this condition.

- It often is referred to as "pigeon fever" or "pigeon breast."
- Most cases have been reported in California and Texas, but cases also have been reported in Washington, Idaho, Montana, and southwestern Canada.
- Abscesses can be identified ultrasonographically.

♦ Definitive diagnosis requires bacterial culture.
  • A hemagglutination inhibition test for occult *C. pseudotuberculosis* abscesses is available.

Treatment
Treatment is as for abscesses in other parts of the body.
♦ Mature ("pointing") abscesses are incised, flushed, and allowed to drain.
  • Most of these lesions heal satisfactorily over a period of weeks with routine wound care, although repeated surgical drainage may be required.
♦ Immature abscesses may be treated with hot compresses to encourage maturity.
  • Administration of antimicrobial agents retards growth of the organism and often leads to recrudescence when the drugs are discontinued.

METABOLIC DISEASES
Hypocalcemia
Hypocalcemia (lactation tetany, transit tetany, eclampsia) is relatively rare in horses.
♦ Clinical signs include increased muscle tone, a stiff, stilted gait, hind limb ataxia, and muscle fasciculations (especially temporal, masseter, triceps muscles).
  • Other signs may include trismus, dysphagia, salivation, anxiety, sweating, tachycardia, fever, arrhythmias, synchronous diaphragmatic flutter, convulsions, coma, and death.
♦ Definitive diagnosis requires laboratory demonstration of hypocalcemia.
  • Serum ionized calcium concentrations of 5 to 8 mg/dL usually produce tetanic spasms and incoordination; concentrations <5 mg/dL usually result in recumbency and stupor.
♦ Treatment involves IV administration of calcium solutions, such as 20% calcium borogluconate at 250 to 500 mL/500 kg, diluted 1:4 with saline or dextrose.
  • *Calcium preparations should be infused slowly* while closely monitoring the cardiovascular response.
  • Relapses of hypocalcemia may occur.

Synchronous Diaphragmatic Flutter
Also known as "thumps," this disorder usually occurs in horses with derangements in fluid and electrolyte balance, most commonly hypocalcemia and hypochloremic metabolic alkalosis.
♦ The characteristic clinical manifestation occurs when the diaphragm contracts in synchrony with the heart, causing rhythmic contractions or twitching of the flank muscles.
♦ In some cases the inciting metabolic derangements are clinically apparent.
  • Endurance horses may be dehydrated, hyperthermic, depressed, anorectic, and have an abnormal sweat response and aperistalsis.
♦ In most cases, "thumps" is a transient event, abating when the underlying cause is resolved.
  • Most horses rapidly improve when given calcium solutions IV.

Malignant Hyperthermia
Malignant hyperthermia is a rare syndrome that is associated with administration of certain volatile anesthetic agents.
♦ Clinical signs develop during anesthesia and include the following:
  • muscle stiffness, cramping, and fasciculations
  • hyperthermia, often to $\geq 42.2°$ C (108° F)
  • sweating, elevated or irregular heart rate, variable blood pressure, and irregular breathing
♦ Discontinuation of anesthesia is advisable in horses with suggestive clinical signs.
  • Alcohol or cold-water baths and ice-water enemas should be used to cool the horse.

Muscle Cramping in Endurance Horses
This disorder commonly occurs in endurance horses during hot weather.
♦ Stiffness, muscle cramping, and pain on palpation of the locomotory muscles are features.

- Dehydration, electrolyte abnormalities, elevations in heart and respiratory rates, depression, hyperthermia, and synchronous diaphragmatic flutter also are common.
  - Serum CK and AST are not markedly elevated, and there is no myoglobinuria.
- Under most circumstances, this condition is self-limiting and signs abate with rest or light exercise, although treatment of concurrent metabolic derangements is indicated.

NUTRITIONAL DISEASES

Nutritional Myodegeneration

Nutritional myodegeneration ("white muscle disease") occurs most commonly in young foals. The disease is caused by a deficiency of selenium and possibly vitamin E. Stress, such as unaccustomed exercise, may precipitate clinical signs.

Clinical signs

The two syndromes are acute myocardial degeneration and subacute skeletal myodegeneration.

- Foals with myocardial degeneration may be found dead, die suddenly, or become severely debilitated.
- The onset of signs of skeletal myodegeneration usually is slower; signs frequently include failure to suckle, muscle weakness, stiffness, trembling, and possibly recumbency.
- Affected muscles may be swollen and myoglobinuria can occur.

Diagnosis

Most cases occur in known selenium-deficient and/or vitamin-E–deficient areas. Diagnosis is aided by:

- finding elevations in serum CK, AST, and LDH
- finding dry, pale or streaked muscles on postmortem examination
- determining the animal's selenium (Se) and possibly vitamin E status
  - Se status is adequate when serum Se is 0.14 to 0.25 µg/mL or RBC glutathione peroxidase activity is 30 to 150 mmol/min/(g Hb).

Treatment

Parenteral administration of Se and vitamin E is indicated, although care must be taken to limit Se supplementation.

- The recommended dosage for selenium is 0.05 to 0.07 mg/kg.
- Vitamin E can be supplemented at a rate of up to 100 IU/kg/day.
- Confinement and nursing care also are important until the foal responds to supplementation.

Supplementing mares with selenium during pregnancy plays a significant role in preventing nutritional myodegeneration. Other measures are discussed in *Equine Medicine and Surgery V*.

Diseases of the Hoof, Distal Phalanx, and Associated Structures

(pages 1496-1546)

William A. Moyer, Joerg A. Auer, Brent A. Hague, G. Kent Carter, Tracy A. Turner, Clifford C. Pollitt, William P. Hay, P.O. Eric Mueller, J. Lane Easter, Jeffrey P. Watkins, Dean W. Richardson, Roger K.W. Smith, Peter M. Webbon, and Patrick T. Colahan

DISEASES WITH PHYSICAL CAUSES

Hoof Wall Cracks

Hoof cracks, especially those in the quarter and heel region, are a common cause of foot lameness. While they do not all create lameness, the potential to do so always is present. Each crack should be examined visually and by careful manipulation with hoof testers to define the degree of instability as well as the presence of pain.

Treatment

Treatment depends on the horse's use, the severity and location of the defect, and whether or not the problem is complicated by infection, hoof wall loss, or exposed sensitive tissue.

- Small superficial cracks beginning at the ground surface generally require little more than careful trimming and perhaps a bar shoe.
- Infected cracks, regardless of location, should be explored with a hoof knife or motorized burr; any defective or separated hoof wall should be trimmed away.

- With heel and quarter cracks, the principle of repair is to eliminate motion by stabilizing the independent portion of the wall.
- Conservative approaches include bar shoes, side clips, rasping a perpendicular notch at the crack's proximal limit, and trimming to eliminate weight bearing at the crack.
- Extensive, painful, bleeding, or infected cracks usually require repair with acrylic materials and/or screws and wire (see *Equine Medicine and Surgery V*).

Keratoma

Keratoma is an uncommon tumor of the keratin-producing cells of the hoof wall. The mass may cause lameness if it impinges on the sensitive laminae and/or. Most often there are no outward signs, but in some cases the hoof wall bulges over the mass, and the white line may be deviated. Keratomas usually are suspected from the radiographic appearance of P3 (focal area of bone loss with a smooth, curved edge). The only effective treatment is excision.

Sole Bruising

Sole bruising is a common but often overlooked and underrated cause of lameness.

- Lameness can be acute or insidious in onset, and the severity can vary from barely perceptible to an inability to bear weight.
- Focal pain usually can be identified with hoof testers.
- The bruise may be visible on the sole, but this is not always the case.
- There usually are no radiographic changes.
- Focal osteolysis of P3 (pedal osteitis) may develop with repetitive focal trauma.

Treatment

Therapy begins by identifying the cause, if possible, and then eliminating or reducing its effects.

- This may require eliminating toe grabs or heel caulks or rebalancing the foot.
- The most successful treatment is to reduce or eliminate weight bearing at the site of the bruise with a cutout rim pad or a shoe with a deeply concave sole surface.
  - If possible, a full bar is used as well.
- Soaking the foot in cold water and giving phenylbutazone is useful for the first few days.

Fractures of the Distal Phalanx

P3 fractures are more common in racing Thoroughbreds and Standardbreds.

- The history typically includes sudden onset of lameness, the degree depending on the type of fracture and duration of the problem.
  - Articular fractures are more painful than nonarticular fractures.
  - Solar margin fractures usually cause only mild lameness.
  - Extensor process fractures may cause subtle lameness evident only at speed or in turns.
- In most cases, hoof testers can be used to localize the problem.

The diagnosis is confirmed via radiography.

  - It is advisable to make several radiographs, including lateromedial, dorsopalmar/plantar, and in selected cases oblique dorsopalmar/plantar views.
  - When no fracture can be detected, yet other acute problems have been ruled out, the hoof should be tightly wrapped and radiographs repeated a few days later.

Treatment and prognosis

Treatment and prognosis depend on the fracture type.

- Conservative treatment is used for most nonarticular and abaxial articular fractures.
  - Balanced trimming and an egg bar or full bar shoe and/or side clips are recommended.
  - The shoe should be refitted every 4 to 6 weeks and worn for 6 to 9 months.
  - Horses with articular fractures may develop degenerative joint disease, so the prognosis for return to full soundness is guarded; some require palmar digital neurectomy.

◆ Sagittal fractures often are amenable to lag screw fixation (see *Equine Medicine and Surgery V*).
  • Generally, the prognosis with good articular alignment is reasonable.
◆ Extensor process fractures can occur unilaterally or bilaterally and may actually be separate centers of ossification.
  • When regional anesthesia confirms that the fracture is the cause of lameness, surgical removal or lag screw fixation is indicated (see *Equine Medicine and Surgery V*).
◆ Solar margin fractures most often occur after penetration of the sole by a sharp object; local osteomyelitis results in formation of a bone sequestrum.
  • Surgical removal of the fragment and debridement of diseased bone is recommended.
  • In most cases, the prognosis is good.

Quittor

Quittor is a lay term for necrosis of the collateral cartilage of P3. It is characterized by intermittent purulent discharge over the affected cartilage and a history of variable lameness. In addition to routine radiographs, a radiopaque probe should be placed into the sinus tract. Treatment involves surgical debridement of the affected tissues. Assuming that the diseased area is removed in its entirety without disturbing healthy tissue, the prognosis is fair.

Sidebone

"Sidebone" is a lay term describing ossification of the collateral cartilages of P3. This is a common aging process. Sidebone often coexists with other foot problems that are of greater significance, so it is important to correlate radiographic appearance with clinical findings. Balanced trimming and shoeing helps most horses in which sidebone is the only problem. Horses with other chronic foot problems usually do not remain sound.

Pedal Osteitis

Pedal osteitis is defined as demineralization of the solar margin of P3.
◆ It generally is secondary to laminitis, severe or chronic sole bruising, submural or subsolar hoof infections, or excessive paring of the soles.
◆ Clinical findings can vary greatly with the cause and severity.
  • Pedal osteitis may be an incidental radiographic finding in a sound horse or associated with an unrelated cause of lameness, such as navicular disease.
◆ Diagnosis involves localizing the pain to the area over P3 with hoof testers and regional anesthesia and examining excellent-quality radiographs (especially a 60-degree dorsoproximal/palmarodistal view).
◆ The aim of treatment is to decrease or eliminate focal impact at the site of pain.

Sheared Heels

Sheared heels is a relatively common cause of foot lameness.
◆ It results from single heel overload and may occur alone or with other foot problems.
◆ The affected heel is displaced above its mate, and the nondisplaced heel and quarter wall generally have a flared (less upright) hoof wall.
  • Hoof testers generally elicit a painful response across the heels.
◆ Lameness may be intermittent and variable but improves with a palmar digital nerve block.
◆ The goal of treatment is to balance the foot by trimming the affected heel so that it does not contact the shoe and supporting the foot with a bar shoe.

Underrun Heels (Low Heel, Long Toe)

The low-heel, long-toe configuration is a common foot abnormality. It is most prevalent in Thoroughbred racehorses but can occur in all breeds and types. It does not cause lameness itself but is a major cause of foot problems (e.g., sole bruising, navicular syndrome, quarter cracks) and a contributor to limb problems. The condition can be difficult to reverse if it is severe and long-standing; generally, it is best to begin with a square-toed egg bar shoe.

INFLAMMATORY, INFECTIOUS, AND IMMUNE DISEASES
Subsolar Abscesses and Foot Infections
Subsolar infections probably are the most common cause of acute lameness in horses.

* Most affected horses show sudden lameness, which can be severe.
* Digital manipulation and hoof testers help identify the area of focal pain.
  * Often the involved foot is markedly warmer and the digital pulse usually is bounding.
  * The coronary band proximal to the infected area may be swollen, tender, or draining if the infection extends into the hoof wall region.
  * Hoof testers usually elicit pain at the site of infection, but a pain response may be found all over the affected foot.
* Radiography is useful to rule out other causes of lameness, identify possible complications (osteomyelitis, foreign material), and localize the abscess cavity.

Treatment and prognosis
The object of therapy is to open and drain the infection.

* The site is pared open with a hoof knife, making the opening of sufficient size to allow drainage but not so extensive as to create further damage.
  * Exploration of deep wounds potentially involving P3, the navicular bone, deep flexor tendon, or coffin joint may necessitate general anesthesia (see *Equine Medicine and Surgery V*).
* The foot should be periodically soaked in a warm solution of Epsom salts until the area is no longer draining or inflamed.
* The bottom of the foot can be protected with a foot bandage and local antiseptic, a treatment plate, or at a later date a plastic or leather pad.

* The horse's tetanus status should be determined; use of antibiotics and analgesics is optional.

The prognosis can vary from excellent with a simple subsolar abscess to grave if deeper structures are involved.

Thrush
Thrush is a degenerative condition of the frog and surrounding tissues.

* It is characterized by necrotic, foul-smelling material originating from the frog sulci.
  * Thrush generally is associated with unhygienic conditions, but this is not always the case.
* Involvement can vary from barely detectable to extensive invasion of the digital cushion, hoof wall degradation, and exudative dermatitis of the heel bulbs.
  * Part or all of the frog may be undermined by the degenerative process.
* Lameness and pain on manipulation of the frog are variable findings.
* Treatment involves topical application of mild caustic materials, such as iodine, methylene blue, or formaldehyde.
  * Severely affected feet may require careful removal of all necrotic material, often to the level of the frog corium.

Infectious Joint Disease of the Distal Interphalangeal Joint
Coffin joint infections usually are induced by puncture wounds, lacerations, and other forms of trauma. Unlike most other joints, swelling generally is not apparent. Principles of diagnosis and treatment of infectious arthritis are discussed on p. 394. Lavage is best accomplished with needles placed in the palmar/plantar pouch and in the dorsal aspect of the joint.

MULTIFACTORIAL DISEASES
Navicular Syndrome
Navicular syndrome is a common and complex foot problem characterized by pain in the caudal half of the foot.

The condition is more common in horses 7 to 14 years old, and the incidence is highest in Quarter Horses, Thoroughbreds, and Standardbreds. Pathophysiology is discussed in *Equine Medicine and Surgery V*.

Clinical evaluation

Diagnosis should be based on the history and clinical findings.

- Typically the history indicates intermittent lameness or inconsistent performance.
  - The lameness often is more noticeable after heavy work and usually improves with rest.
- Classically, navicular syndrome causes bilateral forelimb lameness, but it can occur as a unilateral lameness.
  - The gait is short and choppy, and the horse has a tendency to land toe-first.
  - The lameness usually can be accentuated by turning the horse in a tight circle at the trot and by working the horse on hard or rough surfaces.
- Application of the hoof testers from collateral sulcus to opposite hoof wall, central sulcus to toe, and across the heels is a test for navicular pain.
  - It is important to make sure the horse does not have sore heels, corns, or sole bruising that could account for a positive response.
- A positive response to distal limb flexion could be expected if the problem is related to distal interphalangeal synovitis and possibly navicular ligament or tendinous damage.
- Two wedge tests (inducing coffin joint hyperextension with a toe wedge and applying frog pressure) may be helpful in diagnosing navicular syndrome (see *Equine Medicine and Surgery V*).

It is important to remember that there are no clinical signs that are pathognomonic for navicular syndrome. In fact, none of these tests has a predictive value >53%.

REGIONAL ANESTHESIA. Navicular lameness typically improves at least 90% after a medial and lateral palmar digital nerve block. Important exceptions to this are horses with a sec-

ondary problem, such as pedal osteitis or suspensory desmitis. In some cases, coffin joint and navicular bursa anesthesia add useful information (see *Equine Medicine and Surgery V*).

Radiographic assessment

Radiography should be used to confirm a clinical impression and rule out other osseous causes of lameness. Navicular bone changes can be divided into five categories:

- calcification of the proximal suspensory ligaments ("spurs"), consistent with ligament strain
- remodeling of the proximal and distal borders, also consistent with ligament strain
  - This is the most reliable change, being present in about 50% of horses with navicular syndrome and only about 3% of normal high-risk horses.
- enlarged fossae ("lollipops," "cones"), which may indicate coffin joint synovitis
- cyst formation, which may indicate bone resorption or necrosis
- flexor cortex changes, evident on the "skyline" view and indicative of tendon damage

NOTE: *These radiographic changes are not pathognomonic for navicular syndrome.* Radiographs alone cannot be used to diagnose or predict the problem; in all cases, radiographic findings must be interpreted in light of the clinical picture.

Treatment

The basis of treatment is proper shoeing.

- Shoeing for navicular syndrome involves the following principles:
  - Correct any hoof abnormalities to balance the foot and align the hoof/pastern axis.
  - Use all weight-bearing structures of the hoof and allow for hoof expansion.
  - Ease breakover.
- Rolled-toe egg bar shoes are a good starting point; other options are discussed in *Equine Medicine and Surgery V*.
- Resumption of a regular exercise program is essential.
- Drugs with antiinflammatory and/or vascular effects may be effective when shoeing changes alone

are insufficient to restore functional soundness; phenylbutazone is used most often.

- Warfarin and isoxsuprine have been used with variable success.
- Palmar digital neurectomy usually is saved as a last resort.
  - Desmotomy of the navicular suspensory ligaments has been effective in some horses.

Laminitis

Laminitis is a potentially devastating condition that involves failure of the bond between the lamellae of the inner hoof wall and the surface of P3. Most often the inciting event involves the gastrointestinal tract (e.g., excess consumption of grain or lush pasture, duodenitis/proximal jejunitis, colitis). Other possible causes include retained placenta and septic metritis, pneumonia/pleuritis, and severe rhabdomyolysis. Pathophysiology is discussed in *Equine Medicine and Surgery V*.

Phases of laminitis

The process of laminitis can be divided into three phases.

- *developmental phase:* triggering of lamellar separation
  - This phase lasts as little as 8 hours in cases of laminitis caused by black walnut or up to 40 hours in cases caused by grain overload.
- *acute phase:* from the onset of foot pain to the point when there is clinical (usually radiologic) evidence of displacement of P3
  - If the horse survives, it can make a complete recovery or develop chronic laminitis.
- *chronic phase:* can last indefinitely with signs ranging from persistent, mild lameness to continued severe foot pain, further lamellar degeneration (with or without hoof sloughing), and hoof wall deformation

Clinical signs of acute laminitis

Shifting weight from one foot to the other is the first sign of lamellar degeneration and usually is first noticed in the forefeet. Other findings may include:

- palpable warmth in the affected feet (mostly during the developmental phase)

- bounding digital pulses (Note: This is not pathognomonic for laminitis.).
- pain over the sole at the toe with thumb or hoof tester pressure
- pain when the dorsal hoof wall is tapped with a hammer

Horses with extensive lamellar pathology exhibit more obvious signs.

- Severely affected horses refuse to pick up their feet.
- When standing, the forefeet are placed forward of the normal position. If forced to walk, the horse arches its back and places the hind limbs forward under the abdomen.
  - When the hind feet are more severely affected, the forelimbs are placed under the body and the horse leans over its forequarters, lowering its head and neck.
- With severe lamellar failure in all four feet, the horse is immobile and extremely distressed; it may lie in lateral recumbency with the limbs extended.

Clinical signs of chronic laminitis

When the majority of lamellar attachments fail, as they do in severe cases, P3 displaces within the hoof capsule, causing the following changes:

- a deficit in the coronary band that allows the top of the hoof wall to become palpable
  - If this deficit extends around the coronet to the quarters and heels, the prognosis is grave.
  - Separation of the skin at the coronet and exudation of serum is an extremely grave sign.
- flattening or bulging of the sole (dropped sole)
  - This predisposes to chronic sole bruising and infection, including subsolar abscesses and osteomyelitis of P3.
  - In severe, deteriorating cases, P3 prolapses through the sole.
- deformed hoof growth, especially retarded dorsal hoof wall growth and concentric rings in the hoof wall that are widest apart at the heels
  - In severe cases the disparity of wall growth produces a dramatic upturning of the toe.

Diagnosis

A presumptive diagnosis of laminitis usually is readily made from the history and clinical findings. Whenever possible, the feet should be examined by radiograph as soon as clinical signs appear, checking for the following abnormalities:

- increase in the distance between the dorsal hoof wall and the dorsal cortex of P3
  - For most 400- to 450-kg (880 to 990 lb) horses, the distance normally is 15 to 17 mm on radiographs uncorrected for magnification error.
  - Evaluating this distance using the length of the palmar cortex of P3 as an internal reference gives uniform results irrespective of magnification and body size (see *Equine Medicine and Surgery V*).
  - An increasing distance is an important prognostic indicator.
- radiolucent (gas) line between the dorsal hoof wall and dorsal cortex of P3
  - These lines indicate considerable lamellar stretching and separation.
- increase in the distance between the proximal edge of the hoof wall and the extensor process of P3 (indicating downward displacement of P3, or "sinking")
  - Sinking carries a grave prognosis; euthanasia usually is the most humane option.
- palmar rotation of the tip of P3 and narrowed distance between it and the ground surface

Radiographic changes associated with chronic laminitis are described in *Equine Medicine and Surgery V*.

Treatment

No known therapy is able to arrest or block the triggering of laminitis. Thus treatment centers on symptomatic relief.

- It is *essential* that the primary disease is treated immediately and effectively.
  - Administration of mineral oil (4L/450 kg) or activated charcoal via NG tube may be beneficial in cases of grain overload.
- During the developmental phase, packing the feet in crushed ice or soaking them in cold water can be protective.
  - *Exercise and nerve blocks are contraindicated during this phase.*

- NSAIDs are indicated for pain relief.
  - Flunixin meglumine (0.25 mg/kg IV q8h or 1.1 mg/kg IV q12h) often is used for its antiendotoxic effects.
  - Phenylbutazone (4.4mg/kg IV or PO q12h initially, then 2.2 mg/kg q12h) is effective at controlling foot pain.
- DMSO (≤20% solution given slowly IV) is used by some clinicians.
- Vasodilators, such as isoxuprine, acepromazine, and glyceryl trinitrate (applied as a patch to the pastern), may be beneficial *after* the developmental phase.
- Strict confinement to a stall with a deep bedding of sand or shavings and mechanical support for the distal phalanges are important.
  - Support may comprise a roll of gauze taped to the frog, commercial frog support pads (Lilly Pads), application of dental putty or support foam to the sole, or a heart bar shoe.
  - Dorsal hoof wall resection may be combined with a heart bar shoe to reduce stress on the compromised dorsal lamellae (see *Equine Medicine and Surgery V*).
- Raising the heels 12 to 18 degrees to decrease tension on the deep digital flexor tendon can also reduce stress on the dorsal lamellae and relieve pain in some horses.
  - If radiographs show no rotation of P3, heel wedging can proceed immediately.
  - If rotation is already present, the hoof should trimmed to normalize the position of P3 in relation to the hoof capsule before wedges are applied.
  - Strict stall rest with deep bedding is mandatory when using heel wedges.
- Deep flexor tenotomy can be considered if despite initial therapy, P3 continues to rotate and pain persists (see *Equine Medicine and Surgery V*).

Prognosis

Many horses with acute laminitis completely recover if treated promptly. But if radiographs show displacement of P3, the prognosis must be guarded. Horses with significant displacement are prone to recurrent episodes of foot pain.

Flexural Deformity

Flexural deformity of the coffin joint results from contraction of the deep digital flexor tendon.

* This condition most commonly occurs in foals 1 to 4 months of age.
  * It also may occur in fast-growing weanlings and yearlings and in adult horses secondary to severe lameness.
* The hoof wall is more upright than the pastern, and the length of hoof wall at the heel increases relative to the toe, resulting in the classic "club foot."
  * Chronic cases develop dishing of the dorsal hoof wall.
* The affected limb should be closely examined for signs of developmental joint and physeal disease that may have initiated the flexural deformity.
* Radiographs of the distal phalanx should be obtained.

Treatment and prognosis

Foals with mild or early flexural deformities often respond well to nonsurgical therapy. Any inciting musculoskeletal conditions must be treated and the diet balanced.

In particular, excess carbohydrate and protein should be avoided.

* NSAIDs can be given in low doses, and controlled exercise should be provided.
* Oxytetracycline (44 mg/kg, diluted in 1L polyionic fluids and given slowly IV once; may be repeated in 24 hours) can be effective.
* Corrective trimming and shoeing is important.
  * Options include use of an extended-toe steel shoe or plastic glue-on shoe and direct application of acrylics to the toe.
  * The heel can be gradually shortened in mildly affected foals.
* More severely affected foals and those that do not respond to conservative therapy require distal check desmotomy (see *Equine Medicine and Surgery V*).

* Foals that do not respond to desmotomy may require deep digital flexor tenotomy.

The prognosis for foals requiring distal check desmotomy is determined by the severity of the deformity. The prognosis for an athletic career after deep digital tenotomy is poor.

Osteochondrosis of the Distal Interphalangeal Joint

Osteochondrosis of the coffin joint is uncommon. When it does occur, it usually is in the form of a subchondral bone cyst within P3. The prognosis for such lesions in this location is guarded. Subchondral bone cysts are discussed on p. 397.

Degenerative Joint Disease of the Distal Interphalangeal Joint

Degenerative joint disease of the coffin joint occurs in all breeds but may be more common in hunter-jumpers and western sport horses.

* Diagnosis often is difficult, since many horses simply appear "foot sore"; intraarticular anesthesia is necessary to localize the lameness to the joint.
* The first radiographic signs are lytic and proliferative changes on the extensor process of P3.
  * Corresponding lesions later become apparent on the distal aspect of P2.
  * Bilateral lesions are relatively common.
* Treatment should include evaluation of foot conformation and correction of imbalances.
  * In general, these horses should be shod with a relatively short, rockered toe.
  * NSAIDs usually are used in conjunction with corrective shoeing/trimming.
  * Intraarticular corticosteroids can be quite effective, but rapid deterioration of the joint may occur after repeated injections.

Contracted Heels

Contracted heels is a descriptive term, not a specific cause of lameness. It is important because it signals underlying problems.

- Causes or contributing factors include improper trimming or shoeing, chronic heel pain, lack of exercise, prolonged inability to bear weight, "club foot," and poor conformation.
- The wall of the affected heel(s) and quarter(s) develops a steeper orientation, and the frog appears recessed.
- The horse may or may not be lame at the time of examination.
- Treatment involves identifying the cause and treating it accordingly.
  - The most effective approach in horses showing no obvious cause of lameness may be to allow the horse to go without shoes and allow for plenty of exercise.

IDIOPATHIC DISEASES
Canker
Canker is progressive, chronic hypertrophy of horn-producing tissues.
- It likely is caused by an intracellular gram-negative anaerobe in the basal epidermal layers.
- Canker is most common in the hind feet of draft horses.
- The frog is most often affected; normal frog tissue is replaced by a vegetative growth.
  - The mass may be reasonably defined or may spread to involve the sole, possibly extending up the hoof wall.
- Although canker could be mistaken for severe thrush or excessive granulation tissue, it may be diagnosed by some characteristic findings.
  - numerous, small papillae of soft, off-white material primarily involving the frog
  - a fetid odor and grayish-white material exuding from the area
  - absence of lameness despite lesions that are highly sensitive to the touch and bleed easily

Treatment and prognosis
Treatment involves total excision of the mass and daily aftercare.
- Surgical debridement of infected areas should be limited to removing undermined and poorly keratinized hoof (see *Equine Medicine and Surgery V*).

- Cutting into tissues deeper than the epidermis only delays healing and risks permanent scarring and deformity of the hoof.
- Application of caustic agents before or after debridement is contraindicated.
- Topical tetracycline with or without DMSO often is effective after debridement.
  - Oral metronidazole also may be helpful.

Although many horses respond to proper treatment, canker can be a difficult problem to resolve. Lesions may recur or eventually involve other feet.

Diseases of the Pastern Region *(pages 1546-1558)*
Joerg A. Auer, Roger K.W. Smith, Peter M. Webbon, Brent A. Hague, G. Kent Carter, and Dean W. Richardson

DISEASES WITH PHYSICAL CAUSES
Fractures of the Middle Phalanx
P2 fractures occur most frequently in the rear limbs of working horses, such as polo ponies and cutting and roping horses. These fractures are categorized as *non*articular, *mon*articular, or *bi*articular and range in severity from small chip fractures to complete, comminuted fractures.

Treatment and prognosis
Treatment and prognosis vary with fracture type.
- Nonarticular fractures resulting in a bone fragment are best treated by fragment removal.
  - The prognosis is good, and the horse should be able to return to its previous activity.
  - If the fracture was caused by a penetrating foreign body and resulted in osteomyelitis, the area should be curetted and a culture taken at the time of surgery.
- Chip fractures involving either the pastern or coffin joint may be treated conservatively, but if the horse is to perform as an athlete, surgical removal is indicated.
  - The prognosis after surgery usually is good.

• Fractures involving only the pastern joint can be treated conservatively (immobilization in a cast for 2 to 3 months) or surgically (primary repair and pastern arthrodesis).
  • The prognosis for return to work is good after arthrodesis.
• Biarticular fractures carry a poor prognosis for return to soundness.
  • Treatment, if attempted, comprises internal fixation, pastern arthrodesis, and casting.

Luxations and Subluxations of the Proximal Interphalangeal Joint

Luxation accompanied by an open joint is easily diagnosed. Subluxation may present as abnormal pastern extension or flexion. Most affected animals continue to bear weight on the limb unless subluxation is associated with a fracture. With chronic subluxation, a painful response cannot be elicited during manipulation. Treatment depends on the concomitant problems. Subluxation of the pastern joint should be treated with pastern arthrodesis.

INJURIES TO THE DEEP DIGITAL FLEXOR TENDON

Tendonitis

Deep digital flexor tendonitis is far less common than superficial digital flexor tendonitis.

• It invariably is unilateral and almost always involves the tendon within the digital sheath.
• Moderate-to-severe lameness is a prominent sign, as is pain on palpation and marked subcutaneous swelling and tendon sheath effusion.
• Ultrasonography can confirm the lesion.
• General treatment principles for tendonitis should be employed (see p. 393).
  • Injection of hyaluronan into the digital sheath is advisable.
  • Pain often can be relieved by taping a wooden wedge to the foot.
• The prognosis for return to work is poor.

Tendonitis/Rupture of the Deep Digital Flexor Tendon within the Foot

This problem usually is associated with advanced navicular disease, especially if neurectomy or treatment with intrabursal steroids has been performed.

• Lameness is acute and severe; the toe lifts and the fetlock sinks with weight-bearing.
• If salvage is required, treatment should include a shoe with a caudal extension, a well-padded distal limb bandage, and an extended period of stall rest.
• In most cases euthanasia is justified, since the prognosis is hopeless for return to exercise.

Lacerations or Penetrating Injuries to the Tendons within the Pastern Region

The degree of lameness associated with pastern wounds depends on the amount of damage to the tendons and the extent of infection.

• If the deep flexor tendon has been completely transected, the toe lifts and the fetlock sinks.
• Small skin wounds require careful assessment both by palpation and ultrasonography.
• Swelling and pain over the full extent of the sheath indicate probable tendon sheath sepsis.
• Treatment varies with the type and extent of injury.
• Surgical exploration, debridement, and lavage are recommended for wounds that penetrate the digital sheath.
• If possible, severed tendon ends should be sutured and the limb supported in a cast.
• The prognosis for return to athletic activities is poor after complete transection of the deep flexor tendon within the digital sheath.
  • Partial transection has a better prognosis, although adhesions are a common complication
  • Concurrent digital sheath sepsis worsens the prognosis.

Desmitis of the Distal Sesamoidean Ligaments

Damage to the distal sesamoidean ligaments most often results from sharp trauma to the region distal to the ergot or strenuous athletic competition, especially if it involves jumping.

- Affected horses are moderately lame, and pain on palpation is found during the acute phase.
- Confirmation of the diagnosis requires ultrasonography.
- Radiography is of limited use, although enthesiophyte formation at the insertion of the ligaments, especially the obliques, is consistent with chronic strain.
  - Enthesiophytosis may be found in sound horses, however.

Treatment and prognosis

Horses with acute injuries should be rested from strenuous work.

- Ice packs are applied during the first 2 days and the limb is supported with bandages.
  - In severe cases the distal limb should be placed in a cast for 2 to 4 weeks.
- On return to exercise, work should begin with hand walking, followed by riding at a walk.
  - Affected horses should not be turned out to pasture.
- Careful attention to correct foot balance is important during the healing phase and when the horse resumes regular exercise.

The prognosis is guarded. Some horses require up to 1 year to return to soundness, and reinjury is common.

INFLAMMATORY, INFECTIOUS, AND IMMUNE DISEASES

Infection of the Proximal Interphalangeal Joint

Diagnosis and treatment of infection involving the pastern joint is based on the principles outlined on p. 394. Lavage usually is best accomplished via a needle inserted in the dorsal aspect of the joint and one in the palmar/plantar aspect. Arthrodesis is an option for nonresponsive arthritis or osteomyelitis of the pastern joint. The prognosis for recovery is somewhat better than with infections involving other joints.

MULTIFACTORIAL DISEASES

Degenerative Joint Disease of the Proximal Interphalangeal Joint

Degenerative joint disease involving the pastern joint is more common in horses that do work involving abrupt turns and stops.

- Other inciting causes include fractures, osteochondrosis, and poor conformation.
- Periarticular thickening of the pastern ("ringbone") may be associated with focal pain.
- Circling to the affected side and flexion of the digit exacerbates lameness.
- Regional anesthesia coupled with radiography frequently suffices for diagnosis.
  - Lysis and proliferation are first seen only on the dorsal aspect of distal P1 and proximal P2.
  - Diminished joint space and medial and lateral osteophytic "lipping" develop later.
- Initial treatment includes rest, NSAIDs, and correction of any hoof problems.
  - Intraarticular medications, including corticosteroids, can yield excellent results.
- Arthrodesis of the pastern joint may be performed in horses that cannot be managed by more conservative methods.

Diseases of the Fetlock Region *(pages 1558-1586)*

Dean W. Richardson, Brent A. Hague, G. Kent Carter, Roger K.W. Smith, Peter M. Webbon, Joerg A. Auer, William P. Hay, P.O. Eric Mueller, J. Lane Easter, and Jeffrey P. Watkins

DISEASES WITH PHYSICAL CAUSES

Fractures of the Proximal Phalanx

P1 fractures are one of the most common fractures in racehorses. They range in severity from clinically insignificant chips to life-threatening comminuted fractures.

Chip fractures

Chip fractures of the dorsal proximal rim of P1 are common in Thoroughbred horses.

- Joint effusion develops immediately after a gallop, and forced flexion produces pain.
  - Lameness often resolves quickly, but there may be a subsequent drop in performance.
- Cold therapy and intraarticular medications may keep the horse performing, but continued hard use, especially after administration of corticosteroids, may result in progressive joint deterioration.
- Arthroscopic removal of the fragments can prevent joint deterioration and carries an excellent prognosis.

Palmar/plantar process fractures

Fractures of the proximal plantar/palmar process of P1 may be articular or nonarticular.

- They are more common in the hind limbs, and Standardbreds appear predisposed.
- Nonarticular fractures often are an incidental finding.
- Large articular fractures can be repaired with lag screws; smaller lesions can be removed.
  - The significance of the lesion must be determined preoperatively, since these fractures can be found in horses showing no obvious clinical signs
- The prognosis for performance after fragment removal is good with 3 to 4 months of rest.

Sagittal fractures

Midsagittal P1 fractures vary in their extent.

- Short, incomplete fractures usually occur in young racehorses.
  - Although lameness often is marked, localizing signs can be subtle.
  - Three to four months of rest alone usually is adequate to allow healing.
- Longer incomplete fractures usually cause pronounced lameness that is easily localized by direct palpation and manipulation (twisting of the distal limb).
  - These fractures can be treated with external coaptation, but lag-screw fixation is preferred.
- With complete, displaced fractures, accurate surgical realignment of the joint surface is essential for a good outcome.

- The prognosis is guarded because degenerative joint changes are a common consequence.

Comminuted fractures

Comminuted P1 fractures are life-threatening injuries.

- The diagnosis is immediately obvious. Emergency immobilization with a cast or splint is recommended before the horse is transported.
- Treatment usually is indicated only for salvage purposes.
  - Often the fracture is so comminuted that internal fixation is impossible; these fractures must be treated with external coaptation.
- The prognosis for survival is guarded; collapse of the fragments usually requires euthanasia.

Medial avulsion fractures

Avulsion fractures involving the medial collateral ligament occur in young horses. The fractures have a characteristic triangular shape on dorsopalmar/plantar radiographs. Surgical repair is recommended. The prognosis is guarded because the articular cartilage often is involved.

Fractures of the Proximal Sesamoid Bones

Sesamoid fractures are common injuries in racehorses. They range in severity from nearly asymptomatic to those causing marked instability of the fetlock joint.

Apical fractures

Apical fractures are the most prevalent type of sesamoid fracture.

- They include all transverse fractures involving up to one third of the proximal portion of the bone.
  - Associated injury to the suspensory ligament is common.
- Signs include fetlock effusion and pain on flexion. Lameness is severe immediately after injury but moderates rapidly.
  - Either perineural or intraarticular anesthesia improves the horse's gait.
- Removal of the fragment is the treatment of choice in athletic horses and usually carries a favorable prognosis.

- Concurrent suspensory desmitis worsens the prognosis.

Midbody fractures

Single midbody sesamoid fractures tend to occur more often in the medial sesamoid bone.

- Lameness and swelling generally are more marked than with apical fractures.
- Comminution is common and greatly affects surgical options.
  - Rest is adequate treatment for horses being retired from athletic endeavors.
  - Surgical repair is recommended in athletic horses.
- Even with surgical repair, the prognosis for racing is guarded.
  - At least 1 year of rest is necessary before horses can return to training.

Basilar fractures

Basilar fractures are treated according to their size and shape.

- Small articular fragments can be removed arthroscopically with reasonable success
- Large fractures that involve a major portion of the distal sesamoidean ligaments' origins carry a poor prognosis for return to athletic activities.
  - Surgical realignment of the articular surface and stabilization maximizes the chance of a reasonable outcome.

Abaxial fractures

Abaxial sesamoid fractures involve avulsions of the suspensory ligament.

- Small nonarticular avulsions often can be successfully treated with rest (at least 6 months).
- Fragment removal is recommended with small articular fractures.
- Some larger articular fractures can be repaired with a lag screw.
- The prognosis is largely related to the degree of concurrent suspensory desmitis.

Axial fractures

Axial sesamoid fractures nearly always are associated with displaced lateral condylar fractures.

- They range in size from small slivers to nearly sagittal disruptions of the bone.
- Removal of small fragments and fixation of large fragments can be considered at the time of condylar fracture repair, but the prognosis is poor.
- Lytic lesions involving the axial margins of the sesamoid bones may be due to osteomyelitis or avulsion of the intersesamoidean ligament.

"Breakdown" Injuries

Traumatic disruption of the suspensory apparatus is a devastating athletic injury.

- It primarily involves one of three basic injuries:
  - displaced transverse fractures of both sesamoid bones
  - complete rupture of the distal sesamoidean ligaments
  - failure of the body or both branches of the suspensory ligament
- The radiographic appearance and position of the sesamoid bones are used to determine the type of injury present.
- Loss of fetlock support is accompanied by swelling, pain, and non–weight-bearing lameness.
- Emergency measures to support the limb help prevent further damage to soft tissues, especially the palmar vein and artery (see p. 391 for splinting techniques).
- Treatment is for salvage only.
  - The three options, depending on the type and extent of injury, are primary repair, fetlock arthrodesis, and splinting (see *Equine Medicine and Surgery V*).

Luxation of the Fetlock Joint

Most cases of fetlock luxation occur after unwitnessed trauma at pasture.

- Lameness is immediate and severe.
- Complete luxation must be treated as an emergency.
  - Some fetlock luxations can be reduced in a standing, sedated horse, but often general anesthesia is required.
  - All openly luxated joints should be meticulously debrided and lavaged and, if possible, the damaged collateral ligaments apposed (see *Equine Medicine and Surgery V*).
  - Radiographs should be made to rule out concomitant fractures.

• After the luxation has been corrected, a half-limb fiberglass cast is applied for 4 to 6 weeks.
  • Earlier cast removal, relying on bandaging and splints for support, allows more rapid rehabilitation.
• The prognosis is guarded for athletic function.

Chronic Proliferative (Villonodular) Synovitis

This condition develops when persistent inflammation results in fibrous thickening of the synovial pads in the dorsal proximal part of the fetlock joint.

• Firm swelling often is evident at the front of the fetlock.
  • Most horses show pain on full flexion and decreased range of joint motion.
• Intraarticular anesthesia eliminates the lameness.
• Radiography and ultrasonography can be used to identify the lesion.
  • A lateral projection may reveal an erosive lesion on the dorsum of the distal cannon bone.
  • Dystrophic calcification of the mass also may be evident, as may concurrent chip fractures at the dorsal proximal rim of P1.
• Medical treatment usually involves cold therapy and intraarticular hyaluronan, alone or in combination with corticosteroids.
  • In persistently lame horses, excision of the mass is recommended.

INFLAMMATORY, INFECTIOUS, AND IMMUNE DISEASES

Infectious Joint Disease

Diagnostic and therapeutic principles for managing septic arthritis are covered earlier in this chapter.

Arthroscopy allows evaluation of the cartilage and more effective lavage. The prognosis for athletic function is guarded at best.

Digital Sheath Tenosynovitis
Idiopathic tenosynovitis

Idiopathic tenosynovitis usually is not associated with lameness.

• Diagnosis is based on bilateral effusion, absence of lameness, and lack of ultrasonographic abnormalities within the digital sheath.
  • The palmar annular ligament should be carefully evaluated (see below).
• Treatment is not necessary on clinical grounds but often requested on cosmetic grounds.
  • Intrathecal injection of hyaluronan and/or corticosteroids may have some benefit.

Traumatic tenosynovitis

Fetlock overextension can result in primary tenosynovitis. Secondary inflammatory (nonseptic) tenosynovitis occurs in conjunction with injuries to the soft tissues associated with the sheath (superficial and deep digital flexor tendons, and annular ligament).

• Lameness varies with the degree and site of inflammation and the stage of disease.
• Effusion and some pain on palpation of the sheath are common findings.
  • Intrathecal anesthesia is helpful in localizing the site of lameness.
• Ultrasonography helps to confirm the diagnosis.
  • Careful inspection of the associated soft tissues should be made.
• Management of primary tenosynovitis consists of rest, cold therapy, pressure bandaging, and administration of antiinflammatory agents.
  • Intrathecal hyaluronan with or without corticosteroids may reduce adhesion formation.
• Secondary tenosynovitis requires appropriate treatment for the inciting cause.

Septic tenosynovitis

Sepsis of the digital sheath is a common sequela to penetrating wounds in the palmar/plantar aspect of the distal limb.

• Infection causes painful distention of the sheath. Lameness is severe and unrelenting unless the sheath is open.
• Ultrasonography is essential to assess the integrity of the structures within the sheath.
• Synovial aspiration and analysis is necessary to confirm the diagnosis (total protein >4 g/dL; WBC count >30,000/μL, of which >90% are neutrophils).

- A sample should be submitted for bacterial culture and sensitivity.
- Systemic antibiotics, tetanus prophylaxis, and lavage should be instigated immediately.
  - In more established cases, tenoscopy is recommended for debridement and lavage.
  - Systemic antibiotics should be continued for at least 3 weeks.

The prognosis for return to full function is favorable in horses with simple infection of <24 hours' duration but guarded with established sepsis and/or accompanying soft tissue or bony damage. Adhesions are a common consequence and their presence often precludes soundness.

Palmar Annular Ligament Syndrome

This condition involves relative constriction of the tendons within the fetlock canal.

- There is a characteristic notch at the level of the annular ligament and digital sheath distension.
- Lameness is mild to moderate and persists even after rest.
- Intrathecal anesthesia usually improves the lameness but rarely abolishes it entirely.
- Diagnosis is confirmed ultrasonographically by measuring the annular ligament thickness.
  - The distance between the skin surface and the palmar surface of the superficial digital flexor tendon normally is 3.6 ± 0.7 mm.
  - All other soft tissue structures within the sheath should be carefully evaluated.
- Early cases of *primary* annular ligament syndrome (annular desmitis) are treated with rest, analgesics, and intrathecal corticosteroids and/or hyaluronan.
  - Chronic cases require surgical transection of the annular ligament (see *Equine Medicine and Surgery V*).
- In cases of *secondary* annular ligament syndrome, treatment should be directed at the inciting cause (usually flexor tendonitis at the level of the tendon sheath).

- Symptomatic relief can be achieved by surgical transection of the annular ligament.

MULTIFACTORIAL DISEASES
Angular Limb Deformities

The most commonly diagnosed angular deformity in the fetlock region is varus.

- Attention should be given to the alignment of the carpus relative to the phalangeal region.
  - As long as both are facing the same direction, spontaneous correction may be possible.
  - If, however, the toe points straight forward and the carpus outward, surgical correction should be attempted immediately.
- These deformities do not respond well to stall rest; surgery and corrective trimming are required (see *Equine Medicine and Surgery V*).
- To be successful, *surgery should be carried out before the foal is 2 months old*.
  - After 3 to 4 months of age virtually no growth potential remains in these physes.
- If treated early, the prognosis for correction is good.

Flexural Deformity

Flexural deformity of the fetlock may be congenital or acquired.

- Congenital flexural deformity occurs in newborn foals.
- Acquired flexural deformity is most common in fast-growing yearlings. It also may occur in adult horses secondary to trauma of the flexor tendons or suspensory apparatus.
- Contracture of the superficial digital flexor tendon is most often involved; however, the deep digital flexor tendon, suspensory ligament, and fetlock joint capsule also can contribute.

Diagnosis

The condition is easily identified on physical examination.

- The fetlock is upright and often knuckles forward.
  - In severely affected foals, the fetlock may be fixed in this posi-

tion, with subsequent subluxation of the coffin joint.

- This condition usually is most severe in the forelimbs; however, examination often reveals lesser involvement of the hind limbs.

Treatment

Treatment depends on the age of the animal and the severity of the defect.

- Foals with mild to moderate congenital flexural deformity often respond well to conservative therapy, including support wraps, PVC splints, or casting.
  - Oxytetracycline therapy can facilitate tendon relaxation (see p. 409).
- In severe cases and in foals that do not respond to conservative therapy, surgery is indicated.
  - Many affected foals respond to inferior check desmotomy.
  - Proximal check desmotomy may further improve the fetlock angle, but in severe cases it may be necessary to sever the superficial digital flexor tendon or suspensory ligament.
- Most horses with mild acquired flexural deformity respond to conservative therapy.
  - One of the most important aspects is eliminating excessive dietary carbohydrate and protein and balancing copper and zinc levels.
  - Corrective shoeing, consisting of a mild heel wedge, often improves the fetlock angle.
  - NSAIDs and controlled exercise also are important.
- Surgical intervention is indicated in horses that do not respond to conservative therapy.
  - The procedure used is determined by which structure is primarily involved.
- The prognosis for mildly affected animals is good; however, recurrence can occur, especially in horses that are returned to high levels of nutrition.
  - More severely affected horses have a poor prognosis for obtaining their intended use.

Osteochondrosis of the Fetlock

The fetlock joint is often affected with osteochondrosis, manifested as OCD or subchondral bone cysts. The primary site is the distal cannon bone.

Osteochondritis dissecans

OCD lesions primarily affect the sagittal ridge of the cannon bone.

- Fetlock effusion is typical.
- Lameness is not always evident, but fetlock flexion often elicits a pain response.
- Radiographic lesions vary from mild flattening to extensive, irregular subchondral defects with multiple bony fragments on the dorsoproximal aspect of the sagittal ridge.
- Treatment either is conservative (rest, antiinflammatory drugs) or surgical.
  - When lesions are restricted to flattening or undulation, the prognosis with conservative management is good; other cases respond best to surgery.

Subchondral bone cysts

Subchondral cystic lesions most often are found in the center of the medial condyle of the cannon bone and beneath the proximal joint surface of P1.

- Lameness (with or without joint effusion) usually is the presenting complaint.
  - Lameness is exacerbated by joint flexion and alleviated by intraarticular anesthesia.
- Recommended treatment is surgical enucleation of the cystic lesions.

Degenerative Joint Disease

Treatment of an acutely traumatized fetlock joint involves rest, cold hydrotherapy, and NSAIDs. Intraarticular corticosteroids can be effective in interrupting the inflammatory process but should be followed by a period of rest. Physical factors affecting the fetlock, such as track surface, exercise schedule, and toe length, should be changed to minimize further stress on the fetlock.

Sesamoiditis

Sesamoiditis is a relatively common radiographic diagnosis.

- Radiographic changes include the following:
  - loss of the normal fine trabecular detail

- increased size and apparent number of vascular channels within the bone
- development of enthesiophytes at the site of ligamentous attachments

◆ Pain on palpation of the sesamoids and fetlock manipulation is typical and improves with nerve blocks proximal to the fetlock.

◆ Treatment includes rest and correction of any shoeing problems.

◆ It is important that vascular channels are distinguished from incomplete fractures; a longer rest period (3 to 4 months) should be prescribed for the latter.

◆ Training at a diminished intensity and use of cold therapy and intraarticular medications allow some horses to continue racing.

Diseases of the Metacarpus and Metatarsus *(pages 1586-1626)*

David N. Nunamaker, Nathanial A. White, Michael C. Schramme, Joerg A. Auer, Roger K.W. Webbon, Brent A. Hague, G. Kent Carter

DISEASES WITH PHYSICAL CAUSES

Fractures of the Third Metacarpal and Third Metatarsal Bones

Fractures in foals

Most cannon bone fractures in foals are caused by the dam stepping on the foal. The prognosis depends on initial management, so immediate steps must be taken to immobilize the fracture with a Robert-Jones bandage. Unstable diaphyseal and metaphyseal fractures are best treated by internal fixation using plates and screws.

Condylar fractures in adults

Condylar fractures are common in young racehorses.

◆ The fracture may be complete or merely a crack that originates at the joint surface and disappears as it traverses proximally.
- Complete fractures may be nondisplaced, minimally displaced, or displaced.

◆ Treatment options vary.
- Incomplete and nondisplaced fractures are treated with either rest and immobilization or lag-screw fixation (recommended for all medial condylar fractures).
- Lag-screw fixation is recommended for displaced fractures.

◆ The prognosis for return to racing is best for incomplete fractures (85% in one study, compared with 66% for complete nondisplaced fractures).
- Medial condylar fractures in the hind limb, although almost always incomplete, have the potential for catastrophic failure, even after surgical fixation.

Diaphyseal fractures

Fractures through the third metacarpal/tarsal diaphysis are more common in the forelimb and may be related to a previous stress fracture (see below). Internal fixation with two broad plates is the treatment of choice; few horses have a successful outcome if treated with external immobilization alone.

Fractures of the proximal metacarpus/tarsus

Three types of fracture may be found in the proximal cannon on dorso-palmar radiographs.

◆ Fissure fractures often are missed because the lameness, which often is resolved with intracarpal anesthesia, is assumed to be associated with the carpus.
- Rest alone can be successful in returning the horse to racing.

◆ Avulsion fractures of the proximal palmar surface are associated with the suspensory origin.
- Rest is the treatment of choice.

◆ Frontal fractures are amenable to lag-screw fixation.

Bucked Shins Complex and Stress Fractures

The bucked shins complex involves the dorsal cortex of the cannon bones in young racehorses. It includes "bucked shins" (periosteal new bone production) and cortical fractures ("stress fractures"). Pathogenesis is discussed in *Equine Medicine and Surgery V*.

Diagnosis

The usual history includes a period of race training, with clinical signs developing at or near the time of fast work.

- Pain, which often progresses from minimal to severe lameness, usually precedes clinical or radiographic evidence of periosteal new bone formation.
- Stress fractures typically are manifested acutely and are diagnosed radiographically.
  - An oblique radiolucent line progresses from the outer surface to the middle of the dorsolateral cortex; multiple lesions on the same bone are common.

Treatment

Treatment for *bucked shins* usually is directed at reducing pain and lameness, then revising the training program.

- Acutely painful horses should be rested for a few days and cold therapy and phenylbutazone used until the shins are no longer painful on palpation.
- The horse then is started back in work, with the galloping distance cut in half and short (1 furlong) breezes introduced and gradually increased in distance over several weeks.
- If a raised profile has developed over the dorsal cannon and there is marked periosteal new bone formation on radiographs, the horse should be taken out of training.

Most *stress fractures* are treated conservatively.

- The horse is rested until the area is no longer painful; hand walking may be beneficial.
- A controlled exercise program then slowly progresses through ponying, jogging on the track, slow galloping, and eventual resumption of full training.
- Radiographic reassessment should continue at monthly intervals until healing is complete.

Second and Fourth Metacarpal/Metatarsal Fractures

Splint bone fractures can occur anywhere along the bone.

- Fractures can be either simple or multiple (most common in the upper half of the bone).

- Spontaneous fracture in the distal third often is associated with suspensory desmitis.
  - Clinical signs are determined by the degree of suspensory desmitis.
- Open fractures are caused by trauma and are most common in the lateral splint bone.
  - Osteomyelitis and sequestration are common sequelae and cause persistent lameness accompanied by chronic or intermittent purulent discharge and delayed wound healing.
  - Contamination of the carpometacarpal/tarsometatarsal joint can occur with open fractures involving the proximal aspect of the splint bone.
- Definitive diagnosis is made by radiography.
  - Radiographs should be carefully inspected for hairline fractures of the cannon bone.
  - Ultrasonography also is recommended to evaluate the suspensory ligament.

Treatment

Treatment of *closed* fractures depends on the location and extent of the fracture.

- Some splint bone fractures heal with stall rest and support wraps.
- Surgical removal of distal portion often is recommended, especially for distal fractures.
- Fractures involving the proximal third of the medial splint bone, especially if intraarticular, can be repaired with a small bone plate.

Treatment of *open* fractures comprises the following:

- wound lavage and debridement
- stall rest, daily wound cleaning, and a support wrap
- systemic antibiotic therapy until wound drainage ceases
- surgical removal of sequestra and damaged bone if drainage persists after 7 to 10 days

Prognosis

The prognosis depends on the location and extent of the fracture.

- With simple fractures, the prognosis is good after distal fragment removal unless complicated by suspensory desmitis.

• The prognosis after removal of the majority of a splint bone also is favorable, but persistent lameness may require prolonged rest or use of internal fixation.
• Open fractures generally have a good prognosis unless they are intraarticular.

Exostoses and Splints

Splints (exostoses between the second and third metacarpal bones in the proximal third of the medial metacarpus) are common in young horses. Pain and lameness initially may be moderate; chronic splints usually are not painful but merely are blemishes. Treatment in the first 2 to 3 days includes cold therapy, bandages, and, after a week, sweats.

Tendon Lacerations in the Metacarpal Region: Digital Flexor Tendon Lacerations

The size of the laceration cannot be used to indicate the extent of the injury; rather, the structure lacerated can be deduced from the stance.
• With laceration of the superficial digital flexor tendon, the fetlock overextends and drops when the limb is loaded; at other times, the fetlock angle is normal.
• With laceration of both flexor tendons below the insertion of the inferior check ligament, the fetlock drops and the toe tips up.
  • Concurrent suspensory ligament laceration results in complete loss of fetlock support.
Further evaluation is made during surgical debridement and repair of the tendon (see *Equine Medicine and Surgery V*).

Tendon Lacerations in the Metacarpal Region: Digital Extensor Tendon Lacerations

Complete transection of the digital extensor tendons produces few clinical signs.
• There may initially be knuckling of the fetlock when the horse walks.
• Treatment simply consists of wound debridement; tendon repair is not necessary.
  • A dorsal splint incorporated into a bandage can be used if the horse is knuckling.

• The prognosis for a full return to expected performance is good in most cases.

Tendonitis of the Superficial Digital Flexor Tendon

Diagnosis of superficial digital flexor tendonitis can be made by clinical examination.
• There is heat, swelling ("bow"), and pain associated with the flexor tendon.
  • The most severe damage usually is centered just distal to the mid-metacarpal region.
• Lameness is variable but often is severe in the acute stages.
  • Lameness usually resolves once the acute phase has passed.
Ultrasonography is essential for the best possible outcome.
• The typical ultrasonographic appearance is a concentric ("core") hypoechoic lesion.
• Other changes include an increase in cross-sectional area and alterations in shape of the tendon (see *Equine Medicine and Surgery V*).
Treatment and prognosis
The general principles of treatment are discussed on p. 393. The most important factor determining prognosis is the severity of the original injury. In one study, 100% of mildly affected horses returned to work and 63% raced; 50% of moderately affected horses returned to work and 30% raced; and only 30% of severely affected horses returned to work, with only 23% racing. Another factor is the location of the injury. Lesions within the digital sheath frequently heal poorly.

Desmitis of the Inferior Check Ligament

Desmitis of the accessory ligament of the deep digital flexor tendon (inferior check ligament) is a passive injury associated with overextension of the digit.
• It usually affects only one limb but may occur bilaterally.
• Lameness is mild to moderate. Swelling usually is apparent in the proximal metacarpal region, and pressure on the ligament elicits a pain response.
• Confirmation of the diagnosis is provided by ultrasonographic examination.

- Lesions range from localized hypoechoic regions to thickening of the whole ligament.
- Concurrent superficial digital flexor tendonitis exists in some cases.
- Treatment principles are the same as for tendonitis (see p. 393).
  - An initial period of rest is followed by a gradual controlled ascending exercise regimen over a 3- to 5-month period, with regular repeated ultrasonographic examinations.
- The prognosis is fair to good depending on the quality of healing and the extent of adhesions.

Proximal and High Suspensory Disease

With this condition, lameness is variable and its onset may be insidious or acute.

- In acute cases, swelling and pain may be appreciated dorsal to the digital flexor tendons in the proximal metacarpal region.
  - Many chronic cases show minimal clinical signs.
- Diagnostic local anesthesia is necessary to confirm the site of pain (see p. 387).
- Ultrasonography is the best diagnostic aid.
  - Clinically significant lesions range from poor definition of the ligament's margins through focal hypoechoic lesions to generalized thickening of the ligament.
- Associated sclerotic changes and small avulsion fractures can be identified radiographically.
- Treatment consists of a controlled ascending exercise regimen over a 3-month period for forelimb cases and up to 9 months for hind limb cases.
- The prognosis is good to fair; forelimb lesions carry a better prognosis than hind limb lesions (86% versus 17% in one study).
  - The presence of radiographic changes worsens the prognosis.

Desmitis of the Body of the Suspensory Ligament

This injury is more common in racehorses and affects the forelimbs more frequently than the hind limbs, except in Standardbreds. It may be associated with splint bone fracture (see p. 419). Diagnosis by palpation usually is not difficult, but ultrasonography enables an accurate assessment of the extent and severity. Treatment is similar to that described for tendon injuries (see p. 420). The prognosis is guarded because of the high incidence of reinjury.

Suspensory Branch Injury

Suspensory branch desmitis is the most common suspensory injury.

- Lameness is variable, but there usually is palpable enlargement of the affected branches.
- Diagnosis can be confirmed by ultrasonography.
  - Changes include periligamentar fibrosis, enlargement, shape alterations, focal or generalized hypoechoic regions ("core" lesions), and poor definition of the margins.
  - Enthesiophytosis along the abaxial surface of the sesamoid bone and small avulsion fractures at the insertion of the branches also may be seen.
- Radiography is recommended to assess concurrent bony lesions, such as fractured splint bones and sesamoiditis.
- Treatment is as for tendon injuries (see p. 393).
- The prognosis is guarded because reinjury is common.
  - Persistence of lesions does not preclude successful return to work, but reinjury is more likely in these cases.

Diseases of the Carpal Region *(pages 1626-1643)*

Dean W. Richardson, Carl A. Kirker-Head, Brent A. Hague, G. Kent Carter, Joerg A. Auer, William P. Hay, and P.O. Eric Mueller

DISEASES WITH PHYSICAL CAUSES

Chip Fractures

Radiocarpal fractures

These chip fractures occur almost exclusively in racing Thoroughbreds and Quarter Horses.

- Signs generally are subtle, even with sizable fractures.

- Many horses appear sound within only a few days after injury, but with continued work, there often is decreased performance.
- Swelling over the radiocarpal joint often is observed, and sometimes lateral outpouching of the joint capsule is quite prominent.
- In acute injuries, direct pressure over the site may cause pain.
- Pain on full carpal flexion is helpful for diagnosis but is not always present.
- Intraarticular anesthesia improves the horse's gait, but radiography is necessary for diagnosis.
- Arthroscopic removal of the fragment carries an excellent prognosis for return to racing.
  - In acute fractures with minimal degenerative change, many horses can return to race training in 6 weeks; more severely damaged joints require a longer convalescent period.

Middle carpal fractures

The middle carpal joint is the most common site of carpal lesions in horses that work at speed.

- Lameness usually is more pronounced and effusion is more obvious than with radiocarpal chip fractures.
- Radiographic evaluation of this joint should include dorsopalmar, medial and lateral oblique, "skyline," and flexed and standing lateromedial projections.
- Arthroscopic fragment removal is the treatment of choice.
  - A horse with minor joint damage can begin swimming or a progressive hand-walking program within 2 weeks of surgery and can begin galloping 4 to 6 weeks later.
  - In horses with extensive cartilage damage, 4 to 6 months of rest is recommended.
- The prognosis depends on the degree of degenerative joint disease and fracture location; fractures of the proximal row carry a better prognosis than those of the distal row.

Slab Fractures

Slab fractures are those that involve both the proximal and distal articular surfaces of the cuboidal bones.

- In the carpus, >95% of such fractures involve the third carpal bone.
- There usually is moderate to marked lameness, with obvious middle carpal effusion and pain on flexion; with nondisplaced fractures, signs may be much more subtle.
- Slab fractures should be identified on at least two radiographic projections.
  - They are best seen on a dorsolateral oblique or a standing lateromedial view.
  - A "skyline" view is essential to evaluate the medial to lateral width of the fracture.
- Lag-screw fixation, fragment removal, and rest are the three treatment options.
  - Rest is a reasonable treatment only for nondisplaced fractures; however, screw fixation lessens the chance of later displacement and improves healing of the articular surface.
- Though some horses have raced successfully as soon as 3 months after screw fixation, 6 months is a more realistic goal, and many horses take up to 1 year to return to racing.
- A guarded prognosis must be given, especially if the fracture is severe.
  - A large percentage of horses with simple slab fractures return to racing, although a drop in class and a shortened career can be expected.

Sagittal fractures of the third carpal bone

Sagittal or near-sagittal fractures occur most commonly on the medial side of the bone.

- Identification on views other than the skyline is difficult.
- Lag-screw fixation and rest are the treatment alternatives.
  - Six to twelve months of rest usually results in healing and soundness.
  - An obviously displaced fracture warrants a much worse prognosis.

Accessory Carpal Bone Fractures

Accessory carpal bone fractures typically are longitudinal and seen most easily on lateromedial projections. Most of these fractures are nonarticular, and despite the fibrous nonunion that develops, many heal satisfactorily with extended rest (6 to 12 months). Carpal canal syndrome can develop if the injury and subsequent healing impinge on the carpal canal (see below).

Comminuted Carpal Fractures

Comminuted fractures of the carpus occur as both racing and pasture accidents. Euthanasia often is justified. Reconstruction with lag screws, coupled with external coaptation, may be an option if large fragments are present. External coaptation alone is successful in a few cases, but severe carpal varus often is a long-term consequence. Arthrodesis could be considered for severely comminuted, unstable carpal fractures. But no matter what treatment is selected, laminitis in the contralateral foot is a common complication.

Carpal Canal Syndrome

Fracture of the accessory carpal bone with subsequent fibrosis and bony callus is the most common cause of carpal canal lameness.

- Flexor tendonitis, carpal sheath tenosynovitis, and osteochondroma of the distal radius are other causes.
- Signs include pain on palpation and exacerbation of lameness with carpal flexion; distention of the carpal sheath often is evident proximally.
- Intrasynovial anesthesia of the flexor sheath improves the horse's gait in most cases.
- Ultrasonography and radiography are useful for diagnosis and determining treatment options.
- Treatment is directed at resolution of the primary problem.
  - Acute synovitis is treated with stall rest and intrasynovial injection of corticosteroids.
  - Osteochondromas are treated by excision of the bony protuberance.
  - With accessory carpal bone nonunion or chronically thickened tendon and tendon sheath, relief is afforded by incision of the flexor retinaculum (see *Equine Medicine and Surgery V*).

Rupture of the Extensor Carpi Radialis

Rupture of the extensor carpi radialis tendon may be partial or complete and usually occurs within the tendon sheath.

- Acute injury is accompanied by pain and distention of the tendon sheath; extension and flexion of the carpus are limited, and the toe may be dragged.
- Tendon sheath effusion persists in the chronic injury, but the condition is painless unless inflammatory tenosynovitis remains.
- The site of the rupture usually is palpable over the proximal carpus; ultrasound can help characterize tendon sheath injury and adhesions.
- Acute, complete rupture is treated surgically with tenoscopic debridement and lavage.
  - Return to soundness after surgery is variable.
- Surgical treatment of chronic rupture generally is less successful; tenolysis and partial tenosynovectomy are of benefit in some cases.

Rupture of the Common Digital Extensor Tendon

Rupture of the common digital extensor tendon is most common in neonatal foals and often is bilateral.

- It may be primary or secondary to flexural deformity of the fetlock or carpus.
- Rupture causes swelling of the tendon sheath on the dorsolateral aspect of the carpus; affected foals stand with their carpi slightly flexed and may knuckle over on their fetlocks.
- Carpal radiographs should be obtained to rule out cuboidal bone malformation.
- Treatment involves stall rest and use of a well-padded wrap and PVC splint from elbow to fetlock; the splints are maintained for 2 to 4 weeks.
- Foals with primary tendon rupture have an excellent prognosis.

Carpal Hygroma (Capped Knee)

Carpal hygroma describes a traumatically induced, subcutaneous, synovial-lined, fluid-filled swelling (bursa) overlying the dorsal aspect of the carpus.

◆ Most begin as a hematoma, but with repeated trauma a bursa develops.

◆ Carpal hygromas generally are painless.

◆ Ultrasonography can be used to characterize the lesion.
   • Radiographs can help determine extent of the lesion and identify any joint disease, foreign bodies, and synovial hernias or fistulae.

◆ In the acute phase, subcutaneous hematomas respond well to hydrotherapy, pressure bandaging, and limb immobilization.
   • Larger hematomas may need to be drained ventrally 10 to 14 days after onset.

◆ Established bursae may be treated with surgical excision or cauterization (see *Equine Medicine and Surgery V*).

◆ The prognosis is good with treatment of subcutaneous hematomas; acquired bursitis warrants a guarded prognosis for complete resolution.

INFLAMMATORY, INFECTIOUS, AND IMMUNE DISEASES
Infectious Joint Disease
Guidelines for diagnosis and treatment of infectious arthritis are given on p. 394. The prognosis for septic arthritis of the carpus is guarded at best.

MULTIFACTORIAL DISEASES
Angular Limb Deformities
Most angular limb deformities occur in the carpal region. A dorsopalmar radiograph directed perpendicular to the frontal plane of the distal radius is the most important diagnostic aid (see *Equine Medicine and Surgery V*).
Treatment
Treatment depends on the location and severity of the defect.

◆ Foals with minimal incomplete ossification and straight limbs benefit from stall rest.

◆ Foals with incomplete ossification and angular limb deformities should be treated with splints or tube casts and stall rest.

• Radiographic evaluation at 2-week intervals is indicated until the carpal bones are sufficiently ossified to permit weight bearing without external support.

◆ When an early deformity is primarily caused by soft tissue laxity as a result of the abnormal loading, splinting or casting may be effective.

◆ Periosteal transection and stripping is the treatment of choice for deformities caused by asynchronous growth (see *Equine Medicine and Surgery V*).
   • In severe cases or in older foals, this procedure may be combined with a growth-retardation technique for faster and more complete correction.

Flexural Deformity
Flexural deformity of the carpus in foals generally is a congenital condition, although it may be acquired in foals that are recumbent as a result of severe illness or injury.

◆ The deformity can range from mild buckling of the carpus in the standing foal to severe flexion that results in dystocia and a foal that is unable to stand.

◆ Manual manipulation often results in only partial improvement in the angle of the carpus.

◆ Radiographs should be obtained to rule out bony malformation of the carpus.

◆ Foals with mild contracture often improve without treatment in the first few days of life.

◆ In other foals, a full-limb support wrap and PVC splint, applied on the palmar aspect from elbow to fetlock, can be used to straighten the limb.
   • The leg must be well padded as rub sores can develop quickly.

◆ In foals with severe flexural deformity that does not respond to splinting, surgery may be performed in an attempt to release tension in the palmar aspect of the carpal joints.

◆ The prognosis is guarded for severely affected foals and poor for foals that require surgery.

Osteochondrosis of the Carpus

The most commonly reported manifestation of osteochondrosis in the carpus is a cystlike lesion. These lesions often cause lameness but may be incidental findings. Treatment generally is conservative; rest or controlled exercise in conjunction with NSAIDs is successful in most cases.

Degenerative Joint Disease

Degenerative joint disease of the carpus generally is a consequence of racing.

* Radiographic changes include marginal osteophytes, enthesiophytosis, loss of radiographic joint space, and changes in density of the subchondral bone (either lysis or sclerosis).
  * A common manifestation is subchondral sclerosis of the third carpal bone.
* Chip, central surface, and slab fractures must be identified and treated, but even with early treatment, all that can be hoped for is halting of the degenerative process.
* Intraarticular hyaluronan or polysulfated glycosaminoglycan can be beneficial.
* Proper conditioning and adjustments in shoeing and training surfaces also are important.

Diseases of the Forearm and Elbow Region

(pages 1643-1656)

Joerg A. Auer, Jeffrey P. Watkins, Carl A. Kirker-Head, Brent A. Hague, G. Kent Carter, J. Lane Easter, and Robert D. Welch

DISEASES WITH PHYSICAL CAUSES

Radial Fractures

Epiphyseal fractures

Signs of epiphyseal fracture include acute, non–weight-bearing lameness with regional swelling, heat, and instability. Immediate application of a bandage and splint is indicated (see p. 391). Surgical stabilization is the treatment of choice. Fractures of the distal radial physis have a better prognosis than proximal physeal fractures.

Complete metaphyseal and diaphyseal fractures

Diagnosis of complete fractures is straightforward; emergency treatment is described on p. 391. Distal metaphyseal fractures may be treated conservatively with a splint or cast, although this is merely a salvage procedure; it does not allow resumption of an athletic career. From the diaphysis proximally, conservative treatment with a cast is no longer an option. Internal fixation is necessary if euthanasia is not elected.

Incomplete radial fractures

Occasionally, horses are presented with severe, non–weight-bearing lameness localized to the radial region, but with no definite evidence of a fracture. Such an animal should be managed as if the radius is fractured; the entire limb should be placed under a splint bandage and the horse prevented from lying down in the stall. Radiographic evaluation repeated 3 to 4 days later frequently reveals a fissure fracture. Conservative treatment is appropriate for these fractures.

Impression fractures

Impression fractures resulting from a kick frequently are open fractures. Debridement and drainage of the wound should be performed and the fragment removed, if it is small, to prevent sequestrum formation.

Ulnar Fractures

Olecranon fractures commonly occur in horses that sustain a direct blow to the elbow.

* Characteristically the elbow is dropped and the carpus is maintained in a flexed position, although the horse maybe able to place the foot flat on the ground.
  * Differential diagnoses include radial nerve paralysis (see Chapter 11, Nervous System) and humeral fracture (see p. 426).
* There is a variable degree of soft tissue swelling and crepitation.
* Medial-to-lateral radiographs taken with the limb extended best define the fracture.
* As an emergency measure, a splint should be applied over a padded bandage from the ground

to the proximal forearm to allow the horse to bear weight on the limb.

- Nondisplaced, nonarticular fractures and some nondisplaced articular fractures of the distal olecranon can be managed conservatively (strict stall confinement and possibly splinting).
- Displaced and most articular fractures require internal fixation (see *Equine Medicine and Surgery V*).
- With proper case selection, the prognosis for both conservative and surgical therapy is good.

Hygroma at the Point of the Elbow (Olecranon Bursitis, Capped Elbow, Shoe Boil)

This condition is characterized by soft tissue swelling over the olecranon tuberosity.

- It is most commonly caused by the hoof of the affected limb chronically traumatizing the point of the elbow while the horse is sternally recumbent.
  - Predisposing factors include prolonged recumbency, poor bedding, long heels, and use of shoes with trailers or caulks.
- Lameness generally is not seen, except in the acute stage or if the lesion becomes infected.
- Radiographs can be used to rule out osseous lesions; ultrasonography also may be beneficial.
- Treatment includes removal of the inciting cause and cauterization or excision of the bursa (see *Equine Medicine and Surgery V*).

INFLAMMATORY, INFECTIOUS AND IMMUNE DISEASES
Infectious Joint Disease

Guidelines for diagnosis and treatment of infectious arthritis are discussed on p. 394. Joint distention and periarticular edema often are not readily apparent in this joint. Lavage usually is accomplished with needles rather than with arthroscopy. As diagnosis often is delayed, septic arthritis of the elbow tends to have a poorer prognosis than other joints.

MULTIFACTORIAL DISEASES
Osteochondrosis

Although rare, manifestations of osteochondrosis in the elbow include osteochondrosis dissecans of the lateral humeral condyle, subchondral bone cysts of the proximal medial radius and osteochondrosis-like lesions of the anconeal process. Treatment options include stall rest, intraarticular medication, and surgical treatment. The prognosis for athletic performance is guarded for all methods of therapy.

IDIOPATHIC DISEASES
Osteochondroma (Supracarpal Volar Exostoses)

Osteochondromas are solitary bony exostoses that most often occur at the distal caudal diaphysis or metaphysis of the radius. Findings include a fluctuant swelling of the carpal sheath proximal to the accessory carpal bone and pain on deep palpation of the caudodistal radius. Lameness may be present at the trot. Occasionally the bony protuberance can be palpated, but the diagnosis is made radiographically. Treatment options include stall rest, corticosteroid injections into the carpal sheath, and surgical removal of the exostosis.

Diseases of the Proximal Forearm *(pages 1656-1658)*
Jeffrey P. Watkins

DISEASES WITH PHYSICAL CAUSES
Fractures of the Humerus
Complete diaphyseal fractures

Horses with complete, displaced diaphyseal fractures are unable to bear weight on the limb.

- The elbow drops and the limb is carried in a flexed position.
  - Manipulation elicits a painful response, but soft tissue swelling and the overlying musculature may mask crepitus.
- Some degree of radial nerve injury inevitably accompanies these fractures (see Chapter 11, Nervous System).

◆ Diagnostic radiographs usually can be achieved in the standing, sedated patient.

◆ Stall confinement may be successful in foals with long oblique fractures.
  • Splinting the carpus to facilitate weight bearing can prevent complications.

◆ Short oblique or transverse fractures in foals <250 kg (550 lb) require internal fixation.

◆ Euthanasia usually is recommended with these fractures in larger foals and adult horses.

Incomplete fractures of the proximal humerus

Incomplete metaphyseal ("stress") fractures at the proximocaudal cortex can occur in young Thoroughbred racehorses. The degree of lameness varies greatly. Severe cases may mimic radial nerve paralysis in the acute phase. In more moderate cases, the lameness may resolve after a few days of stall rest. Radiography and/or nuclear scintigraphy are necessary for diagnosis; oblique radiographic views are essential. These fractures usually respond well to stall rest for a minimum of 6 weeks, followed by 6 weeks of controlled walking.

Diseases of the Shoulder

(pages 1658-1669)

Sue J. Dyson

DISEASES WITH PHYSICAL CAUSES

Fracture of the Supraglenoid Tubercle

Fracture of the supraglenoid tubercle usually is a sequela to trauma.

◆ In the acute phase, the horse may bear weight incompletely on the injured limb.
  • Diffuse soft tissue swelling is present, and the horse may resent deep palpation and/or manipulation. Occasionally, crepitus is audible or palpable.
  • Severe lameness is obvious at the walk.

◆ Most horses experience slow but progressive improvement, although moderate lameness usually persists,

and atrophy of supraspinatus and infraspinatus muscles may develop.

◆ The diagnosis is confirmed radiographically.

◆ Treatment depends on whether the fracture is single or multiple, articular or nonarticular.
  • Occasionally, a nondisplaced fracture heals with rest; usually, however, nonunion results and lameness persists.
  • Surgical removal of the fragment(s) is successful in some horses.

◆ Degenerative joint disease and/or calcification in or around the biceps brachii tendon are potential sequelae and warrant a guarded prognosis.

Other Fractures of the Scapula

Fractures of the glenoid cavity or body of the scapula usually are the result of a fall and cause severe and sometimes non–weight-bearing lameness.

◆ Occasionally, crepitus can be detected with articular fractures or complete fractures through the scapular neck.
  • Usually, there is considerable soft tissue swelling with complete, displaced fractures.

◆ Some nondisplaced, nonarticular fractures heal with stall rest, allowing full athletic function.

◆ Complete transverse fractures of the scapular neck have been successfully repaired with bone plates in small, immature horses.

◆ Displaced fractures in adult horses and articular fractures warrant a poor prognosis.

Instability of the Scapulohumeral Joint

Instability of the shoulder joint (shoulder slip) usually is a sequel to traumatic injury that results in suprascapular and/or brachial plexus neuropathy.

◆ Most horses can bear some weight on the limb, but the proximal humerus suddenly moves or "pops" abaxially.

◆ Atrophy of supraspinatus and infraspinatus muscles develops within

7 to 14 days; other muscles also may be affected.

- In the acute stage, antiinflammatory analgesics are recommended.
  - Electrical muscle stimulation helps maintain muscle mass.
- Surgical release of the suprascapular nerve is beneficial in some horses (see *Equine Medicine and Surgery V*).
- Some horses spontaneously improve, though it may be 6 to 9 months before the gait abnormality resolves, and muscle atrophy may persist despite resolution of lameness.

Luxation of the Scapulohumeral Joint

Luxation of the shoulder usually is the result of trauma and causes severe, non–weight-bearing lameness and a variable amount of soft tissue swelling.

- The humerus may be displaced medially or laterally.
  - Fractures of the glenoid cavity and/or humerus may occur concurrently.
- Radiography is necessary to confirm the direction of luxation and identify concurrent fracture(s).
- If major damage to the articular surfaces is detected, treatment should not be attempted.
- In uncomplicated cases, closed reduction under general anesthesia can be successful.

INFLAMMATORY, INFECTIOUS, AND IMMUNE DISEASES

Intertubercular (Bicipital) Bursitis

Inflammation of the intertubercular (bicipital) bursa may arise iatrogenically, secondary to trauma, or as a result of infection.

- Lameness is extremely variable.
  - With acute infection, lameness is moderate to severe and is characterized by a markedly short cranial phase of the stride and low arc of foot flight.
  - Palpation causes pain, and flexion of the shoulder and/or retraction of the limb are strongly resented.
  - With chronic infection and with nonseptic bursitis and/or tendonitis the lameness may be mild

to moderate, with no localizing signs and no pain on palpation or manipulation.

- Diagnosis may involve the use of intrabursal anesthesia (see p. 388), synovial fluid analysis, ultrasonography, and/or radiography.
- In acute nonseptic bursitis, repeated intrabursal administration of corticosteroids and/or hyaluronan may produce good results.
- Biceps brachii tendonitis is treated with extended stall rest and controlled exercise (for 6 to 9 months), intrabursal injection of hyaluronan, and systemic NSAIDs.
  - However, long-term results may be poor.
- The same principles apply to treatment of infectious bursitis as for infectious arthritis.

Infectious Arthritis

Diagnosis and treatment of infectious arthritis are discussed on p. 394. It can be difficult to perform through-and-through lavage in the shoulder joint, but a distention-irrigation technique usually is satisfactory.

MULTIFACTORIAL DISEASES

Osteochondritis Dissecans

OCD of the shoulder joint is more common in Thoroughbreds and usually causes lameness within the first 18 months of life, though occasionally lameness is not recognized until later.

- Typically the lameness is unilateral, though subclinical radiographic abnormalities sometimes are identified in the contralateral limb.
  - The severity of the gait abnormality varies from mild to severe.
- Intraarticular anesthesia is useful in many cases, but lack of response does not preclude the joint as a source of pain.
- Radiography may identify lesions in the scapula and/or humerus, predominantly in the caudal half of the joint (see *Equine Medicine and Surgery V*).
  - Arthrography may be used to highlight subtle lesions and identify cartilage flaps.

- The degree of lameness correlates poorly with the severity of radiographic abnormalities.
- Conservative therapy generally is of limited benefit in horses destined for an athletic career.
- Most young horses improve with surgery, and some become sound enough to train and race.
- Older horses with marked subchondral sclerosis or other extensive degenerative changes have a guarded prognosis.

Osseous Cystlike Lesions

Osseous cystlike lesions (well-defined, discrete radiolucent lesions) in the scapula or humerus are seen most commonly in horses <3 years of age but are an occasional cause of lameness in older horses. With stall rest and possibly intraarticular hyaluronan or polysulfated glycosaminoglycan, some horses have become sound and remained so. A few horses have been treated by curettage of the cysts, with variable results.

Degenerative Joint Disease

Degenerative joint disease of the shoulder generally is a sequela to an articular fracture, luxation or subluxation, infectious arthritis, or osteochondrosis lesion. Lameness varies from mild to moderate and is usually improved, but not alleviated, by intraarticular anesthesia. The prognosis for athletic function is guarded.

Diseases of the Head and Neck *(pages 1669-1676)*
J. Lane Easter and Jeffrey P. Watkins

DIAGNOSTIC CONSIDERATIONS

Physical examination should include complete evaluation of the status of the head and oral cavity. Trauma to the skull often causes swelling, crepitus, and deformity at the site of injury. Certain functions, such as alimentation, vision, and respiration may be disturbed.

Radiography of the equine head can be accomplished by most x-ray machines available to practitioners today, with high-speed screen and film combinations.

CONGENITAL AND FAMILIAL DISEASES

Parrot Mouth (Brachygnathia)

Parrot mouth is the most common congenital oral malformation of horses.

- In this condition the maxilla is relatively longer than the mandible, resulting in lack of contact between the occlusal surfaces of the upper and lower incisors.
- Affected animals exhibit ruptured common digital extensors, underdeveloped pectoral muscles, and goiter. This is considered to be a hereditary condition.
- In foals with severe malocclusion that impairs their ability to eat, growth of the maxilla can be slowed by application of wire braces extending from the upper cheek teeth to the incisors.

Wry Nose

Severe deviation of the nasal septum and premaxilla (wry nose) is an infrequently reported congenital condition in foals. Severely affected foals may be unable to nurse and may have extreme difficulty breathing. Surgical correction has been reported. Because the heritability of the condition is unknown, patients chosen for surgery should be sterilized as well.

DISEASES WITH PHYSICAL CAUSES

Mandibular and Maxillary Fractures

Fractures of the mandible and maxilla are a common equine head injury.

Causes

- direct blow to the head, such as from a kick
- when the mandible is caught in a stationary object and the horse suddenly pulls away
- iatrogenic trauma during repulsion of cheek teeth

Clinical Signs

- history of trauma to the head
- difficult mastication
- malocclusion

• varying degrees of instability.
Nondisplaced fractures of the mandible that include the alveolus of a cheek tooth may go unnoticed until signs of alveolar periostitis become evident.

Diagnosis

• Physical examination reveals varying degrees of soft tissue swelling and mandibular or maxillary instability.
• Manipulation of the area elicits pain and may produce crepitus.
• Oral examination reveals the fracture opening into the oral cavity.

Treatment

Horses with unstable or painful fractures of the mandible or maxilla may suffer severe debility if therapy is delayed. They cannot eat or drink and become dehydrated and emaciated, requiring fluid therapy and special feeding applications.

Conservative treatment is indicated for stable fractures with minimal malocclusion, typical of unilateral body and ramus, as well as some fractures of the maxilla. If radiographic evidence of healing is not present within 6 weeks of the injury, internal fixation should be considered.

Indications for internal fixation
• unstable fractures
• those that cause significant malocclusion
• those that cause pain or disability that prevents eating

Perioperative considerations
• rehydration
• attention to nutritional status
• perioperative antimicrobial therapy
• tetanus prophylaxis

Fixation techniques for rostral mandibular fractures include:
• partial incisor avulsion, including stainless-steel wire fixation alone
• wire fixation in combination with stainless-steel pins and lag-screw fixation

Fractures involving interdental space should not be treated with wire fixation alone, because this may not provide adequate stability. Thus wire fixation should be supplemented with pin or lag-screw fixation across the fracture line.

Fixation of unstable body fractures, particularly bilateral injuries:
• plate application
• use of an intraoral U-bar wired to the cheek teeth and incisors
• intramedullary pinning
• external skeletal fixators.

Treatment for markedly displaced or highly unstable bilateral body fractures:
• bone plating
• U-bar fixation
• external skeletal fixators

Alternative technique: Use of methyl methacrylate as an intraoral splint wired to the teeth or to the body of the mandible or premaxilla. Both U-bar and methyl methacrylate splintage require minimal surgical invasion.

Another option for stabilization of mandibular body fractures is placement in a type II external skeletal fixator.

Fractures into the temporomandibular joint or fractures separating the ramus from the condylar process of the mandible present special problems. Treatment by mandibular condylectomy has been suggested, but this procedure requires further evaluation.

Complications

• Chronic infection and fistula formation caused by sequestration of bone fragments are not common because of the excellent blood supply to the region.
• Alveolar periostitis may develop if the fracture involves an alveolus of a tooth.
• Nonunion may occur, primarily with bilateral mandibular body fractures at the rostral aspect of the alveolus of the first cheek tooth.

Temporomandibular Joint Luxation

• Injuries to the temporomandibular joint are rare in horses.
• Rostral displacement of the mandible results in malocclusion of the caudal cheek teeth, which meet prematurely and prevent contact between the upper and lower incisors.
  • *Therapy:* Increase the occlusal surface area of the teeth and reduce the gap between the incisors by floating the maloccluded molars.

Facial Fractures

Cause

The frontal, nasal, lacrimal, and zygomatic bones are commonly affected, as well as the maxilla. Facial fractures may concurrently affect the paranasal sinuses, nasal cavity, nasal septum, teeth, and globe.

Prevention

* use of padded restraining stocks
* care in securing lead ropes
* use of fences with less potential for causing injury
* removing excessively aggressive horses from the herd
* behavior modification of "head-shy" horse

Clinical Signs

* Deformation of facial contour will be present.
* An open wound occasionally is present.
* Crepitation, instability, and pain on palpation may be present but become less evident as the injury becomes chronic and fibrosis occurs.
* If the fracture enters the nasal cavity or paranasal sinuses, epistaxis is a concomitant sign.

Diagnosis

* Careful deep palpation may be required to identify fracture fragments and crepitation through the overlying hematoma and swollen soft tissue.
* Radiographic evaluation is indicated to confirm fracture location, establish the degree of displacement, and identify nondisplaced fracture lines.

Treatment

* *conservative management:* when the fracture fragments are minimally displaced and vital functions are not impaired (e.g., ocular entrapment, respiratory compromise)
  * protective bandages
  * antimicrobial agents
* *reconstructive surgery:*
  * when facial deformation is significant or vital functions are impaired
  * best performed on an elective basis as soon after fracture as feasible
  * Delays exceeding 72 hours may prevent good realignment of fracture fragments

* *reduction methods:*
  * Strategically place holes in the adjacent bone through which instruments can be introduced to elevate the fragments into place from beneath without disturbing the edges of the fracture.
  * Drill holes in the bone fragments, introduce a bone hook, and elevate the fragments into reduction.
* *perioperative and postoperative care:*
  * Perioperative antimicrobial agents are indicated for fractures that open into the upper respiratory tract or those accompanied by a skin wound.
  * The head should be protected with a padded helmet during recovery from anesthesia to prevent additional trauma.
  * Bandages help prevent subcutaneous emphysema and accumulation of wound fluids.

Complications

* Loss of skin and bone, as may occur with severe injuries, may predispose to development of a mucocutaneous fistula into the affected sinus or nasal cavity.
* Tubes should be positioned to provide for postoperative sinus lavage to prevent sinusitis.
* Fractures that involve the nasal septum may ultimately result in thickening or deformation of this structure and lead to upper respiratory tract obstruction, and nasal septum resection may be required at a later date.

Periorbital Fractures

Periorbital fractures are a type of depression skull fracture that, if left untreated, may result in permanent damage to the eye. There is the potential for displacement of bone fragments into the retrobulbar area, which may cause entrapment of the eye, exophthalmos, and pain. Periorbital fractures are managed in the same manner as other depression fractures of the facial bones.

Fractures of the zygomatic process can usually be reduced by a noninvasive technique in which a bone hook is carefully passed into the conjunctival fornix and positioned beneath the fracture fragments. Care should be exercised when reducing fractures adjacent to the medial canthus to avoid injury to the lacrimal canal.

Neoplasia

Various neoplasms of the maxilla and mandible have been reported, including osteomas, osteosarcomas, fibromas, fibrosarcomas, adamantinomas, and odontomas.

* Osteomas are benign, slow-growing neoplasms composed of trabecular bone.
* Osteosarcomas are rare but can occur in the head region of the horse. They are locally invasive and have a low incidence of metastasis and a long clinical course.
* Fibromas of the head can invade bone and clinically resemble fibrosarcomas or osteosarcomas. Fibrosarcomas are highly malignant and have a higher incidence of metastasis that osteosarcomas.
* Tumors of dental origin include adamantinomas and odontomas. Adamantinomas (ameloblastomas) are of enamel origin. Although they do not metastasize, they are locally invasive, causing destruction of surrounding tissues, and tend to recur.

Therapy for the above neoplasms is directed at debulking the tumor mass and preventing recurrence. With highly invasive osteosarcomas and fibrosarcomas, euthanasia usually is indicated.

Diseases of the Tarsus

(pages 1669-1676)

Kenneth E. Sullins, Carl A. Kirker-Head, Brent A. Hague, G. Kent Carter, Joerg A. Auer, J. Lane Easter, and Jeffrey P. Watkins

DISEASES WITH PHYSICAL CAUSES

Fractures of Tarsal Bones

Slab fractures of the central and third tarsal bones

Fracture of these tarsal bones has been reported in all breeds but predominately in those that race.

* Lameness may be severe or subtle.

* With fracture of the central tarsal bone, tarsocrural distention often is present.
* Radiography is required for diagnosis.
  * A 25-degree plantarolateral oblique view best reveals central tarsal slab fractures, but all projections should be scrutinized for comminution.
* With early diagnosis, lag-screw fixation has a favorable outcome.
  * The outcome for unstable or displaced fractures is poor with conservative therapy.
* Arthrodesis of the involved joints may be necessary to prevent chronic lameness.

Fibular tarsal bone (calcaneal) fractures

Nondisplaced fractures of the calcaneus cause typical signs of tarsal lameness.

* The necessity for surgical intervention depends on accessibility, articular involvement, potential for degenerative sequelae, and required activity of the horse.
* Conservative therapy can have good results in nonathletes, even with sizable fractures.
  * If sequestration of a fragment occurs, it should be removed surgically.

With displaced fractures, superficial flexor and gastrocnemius function is compromised or lost, and surgical repair is necessary to stabilize the tuber calcis. With severe comminution, however, euthanasia is advised.

Fracture/Luxation of the Distal Tarsal Joints

These injuries are easily diagnosed by physical and radiographic examination.

* The proximal intertarsal and tarsometatarsal joints are most often affected.
* Reduction can be quite difficult, particularly if the injury has been present for some time.
* Internal fixation to stabilize the fragments and facilitate arthrodesis should be considered.

Fractures of the Malleoli of the Distal Tibia

Tarsocrural effusion is a feature of these fractures, and pain may be elicited by direct pressure on the injured site.

- Radiographs provide adequate visualization of the bony injury.
- Horses with nonarticular or stable fragments may become sound with conservative therapy.
- Articular or displaced fractures should be removed or repaired.
- In the absence of degenerative changes, the prognosis with adequate fragment removal or stabilization is good.

Hygroma of the Tuber Calcis (Capped Hock)

This condition results from direct trauma, usually self-inflicted, to the point of the hock.

- Distention of the resulting subcutaneous bursa becomes self-perpetuating and can be difficult to resolve.
  - If the hygroma is treated early and further trauma is avoided, local and systemic antiinflammatory agents may be successful.
  - Intrasynovial hyaluronan or corticosteroids may be helpful.
- When the chronic stage has been reached, open drainage or surgical removal of the offending tissue can be successful if postoperative immobilization is adequate.

Lacerations of the Long Digital Extensor Tendon and Lateral Digital Extensor Tendon

Lacerations involving the digital extensor tendons in the hind limb are managed as described for extensor tendon injuries in the forelimb (see p. 420).

Luxation of the Superficial Digital Flexor Tendon

If traumatized or excessively stressed during athletic activity, one or both of the retinacula that anchor the superficial flexor to the tuber calcis may rupture, resulting in luxation of the tendon.

- Lateral luxation in one hind limb is the most common presentation.
- Luxation initially is accompanied by lameness and swelling over the point of the hock.
  - As the swelling subsides, the luxation becomes more apparent visually and on palpation.

- Radiographs should be made to rule out concomitant bone injury.
- Although prolonged rest may allow return to light work or soundness in some cases, surgical stabilization of the tendon is recommended in horses intended for athletic activity.

INFLAMMATORY, INFECTIOUS, AND IMMUNE DISEASES

Tarsal Plantar Desmitis (Curb)

Curb is desmitis of the tarsal plantar ligament.

- Inflammation may result from direct trauma, such as a kick, or from excessive tension (especially in "sickle-hocked" or "cow-hocked" horses).
- In the acute stages the horse may be quite lame, and palpable heat and swelling are noticed on the plantar aspect of the tarsus.
- Ice packs, hydrotherapy, DMSO, and NSAIDs are indicated for acute inflammation.
  - Injection of the ligament with a corticosteroid may be effective.
- The prognosis is good for traumatic desmitis; horses with poor conformation have a guarded prognosis.

Distal Intertarsitis and Tarsometatarsal Synovitis/ Osteoarthritis (Bone Spavin)
Standardbred tarsitis

This condition of young Standardbreds is characterized by subtle lameness that may be evident only when the horse is jogging in harness.

- The lameness is localized by intraarticular anesthesia of the distal intertarsal and tarsometatarsal joints.
- Radiographic changes in the distal tarsal joints frequently are absent or minimal.
- Injection of hyaluronan or a short-acting corticosteroid into the tarsometatarsal and distal intertarsal joints is recommended.
- The horse is allowed light exercise (walking or jogging) for 3 to 4 weeks before continuing training; most have no recurrence of signs.
  - Distal tarsal pain also can be helped by correcting the hoof-pastern angle and applying hind

shoes with a rockered toe to ease breakover.

True bone spavin

True bone spavin (osteoarthritis) is diagnosed more often in mature performance horses, such as jumpers, hitched horses, and those used for roping or reining.

- Radiographic changes, which most often are found in the distal intertarsal joint, are characterized by osteophyte formation, bone lysis, and loss of joint space.
- Daily phenylbutazone therapy allows continuation of work with the hope that exercise will incite enough osteoarthritis to cause ankylosis.
  - Intraarticular injection of long-acting corticosteroid can be successful for variable periods.
- In severe or unresponsive cases, surgical or chemical arthrodesis of the distal tarsal joints may be the only viable option (see *Equine Medicine and Surgery V*).

Deep Digital Flexor Tenosynovitis (Thoroughpin)

Thoroughpin, or distention of the deep digital flexor tendon sheath, develops proximal and plantar to the plantar-lateral pouch of the tarsocrural joint. It rarely causes lameness. When lameness is present, local anti-inflammatory therapy is recommended. Complete evaluation consists of ultrasound of the deep digital flexor tendon and its sheath and tarsal radiographs.

Tarsocrural Synovitis (Bog Spavin)

The initial cause of tarsocrural synovitis may be idiopathic or traumatic.

- The main etiologic consideration should be osteochondrosis (see p. 397).
- Lameness may or may not be present.
- Radiographs should be made to rule out underlying bone lesions.
- When identifiable, the primary condition should be treated.
- When the underlying cause remains obscure, intraarticular corticosteroids may be successful, but repeated injections should be avoided; hyaluronan is another option.

- If effusion returns, exploratory arthroscopy is indicated and reveals a lesion in most cases.

INFECTIOUS JOINT DISEASE

Guidelines for diagnosis and treatment of infectious arthritis are outlined on p. 394. The proximal intertarsal and tarsocrural joints communicate and therefore may be treated as one joint. The distal intertarsal and tarsometatarsal joints require individual therapy. Because of the large size of the tarsocrural joint, fibrin accumulation can be extensive and warrants removal via arthroscopy or arthrotomy. Both dorsal and plantar pouches should be debrided for effective lavage.

MULTIFACTORIAL DISEASES
Angular Limb Deformities

As a rule, if angular limb deformities are present in the carpal region, they also are present in the tarsal region. However, a certain degree of valgus deformity of the hocks is normal. Any obvious angular limb deformity should be treated. Guidelines are similar to those for deformities involving the carpal region (see p. 396).

OSTEOCHONDROSIS OF THE HOCK

The tarsocrural joint is one most commonly affected with osteochondrosis.

- Three clinical syndromes are recognized.
  - The most common involves young horses (4 to 12 months of age) presented for tarsal effusion without associated lameness.
  - The next most common is seen in horses that develop tarsal effusion and mild to moderate lameness soon after training begins.
  - The third is asymptomatic, with the lesion discovered as an incidental finding.
- The most common sites for OCD lesions are the distal intermediate ridge of the tibia, lateral trochlear ridge of the talus, medial malleolus, and medial trochlear ridge of the talus.

- Lesions vary from areas of sub-chondral radiolucency to osteochondral flaps to large osteochondral fragments.

Treatment

Treatment depends on clinical signs and intended use.

- When lameness and effusion are present, surgical removal of cartilage and osteochondral fragments is indicated, especially for horses destined to perform athletically.
- Fragments off the intermediate ridge often become clinically significant once the horse begins training, so many clinicians recommend their removal, even in asymptomatic horses.
  - Asymptomatic lesions of the medial trochlear ridge generally are not treated.
- The prognosis is good for intended use after surgery.

Diseases of the Tibia

(pages 1696-1703)

Joerg A. Auer, Jeffrey P. Watkins, and Robert D. Welch

DISEASES WITH PHYSICAL CAUSES

Tibia Fractures

Epiphyseal fractures

Fractures involving the proximal or distal tibial epiphysis always should be considered in foals with trauma and instability in the stifle or hock region.

- Signs include non–weight-bearing lameness, moderate to severe soft tissue swelling, and with proximal fractures, medial deviation of the stifle and lateral deviation of the distal limb.
- Radiography is necessary to confirm the diagnosis and determine fracture configuration.
- Surgical repair is indicated.
- If stability can be achieved, the prognosis for a functional limb is favorable.

Metaphyseal and diaphyseal fractures

Signs of fracture in the tibial metaphysis or diaphysis vary.

- Horses with incomplete fractures may be very lame, but there is no

crepitation and little swelling, although pain may be elicited on palpation.

- Horses with complete fractures are unable to bear weight; the limb may have an abnormal configuration, usually with the distal portion deviated laterally.
  - These fractures result in considerable edema and often are open medially.
- Radiography is required to identify the location and extent of the fracture.
- Incomplete fractures can be difficult to diagnose initially; repeated radiographs a few days later and/or nuclear scintigraphy may be necessary.
- Incomplete tibial fractures may be treated conservatively with stall rest, although there is a possibility of complete fracture, even if the horse is cross-tied.
  - Internal fixation may be indicated if the fracture is well delineated on radiographs.
  - Provided the fracture completely heals before training resumes, the prognosis is good.
- Complete fractures in foals are best treated with internal fixation
  - The prognosis for future athletic function is guarded to good.
- Complete fractures in adult horses often necessitate euthanasia for humane reasons.

Rupture of the Peroneus Tertius

Peroneus tertius ruptures usually are due to overextension of the hock.

- The tendon may rupture anywhere, but most often it tears just proximal to the tarsus.
- Diagnosis is readily made because the hock can be overextended with normal stifle flexion.
  - The Achilles tendon tends to pucker during walking or when the limb is extended.
  - The stifle flexes jerkily as the limb is advanced, without flexing the hock.
- The horse usually can bear full weight on the limb, with little or no evidence of pain.
  - Avulsion fractures at the tendon's origin usually result in severe lameness (grade 4/5).

- Stall rest for 6 to 8 weeks is recommended; limited exercise may begin after this period.
  - Several months may be required for the fibrous tissue to become a functional structure.
- Rupture near the tarsus tends to heal well; rupture near the origin warrants a guarded prognosis for successful athletic performance.

Rupture of the Achilles Tendon and Gastrocnemius Muscle

Rupture of the gastrocnemius tendon and/or superficial digital flexor tendon is rare in horses. Incomplete ruptures are more common than complete ruptures.

With complete rupture, the limb cannot bear weight and the hock may appear lower and more angled than normal; the hock may be flexed independent of the stifle.

- Partial ruptures and tendonitis can be confirmed and monitored ultrasonographically.
- Therapy for partial ruptures should include at least 8 weeks of stall confinement.
- With complete rupture, a full-limb cast is indicated; surgical repair is difficult (see *Equine Medicine and Surgery V*).
- The prognosis is good to guarded for partial ruptures and poor for complete ruptures.

Diseases of the Stifle

(pages 1703-1715)

Joerg A. Auer, Brent A. Hague, G. Kent Carter, J. Lane Easter, and Jeffrey P. Watkins

CONGENITAL AND FAMILIAL DISEASES

Lateral Luxation of the Patella

Luxations of the patella are most often seen in neonatal pony foals. One or both limbs may be involved; foals with bilateral luxation cannot stand. Unilateral patellar luxation may be seen in adult horses after trauma, but this is rare. Surgical intervention is indicated in both foals and

adults, although in all cases the prognosis is guarded.

DISEASES WITH PHYSICAL CAUSES

Patellar Fractures

Fractures of the patella are uncommon and usually associated with acute trauma.

- Lameness, soft tissue swelling, and femoropatellar effusion vary with the injury.
  - Usually the limb is held in a flexed position, and passive flexion of the stifle is resisted.
  - In most cases, palpation elicits a painful response and crepitus.
- Lateromedial and dorsoplantar radiographs are necessary for diagnosis.
- Treatment varies with the type of fracture.
  - Horizontal fractures must be treated surgically with lag-screw fixation.
  - Vertical or sagittal fractures also can be treated with lag-screw fixation.
  - Small fragments may be removed via arthroscopy or arthrotomy.
  - Conservative treatment may be an option for some avulsion fractures.
  - Comminuted fractures are best treated conservatively with stall rest, although degenerative joint disease is a likely sequela.

Chondromalacia of the Patella

Patellar chondromalacia is characterized by degeneration of the articular cartilage of the patella.

- Possible causes are inflammation and local pressure (e.g., repetitive trauma, malalignment after medial patellar desmotomy).
- Signs include pain and, in some cases, synovial effusion and crepitation.
- Treatment consists of rest and intraarticular hyaluronan or glycosaminoglycans.

Upward Fixation of the Patella

With this condition, the patella is fixed over the medial condyle of the distal femur.

- Predisposing factors include poor conformation (straight limbs), poor conditioning, and in fit horses, a period of stall confinement without exercise.

- Fixation may be maintained over a prolonged period, or it may occur intermittently.
- Acute fixation locks the hind limb in extension, and the stifle and hock cannot be flexed.
  - In intermittent cases, walking the horse up and down a hill may result in a jerky gait.
  - To determine how readily the patella becomes fixed, an attempt should be made to lock it by pushing it proximally and laterally.
- In acute cases, antiinflammatory drugs should be given for a few days and the predisposing or precipitating factors addressed.
  - Corrective shoeing helps some horses.
- Medial patellar desmotomy can be performed if conservative therapy is unsuccessful.
  - However, this procedure may lead to degenerative lesions at the apex of the patella.

Ligamentous and Meniscal Tears

Ligamentous and meniscal injuries are uncommon. Affected horses show stifle lameness that may vary from non–weight-bearing lameness associated with severe instability (caused by rupture of the collateral ligament) to mild, intermittent lameness. Diagnosis is difficult and usually derived through a process of elimination. In selected cases, stall rest may result in some improvement with time. But all ligamentous and meniscal problems of the stifle have a poor prognosis for return to an athletic career.

INFLAMMATORY, INFECTIOUS, AND IMMUNE DISEASES
Infectious Joint Disease

Guidelines for diagnosis and treatment of infectious arthritis are outlined on p. 394. The medial femorotibial joint usually communicates with the femoropatellar joint and generally does not require separate attention. The lateral femorotibial joint requires individual treatment.

MULTIFACTORIAL DISEASES
Osteochondrosis of the Stifle

The stifle is the joint most frequently affected with osteochondrosis. Both OCD and subchondral bone cysts are common causes of lameness.

Osteochondritis dissecans

OCD primarily occurs in the femoropatellar joint, often bilaterally.

- Most affected horses are 6 to 24 months old and presented for lameness and synovial effusion.
  - Lameness varies from mild to severe and may resolve with rest.
  - Significant improvement follows intraarticular anesthesia.
- Radiographically, lesions are located on the lateral trochlear ridge of the femur and less commonly in the trochlear groove, medial trochlear ridge, and patella.
  - Lesions consist of irregularity or flattening of the subchondral bone with or without mineralized cartilage fragments (which, when detached, may be found distally within the joint).
  - Lesions found at surgery tend to be more extensive than predicted by radiographs.
- Surgical removal of fragments and curettage of the articular defect produce satisfactory results more consistently than does conservative therapy.

Subchondral bone cysts

Most horses with subchondral bone cysts of the stifle are presented between 1 and 2 years of age (range, 6 months to 5 years).

- Mild-to-moderate lameness that worsens with work and often resolves with stall confinement is the typical presenting complaint; synovial effusion may not be apparent.
- In many cases the lameness is exacerbated by joint flexion and alleviated by anesthesia of the medial femorotibial joint.
- Lesions are best identified radiographically in the caudocranial view of the femorotibial joint.
  - The lesion most commonly is located in the center of the medial femoral condyle.
  - Radiographic changes vary from flattening of the articular surface to large cystic lesions that com-

municate with the articular surface via a narrow channel.
- Radiographs of the contralateral limb often reveal similar, although usually milder, lesions.
- ◆ Conservative therapy (rest or controlled exercise, and NSAID therapy) reportedly returns 55% to 65% of horses to soundness.
  - Best results are obtained in horses <3 years of age with small lesions.
- ◆ Surgery is recommended for lesions with readily identifiable subchondral lucency.
  - Success rates range from 56% to 74%.

Diseases of the Thigh

(pages 1715-1718)
Jeffrey P. Watkins, Brent A. Hague, G. Kent Carter, and Robert D. Welch

DISEASES WITH PHYSICAL CAUSES
Fractures of the Femur

Fractures of the femur occur as the result of external trauma.
- ◆ Patients with femoral fractures generally are unable to bear weight on the affected limb.
  - Some foals with proximal physeal fractures can bear some weight on the limb.
  - With a discrepancy in hind limb lengths, fracture should be suspected in the shorter limb.
  - Most diaphyseal fractures are accompanied by massive soft tissue swelling.
  - Manipulation of the limb elicits pain and may reveal crepitation.
- ◆ Radiographs are required to confirm the fracture and determine its location and severity.
- ◆ Treatment varies with the type of fracture and size of the patient.
  - Displaced diaphyseal fractures in horses <200 kg warrant euthanasia in most instances.
  - Simple oblique diaphyseal fractures in small foals may be amenable to internal fixation.
  - Fractures of the proximal or distal physis require internal fixation.

Diseases of the Hip and Pelvis *(pages 1719-1723)*
Robert D. Welch, Brent A. Hague, G. Kent Carter, and Dean W. Richardson

DISEASES WITH PHYSICAL CAUSES
Pelvic Fractures

Signs of pelvic fracture depend on the fracture's location and severity.
- ◆ Usually, a fractured tuber coxae is displaced ventrally ("knocked-down" hip).
  - Lameness may be subtle, but the cranial phase of the stride often is shortened.
  - Lacerations and swelling may be present over the tuber coxae.
- ◆ Fractures of the ilium, especially those involving the acetabulum, tend to cause marked lameness with a shortened cranial stride.
  - If overriding of the fragments occurs, the affected limb may appear shorter than the other.
  - Gluteal atrophy can occur as early as 2 weeks after injury.
- ◆ Fractures involving the symphysis pubis or obturator foramen often produce lameness in both hind limbs.
  - With severe or multiple pelvic fractures, the horse may be recumbent and unable to rise.

Diagnosis

The diagnosis is supported by physical and rectal examination, although definitive diagnosis may require radiography.
- ◆ Gently rocking the horse from side to side or pushing on the tuber coxae during rectal examination may reveal obvious bone displacements, crepitation, or hematoma.
- ◆ Pelvic radiography is the most reliable diagnostic aid; however, general anesthesia may be required, with the attendant potential complications of recovery.
- ◆ Nuclear scintigraphy can indicate the location of certain pelvic fractures.

Treatment

Stall confinement and use of analgesics often is the only viable treatment option for pelvic fractures other than those simply involving the tuber coxae.

The horse should be confined for at least 3 months. Some ilial fractures in small foals may be amenable to internal fixation. Excision of necrotic sequestra may be necessary with fractures of the tuber coxae or tuber ischii.

Prognosis

The prognosis for pelvic fractures depends on the type, location, and extent of the fracture.

* Fractures of the tuber coxae, tuber sacrale, and tuber ischii have the best prognosis.
* Minimally displaced fractures of the ilial wing and body of the ischium have a fair prognosis.
* Fractures involving the acetabulum usually cause degenerative arthritis, so the prognosis for soundness is guarded to poor.
* Pubic and ilial shaft fractures have a poor prognosis.
  * In mares with moderate fracture displacement, callus formation during healing may compromise the size of the pelvic canal, necessitating cesarean section at foaling.

Coxofemoral Luxation

Luxation of the hip joint is a rare cause of hind limb lameness.

* Ponies and younger horses are more susceptible to this injury.
* The femur usually is displaced dorsally and cranially, which causes shortening of the affected limb, with outward rotation of the toe and stifle and axial deviation of the hock.
* Radiography is important to identify concurrent fractures of the dorsal acetabular rim and, in foals, to differentiate luxation from a slipped capital femoral epiphysis.
* Reduction is best attempted within the first 24 hours after injury.
  * General anesthesia and muscle relaxants facilitate traction and manipulation of the limb.
* Because of the risk of reluxation and development of degenerative joint disease, the prognosis is guarded to poor.

MULTIFACTORIAL DISEASES

Degenerative Joint Disease

Degenerative joint disease of the hip is uncommon in horses and usually is due to an underlying structural abnormality, such as osteochondrosis, ruptured round ligament, osteomyelitis, or luxation. Localizing signs are gluteal atrophy and persistent lameness. In advanced cases, there may be pain on pressure over the greater trochanter and possibly crepitus if cartilage destruction is extensive. The prognosis for performance is poor.

Diseases of the Thoracolumbar Region

(pages 1723-1730)
Leo B. Jeffcott

DISEASES WITH PHYSICAL CAUSES

Muscle Strain

Damage to the epaxial muscles is the most common back injury in horses.

* Strain or injury to the longissimus muscles most often occurs during ridden exercise as a result of a slip, fall, or poorly executed jump.
* Poor performance and a change in temperament develop acutely.
* Local swelling and heat may be evident, particularly in the lumbar region.
  * The back is kept rigid and there is impairment in the hind limb gait, often with wider than normal hind foot placement.
  * There is obvious pain on palpation and markedly reduced thoracolumbar flexibility.
* In the acute stages, plasma activities of muscle enzymes may be mildly elevated.
* Treatment should involve rest and possibly antiinflammatory medications and physical therapy.

Ligamentous Damage

The supraspinous ligament may be strained or damaged in gallopers and jumpers.

* Signs are similar to those of muscular injury but tend to persist for longer.
* The cranial lumbar region is the most common site; often there is thickening of the ligament. Dorsal

to the spinous summits and pain is easily elicited on palpation.

• Diagnosis is assisted by ultrasonographic examination.

• Management is as described for muscular injuries.

• In general, the prognosis is guarded, largely because of the likelihood of recurrence.

Fractures of the Dorsal Spinous Processes

Multiple fractures of the dorsal spinous processes of the withers (T3-T10) are readily diagnosed by the history and clinical signs, though the extent and number of spines involved can be confirmed only by radiography.

• There invariably is a history of some traumatic incident, such as falling over backward.

• There is local pain, heat, and swelling, with stiffness of the forelimb action.

• Recovery usually is complete within 4 to 6 months; depression of the withers often remains, but with no permanent effect on performance.

Overriding Dorsal Spinous Processes

Impingement of the thoracolumbar spinous summits causes back pain in some horses.

• It mainly occurs beneath the saddle region (T12-T17) but may occur in the caudal withers or cranial lumbar region.

• Onset of signs often is insidious; signs include increasing back stiffness, poor jumping ability, reduction in hind limb impulsion, and a disinclination to work.
  • A temperament change or resentment toward being groomed or shod also may be noticed.

• Back pain usually is mild and, in long-standing cases, may not be evident on palpation, although the back muscles are rigid and the horse resists dipping of the back (extension).

• Local anesthesia of the interspinous spaces results in marked improvement in some horses.

• Most horses respond to rest and antiinflammatory and/or physical therapy, but recurrence of clinical signs can be expected.
  • Surgical resection frequently is no more successful than conservative therapy.

Diseases of the Lumbosacral Region

(pages 1730-1733)

Leo B. Jeffcott

DISEASES WITH PHYSICAL CAUSES

Fractures

Lumbar vertebrae

Fractures of the lumbar vertebrae are common in young foals and result in sudden onset of paraplegia. The diagnosis can be confirmed radiographically; the prognosis is grave.

Sacrum

Fractures of the sacrococcygeal vertebrae usually occur when a horse falls heavily on its rump. If the sacral body is affected, damage to the vertebral canal is associated with signs of cauda equina paralysis, such as tail flaccidity and progressive local muscle atrophy (see Chapter 11, Nervous System). Problems with micturition and defecation are common. The prognosis is poor.

Soft Tissue Injuries

Soft tissue damage to the sacral region is common in harness racing horses.

• Pain on palpation along the croup (S2-Cy1) often is associated with poor performance and impaired hind limb gait.

• The probable cause is strain or damage to the caudal insertion of the longissimus dorsi muscle on the sacral spinous summit and/or dorsal and lateral sacroiliac ligaments.

• The condition usually responds favorably to prolonged periods of rest (6 months), but recurrence is common.

Sacroiliac Damage

Acute sacroiliac injury

Severe injury to the sacroiliac ligaments caused by slipping and falling or by twisting the sacroiliac joint results in moderate to severe hind limb lameness. Exerting pressure over the sacroiliac region sometimes can produce crepitation, and the hindquarters may be asymmetric. Nuclear imaging often is diagnostic. Treatment comprises rest and antiinflammatory medications.

Chronic sacroiliac damage

Horses with chronic sacroiliac damage usually exhibit poor performance.

* Intermittent, sometimes shifting hind limb lameness may be noted, with toe dragging and "plaiting" in the hind limb(s); exercise often induces back stiffness.
* In the early stages, pain can be elicited by applying pressure just cranial to the tubers sacrale, pressing down on the tubers coxae, flexing the hind limb, or by rectal palpation.
* Most horses show some degree of pelvic asymmetry; the tuber coxae are 1 to 2 mm lower on the affected side, and there is some gluteal atrophy.
  * "Hunters' bumps," or prominence of the tips of the lumbar spinous processes and tuber sacrale, are common in these horses (but also can be found in normal horses).
* Many of these animals temporarily respond to NSAIDs, such as phenylbutazone.
* Building up the muscles of the hind quarters and back with regular exercise is important to long-term function; thereafter, the horse must be kept fit and not allowed extended rest.

16

Urinary System

Examination of the Urinary System

(pages 1760-1765)

Thomas J. Divers and Ellen L. Ziemer

PHYSICAL EXAMINATION

After a general physical examination, the urinary system should be assessed by palpation and observation of external structures.

- In males the urethral orifice and penile urethra can be palpated.
- In females the vaginal opening and perineum should be inspected.
- In foals the umbilicus also should be palpated and examined for urine, exudate, or swelling.
  - The abdomen should be ballotted in foals with dysuria or abdominal distention.

Rectal Palpation

The following parts of the urinary system are palpable per rectum:

- The proximal urethra is palpated against the pelvis.
- The bladder is palpated to determine its size and wall thickness and the presence of any masses.
- If enlarged, the ureters can be felt dorsal to the rectum on either side of the dorsal midline.
  - Ureteral calculi most often are felt just cranial to the pelvic brim.
- The caudal half of the left kidney usually can be felt on rectal palpation.
  - A smaller-than-normal kidney indicates chronic renal disease or hypoplasia.

- An enlarged kidney may be found with acute nephrosis or obstructive renal disease.
- The right kidney usually is not palpable unless it is greatly enlarged.

Measuring Water Consumption and Urine Output

Approximation of daily water consumption and urine production is important in evaluating the urinary system. Depending on environmental conditions, the average adult horse consumes 25 to 35 L/day of water and produces 22.5 L/day of urine.

ANCILLARY DIAGNOSTIC AIDS
Urinalysis

Complete urinalysis helps determine the cause of discolored urine, the presence of inflammatory disease, the location of disease, and the kidneys' ability to concentrate or dilute urine.

- Large numbers of white blood cells (WBCs) (pyuria) and bacteria (bacteriuria) suggest urinary tract infection.
- Marked proteinuria without hematuria or pigmenturia usually indicates glomerular disease, but severe tubular disease also may cause proteinuria.
  - Dipstick determination of proteinuria should be confirmed by quantitation of protein.
- Strong hemoprotein reaction on dipstick is consistent with acute renal disease.
- Urinary casts suggest renal tubular disease.

442

- Isosthenuria (specific gravity of 1.007 to 1.012), indicating inability to concentrate or dilute urine, occurs in most horses with renal failure, regardless of the cause.
  - Urine volume may vary, however; there may be an increased amount (polyuria), decreased amount (oliguria), or total absence of urine (anuria).
- Urine pH can be useful in assessing the degree of potassium (K) deficiency (acid urine), systemic acid-base imbalances, and renal tubular acidosis.
- Marked hematuria may be idiopathic (e.g., exercise induced) or indicative of a bleeding lesion of renal or extrarenal origin.

Serum Chemical Analysis

Several serum chemistry abnormalities can occur with renal dysfunction.

- Elevations of creatinine and urea nitrogen often are the first indications of renal dysfunction.
- Electrolyte abnormalities in *acute* renal failure include the following:
  - hyponatremia and hypochloremia (both often severe)
  - tendency toward hypocalcemia (although hypercalcemia has been reported)
  - hypokalemia or normokalemia (most common in subacute or polyuric acute renal failure) or hyperkalemia (peracute disease with oliguria)
- Electrolyte abnormalities in *chronic* renal failure are more variable:
  - Hyponatremia and hypochloremia are found in most cases.
  - Marked hypercalcemia is seen in about 30% of cases, possibly with corresponding hypophosphatemia.
  - Moderate hyperkalemia is common, but hypokalemia may be seen.
  - Hypermagnesemia, often proportional to the severity of azotemia, may be found.
- Postrenal azotemia causes hyponatremia, hypochloremia, and hyperkalemia, with moderate elevations in serum creatinine and urea.
  - It usually is the result of urinary outflow obstruction or rupture of the urinary tract.

- Uroperitoneum can be diagnosed by a *peritoneal fluid* creatinine level at least 2 times that of serum and the presence of calcium carbonate crystals in the fluid (see p. 449).
- Urine accumulation in the retroperitoneal space as a result of ureteral rupture or severe nephrosis causes elevation in peritoneal fluid creatinine but <2 times that of serum.

Prerenal azotemia

Prerenal azotemia is an excess of urea or other nitrogenous products in the blood, primarily as a result of decreased renal blood flow. The serum urea concentration is relatively higher than that of creatinine (which generally is <5 mg/dL), and the urine reflects water and electrolyte conservation (specific gravity $\geq$1.030, osmolality 3 times that of serum, and fractional excretion of sodium [Na] <1%). Prerenal azotemia is readily corrected by fluid therapy.

Fractional Urinary Excretion of Electrolytes

Fractional excretion (FE) of an electrolyte in the urine can be determined by simultaneous collection of urine and blood and measurement of creatinine and the electrolyte in both samples.

- FE (%) = [Serum creatinine/Urine creatinine] × [Urine electrolyte/Serum electrolyte] × 100.
- In a normal adult horse, the FE of sodium and phosphorous (P) should each be <1%.
- The FE of potassium normally ranges from 15% to 65%.

Other Tests

Urinary FE of gamma glutamyl transaminopeptidase (GGT) and clearance rates of creatinine, insulin, and other compounds occasionally are used to further define renal disease. These tests are discussed in *Equine Medicine and Surgery V.*

Diagnostic Imaging

The following diagnostic imaging techniques may be useful in evaluating the urinary system:

- Radiography is limited to foals or the distal urinary tract of adult males.
  - Retrograde contrast studies can be used to detect rupture of the urethra or bladder.
- Ultrasonography is used to evaluate the kidneys, ureters (calculi), bladder, urethra, and umbilical structures.
- Endoscopic examination (cystoscopy) of the urethra, bladder, and ureteral openings can be performed in adult horses.

Renal Biopsy

Renal biopsy should be performed only if the cause of renal failure is not known and biopsy results are likely to influence therapy or prognosis. A strong indication is a renal mass. The technique is described in *Equine Medicine and Surgery V.*

Water Deprivation Test

Water deprivation testing is indicated in nonuremic, well-hydrated, polydipsic, polyuric patients in which the urine specific gravity remains <1.008 and the ability to concentrate urine is in question. The test and its interpretation are described in *Equine Medicine and Surgery V.*

Diseases of the Kidney

(pages 1768-1777)

Thomas J. Divers, William V. Bernard, and Ellen L. Ziemer

DIAGNOSTIC AND THERAPEUTIC CONSIDERATIONS

Acute Renal Failure

Conditions that alter renal blood flow are the most common cause of acute renal failure in horses.

- Causes include acute diarrhea, hemorrhagic crisis, disseminated intravascular coagulation (DIC), heart failure, abdominal crisis, and bacterial toxemia.
- Abnormally high serum creatinine and low urine specific gravity (<1.015) are the most common laboratory findings.
- Systemic effects include diarrhea, generalized or ventral edema, en-

cephalopathy (with severe azotemia), laminitis, and hemolysis.

Treatment

Initial therapy should consist of replacement of fluid deficits and correction of any electrolyte and acid–base abnormalities.

- In nonoliguric patients, normal saline (40 to 80 mL/kg/day intravenously [IV]) with added potassium chloride (KCl) (20 to 40 mEq/L) usually is all that is needed to decrease the serum creatinine level.
  - Serum creatinine should be reevaluated 2 to 4 days after fluid therapy is discontinued.
- Fluid and sodium replacement in oliguric patients must be guided by measurement of body weight, PCV, total plasma protein, and central venous pressure (CVP, normally <8 cm H_2O)
  - Fluid and electrolyte replacement should be followed by IV dopamine (3 to 5 µg/kg/min in 5% dextrose solution) and furosemide (1 mg/kg q2h).
  - Blood pressure should be monitored before and during dopamine infusion (see *Equine Medicine and Surgery V*).
  - If this approach does not increase urine production and the CVP remains elevated, dialysis is the only therapeutic option.
- Adequate caloric intake should be provided, by nasogastric tube feeding if necessary.
  - Addition of 50 to 100 g of dextrose to each liter of IV fluids provides some calories for horses that cannot be fed.

Chronic Renal Failure

Chronic renal failure primarily affects either the glomeruli or the tubules. Chronic glomerular disease is thought to result from immunologic causes, while chronic tubulointerstitial disease most often results from progression of acute nephrosis or from chronic obstruction and/or infection. Melena, oral erosions, and excessive dental tartar may be found in horses with chronic renal failure; weight loss often is marked in these horses. Laboratory abnormalities are described in the earlier section on serum chemical analysis.

Treatment

Treatment is primarily supportive. The most important principle is to provide sufficient fluids, electrolytes, and nutritional support.

- Free-choice water should be available at all times.
- Salt should be provided free-choice unless edema or hypertension is present.
  - If edema develops, salt should be restricted, even in the presence of hyponatremia.
- Weight loss should be addressed by increasing dietary carbohydrates and fats.
  - Protein intake need not be restricted unless serum urea nitrogen:creatinine ratio is >15:1.
- If serum calcium is elevated, calcium-rich feeds such as alfalfa hay should be removed from the diet and vitamin D supplements should be avoided.
- Therapies that may decrease the inflammatory response include aspirin (200 mg orally [PO] every third day) and linseed oil (30 mL added to the feed).

Sudden changes in diet, housing, and exercise and use of nephrotoxic drugs should be avoided. Treatment is likely to be successful only if there is an acute, reversible component exacerbating the chronic condition.

CONGENITAL AND FAMILIAL DISEASES

Congenital diseases involving the kidneys are uncommon and include the following:

- Bilateral renal hypoplasia: Some affected horses live to ≥4 years of age (but are "poor doers"); severely affected foals may die within the first 24 hours of life.
- Unilateral renal agenesis: This is most often an incidental finding.
- Vascular anomalies: Signs other than hematuria usually do not occur unless both kidneys are severely involved.
  - Cystoscopy reveals blood exiting the ureter.
  - An abnormality often can be seen ultrasonographically.

INFLAMMATORY, INFECTIOUS, AND IMMUNE DISEASES

Interstitial Nephritis

Interstitial nephritis usually can be distinguished from glomerular disease by the absence of persistent proteinuria and by indications of defects in tubular function. Causes include infectious, toxic, and metabolic conditions and bilateral obstruction. The most common infectious cause in neonates is *Actinobacillus equuli*.

Immune-Mediated Glomerulonephritis

Glomerulonephritis is a common cause of chronic renal insufficiency in horses >5 years of age.

- Causes are varied, but the underlying mechanism is immune mediated.
  - Endogenous sources of antigen include nuclear and immunoglobulin proteins.
  - Exogenous antigens include bacteria (e.g., *Leptospira pomona*, *Streptococcus equi*), viruses (e.g., equine infectious anemia, herpesvirus), and foreign proteins.
- Signs often include weight loss, depression, anorexia, polyuria, and polydipsia.
- Proteinuria is the most common laboratory finding.
  - Other findings may include azotemia and fluid, electrolyte, and acid-base disorders.
  - Hypercalcemia and hypophosphatemia also may develop.
  - Moderate unresponsive anemia can occur late in the disease.
  - Isosthenuria and elevated plasma creatinine confirm the presence of renal insufficiency.
- Rectal examination may reveal a small, irregularly surfaced kidney, but histopathology and immunofluorescence of renal biopsies are necessary for definitive antemortem diagnosis.

Treatment

Successful treatment requires removal of the underlying cause of the immune process. However, by the time the disease is diagnosed, it usually has progressed to irreversible renal damage. Other than therapy directed toward the underlying disorder, treatment should include supportive care for chronic renal failure; a high-carbohydrate diet containing <10% protein may be useful.

Pyelonephritis

Pyelonephritis is suppurative bacterial infection of the kidney.
* It is relatively rare in horses.
* The usual source is an ascending lower urinary tract infection or obstruction.
  * Common isolates are *Corynebacterium, Escherichia coli, Proteus mirabilis, Enterobacter, Klebsiella, Pseudomonas, Staphylococcus, Actinobacillus, Salmonella,* and *Streptococcus* organisms.
  * Hematogenous infection most often involves *L. interrogans, A. equuli,* and *Salmonella* spp.

Clinical signs and diagnosis

Pyelonephritis is insidious in onset, so it usually is not recognized until it becomes chronic.
* Signs include those of chronic renal disease, such as weight loss, depression, and anorexia.
  * Other signs may include fever, dysuria, pollakiuria, and stranguria; polyuria may occur with tubular dysfunction.
* Pyuria and/or bacteriuria may be present, but their absence does not rule out pyelonephritis.
  * Hematuria may be observed grossly or microscopically; proteinuria usually is minimal.
* Other laboratory findings may include mild anemia, leukocytosis, and hyperfibrinogenemia.
  * Uremia and fluid, electrolyte, and acid–base disturbances occur if the disease progresses to renal failure.
* Rectal examination typically reveals abnormal ureters or an abnormal left kidney.
  * Ultrasonography may show a dilated renal pelvis or ureters and/or parenchymal changes.
  * Cystoscopy can help distinguish unilateral from bilateral involvement.
* An attempt should be made to identify predisposing causes (e.g., obstructions, calculi, abscesses, neoplasia).

* Urine samples should be collected for culture and sensitivity testing.

Treatment

Treatment includes the following:
* identification and elimination of any predisposing cause
* appropriate antimicrobial therapy
* management of renal compromise
  Often a protracted course of therapy (>2 weeks) is required; even then, treatment failure is common because the disease often is well advanced when recognized. Renal calculi should be considered in chronic, unresponsive pyelonephritis.

TOXIC DISEASES

Aminoglycoside Toxicity

Aminoglycoside-induced renal failure usually is precipitated by dehydration.
* Polyuria is a common sign.
* Urinary casts, microscopic hematuria, abnormal enzymuria, or slight increases in serum creatinine are indications that the drug should be discontinued or the interval increased.
* Fractional excretion of GGT will be increased.
* Usually the damage is reversible if aminoglycoside use is stopped, but oliguric failure and death can occur even after the drug is withdrawn.
  * Peritoneal dialysis, leaving the fluid in the abdomen for 2 hours, is recommended for patients with oliguric renal failure and high serum concentrations of the aminoglycoside.
* The best means of preventing nephrotoxicity is by administering polyionic fluids IV and regularly measuring serum aminoglycoside and creatinine levels.
  * Unless trough levels can be monitored (see Chapter 4, Principles of Therapy), aminoglycosides should be used with extreme caution in foals <10 days old.

Pigment Nephropathy

Diseases causing myoglobinuria or hemoglobinuria can cause renal failure.
* The potential for renal failure should be considered in all horses with hemolysis or myopathy.

- If depression is noted after the episode has abated, renal failure should be considered.
- Therapy to decrease this likelihood should include maintaining an adequate flow of alkaline urine and controlling the primary problem.
  - Diuresis with IV polyionic fluids usually is all that is required.
- Generally the prognosis is good if the primary condition is controlled and renal failure has not been present for more than a few days.

Other Toxins

A variety of toxic compounds can cause renal failure in horses, including the following:

- heavy metals: organic and inorganic mercurial compounds and cadmium
- vitamin K_3 (menadione sodium bisulfite)
- vitamin D_2 (ergocalciferol) or D_3 (cholecalciferol), when fed or injected in excessive quantities
  - Stiffness, impaired mobility, weight loss, polydipsia, and polyuria are common signs.
  - The most incriminating laboratory finding is an elevation in both serum phosphorous and calcium.
  - Ultrasonography reveals mineralization of the great arteries, kidneys, and tendons.
  - Treatment comprises decreasing dietary calcium and increasing urinary excretion of calcium with corticosteroids (prednisolone, 1 mg/kg) and furosemide.

Nonsteroidal Antiinflammatory Drug Intoxication

Renal failure may result from prolonged administration of nonsteroidal antiinflammatory drugs (NSAIDs) in volume-depleted animals. NSAID toxicity can cause severe and protracted renal papillary necrosis, although it is much more likely to affect the gastrointestinal (GI) tract (see Chapter 10, Alimentary System). Management of renal failure is discussed on p. 444. Ideally, serum creatinine should be monitored if NSAIDs are to be used for prolonged periods in large doses.

Miscellaneous Drug Toxicities

A few additional drugs have caused renal failure in horses:

- amphotericin B (highly nephrotoxic)
- oxytetracycline in young foals (very uncommon)
- idiosyncratic, presumably allergic reactions to any drug

Treatment should include discontinued use of the drug, with general therapy for acute renal failure as indicated (see p. 444).

Plant Toxicity

Rarely, renal failure is caused by ingestion of toxins found in or on plants.

- Plants containing pyrrolizidine alkaloids frequently cause renal disease but rarely failure.
- *Cestrum diurnum* (flowering jasmine) reportedly causes severe renal disease in horses in the southeastern United States.
- Cantharidin (blister beetle) intoxication, seen in horses fed alfalfa hay harvested in the southwestern United States, can cause severe renal dysfunction and urinary tract inflammation.
  - The inflammatory response may be manifested as dysuria and pollakiuria.
  - The most pronounced clinical signs are a result of intestinal damage and hypocalcemia (see Chapter 10, Alimentary System).

Leptospirosis

L. interrogans serovar *pomona* infections may cause acute renal failure with accompanying fever and leukocytosis. Diagnosis is confirmed by fluorescent antibody assay of the urine for *Leptospira* antigen and presence of an extremely high antibody response to *L. pomona* and other cross-reacting serovars. Specific treatment includes fluid therapy and penicillin or potentiated penicillins. Management of acute renal failure is discussed on p. 444.

NEOPLASIA
Adenocarcinoma and Transitional Cell Carcinoma

Primary renal tumors are rare in horses and include benign renal adenomas and more aggressive renal carcinomas. Disseminated tumors of any type may localize in the kidney. Renal tumors in horses generally do not cause signs of renal insufficiency. Hematuria, colic, weight loss, ascites, and anemia are more common findings.

MULTIFACTORIAL DISEASES
Hydronephrosis
Hydronephrosis is dilation of the renal pelvis and calices caused by obstruction of urine outflow.

* It results in progressive interstitial fibrosis and renal atrophy.
* Causes include urolithiasis, compression of the ureters by surrounding inflammatory or neoplastic conditions, cystitis, and urethral strictures.
* Acute obstruction may cause colic-type pain, but unilateral hydronephrosis may remain clinically inapparent for long periods.
  * Complete bilateral obstruction is rapidly terminal unless the obstruction is relieved.
* Rectal palpation may reveal dilation of the ureters, enlargement of the left kidney, and in some cases the actual obstruction.
* Ultrasonography reveals dilation of the renal pelvis, calices, and/or ureters.
* Treatment requires identification and removal, if possible, of the inciting cause.
* Irreversible renal damage occurs with extended or repeated periods of obstruction.

Amyloidosis
Renal amyloidosis (abnormal deposits of protein in the glomeruli) is rare in horses. It is seen most often either in horses used for antiserum production or secondary to chronic infection. Large amounts of protein may be lost through the glomeruli.

IDIOPATHIC DISEASES
Renal Tubular Acidosis
Renal tubular acidosis involves tubular loss of bicarbonate and re-

placement by chloride, resulting in hyperchloremic metabolic acidosis.

* ***Type-1 disease*** is characterized by persistently alkaline urine and inability to acidify the urine during episodes of severe acidosis or after ammonium chloride loading (see *Equine Medicine and Surgery V*).
* ***Type-2 disease*** is characterized by alkaline urine during mild-to-moderate metabolic acidosis, but the urine becomes acidic during episodes of severe acidosis.
* Signs include anorexia, depression, and weakness.
* Azotemia and uremia are minimal or absent.

Treatment
Treatment involves fluid and electrolyte therapy.

* Gradual bicarbonate replacement, either PO or IV, is important.
* Careful monitoring of serum potassium is essential during correction of acidosis because it can rapidly decline to potentially life-threatening levels.
  * Oral potassium chloride therapy frequently is required during the initial treatment period.
* Maintenance therapy involves oral sodium bicarbonate (50 to 150 g PO q12h).
  * Plasma bicarbonate is periodically measured and supplementation adjusted accordingly.

Recovery may occur in anywhere from several days to >2 years.

Diabetes Insipidus
Diabetes insipidus is a rare condition characterized by polyuria, polydipsia, and rapid dehydration after water deprivation. It is caused by either damage to the neurohypophysis or lack of responsiveness of the distal nephron to antidiuretic hormone (vasopressin). Low urinary specific gravity (1.001 to 1.005) with a urine osmolarity of 50 to 200 mOsm/kg suggests diabetes insipidus. A vasopressin challenge test may be done to confirm the diagnosis in nonuremic patients (see *Equine Medicine and Surgery V*). This condition is discussed further in Chapter 18, Endocrine System.

Diseases of the Ureter

(page 1777)
David G. Wilson and Mark D. Markel

CONGENITAL AND FAMILIAL DISEASES

Ectopic Ureters
Ectopic ureters are extremely uncommon in horses. Affected animals have a history of dribbling urine since birth. Examination of the vagina and bladder through a speculum and endoscope may reveal the orifice of the ectopic ureter in females; in males, endoscopic examination of the pelvic urethra is necessary. Correction is by surgical means.

DISEASES WITH PHYSICAL CAUSES

Ureterolithiasis
Ureterolithiasis is a serious but rare problem in horses. Clinical signs vary but often include mild to moderate lumbar pain. Rectal palpation or ultrasonography may confirm diagnosis. Both kidneys should be scanned for calculi and renal pelvis dilation. The calculi can be removed via an abdominal incision or with a device inserted into the ureter via the urethra and bladder (see the section on hydronephrosis).

Diseases of the Bladder

(pages 1778-1782)
Johanna M. Reimer and Mark D. Markel

DISEASES WITH PHYSICAL CAUSES

Bladder Rupture
Urinary bladder rupture is most common in neonatal foals, although it has been reported in postparturient mares. A sex predilection for male foals has been reported. Bladder rupture in foals most often occurs during parturition, though it has occurred in association with trauma, recumbency, urachal abscesses, and severe sepsis.

Clinical and laboratory findings
Clinical signs in foals may not become apparent until at least 24 hours after birth.

- Signs include depression, abdominal distention, colic, inappetance, and dysuria.
- Serum electrolyte abnormalities include hyponatremia, hypochloremia, hyperkalemia, and occasionally, metabolic acidosis.
  - Hyperkalemia is a less consistent finding in adults.
- Serum creatinine levels increase as the problem persists.

Diagnosis
Ultrasonography is of greatest value in the diagnosis of uroperitoneum.

- Occasionally the defect in the bladder wall can be seen, but the most common finding is a very small bladder surrounded by excessive peritoneal fluid.
- A full, grossly intact bladder often is seen with small urachal tears.
  - In such cases, injection of air or agitated saline into the bladder via a urethral catheter results in gas echoes in the peritoneal fluid.
- If the diagnosis is in doubt, abdominocentesis can be used to confirm uroperitoneum.
  - A ratio of peritoneal fluid to serum creatinine of ≥2:1 strongly suggests uroperitoneum.
  - The presence of calcium carbonate crystals in the peritoneal fluid also is a strong indicator.
  - If necessary, 10 mL of new methylene blue can be infused into the bladder via a urethral catheter; appearance of dye in the peritoneal fluid indicates a lower urinary tract tear.

Treatment
Before surgical repair, fluid, electrolyte, and acid-base disturbances must be corrected.

- Physiologic saline is the IV fluid of choice; potassium-containing fluids should be avoided.
- Attempts must be made to correct hyperkalemia before induction of anesthesia.
  - Correction of metabolic acidosis, if present, causes some reduction in serum potassium.
  - In foals with life-threatening hyperkalemia, further reduction in serum potassium may be

achieved with IV infusion of dextrose at 0.5 g/kg and crystalline insulin at 0.1 U/kg.

- Mare's milk should be withheld if serum potassium is >7.5 mg/dL.

◆ Fluid should be *slowly* drained from the peritoneal cavity; too rapid drainage may result in circulatory collapse.

- Xylazine should be used with caution in hyperkalemic foals; diazepam and butorphanol generally is a safe combination.

◆ A broad-spectrum antimicrobial is given before surgery.

INFLAMMATORY, INFECTIOUS, AND IMMUNE DISEASES
Bacterial Cystitis

Bacterial cystitis rarely is a primary disease in horses.

◆ Most often it is secondary to urine stasis (paralytic bladder), prolonged urinary catheterization, cystic calculi, or neoplasia.

- The most common isolates are *E. coli, Proteus, Klebsiella, Pseudomonas, Streptococcus,* and *Staphylococcus* spp.

◆ Signs may include dysuria, stranguria, pollakiuria, and discolored or blood-tinged urine.

◆ Urinalysis and urine culture are necessary to confirm cystitis.

- Bacteriuria and pyuria (>5 WBC/high-power field) strongly suggest urinary tract infection.
- Coliform counts of ≥10,000/mL in a free-catch sample are significant; counts of ≥1,000/mL are significant in a catheterized sample.

◆ Ultrasonography and/or cystoscopy should be performed to rule out predisposing causes.

◆ Successful treatment involves correction of any predisposing causes and use of appropriate antimicrobial agents.

◆ Treatment should be continued for at least 7 days.

- If there is no improvement in that time, urinalysis and culture should be repeated.

TOXIC DISEASES

Cystitis can be induced by cantharidin (blister beetle) and sorghum/Sudan grass toxicosis.

NEOPLASIA

Neoplasia of the urinary bladder is uncommon and seen most often in horses >10 years of age. Squamous cell carcinoma is the most common bladder tumor.

◆ Clinical signs include hematuria, stranguria, dysuria, weight loss, and depression.

◆ Rectal examination, cystoscopy, and ultrasonography are useful for diagnosis.

◆ Urinalysis often is indicative of secondary bacterial cystitis.

- Urine sediment or peritoneal fluid should be evaluated for neoplastic cells, though exfoliation from the tumor is uncommon.

◆ If cystoscopy or ultrasonography reveals a localized mass, resection may be attempted, but even with removal of a well-localized tumor, the long-term prognosis is grave.

MULTIFACTORIAL DISEASES
Bladder Paralysis

Bladder paralysis causes urine dribbling and bladder distention that is palpable per rectum.

◆ It most often is observed with other neurologic signs, such as perineal analgesia, tail or anal sphincter paralysis, and hind limb ataxia.

◆ Causes include equine herpesvirus 1 (EHV-1), myelitis, sorghum or Sudan grass poisoning, cauda equina neuritis, lumbosacral vertebral fractures or osteomyelitis, and vertebral or meningeal neoplasia.

- With lower motor neuron lesions (sacral spinal cord or sacral plexus), manual expression of the bladder per rectum generally is easily accomplished.
- With severe upper motor neuron lesions (most commonly thoracolumbar spinal cord), manual evacuation is difficult.

Treatment involves appropriate therapy for the underlying neurologic disease, bladder catheterization, prophylactic antibiotics, and nursing care.
  • Bethanechol sometimes is used to stimulate bladder emptying and phenoxybenzamine to relax urethral musculature.

Cystic Calculi

Cystic calculi are most frequently diagnosed in adult horses.

♦ Most calculi are composed of calcium carbonate salts.
♦ Signs include hematuria, stranguria, dysuria, and pollakiuria.
  • Additional signs include urine scalding, urine dribbling, abdominal pain, and weight loss.
♦ Diagnosis is based on clinical signs, rectal palpation, ultrasonography, and cystoscopy.
♦ Surgical removal of the calculi is necessary; appropriate antimicrobials (e.g., trimethoprim-sulfa) should be given perioperatively.
  • Some calculi in mares can be removed via the urethra, under epidural anesthesia and tranquilization, by gentle dilation and simultaneous rectal and urethral manipulation.

Diseases of the Urachus and Umbilicus

(pages 1782-1784)
David G. Wilson and Mark D. Markel

CONGENITAL AND FAMILIAL DISEASES

Patent Urachus

Patent urachus may be present at birth or develop after birth.

♦ Moisture may be present in the hair around the umbilicus, or urine may pass through the umbilicus in the resting or micturating foal.
♦ A patent urachus may serve as a source of hematogenous infection, so it should be corrected as quickly as possible.

  • Silver nitrate or 2% iodine solution on sterile swabs inserted about 2 cm into the urachus twice daily usually causes closure in 3 to 4 days.
  • Resection of the urachus is indicated when it does not close with conservative therapy.
♦ With acquired patent urachus, the previously closed urachus opens as a result of infection in one of the umbilical remnants (see below).
  • Debilitated and septicemic foals are most at risk.
  • It is necessary to surgically resect the urachus and any infected umbilical remnants. Broad-spectrum antimicrobial therapy should be started before surgery.

DISEASES WITH PHYSICAL CAUSES

Rupture of the Urachus

Rupture of the urachus most often occurs in neonates but also may occur in foals up to 8 weeks old secondary to urachal abscessation.

♦ If the urachus ruptures within the abdominal cavity, the foal shows signs of uroperitoneum.
♦ If the urachus ruptures within the subcutaneous space, the foal develops subcutaneous edema soon after birth, which often results in sloughing skin around the umbilicus.
♦ The urachus should be surgically resected after stabilizing the foal.

Umbilical Hematoma

Umbilical hematomas usually develop immediately after birth. They can be differentiated from umbilical abscesses by the absence of heat or pain on palpation. These hematomas gradually reduce in size over the first few weeks of life, with no treatment.

INFLAMMATORY, INFECTIOUS, AND IMMUNE DISEASES

Umbilical/Urachal Abscess (Omphalitis)

Umbilical abscessation is relatively common in foals.

♦ Affected foals may have depression, fever, and an inflammatory hemogram; often the umbilicus is enlarged or edematous.

- An apparently normal umbilicus does not rule out the possibility of umbilical vein, urachal, or umbilical artery abscessation.
  - Ultrasonography should be used to examine these structures if the foal is exhibiting signs associated with infection but the source of infection is not obvious.
- Surgical resection of the affected structures is required.
  - Before surgery, the foal should be thoroughly evaluated for other sites of infection, such as septic physitis or arthritis, and broad-spectrum antimicrobial therapy initiated.

The prognosis depends on the extent of infection locally and/or systemically.

Diseases of the Urethra
(page 1784)

Diseases of the urethra are discussed in Chapter 12, Reproductive System: The Stallion and Chapter 13, Reproductive System: The Mare.

17

Integumentary System

Examination of the Skin *(pages 1789-1793)*

Dawn B. Logas and Joy L. Barbet

DERMATOLOGIC EXAMINATION

History

A complete history is vital in diagnosing skin disease and should include signalment, lesion progression, appetite, behavior, environment, types of feed and bedding, contact with other animals, previous treatment for the condition, and general disease history.

Physical Examination

A general physical examination should be performed before attention is focused on the skin.

- Initially, the horse is examined at a distance to get a general idea of the distribution and extent of the disease.
- The skin is examined by sight and touch.
  - Note the general impression of the hair coat (gloss and condition).
  - Record the location, distribution, and configuration of the primary lesions and note the nature and location of any secondary lesions.
  - Record the character of the skin, considering thickness, sensitivity, pruritus, pliability, and any odor.
- Examination should include the mucous membranes and mucocutaneous junctions (nostrils, conjunctiva, oral cavity, anus, and vulva).

Ancillary Diagnostic Aids *(pages 1793-1799)*

Dawn B. Logas and Joy L. Barbet

LABORATORY AIDS

Skin Scrapings

Skin scrapings are indicated in most cases of skin disease.

- Active lesions and those not altered by treatment or excoriation should be selected.
  - Scrapings should be done at multiple sites if there are multiple lesions.
- The scraping should be performed using a dull no. 10 or 12 scalpel blade, held perpendicular to the skin.
- Both superficial and deep scrapings should be performed; for deep scrapings, the site should be gently squeezed, then released and scraped until capillary bleeding results.

Other Superficial Samples

Collected hair, crusts, and scales can be examined for ectoparasites and endoparasites, *Dermatophilus* spp., and dermatophytes.

- Samples can be taken by plucking, scraping, or applying cellophane tape.
- Direct examination of the hair for fungal elements can be performed by placing a few broken hairs from the periphery of a suspicious lesion on a microscope slide.

- A few drops of clearing agent, such as 10% to 20% KOH, KOH + DMSO, or chlorphenolac (50 g chloral hydrate, 25 mL phenol, and 25 mL lactic acid), are placed on the sample.
- The slide is examined for hyphae penetrating the hair shaft and arthrospores on its surface.
- ◆ When dermatophilosis is suspected, crusts are collected and touch impressions made from both the underside of the crust and the skin underlying the crust.
  - These impressions can be stained with new methylene blue, Diff-Quik, or Gram's stain.
  - Microscopic examination reveals branching, parallel rows of gram-positive coccoid cells sometimes described as "railroad tracks."
- ◆ Wood's lamp examination often yields false-negative results because infections by fluorescing dermatophytes are uncommon in horses.

Cultures

Bacterial culture

Samples for bacterial culture should be obtained from pustules or purulent tracts.

- ◆ Areas with pustules should not be scrubbed with alcohol before sampling; gentle cleansing with water alone or mild soap and water is all that is necessary.
- ◆ Areas with deep bacterial infection should be lightly washed with a mild disinfectant soap and rinsed with alcohol, then allowed to completely dry before culturing.
  - The surrounding area is squeezed and a sterile swab is applied to the fresh discharge.
  - If this approach is inadequate, a sterile biopsy sample should be submitted.

Fungal culture

Fungal culture and identification are the most reliable methods for diagnosis of dermatophytosis. Skin grossly contaminated with dirt and manure should be gently washed with a bland soap, rinsed and dried, then gently swabbed with alcohol. Several peripheral and broken hairs and scraped keratin are submitted for culture.

Skin Biopsy

Lesions that should be biopsied include papules and nodules, any suspected neoplastic lesion, persistent ulcers, any dermatosis not responding to appropriate therapy, and any unusual or serious dermatosis.

General considerations

A fully developed primary lesion and several lesions at different stages of development should be selected.

- ◆ Local anesthetic should not be injected into the lesion; rather, SC infiltration of 2% lidocaine beneath or around the site is recommended.
  - Vigorous scrubbing and preparation of the skin surface should be avoided.
- ◆ After collection, the sample should be blotted on absorbent paper then placed on a piece of wooden tongue depressor or cardboard, subcutaneous-side down.
  - After a few minutes, the wood or cardboard and sample are placed upside down in fixative.
- ◆ The most universal fixative for skin biopsies is 10% buffered neutral formalin in a 10:1 fixative-tissue ratio.
  - Biopsies for immunofluorescent tests should be placed in Michel's medium.
  - The fixative of choice for electron microscopy is 3% glutaraldehyde.
- ◆ Biopsies should be sent to a pathologist with expertise in veterinary dermatopathology.

Biopsy methods

The method selected depends on the type, size, location, and probable depth of the lesion; the sample should include skin and subcutaneous fat.

- ◆ With *punch biopsy,* a minimum 6- to 8-mm-diameter sample is required for histopathologic examination; a portion of normal skin need not be included.
  - Punch biopsies are inappropriate for vesicular, bullous, and ulcerous lesions; samples of these lesions are best obtained by elliptic excisional biopsy.
- ◆ When taking *partial excisional* (wedge or elliptic) biopsies, a section of normal tissue should be included.
- ◆ *Complete excisional biopsies* are useful for both diagnostic and therapeutic purposes

Cytologic Examination

Samples for cytologic examination include needle aspirates, tissue imprints, tissue scrapings, and smears of exudates. Tumors, draining tracts, deep fungal infections, or any lesion containing an exudate can be examined.

Intradermal Skin Testing

Intradermal skin testing is useful for identifying substances that cause allergic disease. Insect and inhalant antigens should be selected by prevalent insect and plant types in the area; feed pollens, molds, and dusts also should be considered. Before testing, any glucocorticoids and antihistamines should be withheld for 7 to 10 days (at least 30 days for long-acting glucocorticoids). Techniques and interpretation of results are described in *Equine Medicine and Surgery V*.

Other Tests for Allergic Dermatitis

Other diagnostic methods applicable to suspected allergic dermatitis include:
* *provocative exposure:* The horse is moved to an "inert" isolation area and maintained until free of signs; materials from the previous environment are then added singly and the horse observed for reappearance of signs.
* *environmental control:* One element, such as bedding or hay, is removed singly and the horse observed for improvement.
* *hypoallergenic diet:* See *Equine Medicine and Surgery V*.

Immunologic Tests

Various laboratory tests are available for detection of autoimmune conditions, including antinuclear antibody test, lupus erythematosus cell test, rheumatoid factor test, serum electrophoresis, antibody class quantitation, lymphocyte blastogenesis, and direct immunofluorescence (see *Equine Medicine and Surgery V*).

Tests of Endocrine Function

Tests of thyroid function and of the hypothalamic/pituitary/adrenal axis are the most common endocrine function tests used in equine dermatology. They are discussed in Chapter 18, Endocrine System.

Response to Therapy

Sometimes a therapeutic trial can confirm a clinical diagnosis, relieve animal suffering, and save time and money.

Principles of Therapy

(pages 1800-1868)

Gary M. Baxter, Louise L. Southwood, Dawn B. Logas, and Joy L. Barbet

WOUND MANAGEMENT

Wound healing is described in detail in *Equine Medicine and Surgery V*. Following are guidelines for management of basic wound types.

Closed Wounds

Abrasions

Abrasions are wounds that remove only the superficial layers of the skin. Bleeding usually is minimal, although serum may ooze from the underlying dermis. These wounds can be painful to touch. Treatment principles are as follows:
* The wound should be gently cleansed with an antiseptic soap and rinsed with water or sterile fluid; all debris embedded in the wound should be removed.
* Topical antiseptic ointments may be applied to the wound.

Infection is uncommon and most abrasions heal completely, although often they heal more slowly than anticipated. During fly season, habronemiasis is a possible complication. Severe abrasions, such as rope burns on the pastern, may be complicated by excessive fibrosis and keloid formation.

Contusions

Contusions are traumatic bruises under intact skin, usually accompanied by swelling and pain. Minor contusions heal with minimal care. More severe contusions may benefit from:
* cold-water hydrotherapy, followed by heat therapy after 3 to 4 days
* topical DMSO
* a pressure bandage

If the skin vasculature is severely compromised, the skin may slough 5 to 14 days after injury. In most instances, however, the blood and serum that initially accumulate beneath the skin are absorbed and the area heals without complications.

Hematomas/seromas

Hematomas and seromas are similar to contusions, except that there is a more obvious accumulation of fluid under the skin. Small hematomas are completely resorbed, with no need for surgical intervention. Treatment of larger hematomas is as follows:

* Initial treatment should include cold-water hydrotherapy and topical DMSO ± prophylactic antibiotics; tetanus prophylaxis is mandatory.
* Removal of the blood clots or serum usually is required to permit more rapid healing, but hematomas should not be opened until 7 to 10 days after the initial injury.
* Seromas may be drained by needle aspiration or through a small, ventrally placed incision.
* Inspissated blood clots require manual removal through a ventrally placed incision.
  * In most cases this can be performed under sedation and local anesthesia.
  * The cavity is flushed daily with warm water or antiseptic solutions until the wound closes.

Open Wounds

With traumatically induced wounds, any hemorrhage should be controlled before the wound is examined. *All horses with traumatic wounds should receive tetanus prophylaxis.*

Incisions

Incisions are wounds with cleanly incised skin edges and minimal soft tissue trauma. If the incision is traumatic and there is minimal contamination, the wound is an ideal candidate for primary closure (see below). A major concern with these wounds is whether underlying structures, such as tendons or joint capsules, are involved.

Lacerations

Lacerations are the most common wounds sustained by horses. The wound edges often are irregular, there is surrounding soft tissue trauma, and invariably there is some degree of wound contamination. Consequently, many lacerations that are su-

tured ultimately dehisce. Thorough lavage and debridement are essential in managing these wounds, whether or not primary closure is to be used. These wounds often are best managed by delayed closure or second-intention healing (see below).

Avulsions

Avulsions are lacerations in which tissue has been torn away. These wounds result in extensive soft tissue damage and, on the distal limb, secondary damage to underlying tendons and bone. Sequestrum formation is highly probable. These wounds nearly always are managed by second-intention healing and often require skin grafting for complete healing.

Punctures

Puncture wounds result from sharp objects penetrating to a variable depth, with minimal superficial damage. Severe complications can result from what was thought to be a small, benign, superficial wound. Management is as follows:

* The puncture site should be clipped, surgically prepared, and irrigated.
* The tract should be gently explored with a flexible probe or gloved finger to determine the depth of the wound and involvement of deeper structures.
  * Radiographs should be made with the probe in place, or a fistulogram may be performed to determine the depth of the wound and presence of foreign bodies.
* Ventral drainage should be established and any foreign bodies removed; *puncture wounds should not be closed.*
* With skin wounds, the outer opening may be enlarged to permit drainage and prevent an anaerobic environment.
* If the puncture wound enters a synovial structure, aggressive therapy should be instituted (see p. 458).
* If the puncture involves the foot, the more superficial tissue should be removed so that the puncture hole does not close before the underlying tissue heals.
  * If the navicular bursa is known to be involved, a "street nail" procedure should be performed to permit drainage.

Methods of Wound Closure

There are four basic methods of treating incisions, lacerations, and avulsions.

Primary closure

Primary closure, or first-intention healing, involves direct apposition of the wound edges within 6 to 8 hours of injury.

- The decision to use primary closure should be based more on clinical assessment (extent of tissue damage, adequacy of blood supply, degree of contamination) than on the time elapsed.
  - Other important factors are location of the wound, active stress in the area (movement of wound edges), and the mechanical object that created the injury.
- *If wound infection is likely, the laceration should not be closed.*
- Thorough wound lavage and debridement are essential before primary closure.
  - Suitable solutions include povidone iodine (0.1% to 1%), chlorhexidine (0.05%), saline, balanced electrolyte solutions, neomycin (0.25% to 5%), and Na-hypochlorite (0.125% to 0.25%)
- In most cases, systemic antibiotics should be given, and if possible, the wound should be protected by a bandage or cast.
- Most skin sutures can be removed 10 to 14 days postoperatively.

Delayed primary closure

Delayed primary closure involves wound closure after the 6-hour "golden period" but before the appearance of granulation tissue.

- Initially, the wound should be lavaged, debrided, and bandaged if possible; systemic antibiotics may or may not be indicated.
- Lavage, debridement, and bandaging should be repeated daily until the wound is free of signs of infection; the wound can then be closed.
  - With wounds that are not badly contaminated, closure usually can be performed 2 to 4 days after injury.

The main advantages of this technique are that the risk of wound infection and healing time both are decreased.

Delayed secondary closure

Delayed secondary closure, or third-intention healing, involves apposition of the wound edges after the appearance of granulation tissue (after days 4 to 5). Wounds and lacerations managed by this technique usually are more contaminated and have more associated soft tissue damage.

- The wound is managed as if second-intention healing is to occur, until the wound appears healthy, has minimal exudate, and is free of signs of infection.
- Methods of wound debridement include bandaging, chemical agents, high-pressure lavage, and excision.
- To avoid the risk of subsequent infection, delayed closure is best performed 4 days after injury; however, many wounds of the distal limb require 7 to 10 days before closure.

Second-intention healing

Second-intention healing is wound healing by contraction and epithelialization. The initial goal is to completely fill or cover the wound with healthy granulation tissue.

- Agents that stimulate granulation tissue formation include daily hosing, copolymer flake dressing, and scarlet oil.
- A sequestrum should be suspected if granulation tissue does not form 10 to 14 days after any injury that exposes underlying bone.

Excessive granulation tissue is a common complication of second-intention healing; in most cases, it can be prevented or minimized with good wound care.

- Methods to prevent, control, or remove exuberant granulation tissue include excision, chemical cauterization, immobilization with a cast or bandage, chemical debridement, topical corticosteroids, cryosurgery, and irradiation.
- Topical agents that may decrease formation of exuberant granulation tissue include corticosteroids, collagen gel, caustic chemical agents (copper sulfate, zinc sulfate, salicylic acid), N-butyl cyanoacrylate, protein-denaturing agents, and antiseptic sprays.

Probably the best treatment for exuberant granulation tissue is prevention through use of nonadherent dressings, immobilization, delayed secondary closure, and skin grafts.

Managing Specific Wounds

Wounds in the axilla or groin

Wounds in the axilla or groin are prone to development of subcutaneous emphysema. This is best prevented by confining the horse to a stall, temporarily covering the wound with towels, or packing the entire wound with gauze. As the wound fills with granulation tissue, less gauze is used each time the packing is replaced.

Wounds involving tendons

Current recommendations for management of flexor tendon lacerations include primary or delayed primary closure of the tendons followed by limb immobilization for 4 to 6 weeks and continued support with bandaging and corrective shoeing for an additional 4 to 6 weeks. Management of wounds that involve lacerated extensor tendons is discussed in Chapter 15, Musculoskeletal System.

Wounds involving synovial structures

Puncture wounds or lacerations that involve a joint, tendon sheath, or bursa often go undiagnosed until the animal is severely lame.

- Wounds in the proximity of a synovial structure should be carefully assessed.
  - The wound can be gently probed or the joint capsule or tendon sheath distended (distant to the wound) with sterile fluid while checking for fluid leakage from the wound.
- If the wound communicates with a synovial structure, it is best to lavage the structure and administer broad-spectrum antibiotics for a minimum of 10 to 14 days.
  - Intrasynovial antibiotics (gentamicin, amikacin, or penicillin) also are recommended.
  - Chlorhexidine is detrimental to articular cartilage and should not be used to lavage joints or wounds that enter joints.
- Many of these wounds, when treated appropriately soon after in-

jury, can be closed with minimal risk of synovial infection.

- When in doubt, it probably is best to leave the wound open until the risk of synovial infection is minimal.
  - Delayed closure can then be performed or the wound left to heal by second intention.
- If severe synovial infection develops, more aggressive treatment is warranted (see discussion of infectious arthritis in Chapter 15, Musculoskeletal System).

Wounds involving the thoracic cavity

Wounds that extend into the thoracic cavity can be life-threatening injuries, potentially leading to pneumothorax and lung collapse.

- Rapid closure by suturing or covering with a sterile bandage minimizes pneumothorax.
- A closed-suction drain should be placed in the thoracic cavity after wound closure.
- Pleuritis and wound infection are the main postoperative concerns with these wounds.

Wounds involving the abdominal cavity

Wounds that enter the abdomen and result in eventration of intestines should be closed immediately.

- All herniated abdominal contents should be thoroughly lavaged before being replaced.
  - They should be maintained within the abdomen by a large bandage until general anesthesia can be induced.
- Blunt trauma to the abdomen can result in rupture of the abdominal muscles and fascia, allowing intestine to herniate through the rent and become entrapped along the body wall.
  - These horses usually are presented with signs of abdominal pain.
  - Ventral midline laparotomy should be performed.

SKIN GRAFTING

Skin grafting can be useful in management of large avulsion injuries with considerable skin loss. Skin grafts also are used to promote early epithelialization of burns and to prevent exuberant granulation tissue formation.

Types of grafts, preparation of the graft bed and donor site, the physiology of graft survival, and specific grafting techniques are discussed in *Equine Medicine and Surgery V.*

NEW RECONSTRUCTIVE TECHNIQUES

Reconstructive techniques, including silicone implants, skin expansion techniques, pedicle grafts, and free microvascular grafts, are discussed in *Equine Medicine and Surgery V.*

MANAGEMENT OF BURNS

Types of Burns

The severity of a burn depends on both the size of the area exposed and the depth of the burn.

- Superficial burns are characterized by thickened, erythematous epidermis; they heal rapidly.
- Partial-thickness burns cause massive subcutaneous edema and inflammation.
- Full-thickness burns completely penetrate the dermis and damage the underlying structures.

In general, the prognosis for full-thickness burns is 4 times worse than that for partial-thickness burns. But in many cases, the extent and depth of thermal burns cannot be accurately evaluated immediately after the injury.

Determining severity and prognosis
An approximation of the extent of the burn can be used to estimate the prognosis. Using this technique, each forelimb represents 9%, each hind limb 18%, the head and neck 9%, and the thorax and abdomen each 18% of the body surface. In dogs, burns involving >50% of the total body surface area dictate a grave prognosis, and euthanasia is warranted.

Local and Systemic Effects

With severe burns, life-threatening systemic changes ("burn shock") can occur concomitantly with local damage to the burned tissue.

- Systemic alterations include hypovolemia, electrolyte and protein losses, pulmonary edema, anemia, increased basal metabolic rate and caloric need, and immunocompromise.
- Progressive dermal ischemia, resulting in advancing cell injury and death, is a hallmark of burn wounds for 24 to 48 hours following the thermal insult.
- Local infection and septicemia are potential complications.

Managing Burn Patients

A complete physical examination should be performed and the patient's condition stabilized before the burn wound is assessed. The four primary objectives of treating burns are to:

- save the life of the patient
  - The patient should be monitored for serious systemic alterations.
- relieve pain and suffering
- close or cover the wound
- minimize or correct deformities (scarring) that may occur during healing

Superficial and partial-thickness burns
Superficial and partial-thickness burns usually are not life-threatening and are not difficult to manage.

- Initial treatment includes application of ice or cold water to prevent further dermal necrosis.
- Aloe vera or a water-soluble antibacterial cream may be applied topically.
- Nonsteroidal analgesics, such as flunixin meglumine or phenylbutazone, are useful in alleviating pain and preventing further dermal ischemia.
  - Aspirin at 10 to 20 mg/kg PO also may halt progression of dermal ischemia.
- Partial-thickness burns form vesicles that should be left intact for 24 to 36 hours.
- After 36 hours, the top of the blister can be excised and the area protected with an antibacterial dressing or xenograft (porcine), or an eschar should be allowed to form.
- The bandage should permit drainage but not adhere to the burned surface and should be changed at least daily, depending on the amount of exudate.

Full-thickness burns

Full-thickness burns can be managed with occlusive dressings, eschar formation, continuous wet dressings, or excision and grafting. The most effective and practical therapy for large burns involves leaving the eschar intact and applying moist bandages and antibacterial agents.

◆ Initially, the hair is clipped from the burned area and all devitalized tissue is debrided.
◆ The area is irrigated with antiseptic solution or sterile fluid, and a moist dressing with antibacterial cream is applied.
  • Silver sulfadiazine and aloe vera creams are most effective.
◆ Frequent bandage changes are required to complete the debridement process.
◆ Although topical antibiotic medications always are warranted, debate exists as to whether systemic antibiotics are necessary.

MANAGEMENT OF SKIN TUMORS

Common skin tumors in horses include sarcoid, fibroma, papilloma, squamous cell carcinoma, and melanoma. Although the type of tumor may be tentatively diagnosed by its location and behavior, a histologic diagnosis should be made to determine appropriate treatment and prognosis. Samples may be collected via needle punch (needle-core) biopsy or by incisional or excisional biopsy. Metastasis of skin tumors is uncommon; nevertheless, the draining lymph nodes should be palpated for enlargement, and a fine-needle aspirate or biopsy taken if lymph node involvement is suspected.

Surgical Excision

Surgical excision may be elected for diagnosis, cure, palliation, or debulking to enhance and compliment ancillary treatments.

◆ 2- to 3-cm margins or radical excision (e.g., removal of the eye) may be required for aggressive, locally invasive tumors, such as fibrosarcoma and squamous cell carcinoma.
  • Mastocytomas and papillomas may require marginal excision (1-cm margins) only.

◆ The excised tissue should be examined histologically to determine tumor type, grade, and margins.
  • Incomplete removal of some tumors, such as squamous cell carcinoma and sarcoids, without adjunctive therapy may hasten local recurrence and metastasis.

Adjunctive Therapy

Cryotherapy

Cryotherapy or cryosurgery involves destruction of tissue by controlled freezing.

◆ Cryogens used to produce cryonecrosis include liquid nitrogen (most common), nitrous oxide, carbon dioxide, and freon.
◆ Maximum lethal effects are achieved using a fast freeze followed by a slow, unassisted thaw (see *Equine Medicine and Surgery V*); the freeze-thaw cycle should be performed at least twice.
  • It is best to freeze a 5- to 10-mm margin of normal tissue around most malignancies.
  • The surrounding healthy tissue must be protected from the cryogen.
◆ Care following cryosurgery usually is minimal; tetanus prophylaxis is mandatory but antibiotics usually are not required.

Hyperthermia

Intralesional hyperthermia induced by 2-MHz radiofrequency current (RF Thermaprobe) has been successfully used in treating squamous cell carcinoma in horses. This mode of therapy is particularly helpful for tumors on or around the eye. It is most effective for lesions <5 cm in diameter. To improve the response, surgical debulking is advised before treatment.

Immunotherapy

Immunotherapy for treatment of skin tumors generally is reserved for sarcoids.

◆ The vaccines are purified derivatives of the cell walls of *Mycobacterium bovis, Bacillus* Calmette-Guerin (BCG), or *Mycobacterium phlei* (Regressin V).
◆ Premedication with flunixin meglumine and an antihistamine, with or without corticosteroids, sometimes is recommended.

- In general, 1 mL of the vaccine should be injected per 1 to 2 cc of tumor.
  - No more than 10 mL should be injected into any tumor.
- Treatment is repeated every 2 to 3 weeks as necessary (usually two to five treatments).
- Marked swelling and apparent enlargement of the tumor may precede regression, and
- complete remission may not occur for several months after the last treatment.
- The regimen for Regressin V is 1 mL/cm every 7 to 10 days for up to four treatments.
  - Slight fever, malaise, and inappetence may occur 1 to 2 days following treatment.
- Equistim (a nonviable preparation of *Propionibacterium acnes*) can be effective IV at 4 mL/450kg once a week for 4 to 6 weeks, up to a maximum of 10 weeks.
  - Anecdotal reports indicate success rates equal to or better than *Mycobacterium* vaccines, particularly in horses with multiple sarcoids.

Radiotherapy
Radiotherapy is the preferred method of treatment for most cutaneous neoplasms in horses, although it is currently available at only a few veterinary teaching institutions. Brachytherapy (placing the radiation source on or in the tumor) is the method used almost exclusively in large animals. Use of iridium-192 should be limited to tumors <15 cm in diameter (including a 1- to 2-cm perimeter of normal tissue). Tumor regression may be slow (up to 1 year for large tumors).

Chemotherapy
Local chemotherapy
Chemotherapy is most effective either early in the course of the disease when the tumor is small or at the time of tumor debulking.

- *Cisplatin* is used as a suspension in purified sesame oil (see *Equine Medicine and Surgery V*).
  - The dosage is 1 mg of cisplatin/cm of tumor, including a 1- to 2-cm margin.

- Treatments are repeated at 2-week intervals until tumor resolution (which is gradual).
- Local inflammatory reactions are treated with phenylbutazone.
- *5-fluorouracil* (5-FU) is most effective against rapidly growing, verrucose, necrotic tumors.
  - Efudex cream (5-FU, 5%) is applied topically, daily for lesions that are easily accessible (e.g., labia, vulva, anus) or every 14 days for lesions on the penis and prepuce.
  - Treatment is continued until tumor resolution, which may take 1 to 8 months.

Systemic chemotherapy
Clinical use of systemic chemotherapeutic agents in horses is limited. Drugs that have been used include chlorambucil, cyclophosphamide, cytosine arabinoside, doxorubicin, dactinomycin, l-asparaginase, prednisone, and vincristine.

PRINCIPLES OF DERMATOLOGIC THERAPY
Topical Therapy
Topical therapies (shampoos, lotions, ointments, etc.) are discussed in *Equine Medicine and Surgery V*. Specific recommendations are found in later sections on particular skin conditions.

Systemic Therapy
Antiinflammatories and antipruritics
Antiinflammatory and antipruritic drugs used to treat skin conditions in horses include corticosteroids, antihistamines, and sometimes NSAIDs.

- *Prednisone* is the safest of the corticosteroids.
  - The total daily dosage is 0.25 to 1 mg/kg PO, once daily or divided q12h.
  - It is most effective at the higher dosages for initial control; the dosage then should be gradually decreased for maintenance.
  - If the horse is to be maintained on prednisone long-term, it is best to aim for alternate-day or every-third-day therapy.
- *Dexamethasone* and *triamcinolone* are more potent than prednisone; laminitis and pituitary/adrenal

suppression are more likely with their use.

- The recommended dosage of dexamethasone is 0.04 to 0.08 mg/kg initially, followed by a total dose of 5 to 15 mg every second or third day.
- Prolonged use should be avoided.

◆ *Antihistamines* may be used alone or as an adjunct to corticosteroid therapy.

- Hydroxyzine initially is given at 1 to 1.5 mg/kg q8-12h, then tapered to the lowest effective dose; mild sedation and personality changes may occur.

◆ *NSAIDs* do not completely control pruritus but may be useful in combating pain and discomfort associated with particularly severe conditions.

Antibacterial drugs

Systemic antibacterial therapy occasionally is required in treatment of skin conditions in horses.

◆ Penicillins and trimethoprim-sulfonamides are the most useful; however, culture and sensitivity tests should guide treatment when the infection is deep or initial therapy fails.

- *Procaine penicillin G* is given at 20,000 to 22,000 IU/kg IM q12-24h.
- Alternatively, *ampicillin* may be given at 10 to 20 mg/kg IM q12h.
- *Trimethoprim-sulfonamides* are given PO between feedings at 15 mg/kg q12h; if diarrhea develops, use of this drug should be discontinued.

◆ First-generation cephalosporins have excellent activity against *Staphylococcus* spp. and *Streptococcus* spp.; dosages commonly used are as follows:

- cefazolin, 15 mg/kg IV or IM q8h
- cephalexin, 15 to 30 mg/kg PO q8h
- cefadroxil, 22 mg/kg PO q12h

◆ *Ceftiofur* (a third-generation cephalosporin) at 5 to 10 mg/kg q6-12h, also is effective.

Antifungal drugs

Systemic antifungal drugs generally are required only for deep or persistent fungal infections.

◆ The *iodides* are the most commonly used agents.

- Na-iodide is given as a 20% solution at 40 mg/kg IV daily for 2 to 5 days and then PO.
- K-iodide or iodate is given at 1 to 2 mg/kg PO q12-24h for 1 wk, and then at half the original dosage once daily.
- Iodism may result from therapy with these agents (see p. 472).

◆ *Amphotericin B* has been used in treatment of deep mycoses.

- The initial daily dosage is 150 mg/450 kg IV in 1 L of 5% dextrose solution.
- The dose is increased by 50 mg every third day until a maximum daily dose of 350 to 400 mg is reached.
- Treatment is continued daily or every other day for a total of 30 days.
- Renal function and hematocrit should be monitored weekly; if the horse becomes depressed or anorectic and/or the BUN exceeds 40 mg/dL, therapy should be discontinued.

◆ *Griseofulvin* is occasionally used in treatment of equine dermatophytosis.

- The daily dosage is 5.5 mg/kg PO.
- Because of its teratogenicity, griseofulvin should never be used in pregnant animals.

◆ *Ketoconazole* has been used topically with DMSO and hydrochloric acid for debulking of phycomycotic and pythiotic lesions before surgical therapy

For most deep fungal infections, treatment must be continued for at least 3 weeks after complete healing.

Antiparasitic drugs

Ivermectin is the major systemic antiparasitic in use for equine dermatoses. The oral paste is effective against mange mites, sucking lice, *Onchocerca* microfilariae, *Habronema*, *Hypoderma*, and some species of ticks. The dosage is 200 µg/kg PO. If treating mange mites, it is advisable to repeat treatment in 2 to 3 weeks. Moxidectin and avermectin B$_1$ also are effective against *Onchocerca* microfilariae.

Immunosuppressant drugs

Corticosteroids and aurothioglucose (gold salts) are used to treat autoimmune skin diseases.

- Prednisone is given at 1 to 2 mg/kg PO q12h for immunosuppression.
  - Once the disease responds, usually in 7 to 10 days, the dosage should be gradually tapered to the lowest alternate-day dosage that controls the disease.
  - Dexamethasone also is useful at 0.2 mg/kg/day PO; the dose must be tapered or prednisone substituted for maintenance therapy.
- Aurothioglucose initially is given as a test dose of 20 mg IM, followed 1 week later with another test dose of 40 to 50 mg.
  - If there are no adverse reactions (urticaria and pruritus), therapy is initiated at 1 mg/kg weekly until remission is noted (usually by 6 to 12 weeks).
  - Systemic corticosteroids may be given in the interim, if needed.
  - Once remission is achieved, maintenance injections are given at 2- to 4-week intervals.
  - Weekly examinations, hemograms, urinalyses, and blood chemistry panels should be performed at the onset of therapy and every 1 to 3 months during maintenance therapy.

Immunostimulant compounds

Immunostimulant therapy is primarily used for treatment of neoplastic diseases and pythiosis. BCG has been recommended for treatment of equine sarcoid (see p. 466). Autogenous vaccines occasionally are used for treatment of equine papillomatosis and melanoma. Autogenous vaccines produced from cultures of *Pythium* have been used with variable success in cases of pythiosis in which surgery was not curative.

Immunomodulation therapy

Hyposensitization with specific allergens in treatment of dermatoses resulting from type I hypersensitivity reactions has shown some success. Identification of the offending allergen(s) by intradermal skin testing is required before instituting such therapy (see *Equine Medicine and Surgery V*).

Diseases Characterized by Wheals, Papules, or Small Nodules

(pages 1868-1872)

Dawn B. Logas and Joy L. Barbet

DIFFERENTIAL DIAGNOSES

Possible causes of wheals, papules, or small nodules include:

- foreign bodies (plant material or other foreign matter imbedded in the dermis)
  - Occasionally, draining tracts form.
- fly bites (horsefly, deer fly, stable fly)
  - The papules or wheals have a central ulcer and a hemorrhagic crust.
  - Hypersensitivity reactions, manifested as pruritus or nodules, also may occur.
- mosquito bites
  - Lesions are similar to those of biting flies but have no central crust; heavy attacks may result in urticaria or urticaria-like lesions.
- tick bites
  - Lesions include papules, pustules, wheals, and sometimes nodules; they may crust over, erode, or ulcerate, and foci of alopecia can result.
- nodular collagenolytic granuloma (see below)
- urticaria (see below)
- atopy (IgE-mediated allergic response to environmental allergens)
  - Urticarial lesions are typical; alopecia, excoriations, lichenification, and hyperpigmentation result from chronic pruritus.
  - Ideally, the allergen is identified and avoided; an alternative is long-term maintenance with low-dose oral prednisone and/or hydroxyzine.
  - Hyposensitization may be effective.
- food allergy

- Diagnosis is made by ruling out other more common causes of pruritic dermatoses, such as ectoparasitism, onchocerciasis, and atopy.
- A dietary elimination trial can confirm food allergy and identify the offending feed.
- drug eruptions (urticarial or vesicular dermatitis associated with a particular drug)
  - The reaction can occur any time the drug is used; pruritus is variable.
  - Withdrawal of the suspected drug results in clinical improvement in 10 to 14 days.
- erythema multiforme (uncommon)
  - This is benign, self-limiting condition characterized by persistent urticaria-like lesions that develop into annular, arciform, and polycyclic configurations.
  - Spontaneous resolution usually occurs within 3 months; therapy is aimed at removal of the cause (e.g., infectious agents, pregnancy, drugs, neoplasia, contact reactions).
- unilateral papular dermatosis (uncommon)
  - This is characterized by multiple (30 to 300), nonalopecic, nonpruritic, nonpainful, nonulcerated nodules on one side of the body, most often on the lateral thorax.
  - Treatment is unnecessary, but corticosteroids can shorten the disease course.

MANAGEMENT OF SELECTED CONDITIONS

Nodular Collagenolytic Granuloma

Nodular collagenolytic granuloma, a common condition, is also known as *nodular necrobiosis,* and is thought to be a hypersensitivity reaction, possibly to insect bites.

- Single or multiple nodules are found on the sides of the neck, withers, and back; the nodules are neither pruritic nor painful.
  - The hair and overlying skin seldom are affected unless subjected to trauma.
- Diagnosis is based on histopathologic findings (foci of collagen degeneration surrounded by a granulomatous reaction containing numerous eosinophils).

Treatment

Treatment comprises either surgical removal or corticosteroid therapy.

- Single lesions may be excised or treated with sublesional triamcinolone acetonide (3 to 5 mg/lesion, not to exceed 20 mg total) or methylprednisolone acetate (5 to 10 mg/lesion).
- When multiple lesions are present, systemic corticosteroids may be used.
  - Oral prednisolone is recommended, starting at 1 mg/kg/day for 2 to 3 weeks, followed by alternate-day therapy and gradual reduction of dosage.
  - Older and larger lesions, especially mineralized lesions, may require surgical removal.

Relapses can occur with repeated exposure to the inciting agent; occasionally, lesions resolve without therapy.

Urticaria

Urticaria is characterized by localized or generalized wheals, which are edematous plaques with flat tops and steep sides that appear and often disappear rapidly; in acute cases they pit with pressure. In the early stages, wheals are 0.5 to 3 cm in diameter, but may become large when several lesions coalesce.

Causes

Causes of urticaria are innumerable and include:

- drugs or biologic products and their carriers
  - The more commonly implicated drugs are antibiotics, hormones, insecticides, biologics, phenothiazine, acepromazine, phenylbutazone, and procaine.
  - Wheals commonly develop in a bilaterally symmetric pattern minutes or hours after exposure to the drug, and usually subside in several hours.
- feeds—grains with a high protein content often are implicated ("protein bumps")
  - Others include potatoes, distillery wastes, malt, coconut cake,

beet pulp, buckwheat, clover, alfalfa, St. John's wort, glucose, wheat, oats, tonics, barley, bran, and chicory.

- infectious diseases–strangles, contagious equine pleuropneumonia, horsepox, and dourine (*Trypanosoma equiperdum*)
- inhaled pollens, dusts, or molds
- contactants
- physical urticaria (dermographism or dermatographism)
- endoparasites and ectoparasites
- immunologic diseases, toxic hepatitis, and neoplastic diseases

Single or sporadic episodes of urticaria without a clear cause do not warrant major investigation, but recurrent episodes require a thorough search for the underlying cause. Biopsy, intradermal skin testing, dietary elimination trials, environmental alterations, and a thorough workup for underlying systemic disease may be indicated.

Treatment

Treatment with corticosteroids usually is effective. NSAIDs also may be useful. Antihistamines may not be effective, although hydroxyzine is useful in some cases of chronic urticaria. In severe cases and in cases accompanied by respiratory or cardiac distress, parenteral administration of epinephrine may be necessary. Once an allergic cause is established, it may be treated by avoidance of the offending allergen, low-dose corticosteroid therapy, or hyposensitization.

Diseases Characterized by Nodules or Tumors

(pages 1873-1883)

Gary M. Baxter, Dawn B. Logas, and Joy L. Barbet

DIFFERENTIAL DIAGNOSES

Diagnosis of nodules and skin tumors is aided by the lesions' appearance and location or distribution, but definitive diagnosis generally requires biopsy and histopathologic examination. Possible causes include:

- dermoid cysts (single or multiple, and most common on the dorsal midline)
- heterotopic polyodontia (temporal teratomas, dentigerous cysts, conchal cysts, ear teeth)
  - The lesion consists of a cyst at the base of one ear; in most cases a fistulous tract exudes material through a sinus opening on the rostral border of the pinna.
  - Cysts contain all or part of a tooth; radiography is required to confirm the diagnosis.
  - Treatment involves surgical extirpation of the cyst and curettage of the alveolar socket.
- integumentary mycobacteriosis (rare; more likely in imported horses)
  - Affected horses tend to be emaciated and often have vertebral involvement.
  - Diagnosis is by demonstration of acid-fast organisms in cytologic smears of nodule contents or in biopsy sections; definitive diagnosis requires culture.
  - Treatment is not recommended.
- ermiasis ("warbles"; see below)
- warts (viral papillomatosis; see below)
- neoplasia (see below)
  - The more common skin tumors include sarcoid, squamous cell carcinoma, melanoma, basal cell tumor, cutaneous lymphosarcoma, mast cell tumor, and fibroma.
- keloid (hypertrophic scars, most common on the flexor surfaces of distal limb joints)
  - These hard, raised lesions develop gradually and have a keratinized surface.
  - They often recur following surgical removal, so small benign lesions are best left untreated; podophyllum or 5-FU can be used topically.
- cutaneous amyloidosis (rare)
  - This condition is characterized by multiple cutaneous and subcutaneous, firm, painless nodules 0.5 to >10 cm in diameter, mostly on the head, neck, and pectoral region; overlying skin is normal.

- Nodules may regress spontaneously or in conjunction with corticosteroid therapy, only to return and assume a chronic, progressive nature; no successful treatment is known.
- axillary nodular necrosis (rare)
  - One or two large nodules are found near the girth area or axilla; the nodules are not ulcerated, alopecic, painful, nor pruritic, and respond to sublesional corticosteroids or excision.
- calcinosis circumscripta (see below)

MANAGEMENT OF SELECTED CONDITIONS
Hypodermiasis (Warbles)

Larvae of *Hypoderma bovis* and *H. lineatum* are a sporadic cause of subcutaneous nodules in equidae in the northern hemisphere.

- High-risk horses are young and poorly conditioned, and graze with cattle.
- In horses, the larvae often undertake aberrant migrations to the brain and cause acute neurologic disease, with or without concurrent skin nodules.
- Some larvae migrate to the dorsum and either develop a breathing pore and eventually drop out of the cyst or become encysted and die (nodules become mineralized and permanent).

Dorsal subcutaneous nodules arising in the spring with the characteristic breathing pore are highly suggestive of hypodermiasis. Demonstration of the larva within the cyst is diagnostic.

Treatment

One or two lesions can be treated simply by enlarging the breathing hole with a scalpel blade and removing the larva with a hemostat; care must be taken to avoid larval rupture. Early treatment of suspected *Hypoderma* nodules with intralesional triamcinolone acetonide (4 mg) and fenthion (0.5 mL) may kill the developing larvae and minimize local reaction. In areas of high incidence, pour-on insecticide, such as 13.5% crufomate at 75 mL/100 kg, prevents development of cattle grubs.

Warts (Viral Papillomatosis)

Warts are caused by the equine papilloma virus.

- Warts usually affect young horses (<3 years old), especially when they are housed in groups.
- Lesions most often appear on the muzzle and lips; occasionally they are found on the ears, eyelids, genitalia, or distal limbs.
- In most cases, treatment is unnecessary; natural immunity develops and the warts spontaneously disappear, usually within 60 to 100 days.
- Severe cases may require treatment.
  - Cryosurgery with a 2-cycle freeze-thaw technique is the treatment of choice.
  - Topical trifluoroacetic acid (25 g anhydrous trifluoroacetic acid, 20 g glacial acetic acid, and 3 mL water), on days 1, 4, and 7, is safe and effective.
  - 25% salicylic acid with podophyllin cream also has been used to cauterize warts.
  - Autogenous vaccines can be effective.

Sarcoid

Sarcoid is a locally aggressive, nonmalignant fibroblastic tumor of equine skin. A viral etiology (bovine papilloma virus or a closely related virus) is suspected. Sarcoids most frequently occur on the head (especially on the ears and eyelids), legs, ventral abdomen, groin, and axilla. The lesions are seldom, if ever, pruritic but can vary considerably in appearance. There are four types:

- *Verrucous* (warty) sarcoids rarely are >6 cm in diameter and may remain static for years.
- *Fibroblastic* (proud-flesh–like) sarcoids vary from small dermal nodules to large ulcerated masses; larger sarcoids often have a cauliflower-like appearance.
- Trauma and/or infection may induce transformation from the verrucous to the fibroblastic type, resulting in a third type, the *mixed* lesion.
- A fourth type, the *occult* sarcoid, is flat or slightly raised, with variable degrees of alopecia, crusting, and/or scaling; it remains static for

extended periods before nodules develop.

Histologic examination of biopsy specimens is necessary for diagnosis (see *Equine Medicine and Surgery V*). Wide excision of the entire mass is recommended to decrease the chance of recurrence.

Treatment

Many treatments have been tried, but few are without potential complications, and success rates vary tremendously.

* Static verrucous and occult sarcoids usually are best left untreated, because intervention may prompt transformation to an aggressive fibroblastic type.
  * Some sarcoids undergo spontaneous remission, usually after several years.
* Excision with concurrent use of electrocautery, cryosurgery, hyperthermia, irradiation, or BCG therapy is the most common treatment approach.
* Topical application of cytotoxic agents also can be effective.
  * After tumor excision, 5-FU cream is applied to the tumor base daily for 1 to 3 months, or until the lesion heals; the surrounding skin must be protected with petrolatum.
  * Alternatively, podophyllin can be applied daily with a cotton-tipped applicator until a black scab forms; treatment is discontinued until the scab loosens, and is then repeated.
* Intratumoral injections of cisplatin also appear to be safe and effective

These treatments are discussed in the earlier section on management of skin tumors.

Squamous Cell Carcinoma

Squamous cell carcinoma is a malignant tumor arising from epidermal cells.

* It tends to develop in nonpigmented skin at mucocutaneous junctions, such as the eyelids, lips, nose, vulva, prepuce, and penis.
* Initially, the lesion may be papillomatous or appear as a nonhealing ulcer; as the lesion progresses, it develops scaling and ulceration, and becomes granulomatous.

* Many of these tumors bleed easily.
* Those involving the glans penis often are cauliflower-like.
* These tumors do not readily metastasize, despite their local invasiveness; when they do metastasize, they usually go no further than the local lymph nodes.
* Diagnosis is based on histologic examination of biopsy specimens (see *Equine Medicine and Surgery V*).
* Radical excision and/or radiation therapy is commonly used.
  * Cryosurgery ± cesium-37 needle implants has produced good results.
  * Hyperthermia also has been effective.
* Intratumoral cisplatin appears to be safe and effective.

Melanoma

Melanoma (dermal melanocytosis) is a common equine tumor, especially in older gray horses.

* Melanomas may be hard or soft, solitary or multiple, and dark brown or black.
  * They usually are 1 to 2 cm in diameter, but can be larger.
* The nodules are most often found on the perineum, vulva, and under surface of the tail, but they also occur on the male genitalia, limbs, neck, and ears.
* Three growth patterns have been described.
  * Prolonged and slow, without metastasis.
  * Prolonged and slow, followed by sudden, rapid growth and apparent metastasis.
  * Rapid, with malignant behavior from the onset (the most common type in nongray horses).
* Diagnosis usually is by physical examination; cytologic and histopathologic examinations are useful adjuncts.
  * Whenever possible, lesions in nongray horses should be biopsied by complete excision.
* Treatment of early solitary nodules is by excision or cryosurgery; treatment in advanced cases usually is unrewarding.

* Cimetidine (initially at 2.5 mg/kg PO q8h) may cause partial or complete regression.
  * The dosage is reduced for maintenance after a response is noted.

Basal Cell Tumor

Basal cell tumors are uncommon in horses. They tend to be found on the neck, thorax, and tail. The tumor may be solid or cystic, but most are ulcerated nodules. Excision is the treatment of choice.

Cutaneous Lymphosarcoma

Lymphosarcoma can be manifested as dermoepidermal or subcutaneous nodules that may appear as discrete masses or as multiple bumps resembling urticaria.

* Alopecia, sores over the bridge of the nose, subcutaneous nodular swellings on the neck, shoulder, forelegs, and perineum, and ulcerations of the vulva and cervix also may occur.
* Signs of systemic involvement (depression, weight loss, lymphadenopathy, anemia) usually occur as the disease progresses.
* The disease generally results in death or euthanasia.

Mast Cell Tumor

Mast cell tumors (cutaneous mastocytoma, cutaneous mastocytosis) are rare in horses.

* These tumors are 5 times more likely in males than in females.
* The most common form is a single 2- to 20-cm (0.75 to 7.75 inch) cutaneous/subcutaneous nodule on the head, neck, or distal extremities.
  * The surface of the nodule may be normal or either hairless or ulcerated.
  * Some of these tumors become mineralized.
  * Metastasis has not been reported.
* Total excisional biopsy is the best method of diagnosis and treatment.
  * Intralesional injection of corticosteroids may be useful when surgery is not possible.
* Recurrence, even after incomplete surgical removal, is rare.

Fibroma

Fibromas most commonly occur on the nictitating membrane, conjunctiva, and cornea, but they also occur on the neck, flanks, and legs. Histologically, fibromas can be distinguished from sarcoids, although some authors consider both tumors as sarcoids. Excision is the recommended treatment. Radiation therapy may be useful when adjacent structures do not allow complete excision.

Calcinosis Circumscripta

Calcinosis circumscripta (tumoral calcinosis) primarily occurs in young horses.

* The characteristic lesion is a large (3 to 12 cm [1.25 to 4.75 inch), dense, subcutaneous nodule on the lateral aspect of the stifle; the overlying skin is normal.
  * Lesions can be bilateral.
* Rarely is lameness or pain associated with the condition, which is not progressive.
* Radiography reveals an oval mass irregularly infiltrated with radiopaque deposits.
* Lesions may be intimately associated with the joint capsule, making surgical removal difficult; surgery is recommended only in lame horses or for cosmetic reasons.

Diseases Characterized by Granulomatous Draining Nodules or Masses *(pages 1883-1894)*

Dawn B. Logas and Joy L. Barbet

DIFFERENTIAL DIAGNOSES

In most cases, granulomatous draining masses are associated with an infectious process, whether bacterial, fungal, or parasitic. Consideration of the history, appearance and distribution of the lesions, and results of biopsy and bacterial and/or fungal culture are important for accurate diagnosis. Possible causes include:

* foreign bodies
* necrotic neoplasms

- bacterial infection/abscessation
  - Any organism can cause draining nodules or abscesses when introduced beneath the skin.
  - Botryomycosis (*Staphylococcus aureus* granuloma) consists of painless nodules that ulcerate and discharge pus; treatment involves drainage and/or excision.
  - *Corynebacterium pseudotuberculosis* causes large, deep, slowly developing, thick-walled abscesses, most often in the pectoral area (pigeon breast; see Chapter 15, Musculoskeletal System).
  - Other bacterial infections with specific clinical presentations are described below.
- fungal infection (see below)
  - *Conidiobolus coronataus* has a predilection for the nasal skin and mucosa.
  - *Basidiobolus haptosporus* causes solitary lesions on the trunk, chest, neck, and head.
  - Pythiosis typically occurs on the limbs or ventral chest and abdomen.
- habronemiasis (see below)
- screwworm myiasis (see below)
- parafilariasis (seen in Eastern Europe and Great Britain)
  - Subcutaneous nodules open and discharge a bloody exudate containing microfilariae and embryonated eggs; ivermectin is effective.
- panniculus (inflammation of the subcutaneous fat)
  - This condition is characterized by firm or soft nodules and plaques that may be painful.
  - Lesions may be single or multiple, localized or generalized; they may ulcerate and drain an oily yellow or brown exudate.
  - Glucocorticoids may be effective; relapse necessitates long-term maintenance therapy.

MANAGEMENT OF SELECTED CONDITIONS
Bacterial Infections
Ulcerative lymphangitis
Ulcerative lymphangitis is an uncommon but serious condition that most often occurs on the distal hind legs of horses kept in unsanitary conditions.

- *Corynebacterium pseudotuberculosis* is the most common organism involved.
  - Pyogenic *Streptococcus* spp., *Staphylococcus* spp., *Pseudomonas aeruginosa*, and *Rhodococcus equi* occasionally are isolated.
- Fever and edema of the affected limb often are the first signs.
- Small, well-defined, painful nodules develop, ulcerate, and discharge greenish, creamy pus.
- The regional lymphatics become corded and may ulcerate; lymphatic drainage may become compromised, causing the limb to remain swollen.
  - Cauliflower-like masses may develop on the distal limb.
- Treatment includes improving hygiene, daily cleansing of lesions with povidone iodine, and administration of systemic antibacterials, such as penicillin or trimethoprim-sulfonamides.
- Advanced cases may not respond well to treatment.

Bacterial bursitis
Fistulous withers and poll evil are infections of the supraspinous bursa and cranial nuchal bursa, respectively.

- Traditionally, *Brucella abortus* and *Actinomyces bovis* are most commonly implicated, although in recent reports *Streptococcus zooepidemicus* is isolated most often.
- Radical excision combined with systemic antibiotic therapy is the treatment of choice; further surgery is required in recurrent cases.
  - Deep tissue samples should be submitted for cultures if treatment is attempted.
- All affected horses should undergo serologic testing for brucellosis, and appropriate precautions taken until results are known.

Glanders
Also known as "farcy" or *enzootic lymphangitis,* glanders is caused by the gram-negative bacillus, *Pseudomonas mallei.* It has been eradicated from North America and much of Europe and currently is found pri-

marily in Eastern Europe, Asia, and North Africa. Cutaneous lesions include rapidly spreading ulcers of the nasal mucosa and nodules on the skin of the distal limbs (most often the hind limbs) or abdomen. The nodules ulcerate and rupture, discharging a thick, brown, honey-like exudate. Treatment is not recommended.

Fungal Infections

The most notable fungal infections are zygomycoses (*Conidiobolus* and *Basidiobolus* organisms) and pythiosis. Granulomas may be single or multiple and may have necrotic draining tracts. Most contain granules ("leeches" or "kunkers") throughout the granulation tissue; several are pruritic to the point of inducing self-mutilation. General treatment principles are as follows:

- Radical excision of all foci of infection is essential for effective treatment; nevertheless, recurrence is common.
- Systemic iodides are variably effective and may be most successful when used in conjunction with surgery.
- Topical preparations also can be used in conjunction with surgery.
  - This preparation consists of 400 mL of DMSO, 100 mL of 0.2-N HCl, 7.5 g of ketoconazole, and 4.8 g of rifampin (Phyco fixer).

Some of these fungi have zoonotic potential, so due care should be taken when managing these lesions.

Pythiosis

Pythiosis (Florida horse leeches, Gulf Coast fungus, swamp cancer, bursatti) is caused by *Pythium insidiosum,* formerly *Hyphomyces destruens,* a plant parasite.

- Lesions usually develop at the site of an injury, such as a wire cut or ventral midline dermatitis, and result from exposure of the wound to standing fresh water.
- A rapidly expanding, granulomatous, highly pruritic, draining lesion containing "leeches" is highly suggestive of pythiosis.
  - Invasion of regional lymph nodes may occur with long-standing lesions.

- Washed "leeches" should be submitted to a laboratory experienced in culture and identification of *Pythium* spp.
- Lesions that are too large for complete excision or in which adjacent tissues limit excision often are treated with surgery plus topical or systemic antifungal preparations.
  - Topical preparations include "Phyco Fixer," and amphotericin B mixed with either DMSO or 5% dextrose (see *Equine Medicine and Surgery V*).
  - Amphotericin B also may be injected intralesionally or given systemically (see p. 462)
- The prognosis is guarded in all cases.

Sporotrichosis

Sporothrix schenckii causes sporadic infection primarily of the skin and subcutaneous tissues.

- The organism spreads via the lymphatics, forming firm, subcutaneous 1- to 5-cm diameter nodules, usually on the medial surface of the limb(s).
  - Nodules are most numerous on the thigh or forearm and chest; they also may develop in the jugular groove.
  - Early lesions are small, red nodules that may exude seropurulent material; the nodules later ulcerate and discharge a small amount of thick pus.
- The lymphatics may become thickened and corded; persistent limb edema develops if lymph drainage is compromised.
- Giemsa-stained smears of exudate may demonstrate the round or cigar-shaped yeast form in macrophages or neutrophils.
- Iodides given IV and PO, combined with local wound care using iodine scrubs, usually yield good results.
  - Treatment should be continued for 3 to 4 weeks past clinical resolution.
- Griseofulvin (10 g/day for 2 weeks, then 6 g/day until lesions disappear) can be effective when iodine treatment fails.
  - Itraconazole is very effective in the treatment of sporotrichosis in humans.

Habronemiasis

Habronemiasis (summer sores) is a seasonal, sporadic disease that likely is a hypersensitivity reaction to larvae of the stomach worms *Habronema* spp. and *Draschia megastoma.*

- Larvae are deposited in skin wounds and moist places (e.g., eye, sheath, penis) by flies.
- Lesions usually are first apparent as slowly healing wounds that enlarge and develop exuberant granulation tissue; there often is a serosanguineous exudate.
  - Pruritus is mild to severe.
- Larvae deposited in the eye may produce granular conjunctivitis, most noticeable at the medial canthus.
- Biopsies should be taken from caseous and more granular areas for histopathologic examination (see *Equine Medicine and Surgery V*).
  - Peripheral eosinophilia may reach 15% to 20% of the total WBC count.

Treatment

Most cases can be treated medically, but large or refractory lesions may respond better if surgery or cryosurgery is used for debulking before medical therapy.

- Effective topical preparations contain a combination of organophosphates plus corticosteroids and/or DMSO; some also contain thiabendazole and/or antibacterials.
- Injectable or oral ivermectin also is effective, as are orally administered organophosphates and diethylcarbamazine (see *Equine Medicine and Surgery V*).
- Systemic corticosteroids can be effective as the sole therapy.
  - With prednisone at 1 mg/kg/day PO, improvement should occur within 7 to 14 days; the dosage can then be gradually reduced for withdrawal over the next 2 weeks.
- Ocular habronemiasis is treated with a corticosteroid-antibiotic ophthalmic ointment; conjunctival granulomas may require excision or curettage.
- Fly repellents, environmental insect control, and proper wound care are necessary to prevent recurrence, and all horses on the farm should be treated with ivermectin.

Screwworm Myiasis

In the United States, screwworm infestation sporadically occurs along the Texas-Mexico border.

- Larval invasion of wounds or natural body openings causes extensive liquefaction necrosis.
- Lesions are painful, pruritic, and foul smelling; resulting toxemia and/or septicemia can be fatal.
- Treatment involves thorough debridement and cleansing of the affected area, application of topical insecticides, such as malathion or coumaphos, and antibiotics as needed.

NOTE: *In the United States, screwworm myiasis is a reportable disease.*

Diseases Characterized by Diffuse Swelling or Edema *(pages 1895-1897)*

Dawn B. Logas and Joy L. Barbet

DIFFERENTIAL DIAGNOSES

Possible causes of diffuse swelling or edema include:

- subcutaneous emphysema (crepitus beneath the skin)
  - Causes include leakage from an airway, wounds in the axilla or groin, and infection with gas-forming bacteria (e.g., clostridia).
- bacterial cellulitis (see below)
- equine viral arteritis (see Chapter 19, Hemolymphatic System)
  - Painful edema of the ventrum, distal limbs, and eyelids can be prominent findings.
- bee stings
  - Stings of wasps, hornets, honey bees, or bumble bees cause local pain and edema.
  - Sensitized animals or those subject to a massive attack may develop urticaria, angioedema, or, rarely, death from a shocklike syndrome.
  - Treatment involves removal of the stingers and administration of glucocorticoids; topical application of Na-bicarbonate paste has been suggested.
- spider bites

- Spider bites are characterized by hot, edematous, painful swellings, frequently on the head and neck; bites of the brown recluse spider can cause severe dermal necrosis.
- Treatment includes application of cold packs and administration of systemic glucocorticoids and antihistamines.

◆ Angioedema (localized or generalized edematous swelling, most often involving the head).
- Corticosteroids usually are effective; NSAIDs also may be useful.
- Avoidance of the offending allergen, long-term low-dose corticosteroid therapy, or hyposensitization is indicated.

MANAGEMENT OF SELECTED CONDITIONS
Bacterial Cellulitis
Cellulitis is a serious condition, usually resulting from wound infection that rapidly spreads along tissue planes.
- It can result in skin loss, osteomyelitis, laminitis, and/or loss of function of the affected limb.
- A number of bacteria can cause cellulitis, including staphylococci, streptococci, corynebacteria, and clostridia.
- Treatment should include drainage and debridement of any abscesses, IV antibiotics, NSAIDs, hot packs, hydrotherapy, and support wraps.
  - Antibiotic therapy should include β-lactamase-resistant drugs, such as methicillin, cloxacillin, and ceftiofur.
Clostridial cellulitis
Clostridial cellulitis (malignant edema, gas gangrene) occurs secondary to injection or wound infection. Edema develops at the site of introduction and rapidly progresses to a hot, painful swelling. The skin becomes dark red or black and emphysema may be present. The animal usually is depressed, anorectic, and febrile. Aggressive treatment must be given early to save the animal (see Chapter 15, Musculoskeletal System).

Diseases Characterized by Nonpruritic Alopecia and Scaling
(pages 1897-1901)
Dawn B. Logas and Joy L. Barbet

DIFFERENTIAL DIAGNOSES
Possible causes of alopecia and scaling without pruritus include:
◆ hair follicle dystrophy
  - Hair in affected areas is stubbled, dull, and brittle.
◆ white piedra (infection with the fungus *Trichosporon beigelii*)
  - Affected hairs in the mane, tail, and forelock tend to break off easily.
  - Microscopic examination reveals whitish nodules in the hair shaft above the level of the hair follicle; clipping the hair proximal to the nodules is curative.
◆ demodectic mange (see below)
◆ hypothyroidism (see Chapter 18, Endocrine System)
  - Skin changes include dull hair coat, delayed shedding, and edema of the face and limbs.
◆ chronic selenium poisoning (see below)
◆ iodism
  - Signs include alopecia that spares the mane, tail, and distal limbs, and diffuse scaliness.
  - Removal of the iodine source results in rapid recovery.
◆ mercury poisoning (see below)
◆ leucinosis (toxicosis caused by *Leucaena* spp., or jumby tree)
  - The long hairs of the mane, tail, and fetlocks is lost, and disturbed growth at the coronary band and periople causes hoof dystrophies.
  - Preventing further access to the plant and adding 1% ferrous sulfate to the feed reduces the severity of the problem.
◆ anagen defluxion (hair loss that occurs within days of physiologic stress, such as high fever, systemic illness, or malnutrition)
  - Pressure points and frictional areas are affected first; the mane and tail are spared.

- telogen effluvium or defluxion (stress-related abrupt cessation of hair growth)
  - Large amounts of hair are shed 2 to 3 months after stresses such as fever, pregnancy, shock, and severe illness.
- anhidrosis (see below)
- alopecia areata (rare)
  - Alopecia areata is characterized by sharply circumscribed areas of alopecia with normal skin underneath.

MANAGEMENT OF SELECTED CONDITIONS

Demodectic Mange

Demodectic mange is caused by *Demodex equi.*

- It is rare in horses; clinical disease primarily occurs in immunocompromised animals.
- Lesions are most often found on the forelimbs, neck, and head.
- Alopecic patches covered with branlike scales are typical; secondary bacterial folliculitis and furunculosis may be present.
- Demonstration of mites in multiple, deep skin scrapings from lesions is diagnostic.
  - Biopsies also aid diagnosis.
- General supportive care, such as good nutrition and hygiene, and correction of underlying medical problems are important and may induce spontaneous regression.
  - Bathing the horse and applying a miticide may be helpful in refractory cases (see *Equine Medicine and Surgery V*).
- The condition is not contagious.

Selenium Poisoning

Chronic selenium poisoning ("alkali disease") results from long-term consumption of selenium-accumulating plants or cereal grains or grasses grown in seleniferous soils.

- Seleniferous soils and vegetation are found in much of the western United States and plains states.
- Selenosis causes transverse hoof wall cracks and loss of mane, tail, and fetlock hairs.
- History of exposure, physical findings, and measurement of selenium in tissues, soil, feeds, and water aid definitive diagnosis.
  - Abnormal amounts of selenium in the blood (>1 ppm or >100 mg/dl in blood, >11 ppm in hair, and >3 ppm in hooves) are characteristic of alkali disease.
- Good nursing care and preventing access to high-selenium feeds are important for treatment.
  - Increasing dietary protein, especially sulfur-containing amino acids, is beneficial.
  - Naphthalene (4 to 5 g PO for 5 days, repeated after a 5-day rest) and d,l-methionine (2 to 3 g/day PO) are sometimes recommended.
- Recovery is prolonged.

Mercury Poisoning

The major cause of systemic mercury poisoning is ingestion of mercury-treated seed grain.

- Signs include loss of hair (including the mane and tail) and slight scaling of the skin.
  - Systemic signs include gastroenteritis, anorexia, depression, and emaciation.
- History, physical findings, and urinary or fecal mercury concentrations aid diagnosis.
- K-iodide at 4 g/day for 14 days, coupled with stabling and blanketing, is beneficial.

Topical preparations and blisters containing mercury may cause contact dermatitis, characterized by vesicles that progress to crusted, pruritic lesions.

Anhidrosis

Anhidrosis (dry coat, nonsweating) is a problem in hot, humid climates.

- Affected horses cease to sweat during exercise.
  - Onset of anhidrosis often is preceded by profuse sweating and excessive "blowing."
  - Depending on the degree of anhidrosis, horses may have rectal temperatures of up to 38.9° C (102° F) at rest, and up to 42.2° C (108° F) after exercise.
  - Fatigue, anorexia, and decreased water consumption also may be present.

- Horses affected for several months tend to have a dull, rough, flaky hair coat and alopecia of the face and body friction areas.
- The diagnosis is confirmed by demonstrating a lack of sweating in response to intradermal epinephrine.
  - 0.1 mL of epinephrine is injected under the mane or over the dorsal rib cage at dilutions of 1:1000, 1:10,000, 1:100,000 and 1:1,000,000.
  - Normal horses sweat within minutes of injection at any dilution.
- The most logical treatment is to move the horse to a cooler, more arid climate.
  - When this is not feasible, an air-conditioned stall is the best solution, along with limiting exercise to the cool part of the day.
  - No medical treatments have been consistently beneficial.

Diseases Characterized by Pruritus and Hair Loss *(pages 1901-1909)*
Dawn B. Logas and Joy L. Barbet

DIFFERENTIAL DIAGNOSES

Pruritus and alopecia usually are caused by a hypersensitivity reaction, most often to an ectoparasite. Possible causes, in approximate order of occurrence, include:

- *Culicoides* hypersensitivity (see below)
- cutaneous onchocerciasis (see below)
- horn fly dermatitis
  - Lesions may be found on the shoulders, neck, withers, and abdomen (most common site).
  - Lesions consist of papules and wheals with a central crust; they progress to areas of alopecia, excoriation, crusting, and lichenification; leukoderma may result.
  - Treatment with an corticosteroid-antibiotic ointment may be required in severe cases, but use of insecticides and repellents and separating horses and cattle usually suffice.

- fly (buffalo gnat) dermatitis
  - The head, insides of the ears, neck, pectoral region, and ventrum are favored sites.
  - Papules and wheals may be followed by vesicle formation, hemorrhage, and necrosis; alopecia, excoriations, and lichenification result from chronic scratching.
  - Heavy attacks can result in death from a toxin in the flies' saliva.
  - Treatment includes stabling during daylight hours, use of systemic corticosteroids until fly populations are controlled, and application of fly repellents at least daily.
- oxyuriasis (infestation with *Oxyuris equi*, or pinworms)
  - *Oxyuris equi* infestation causes anal pruritus, primarily in stabled horses; severe rubbing limited to the tail and perineum is the primary feature.
  - Diagnosis is made by applying clear acetate tape to the perineal region and examining the tape microscopically for pinworm eggs.
  - Good stable management and deworming with ivermectin, benzimidazoles, or pyrantel pamoate are effective.
- pediculosis (louse infestation; see below)
- mange (sarcoptic, psoroptic, chorioptic; see below)
- trombiculid infestation (chiggers, heel bugs, harvest mites; see below)

MANAGEMENT OF SELECTED CONDITIONS
Culicoides Hypersensitivity

Dermatitis caused by hypersensitivity to biting gnats in the genus *Culicoides* has been reported in many parts of the world.

- In the early stages, small papules with erect hair may be seen at the favored feeding sites, classically the ears, poll, mane, withers, tail head, and ventral abdomen.
- Severe pruritus causes self-mutilation, resulting in broken hairs, scattered areas of alopecia, fresh excoriations, and scabs.
- Lesions heal and hair grows back during the winter, but the problem

returns the following spring or summer.

Treatment

Treatment involves protecting affected horses from the gnats.

- Stabling the horse from before sundown to well after sunrise is critical.
  - Fine-mesh screens, fans to create a breeze, insecticides applied to the screens, and time-operated spray-mist insecticide systems also help.
- Insecticides and repellents applied at least once daily are useful; the most effective products are synergized pyrethrins or long-acting synthetic pyrethroids.
- Destroying the larval habitat by draining nearby ponds and improving pasture drainage also is important in reducing gnat numbers.

Corticosteroid administration often is necessary while insect-control measures are being implemented. Oral prednisone is recommended. Hydroxyzine is the only antihistamine with reported efficacy in these horses, and is helpful only in some cases.

Cutaneous Onchocerciasis

Onchocerciasis is a nonseasonal dermatitis caused by microfilariae of *Onchocerca cervicalis*.

- Microfilarial numbers in the dermis are highest along the ventral midline, pectoral region, withers, inguinal region, and eyelids.
- Initial lesions consist of thinning hair, ± mild scaling or crusting, and mild-to-severe pruritus.
  - Lesions in the center of the forehead are a hallmark of cutaneous onchocerciasis.
- As the disease progresses, lesions become ulcerated, erythematous, and crusted; lichenification occurs with chronicity.
  - Leukoderma (depigmentation) often occurs and usually is irreversible.
- Ocular lesions also occur; most common is conjunctival depigmentation at the temporal limbus (see Chapter 14, Ocular System).
- Diagnosis is confirmed by response to therapy; finding microfilariae in skin biopsies or deep

scrapings is nondiagnostic because many unaffected horses have microfilariae.

Treatment

Ivermectin is the treatment of choice.

- Improvement is seen in 21 days, and resolution should be nearly complete by 2 months.
  - Retreatment at 2- to 8-month intervals may be required.
- Edema ± pruritus at lesion sites after treatment occurs in about 10% of horses.
  - The response tends to resolve in 24 to 72 hours, whether or not corticosteroids are used.
- If significant ocular disease is present, especially uveitis, it should be controlled before treatment to control microfilariae is instituted.
  - Systemic glucocorticoids should be used during microfilaricidal treatment in these cases.

Use of microfilaricides other than ivermectin (e.g., diethylcarbamazine and levamisole) is discussed in *Equine Medicine and Surgery V*.

Pediculosis

Louse infestation is most common during winter and early spring, when horses have long coats.

- Affected horses rub and bite at their head, neck, mane, flanks, and tail; a rough coat with varying degrees of alopecia and self-inflicted lesions is typical.
- Examination of the skin and parted hairs reveals nits (eggs) attached to hair.
- Two treatments with water-based insecticide sprays or powders 2 weeks apart usually eradicate lice; fomites, such as tack and grooming equipment, should be similarly treated.

Sarcoptic Mange

Sarcoptic mange (scabies, barn itch) is caused by *Sarcoptes scabei* var *equi*.

- Infestation causes intense pruritus; papules appear on the neck, shoulders, and head, gradually progressing to the entire body in untreated cases.
  - Severe itching causes scaly, crusted, excoriated, alopecic, and lichenified skin.

- Multiple superficial and deep skin scrapings must be performed in suspected cases, but negative results do not rule out the disease.
- Sarcoptic mange is treated with topical organophosphates or lime sulfur solution.
  - Thorough wetting of the skin surface is required.
  - Treatments should be repeated at 7- to 14-day intervals at least 3 times.
  - All in-contact horses and contaminated equipment also should be treated.
- Ivermectin PO at least twice, 2 to 3 weeks apart, may be effective.
- Spraying of the premises with a residual acaricide may help prevent reinfestation.
  NOTE: Sarcoptic mange is a reportable disease; infested horses should be quarantined until deemed disease-free.

Psoroptic Mange

Psoroptic mange, caused by *Psoroptes equi,* is highly contagious.
- Intensely pruritic lesions usually are first noticed at the base of the mane, under the forelock, and at the tail base.
- Initial lesions are papules and alopecia, followed by moist, hemorrhagic crusts, scaling, excoriations, and lichenification.
- Scrapings made from the edges of crusts are likely to yield mites.
- Treatment is similar to that described for sarcoptic mange.

Chorioptic Mange

Chorioptic mange (leg or foot mange) is caused by *Chorioptes equi.*
- The disease is most common in winter; draft horses are particularly susceptible.
- Lesions usually develop around the foot and fetlock, causing the horse to stomp and bite.
  - Lesions tend to begin on the hind limbs and extend to the thighs, tail, and abdomen.
- A fine, papular eruption may be noted early in the course, followed by alopecia, crusting, and lichenification.
- Mites usually are found in skin scrapings.

- It may be useful to mix rotenone with mineral oil (1:3) for the scrapings.
- Treatment is similar to that for sarcoptic mange.

Trombiculid and Forage Mite Infestations

Trombiculid mites cause mangelike lesions on the head, neck, chest, and legs.
- Populations tend to be highest in the spring and again in the late summer and fall.
- The papular or wheal-like lesions become encrusted and tufts of hair may be lost; pruritus is variable.
- Close inspection of early lesions reveals red or orange clusters of larval mites.
  - Mites may be identified in skin scrapings from typical lesions, but because mites drop off after a few days, they may not be found if it has been several days since exposure.
- Treatment with 5% lime sulfur washes or acaricides, and removal or insecticidal treatment of contaminated bedding are effective.
  - Addition of detergent to acaricides may increase penetration of the mite's cuticle.
- Infestations are self-limiting when exposure ceases.

Diseases Characterized by Multifocal-to-Diffuse Alopecia, Crusts, and Papules *(pages 1909-1917)*
Dawn B. Logas and Joy L. Barbet

DIFFERENTIAL DIAGNOSES

Causes of multifocal or diffuse alopecia, crusts, and papules are diverse, and include:
- solar keratosis
  - Lesions occur in sparsely haired and lightly pigmented skin; appearance varies from erythematous, scaly patches to hard plaques covered with hyperkeratotic crusts.

- These lesions are premalignant, capable of transforming into squamous cell carcinoma.
  - Treatment is surgical.
- dermatophilosis ("rain scald"; see below)
- bacterial folliculitis (see below)
- dermatophytosis (ringworm; see below)
- viral papular dermatitis
  - Viral papular dermatitis is characterized by numerous firm papules or nodules, 0.5 to 2 cm in diameter, that within 1 week develop crusts that later drop off, leaving circumscribed scaly and hairless areas.
  - The course of the disease varies from 2 to 6 weeks (average, 3 weeks).
- molluscum contagiosum (rare)
  - Well circumscribed, smooth, gray or white papules with a waxy surface develop on the penis, prepuce, scrotum, udder, groin, axilla, and muzzle.
  - They umbilicate and develop a central pore from which a caseous plug is extruded.
  - The disease usually is self-limiting and requires no treatment.
- horse pox (rare, usually benign, and occurs only in Europe)
- pemphigus foliaceus (see below)

MANAGEMENT OF SELECTED CONDITIONS

Dermatophilosis

Dermatophilosis ("rain scald") is an exudative dermatitis caused by the actinomycete *Dermatophilus congolensis*.

- It is more common following prolonged periods of overcast and rainy weather.
- Lesions are most common on the rump, loins, and back, but also occur on the distal limbs.
- Exudate mats the hair together to form plaques that may be tender to the touch.
  - Removal of a matted tuft of hair reveals a moist, pink, bleeding lesion and exudate on the underside of the crust.
- The organism usually is readily identified in smears from exudate on the

underside of the crusts or from crusts crushed on a slide (see p. 454).

- Treatment involves keeping the animal dry, removal and appropriate disposal of the crusts, and, in severe or chronic cases, procaine penicillin at 22,000 IU/kg IM for 5 to 7 days.
  - If crust removal is painful, systemic antibiotics and iodophor or chlorhexidine shampoos should be used for several days before crust removal.
- In mild cases, only topical therapy may be necessary.
  - Solutions of lime sulfur (2% to 5%), captan (3%), or povidone iodine (1:10) may be applied daily as a spray or a dip for the first 5 to 7 days, and weekly thereafter.
  - Many horses spontaneously recover in about 4 weeks.
- Infections in humans may result from contact with infected animals and crusts.

Staphylococcal Folliculitis

Folliculitis caused by *Staphylococcus aureus* is the most common type of bacterial folliculitis.

- Cutaneous trauma, excessive sweating, friction from tack, and stress are involved.
- Lesions occur on the thorax, pasterns, and/or tail.
- The primary lesion is a papule centered around a hair follicle, which causes the hairs to stand up; lesions usually are quite painful when palpated.
  - Pustules may extend into the dermis and subcutis to produce more severe inflammation (furunculosis), with nodules, ulceration, crusting, and draining tracts.
- In the tail form of the disease, pustules arise on the dorsal surface of the tail; severe pruritus leads to self-mutilation, resulting in a chronic condition that responds poorly to treatment.
- Skin scrapings and bacterial and fungal cultures are necessary in the diagnostic workup.
  - Preparations of crusts should be examined for the presence of *Dermatophilus* organisms.

Treatment

Treatment varies somewhat with the severity.

◆ Mild or early infections may respond to iodophor, benzoyl peroxide, or chlorhexidine shampoos, plus rest from the inciting trauma.
◆ If only a few furuncles are present, mupirocin may be applied daily for 5 to 10 days.
◆ More widespread infections and furunculosis require treatment with systemic antibiotics, daily baths with antibacterial shampoos, and rest.
  • Suitable antibiotics include cephalexin (15 to 30 mg/kg q8h), ceftiofur (10 mg/kg q12h), and trimethoprim-sulfamethoxazole (15 mg/kg q12h).
  • Treatment should continue for 2 to 3 weeks.
◆ For tail pyoderma, treatment involves systemic antibiotic therapy and clipping, washing, and application of antibiotic soaks; sublesional antibiotics also may be beneficial.

Corynebacterial Folliculitis

Corynebacterium pseudotuberculosis infection sometimes causes folliculitis (contagious acne, Canadian horse pox, contagious pustular dermatitis).

◆ Painful or pruritic papules develop into pustules and then into furuncles in areas of the skin that contact the harness or tack.
◆ Diagnosis and treatment are similar to that for staphylococcal folliculitis.
  • Some lesions coalesce to develop craterlike ulcers that are poorly responsive to antibiotics and may require surgical excision.

Dermatophytosis (Ringworm)

Dermatophytosis (ringworm, girth itch) is a superficial fungal infection mainly caused by fungi of the genera *Microsporum* and *Trichophyton*.

◆ Young horses are particularly prone to ringworm; warm, damp, dirty, overcrowded, poorly ventilated stables encourage mycotic infection.
◆ Typical features include multiple foci of scaling, crusting, and alopecia, primarily in areas that contact the tack; the lesions spread in a characteristic centrifugal fashion.
  • Very early lesions may be papular, resembling fly bites or urticaria.
  • About 30% of affected horses manifest pruritus and about 20% manifest some pain.
◆ Microscopic examination and fungal culture are best for definitive diagnosis.

Treatment

Most cases spontaneously regress in 2 to 3 months, unless the horse is immunodeficient. Topical and/or systemic treatments can be used to reduce the chances of spread and shorten the course.

◆ If possible, all lesions and a 2.5-cm area surrounding each lesion should be clipped.
◆ The entire horse is bathed with povidone iodine or chlorhexidine shampoo.
◆ After rinsing, a solution of captan (3%), lime sulfur (2% to 5%), chlorhexidine (2% to 3%), or Na-hypochlorite (1:10) is applied to the lesions and sponged on the rest of the body.
  • Treatment should be repeated daily for 1 week, then once or twice weekly.
◆ Griseofulvin (5 to 10 mg/kg PO daily for 1 to 2 months) may be used in refractory cases, although clipping and topical therapy are still necessary.
◆ Adverse environmental factors, such as overcrowding and filth, should be corrected.
  • Disinfection of equipment, pens, and feed bunks is vital.
  • Povidone iodine, 6% Nahypochlorite, 3% cresol, 5% lime sulfur, benzalkonium-Cl, 3% captan, and a solution of 1% lime and 1.5% copper sulfate each are effective.

Handlers should be warned of the zoonotic potential.

Pemphigus Foliaceus

Pemphigus foliaceus is an autoimmune disease that is characterized by autoantibodies directed against components of the epidermis.

- A juvenile form and an adult form have been reported in horses; Appaloosas are predisposed.
- Generalized scaling, crusting, and exudation are the most outstanding signs.
  - Usually these lesions are preceded by transient, often undetected, vesicle and pustule formation; pain or pruritus may be present.
  - Scaling and crusting usually are first apparent on the head, dorsal neck, and sometimes the limbs; occasionally only the coronary bands are affected.
  - Mucocutaneous junctions usually are not involved.
- Limb edema is common and more prominent over the joints; ventral midline edema and edema of the male genitalia also occur.
- Depression occurs in 80% of affected horses, and many are intermittently febrile.
- Signs may wax and wane in a cyclic manner, without apparent cause; signs persist for life, except in the juvenile form.

Diagnosis

Definitive diagnosis is based on histopathologic examination.

- Multiple biopsies should be taken from perilesional and lesional skin, especially from any intact pustules or vesicles.
- Supportive evidence may be derived from direct immunofluorescent of biopsy specimens preserved in Michel's medium.
  - Diagnosis should not be based entirely on results of direct immunofluorescence, however.

Treatment

Long-term immunosuppressive doses of corticosteroids (e.g., oral prednisolone) or gold salts are required (see p. 463). After several months of treatment, gradual withdrawal from immunosuppressive therapy may be attempted; however, most adult horses require medication indefinitely. The juvenile form carries a better prognosis, as remission may be achieved in most cases.

Diseases Characterized by Focal Erythema, Exudation, Crusting, Scaling, and Alopecia

(pages 1917-1920)

Dawn B. Logas and Joy L. Barbet

DIFFERENTIAL DIAGNOSES

Causes of focal erythema, exudation, crusting, scaling, and alopecia include:

- contact irritant dermatitis
  - Lesions range from erythematous and edematous papular and/or scaly eruptions to severe irritation manifested as vesicles, erosions, ulcerations, crusting, and necrosis.
  - Treatment involves cleansing the area and avoiding further contact with the substance.
- fire ant stings
  - Lesions are characterized by pain, swelling, and exudation; the initial lesion is a pustule that quickly ruptures, forming a crust.
  - Treatment may include cleansing followed by application of astringent rinses, systemic glucocorticoids, and NSAIDs; systemic antibiotics may prevent secondary infection.
- contact hypersensitivity (see below)
- photosensitization (see below)

MANAGEMENT OF SELECTED CONDITIONS

Contact Hypersensitivity

Unlike contact irritant dermatitis, which may occur on the first exposure to the offending agent, contact hypersensitivity requires previous exposure.

- Haptens that may be involved include ions, such as nickel or iodine, and plant oleoresins.
  - These substances may be liberated from dyes, rubber, or plants contacting a wet or sweaty skin surface or nonhaired area.
- Lesions are similar to those of contact irritant dermatitis; chronic cases are characterized by alopecia,

lichenification, and pigment changes.
* Provocative exposure and/or patch testing help identify the offending substance.
* Treatment of acutely affected horses includes ceasing contact with the allergen and gentle cleansing, followed by topical and/or systemic glucocorticoid therapy.
* Long- term, low-dose glucocorticoid therapy may be necessary if contact with the allergen cannot be eliminated.

Photosensitization

Photosensitization occurs by one of two mechanisms:
* Primary photosensitization is caused by substances containing a photodynamic agent.
  · Incriminated plants include buckwheat, St. John's wort, perennial rye grass, and burr trefoil.
  · Photosensitizing chemicals include tetracyclines, chlorothiazides, acriflavines, rose bengal, methylene blue, and sulfonamides.
* Secondary photosensitization is associated with liver dysfunction, caused by such insults as toxic plants, mycotoxins, infection, neoplasia, and hepatotoxic chemicals.
  · Of particular importance are plants containing pyrrolizidine alkaloids (*Senecio* spp., *Amsinckia* spp., *Crotalaria* spp.), unknown agents in burning bush (*Kochia* spp.), toxins produced by blue-green algae, and serum or antiserum.
  · Photosensitization resulting from phenothiazines is a primary effect, but it results from liver dysfunction that causes accumulation of the photodynamic agent.
  · Secondary photosensitization is the most common form in large animals.
* Some other agents that can cause photosensitization by unknown mechanisms include oats, clover, vetch, alfalfa, and *Dermatophilus* organisms.

Clinical signs and diagnosis

Nonpigmented skin and thinly haired areas, such as the face, eyelids, ears, lips, coronary band, and perineum, are the primary sites of lesions.
* Edema, erythema, crusting, fissuring, and peeling of superficial skin layers are seen.
* In severe cases, vesicles form, the skin is swollen and painful, and exudation is prominent; patches of skin may necrose and slough completely.
* Pruritus is more common with the hepatogenous form; weight loss, icterus, or signs of CNS dysfunction also may be present if hepatic failure is the cause.
* Liver function tests and careful investigation into the animal's dietary and drug history are essential for diagnosis.

Treatment and prognosis

Treatment involves removal of the offending substance and stabling the horse during daylight hours. Systemic corticosteroids, as well as application of topical antibiotic/corticosteroid ointments, may be beneficial. Symptomatic therapy, such as cleansing and debridement of sloughing skin, may be necessary. Treatment for hepatic insufficiency often is unsuccessful (see Chapter 10, Alimentary System). The prognosis for primary photosensitization usually is good, whereas the prognosis for photosensitization secondary to liver damage usually is poor.

Diseases Characterized by Ulceration and Crusting of Mucocutaneous Regions *(pages 1920-1922)*

Dawn B. Logas and Joy L. Barbet

DIFFERENTIAL DIAGNOSES

Identification of the cause of ulceration and crusting in mucocutaneous regions depends on the location or distribution of the lesions, presence of systemic signs, and the immune status of the animal. Possible causes include:

- candidiasis (rare; can cause oral lesions in immunodeficient foals)
  - Lesions comprise ulcerative patches in the oral cavity, especially on the tongue, and at mucocutaneous junctions; lesions may be covered with a thick, whitish exudate.
  - Treatment involves correction of the underlying condition and topical nystatin, miconazole, clotrimazole, K-permanganate, or gentian violet (1:10,000 in 10% alcohol).
- coital exanthema (equine herpesvirus 3)
  - Lesions consist of papules, vesicles, pustules, and sometimes bullae on the perineum and vulva of the mare and on the penis and prepuce of the stallion (see Chapter 12, Reproductive System: The Stallion, and Chapter 13, Reproductive System: The Mare).
- vesicular stomatitis (see below)
- bullous pemphigoid (see below)
- stachybotryotoxicosis (fungal toxicosis caused by *Stachybotrys* spp. in hay and straw)
  - It primarily occurs in Eastern Europe.
  - Mucocutaneous ulceration and necrosis ± mucosal petechiae are characteristic; catarrhal rhinitis, suppurative rhinopharyngitis, and laryngitis follow.
- pentachlorophenol toxicosis (e.g., waste motor oil, fungicides, mothproofing agents, molluscicides, and wood preservatives)
  - Pentachlorophenol causes generalized ulcerative dermatitis, anorexia, listlessness, weight loss, weakness, unsteady gait, chronic coughing, lacrimation, serous nasal discharge, and death.
  - There is no treatment.

MANAGEMENT OF SELECTED CONDITIONS

Vesicular Stomatitis

Vesicular stomatitis is a *reportable* vesicular disease affecting horses, donkeys, cattle, swine, and several wild species.

- It is characterized by salivation, slight depression, reluctance to eat, and polydipsia develop following a 1- to 3-day incubation.
  - 90% of reported cases occurred in August and September.
- Lesions include macules, vesicles, and erosions successively appearing on the buccal mucosa, dorsum of the tongue, lips, muzzle, prepuce, udder, teats, and/or coronary band.
  - Vesicles tend to be transient and lesions may first be noticed as erosions.
  - Vesicles on the coronary band may be painful enough to cause lameness.
- A small amount of epithelium, saliva, or vesicular fluid can be submitted for virus isolation, or fluid from lesions can be submitted for a complement-fixation test; serology also is used.
- Treatment is mainly supportive, unless secondary infection necessitates antibiotic therapy.
  - Recovery takes 3 to 9 days.
- Stabling and insect eradication drastically reduce the incidence; contact with outside animals should be prevented.

Bullous Pemphigoid

Bullous pemphigoid is an immune-mediated, blistering dermatosis.

- Intact vesicles and bullae rarely are seen, but instead, ulceration and crusting occur.
- Lesions usually occur at mucocutaneous junctions or in the oral, axillary, and/or inguinal regions; the lesions may be painful or pruritic.
  - Anorexia can result from painful oral cavity lesions or systemic illness.
- Biopsy of intact vesicles or bullae is essential for diagnosis; multiple biopsies may be required at different times to arrive at the diagnosis.
  - Direct immunofluorescence provides supporting evidence, although negative results do not rule out the disease.
- Immunosuppressive doses of glucocorticoids are necessary to control the disease.

- Azathioprine or gold salts may be needed in combination with glucocorticoids.
- The prognosis is poor.

Diseases Characterized by Ulceration, Exudation, and Crusting of the Distal Extremities *(pages 1922–1925)*

Dawn B. Logas and Joy L. Barbet

DIFFERENTIAL DIAGNOSES

Causes of ulceration, exudation, and crusting of the extremities include:

- frostbite (from extreme cold weather or cryotherapy)
  - Affected skin becomes pale, then erythematous and swollen; later, hair and superficial layers of the skin are shed, and necrosis and dry gangrene may occur.
  - Treatment involves rapid thawing in warm water, use of bland ointments, and routine wound care.
- rhabditic dermatitis (see below)
- cutaneous vasculitis (hypersensitivity reaction)
  - Manifested as dependent edema, pain or reluctance to move, exudation, crusting, erosion, and ulceration.
  - Treatment consists of systemic glucocorticoids, antibiotics, limb wraps, hydrotherapy, and supportive care as needed.
- purpura hemorrhagica (see below)
- ergotism (see below)
- pastern dermatitis (see below)

MANAGEMENT OF SELECTED CONDITIONS

Rhabditic Dermatitis

Pelodera (*Rhabditis*) *strongyloides,* a nematode that lives in moist soil and decaying organic material, can penetrate the skin of animals kept in unclean environments.

- Signs include alopecia, papules, pustules, ulcers, crusts, scaling, erythema, and pruritus on areas in contact with contaminated bedding, usually the limbs and ventrum.
- Deep skin scrapings reveal small, motile nematode larvae; bedding or soil samples also may contain adult and larval nematodes.
- Infection usually is self-limiting if the animal is moved to clean, dry quarters or if contaminated material is removed from the environment.
  - Spraying the premises with an insecticide, such as malathion, has been recommended.
  - In severe cases, bathing with medicated shampoos, along with topical thiabendazole solution or PO ivermectin, may be effective.
  - Small doses of glucocorticoids may be useful if pruritus is severe.

Purpura Hemorrhagica

Purpura hemorrhagica most often is a sequela to *Streptococcus equi* infection.

- It also can follow infections with *Rhodococcus equi,* equine influenza virus, and other infectious agents.
- Onset of disease usually is 2 to 4 weeks after a respiratory infection.
- It may begin with urticaria, followed by edema of the limbs, ventrum, and head.
- Edema can progress to sanguineous exudation, ulceration, crusting and, finally, sloughing.
  - Mucosal petechiae and ecchymoses may be seen, but fever and anorexia are uncommon.
- Mild-to-moderate anemia and neutrophilia with hypergammaglobulinemia and hyperfibrinogenemia are common; platelet counts and clotting profiles are normal.
- Complications (pyoderma, pneumonia, myositis, renal failure) frequently result in death, so early and aggressive therapy is warranted.
  - Penicillin is given for 5 to 7 days.
  - Furosemide (1 mg/kg q12h) may be useful to reduce edema for the first 2 to 4 days.
  - Prednisone is given at 0.5 to 1 mg/kg PO or IM q12h until remission.
  - Hydrotherapy or gentle exercise may help reduce edema.

* Relapse can occur during recovery, despite therapy.

Ergotism

Claviceps purpurea (ergot), a fungus of rye and many other cereal grains, can cause persistent arteriolar spasm and capillary endothelial damage.

* Lameness, particularly involving the hind limbs, often is the first sign.
* Examination reveals erythema, swelling, coldness, alopecia, and lack of sensation in affected areas, including the teats, tail, and ears.
  * There usually is a distinct demarcation between affected and unaffected areas.
  * With progression, the skin appears dry, turns bluish-black, and eventually sloughs.
  * Fever, anorexia, and weight loss may be present.
* History, physical findings, and examination of feed for the ergot are sufficient for diagnosis.
* Treatment requires removal of contaminated feed and such supportive care as hot soaks, gentle cleansing, and antibiotics.
* Close grazing or mowing of pastures, especially in wet years, prevents formation of seed heads where the fungus grows.

Pastern Dermatitis

"Scratches," "grease heel," "mud fever," and "cracked heels" are common terms for crusting and seborrheic dermatitis of the heel and palmar/plantar pastern regions.

* It occurs most often in breeds with long fetlock hair or horses kept in muddy paddocks, unsanitary conditions, or rough, stubbled pastures.
  * Grit particles on some track surfaces also can precipitate the condition.
* Lesions tend to be bilateral, with the hind limbs affected more often.
* The pain, swelling, alopecia, exudation, and ulceration cause lameness in some horses.
  * Secondary bacterial infection is common.
  * In chronic cases, foul odor and fissures may be present; granulomatous growths ("grapes") occasionally result.

Treatment

Therapy begins with clipping and cleansing with benzoyl peroxide shampoo and warm water.

* Soaking may be necessary to remove crusts and mats.
* Astringents, such as aluminum acetate, white lotion (zinc and lead sulfate), and calamine lotion, are applied when the dermatitis is in the acute, exudative stage.
* In chronic cases, where there is lichenification and fissuring, antibiotic-corticosteroid creams or ointments should be used.
  * Granulomatous masses should be removed by resection, electrocautery, or cryosurgery.
* Systemic antibiotics are beneficial when secondary pyoderma is present.
* The horse should be kept in dry, clean quarters.

Recurrence may be prevented by keeping heel and pastern hair short, maintaining the horse in a clean, dry environment, and application of udder ointments, petrolatum, or other emollients.

Diseases Characterized by Focal or Diffuse Scaling, Crusting, and Alopecia *(pages 1925-1928)*

Dawn B. Logas and Joy L. Barbet

DIFFERENTIAL DIAGNOSES

Focal scaling, crusting, and alopecia may be caused by a wide variety of conditions, including:

* linear keratosis
* Lesions consist of one or more linear areas of alopecia, crusting, and hyperkeratosis, 0.5 to 1 cm wide and 5 to 50 cm (2 to 20 inches) long, on the lateral neck or thorax.
  * Inflammation is minimal and there is no pruritus; lesions persist indefinitely.
  * Most cases occur in young Quarter Horses.

- Keratolytic preparations (coal tar, sulfur ointments and shampoo, salicylic acid, undecylenic acid) and corticosteroid ointments may reduce scaling.
- cannon keratosis
  - Lesions comprise scaling, alopecia, crusting, and seborrhea on the dorsal surface of the hind cannons.
  - Antiseborrheic shampoos may be used locally to control scaling; glucocorticoid creams applied twice daily are useful in severe cases.
- besnoitiosis (rare disease caused by the protozoan *Besnoitia bennetti*)
  - Seen in horses in Sudan and in Mexican burros.
  - Lesions comprise generalized thickening, lichenification, and scaling of the skin; the subcutis of the perineal, genital, and abdominal regions may contain multiple papules.
- systemic lupus erythematosus (see below)
- eosinophilic dermatitis (see below)
- generalized granulomatous disease (see below)
- arsenic poisoning (see below)
- seborrhea (see below)

MANAGEMENT OF SELECTED CONDITIONS

Systemic Lupus Erythematosus

Systemic lupus erythematosus is an autoimmune disease that is rare in horses.

- Cutaneous lesions include alopecia; leukoderma; scaling of the head, neck, and trunk; lymphedema of the extremities; and panniculitis.
  - Polyarthritis, fever, depression, and weight loss also may be seen.
- CBC, serum biochemistry, urinalysis, antinuclear antibody test, and biopsy for histopathologic examination and immunofluorescence are necessary for diagnosis (see *Equine Medicine and Surgery V*).
- Treatment involves immunosuppressive doses of glucocorticoids.
- The prognosis is guarded to poor.

Eosinophilic Dermatitis

This condition also is known as *eosinophilic granulomatosis* and *eosinophilic epitheliotropic* disease.

- Proposed causes include hypersensitivity to *Strongylus equinus* larvae or involvement of an epitheliotropic virus.
- Scaling, crusting, and exudation are the major clinical findings.
  - Oral ulcerations may develop early in the disease, followed by exfoliative dermatitis with alopecia and ulcerations; fissuring at the coronary band and on the face may occur.
  - Affected animals may be pruritic.
  - Cutaneous nodules occur and lymph nodes may be enlarged.
- Weight loss is characteristic and diarrhea sometimes is present.
- Diagnosis is based on the history, physical findings, and skin biopsy; some horses have peripheral eosinophilia.
- Systemic glucocorticoid therapy is recommended, although results are variable.
  - A suggested regimen comprises dexamethasone at 0.2 mg/kg IM for 5 days, followed by prednisolone at 0.55 mg/kg PO q12h for 1 week, 1.1 mg/kg q24h for 1 week, and then 1.1 mg/kg or less on alternate days to control the condition.
- The prognosis is poor.

Generalized Granulomatous Disease (Equine Sarcoidosis)

Generalized granulomatous disease is thought to be a reaction to a persistent antigen.

- Scaling and crusting with various amounts of alopecia are the primary complaints; the disease can be focal or multifocal.
  - Less commonly, nodules or tumors are present.
- Poor appetite, weight loss, low-grade fever, exercise intolerance, resting tachypnea, and mild dyspnea are common.
  - Peripheral lymphadenopathy, icterus, or diarrhea also may occur.
- Diagnosis requires skin biopsy.

- Blood studies may reveal leukocytosis, hyperfibrinogenemia, and either hyperglobulinemia or hypoglobulinemia.
- Results of liver and kidney function tests sometimes are abnormal.
- Lung lesions may be identified radiographically.
- The prognosis is poor; some animals respond to immunosuppressive doses of corticosteroids if treated early.

Arsenic Poisoning

In most cases of arsenic poisoning, gastroenteric signs predominate, but exfoliative dermatitis also can occur.

- Sources of arsenic include parasiticidal dips, insect baits, weed and orchard sprays, pressure-treated wood, and some drugs.
- Skin lesions include alopecia and seborrhea; focal necrosis and ulcers that heal slowly are sometimes present.
  - Some horses become hirsute instead of alopecic.
- Diagnosis is based on a history of exposure, physical findings, and measurement of tissue arsenic levels.
- Treatment options include D-penicillamine, sodium thiosulfate, dimercaprol (BAL), and thioctic acid; removal of the source of arsenic is essential.

Seborrhea

Seborrhea usually is a secondary manifestation of primary disease.

- *Seborrhea oleosa* is characterized by focal or diffuse scaling and excessive lipid accumulation.
- *Seborrhea sicca* consists of dry, scaly skin with accumulation of dry scales.
- *Seborrheic dermatitis* is characterized by scaling and lipid accumulation with evidence of inflammation.
  - The inflammation is due to an underlying skin disease, such as ectoparasitism, bacterial or fungal skin infection, or immune-mediated disease.
- In severe cases, the scales and sebum form heavy crusts; thick, hyperkeratotic crusts frequently are seen in chronic cases.
- Generalized seborrhea tends to be bilaterally symmetrical and usually spares the limbs; pruritus is absent or mild.

Treatment

If a primary disease has been identified, therapy should be directed accordingly. In addition, topical therapy is indicated if severe skin disease is present.

- Topical therapy for seborrhea oleosa involves regular use of keratolytic shampoos (e.g., tar and sulfur or sulfur-salicylic acid combinations, and selenium-containing products).
  - Potent degreasing shampoos containing benzoyl peroxide may be required.
- Seborrhea sicca responds best to emollient shampoos and rinses.
  - The horse should be bathed twice weekly for initial control.
  - Regular and thorough brushing is helpful in removing excess scale.

Diseases Characterized by Pigmentary Changes in the Skin or Hair

(pages 1929-1931)

Dawn B. Logas and Joy L. Barbet

DIFFERENTIAL DIAGNOSES

Changes in skin or hair color generally involve leukotrichia (white hair) with or without leukoderma (white skin). Possible causes include:

- skin injury
- vitiligo (Arabian fading syndrome)
  - This is an idiopathic, nonpruritic depigmentation of Arabians and occasionally other breeds.
  - Varying amounts of skin pigment are lost around the eyes, muzzle and, in some cases, the anus, vulva, sheath, and hooves.
  - Repigmentation varies from none to complete; most cases are refractory to treatment, but dietary supplementation, particularly of

copper, iodine, or fish meal can be helpful.

- spotted leukotrichia
  - This is an idiopathic condition primarily seen in Arabians.
  - Spots of white hair ± leuko-derma appear and may regress spontaneously; there is no treatment.
- reticulated leukotrichia
  - This primarily occurs in yearling Quarter Horses.
  - It begins as a crusting, non-painful dermatitis on the dorsum; hair is lost and regrows white in a cross-hatched pattern, but the skin remains pigmented.
- hyperesthetic leukotrichia
  - This condition is reported only in mature horses in California.
  - Initial lesions are focal crusts that are extremely painful, primarily occurring on the dorsal midline, from withers to tail; white hairs regrow at lesion sites.
  - The disease lasts 1 to 3 months, but may recur; there is no effective treatment.

Diseases Characterized by Abnormalities of the Hair Coat *(pages 1931-1932)*
Dawn B. Logas and Joy L. Barbet

DIFFERENTIAL DIAGNOSES

Possible causes of hair coat changes in horses are limited to a few conditions.

- congenital curly coat
  - This is a recessive trait in Percherons and a breed characteristic in Missouri Fox Trotters and small Bashkin horses.
- pituitary pars intermedia dysfunction (see Chapter 18, Endocrine System)
  - Hirsutism or failure to shed the winter coat often is a prominent sign.
  - The skin may be greasy or dry and scaly; recurrent or chronic skin infections, such as dermatophilosis, may become a problem.
- hypertrichosis

- Causes include local irritation or injury, chronic illness, and arsenic poisoning.
- Hypertrichosis resulting from local irritation or injury may not resolve.
- patchy shedding in the spring
  - Unless accompanied by pruritus, it is of little consequence; new hair grows in about 3 weeks.

Diseases of the External Ear *(pages 1932-1933)*
Dawn B. Logas and Joy L. Barbet

Ear Tick Infestation

Head shaking and rubbing of the ears, head tilt, and excessive waxy discharge are the common signs of ear tick infestation.

- The ears commonly are held in a droopy or flattened position because of the discomfort.
- Rarely, ataxia and other neurologic signs of inflammation and/or secondary infection affecting deeper structures in the ear are seen.
  - A syndrome of intermittent muscle spasms has been associated with the spinose ear tick.
- Thorough otoscopic examination demonstrating the tick is diagnostic; a thick, odoriferous, purulent discharge indicates secondary bacterial infection.
- 1% dioxathion in cottonseed oil or permethrin and rotenone in mineral oil is effective when delivered deep into the ear canal.
  - Malathion, coumaphos, and ronnel also are effective.
- Ear tags or insecticide strips braided into the mane or forelock or attached to the halter, reportedly are effective in preventing spinose ear tick infestation.

Psoroptic Otitis Externa

The mite *Psoroptes cuniculi* causes head shaking and ear rubbing when it invades the ear canal.

- Affected horses often hold their ears in a droopy or lop-eared position.

- Otoscopic examination and collection of wax from deep in the ear canal are needed for diagnosis.
- The ear canal must be thoroughly cleaned with a mild soapy solution or ceruminolytic to remove excessive wax.
  - Effective medications include organophosphates in a topical vehicle, thiabendazole, and rotenone (1:3) with mineral oil.
  - Affected ears should be treated twice per week for 3 weeks.
  - Oral ivermectin likely is effective.

Aural Plaques

Aural plaques (papillary acanthoma, "ear fungus") are flat papillomas or warts caused by equine papilloma virus. The lesions usually are bilateral and consist of small, smooth, raised, depigmented plaques, or large, confluent, hyperkeratotic plaques on the inner aspect of the pinna. The plaques are not sensitive, but persist for life. Similar plaques also may occur around the anus and vulva. There is no specific treatment beyond application of repellents and insecticides during fly season to minimize secondary irritation and infection.

Miscellaneous Dermatoses

Dawn B. Logas and Joy L. Barbet

Aplasia Cutis (Epitheliogenesis Imperfecta)

Aplasia cutis, a rare congenital, possibly autosomal recessive defect is characterized by areas of the body lacking epithelial covering. The hooves, limbs, tongue, and proximal esophagus are most commonly affected. Small lesions may heal adequately, but larger lesions may necessitate euthanasia. Surviving animals should not be used for breeding.

Hyperelastosis Cutis

Hyperelastosis cutis has been reported in Quarter Horses and in an Arabian-cross. This rare collagen disorder is easily recognized because affected animals have skin that is loosely attached to the subcutis and easily traumatized. The skin may tear open from what would normally be insignificant tension, such as innocuous bites or abrasions. Management involves basic wound care. Affected horses should not be bred and often are euthanized.

Pressure Sores

Pressure sores (decubital ulcers, saddle sores) result from prolonged pressure over a small surface area, causing loss of circulation, necrosis, and sloughing. Secondary infection is common. Scarring and leukotrichia are typical sequelae. Treatment involves routine wound care and relief of the inciting pressure.

Hyperhidrosis and Hematidrosis

Hyperhidrosis is excessive sweating. Exercise, severe pain, high ambient temperatures, some drugs, and hyperadrenocorticism are the more common causes of generalized hyperhidrosis. Localized hyperhidrosis may be seen with Horner's syndrome, local injections of epinephrine, and dourine. Hematidrosis refers to blood in the sweat. It may be seen with equine infectious anemia, purpura hemorrhagica, and bleeding diatheses.

18

Endocrine System

Endocrine Disorders

(pages 1948-1950)
Jill Beech

Examination of a horse suspected of having an endocrine disorder should begin with a detailed history, including:

- initial signs, progression of signs, and time course
- changes in body weight, fat distribution, and appetite
- water intake and urine output
- demeanor, behavior (sexual or otherwise)
- shedding and character of the hair coat
- recent illnesses such as infections, bouts of laminitis, seizures, and altered vision

A thorough physical examination should then be performed, including an ophthalmic examination in horses with suspected vision problems (see Chapter 14, Ocular System).

Diseases of the Pituitary Gland *(pages 1951-1956)*
Jill Beech

IDIOPATHIC DISEASES

Hyperplasia of the Pars Intermedia

Pituitary pars intermedia hyperplasia (pituitary adenoma) should be suspected in middle-aged or older horses and ponies variously manifesting the following signs:

- lethargy and weight loss (may appear "pot-bellied")

- Despite poor condition the supraorbital fat pad remains and may even bulge.
- polyuria and/or polydipsia
- abnormal hair coat (failure to shed, sometimes a long, wavy hair coat)
  - Some horses have only subtle hair coat changes.
- recurrent laminitis or laminitis that is refractory to routine therapy
- recurrent infections (e.g., *Dermatophilus* organisms, upper respiratory tract infections)
- abnormal estrous cycles in mares
- altered vision or blindness (uncommon)

Laboratory diagnosis

There is no definitive test for this condition, although the following findings and provocative tests are supportive of the diagnosis.

SERUM BIOCHEMISTRY. Serum biochemistry abnormalities variably include the following:

- elevated serum alkaline phosphatase and in some ponies and occasional horses elevated serum triglycerides or cholesterol
- mild-to-moderate hyperglycemia, although many affected horses are normoglycemic
- hyperinsulinemia, even in normoglycemic horses indicating insulin resistance, although the elevation is greater in hyperglycemic horses
  - Basal insulin concentrations typically are higher in ponies than in horses.
  - Hyperglycemia with hyperinsulinemia is more supportive of the diagnosis.

INSULIN TOLERANCE TEST. Single samples do not adequately reflect the insulin status unless greatly elevated. Insulin tolerance testing may be more revealing.

+ Crystalline insulin is given intravenously (IV) at 0.5 U/kg.
  + An IV source of glucose should be on hand before performing this test.
+ In normal horses blood glucose decreases 30% to 40% at 15 minutes and 60% at 30 minutes.

Horses with pars intermedia hyperplasia appear to be insulin resistant.

DEXAMETHASONE SUPPRESSION TEST. Baseline plasma cortisol can be highly variable in affected horses and is unreliable for diagnosis. Dexamethasone suppression is a sensitive and specific test.

+ Dexamethasone is given at 40 μg/kg intramuscularly (IM) and plasma cortisol is measured 16 to 24 hours later.
+ In normal horses plasma cortisol should be <1 μg/dL at this time.

ACTH. The cortisol response to adrenocorticotropic hormone (ACTH) is helpful but not definitive, since plasma cortisol increases in both normal horses and those with pars intermedia hyperplasia. The most accurate test is measurement of serum ACTH.

+ The normal range is 6.5 to 30.8 pg/mL in horses and 4.9 to 13.6 pg/mL in ponies.
+ The range for clinical hyperadrenocorticism is 40.8 to 669.9 pg/mL in horses and 23 to 1018 pg/mL in ponies.
+ Stressed horses without pituitary dysfunction can have abnormally elevated values (in one study, 16 to 68 pg/mL), and a range of 25 to 102 pg/mL is reported for mares.

URINARY CORTICOIDS. Urinary corticoid levels and urine corticoid:creatinine ratios are higher in horses with hyperadrenocorticism, but there can be overlap and both false positive and false negative results. Reported normal values are 102 to 275 mmol/L for urine corticoids and 4.7 to 16 × 10^{-6} for urine corticoid:creatinine.

Treatment
Some horses and ponies do well for years despite pituitary dysfunction.

Treatment, when elected, involves long-term administration of cyproheptadine or pergolide.

+ *cyproheptadine:* A dosage of 0.25 mg/kg by mouth (PO) once daily (increased to twice daily if no effect) is suggested; the response is variable.
+ *pergolide:* A starting dose of 0.5 mg PO once daily is increased by 0.5 mg every 2 to 3 days to a maintenance level of 2 to 3 mg/day for a 400- to 500-kg horse.
  + This dose is maintained for several weeks before deciding whether an increase is needed.
  + Some ponies do well on 0.5 to 1 mg/day.
  + Low-dose (0.75 mg/day) pergolide treatment reportedly is effective in many horses, although some horses experience clinical relapse on doses <2 mg/day.
  + Clinical improvement takes a variable period of time, but decreased lethargy should be noticed within several weeks.
  + Despite clinical improvement, plasma insulin and the cortisol response to dexamethasone may remain abnormal.

Regardless of whether drug therapy is used, excellent management is a major factor in successful maintenance.

+ Affected horses should be clipped during warm weather and access to fresh water ensured.
+ Appropriate foot care is important, as is regular dental care and deworming.
+ Recurrent infections require treatment.
+ Many affected horses need a higher plane of nutrition.

Diseases of the Thyroid Gland *(pages 1956-1959)*
Jill Beech

DIAGNOSTIC CONSIDERATIONS

Well-documented cases of thyroid dysfunction in horses are rare. Diagnosis is based on clinical signs (see below) and on serum T_3 and T_4 concentrations and their response to provocative testing. Effects of drugs, training status, weather, diurnal variation, and the horse's sex and age must be considered when interpreting results.

Thyroid Function Tests
Serum T_3 and T_4
Reported normal values for serum T_3 in mature horses range from 13.3 to 97.4 ng/dL; values for T_4 range from 0.93 to 4.3 µg/dL. Because of the wide ranges, low concentrations in apparently healthy horses, and various factors that can affect hormone concentrations, thyroid dysfunction should not be diagnosed solely on resting T_3 and T_4 levels.
TSH response
A thyroid-stimulating hormone (TSH) response test involves injection of 2.5 to 5 IU of TSH IV or IM and measurement of serum T_3 and T_4 at 2 to 6 hours. Normal horses exhibit at least a twofold increase in serum T_3 and T_4 over baseline.
TRH response
If a horse has significantly low serum T_3 and T_4 levels but responds to TSH and has no history of drug administration, a thyroid-releasing hormone (TRH) test should be performed to evaluate whether the horse can secrete endogenous TSH. The test involves giving 1 mg of TRH (0.5 mg in ponies) IV and measuring serum T_3 and T_4 at 4 hours. Both T_3 and T_4 significantly increase in normal horses.

CONGENITAL AND FAMILIAL DISEASES
Hypothyroidism in Foals
Ingestion of plant goitrogens or substances containing iodine (e.g., iodinated drugs, excess dietary iodine) by pregnant mares can cause hypothyroidism in neonatal foals. Signs may include incoordination, poor suckling and righting reflexes, hypothermia, goiter, skeletal disproportion, carpal and fetlock joint contracture, delayed ossification of tarsal and carpal bones, ruptured common digital extensor tendons, and sometimes mandibular prognathism. Stunting without limb

deformities also should prompt one to consider hypothyroidism. The thyroid glands may be of normal size.

IDIOPATHIC DISEASES
Acquired Hypothyroidism
Stunting; dull, coarse hair coat not shed normally; wrinkled skin; edema of the distal hind limbs; lethargy; oversensitivity to cold weather; and hypophagia in young horses (1 to 2 years of age) should prompt consideration of hypothyroidism. If chronic diseases, parasitism, and neoplasia are ruled out, serum T_3 and T_4 measurements and a TSH or TRH response test should be performed.
Therapy
If clinical signs and laboratory findings support a diagnosis of hypothyroidism, either iodinated casein (5 g PO once daily for an adult horse) or synthetic L-thyroxine (20 µg/kg PO once daily) may be used for treatment.
- Periodic monitoring of serum T_3 and T_4 is advisable.
- Long-term administration might suppress pituitary TSH production, suggesting that gradual withdrawal of the drug may be prudent.
- Surgical removal of the thyroid gland is indicated with malignant neoplasia or if a benign neoplasm becomes grossly enlarged.
  - Horses can function satisfactorily after unilateral thyroidectomy, but bilateral thyroidectomy necessitates thyroid supplementation for the duration of the horse's life.

Diseases of the Adrenal Gland *(pages 1959-1961)*
Jill Beech

MULTIFACTORIAL DISEASES
Hyperadrenocorticism
Clinical signs of hyperadrenocorticism are described in the section on pars intermedia hyperplasia. All reported cases of equine hyperadrenocorticism have been secondary to pituitary dysfunction, but not all horses

with pars intermedia hyperplasia have classic hyperadrenocorticism. Prolonged use of high doses of corticosteroids can cause similar signs.

Hypoadrenocorticism

When other, more common causes have been ruled out, hypoadrenocorticism should be considered in horses with lethargy, exercise intolerance, decreased appetite, poor hair coat, and poor body condition.

- The history should be reviewed for chronic stresses and drugs that suppress adrenal function (e.g., corticosteroids, chronic administration of anabolic steroids).
- Affected horses often have low plasma cortisol levels that do not show the expected rise after ACTH administration (see *Equine Medicine and Surgery V*).
  - A single low baseline cortisol level does not suffice for diagnosis.
- Measurement of serum ACTH is helpful in determining whether the hypoadrenocorticism is primary or secondary (e.g., drug induced).
  - In primary hypoadrenocorticism, ACTH levels are increased.
- Rest and elimination of stress appear to be the most effective treatment.
- Low-dose corticosteroid administration may be needed if the horse is inappetant and unresponsive to conservative therapy.
  - Prednisone (0.1 to 0.3 mg/kg PO) is given on alternate days and gradually decreased in as short a time as possible.
  - Plasma cortisol levels (baseline and in response to ACTH) should be monitored.

NEOPLASTIC DISEASES
Diseases of the Adrenal Medulla

Pheochromocytomas (tumors of chromaffin cells of the medulla) may be asymptomatic or cause signs associated with excessive secretion of catecholamines. Most affected horses are >12 years of age. The most common signs are tachycardia, tachypnea, sweating, muscle tremor, and anxiety. Hyperglycemia has been reported in some cases. Usually the diagnosis is made postmortem.

Diseases of the Pancreas *(pages 1961-1962)*
Jill Beech

INFECTIONS, INFLAMMATORY, AND IMMUNE DISEASES
Chronic Pancreatitis (Diabetes Mellitus)

Primary pancreatic endocrine dysfunction is rarely diagnosed in horses; most cases of hyperglycemia are associated with pars intermedia hyperplasia. Diagnosis of diabetes mellitus is based on clinical signs, plasma insulin and glucose concentrations (usually >500 mg/dL), rule out of pituitary gland dysfunction, and response to exogenous insulin and glucose administration. In one report a diabetic pony was maintained on 0.5 U/kg of protamine zinc insulin IM twice daily.

NEOPLASTIC DISEASES

Functional insulin-secreting tumors of the pancreas are rare in horses. Manifestations of resulting hypoglycemia include disorientation, loss of awareness, hyperexcitability, sweating, ear twitching, chewing motions, ataxia, dilated pupils, muscle spasms, clonus, and sometimes tetany and head tremor. Hypoglycemia and hyperinsulinemia are marked during episodes.

Miscellaneous Conditions *(pages 1962-1964)*
Tony Mogg

Hyperlipidemia

Hyperlipidemia (elevation of serum triglycerides up to 500 mg/dL without milky plasma or hepatic lipidosis) is a physiologic response to a negative energy balance in all equids. Diagnosis is made by measuring serum triglycerides. Therapy should aim to correct the negative energy balance.

Hyperlipemia

Hyperlipemia (serum triglycerides >500 mg/dL, milky plasma, and hepatic lipidosis) has primarily been reported in ponies, donkeys, and Miniature Horses. It is associated with a negative energy balance caused by pregnancy, lactation, feed restriction, stress (e.g., transport), or disease-induced anorexia. Most affected animals are overweight and insulin resistant. Hyperlipemia can occur in other horse breeds when a negative energy balance *and* azotemia are present and in horses and ponies with pars intermedia hyperplasia.

Clinical signs and diagnosis

The most common signs are anorexia and lethargy. Diarrhea, icterus, weakness, and terminal recumbency also may be seen. In fasted ponies, hyperlipemia can develop within 2 to 3 days and the interval between recognition and death can be as little as 3 days. Laboratory abnormalities include hypertriglyceridemia with or without hypercholesterolemia, elevated hepatic enzymes, and possibly metabolic acidosis, hypoglycemia, and azotemia.

Treatment and prognosis

The aims of treatment are to correct the negative energy balance, treat any underlying disease, and enhance removal of triglycerides from the blood with insulin and heparin.

- Nutritional support may comprise force feeding high-carbohydrate gruels, commercial enteral feeding preparations, or oral glucose or glucose/galactose combinations.
  - Parenteral nutrition with IV glucose and/or amino acids may be necessary in critical cases.
- Protamine zinc or ultralente insulin may be given at 0.075 to 0.4 IU/kg SC or IM q12-24h.
  - An initial dose of 0.4 IU/kg of rapid-acting insulin has been suggested.
  - Insulin therapy should not be used without adequate caloric support.
- Heparin may be given at 30 to 250 IU/kg IV or SC q6-12h.

Mortality rates of up to 80% are reported. The nature and severity of the primary disease may be the major determinate of survival; serum triglyceride concentrations are not prognostic.

Prevention

States of negative energy balance, obesity, and stress should be avoided, and anorectic animals should be provided with nutritional support. Regular exercise may reduce the risk of hyperlipemia. Ponies, donkeys, and Miniature Horses intentionally feed-deprived (e.g., for treatment of colic) should receive IV glucose. Routine blood screening of animals at high risk, such as pregnant or lactating mares, has been advocated.

Diabetes Insipidus

Diabetes insipidus occurs when there is insufficient secretion of antidiuretic hormone (ADH) from the neurohypophysis. It is rarely diagnosed in horses. The usual complaint is polyuria and polydipsia without other abnormalities. Diagnosis is based on low plasma ADH and its failure to increase with water deprivation; low urine specific gravity and osmolarity, with inability to concentrate urine; and dehydration after water deprivation (see *Equine Medicine and Surgery V*).

Parathyroid Gland Dysfunction

Secondary nutritional hyperparathyroidism is a well-recognized consequence of a high-phosphorus diet. Parathyroid dysfunction should be considered in horses showing signs of hypercalcemia or are being maintained on high-phosphorous/low-calcium diets. Primary parathyroid dysfunction is rare and other causes (e.g., neoplasia, renal disease, toxic plants, excess vitamin D) are more likely.

19

Hemolymphatic System

Clinical Evaluation of the Hemolymphatic System *(pages 1970-1973)*

Debra D. Morris and Michelle H. Barton

INTERPRETATION OF PHYSICAL FINDINGS

The following clinical signs may indicate disease referable to the hemolymphatic system:

- ◆ *Mucous membrane pallor* suggests anemia, especially when accompanied by weakness and exercise intolerance.
- ◆ *Icterus* may indicate a hemolytic process; other causes are liver dysfunction and anorexia.
  - Intense icterus usually is caused by intravascular hemolysis.
  - Normal foals may be mildly icteric (physiologic hyperbilirubinemia); prematurity or concurrent illness may worsen the degree of icterus.
- ◆ *Brown mucous membranes* indicate methemoglobinemia, most commonly associated with ingestion of wilted red maple leaves (see p. 506).
- ◆ *Mucosal petechial hemorrhages* indicate thrombocytopenia, severe platelet dysfunction, vasculitis, or septicemia.
  - Thrombocytopenia usually is attended by spontaneous epistaxis, melena, hematuria, hematomas, or bleeding after trauma or venipuncture.
  - Vasculitis causes hot, painful, pitting edema, usually distributed ventrally.

- Petechiation in neonates is a sensitive indicator of septicemia; it is most readily seen in the pinnae of the ears.
- *Ecchymotic hemorrhages* are indicative of clotting factor deficiencies.
  - Disseminated intravascular coagulopathy (DIC) is the most common cause.
- ◆ *Venous thrombosis* may indicate coagulation dysfunction.
  - Thrombotic disease is a clinical manifestation of DIC but also may accompany severe hypoproteinemia secondary to protein-losing states.
- ◆ *Ventral edema* that is not hot or painful may indicate hypoproteinemia.
  - Other causes include lymphatic obstruction secondary to lymphosarcoma or other neoplasms, severe thrombocytopenia, and congestive heart failure.
- ◆ *Hot, painful edema,* often progressing to skin fissures that exude serum, is a sign of vasculitis.
- ◆ *Fever* most often indicates microbial infection; long-standing or repeated infections that do not respond to routine therapy are suggestive of immunodeficiency.
  - Hemolysis often causes fever, especially when red cell destruction is acute and intravascular.
  - Tissue necrosis in large tumor masses or secondary immune suppression and subsequent infections also may produce fever.
- ◆ *Tachycardia* can be a sign of anemia, shock, sepsis, pain, or cardiac disease.

493

- Severe anemia (PCV <15%) also causes a pansystolic murmur.
- *Tachypnea* is a nonspecific sign that accompanies pain, acidosis, apprehension, and respiratory or cardiac insufficiency; rarely is it a primary sign of hemolymphatic disease.
- *Peripheral lymphadenopathy* that is not hot or painful should prompt consideration of lymphosarcoma.
- *Depression, anorexia, and weight loss* accompany a wide variety of chronic infectious, metabolic, neoplastic, and immune-mediated disorders.

CLINICAL INDICATORS OF SPECIFIC DYSFUNCTION
Erythrocyte Dysfunction
Clinical signs referable to decreased red cell mass depend on the severity of the anemia and the speed with which it progresses.
- With mild anemia in an unstressed individual, no obvious signs may be present, although pale or icteric mucous membranes may be noted on physical examination.
  - A performance animal may have reduced exercise tolerance.
- With more profound or rapidly developing anemia, the horse may be obviously depressed and weak; with severe and acute blood loss, hypovolemic shock may occur.
- Other signs of anemia include tachycardia, tachypnea, and a low-grade systolic murmur (mitral valve murmur secondary to decreased blood viscosity).
- Melena or epistaxis may be seen with blood loss anemia; icterus, fever, and hemoglobinuria may be present with hemolytic disease.
  Methemoglobinemia causes decreased *functional* mass and muddy red-brown mucous membranes. Oxidative red cell damage of any cause leads to formation of Heinz bodies within erythrocytes. Intravascular hemolysis and hemo-globinuria subsequently develop. Hemoglobinuria must be distinguished from myoglobinuria because both produce positive tests for blood on urine indicator strips.
- If urine contains dark brown pigment and tests positive for blood, 2.8 g of ammonium sulfate should be dissolved in 5 mL of urine and the solution centrifuged or filtered.
- If the supernatant or filtrate is of normal urine color, the pigment is hemoglobin; if it remains dark brown, the pigment is myoglobin.

Leukocyte Dysfunction
The most important clinical consequence of *leukopenia* is bacterial infection, which may be manifested as fever with signs of regional or localized infection (e.g., abscesses, increased lung sounds, nasal discharge). In rare instances, *leukocytosis* causes clinical signs of illness. Leukemias may produce nonspecific signs, such as rapid weight loss, anorexia, colic, and fever, or may cause unique signs, such as petechiae, paralysis, or lameness involving a single limb.

Platelet Dysfunction
With thrombocytopenia, especially when the platelet count is <40,000/µL, petechial hemorrhages may be visible on the mucous membranes and skin. Ecchymotic or suffusive hemorrhage involving body orifices, tissue planes, and joints is more suggestive of a clotting factor deficiency.

Ancillary Diagnostic Aids *(pages 1973-1990)*
Kenneth S. Latimer, Edward A. Mahaffey, Michelle H. Barton, Debra D. Morris, and Susan Clark Eades

SAMPLE COLLECTION AND HANDLING
Blood
Ethylenediaminetetraacetic acid (EDTA) is the anticoagulant recommended for routine hematology (CBC). Use of excessive EDTA can lead to erythrocyte shrinkage, which decreases the PCV and alters red cell indices. Samples should be processed within 1 to 2 hours, because prolonged contact with EDTA can cause changes in leukocyte morphology, most notably causing neutrophils to appear vacuolated and ragged, which

could be mistaken for toxic changes. If the blood sample cannot be processed within a reasonable time, air dried blood smears should be made.

Bone Marrow

The primary indications for bone marrow examination are anemia, persistent leukopenia, persistent thrombocytopenia, and suspected hematopoietic neoplasia.

- Marrow can be collected from the sternum, ribs, or ilium with an 18-gauge spinal needle.
- The overlying skin is surgically prepared, and the subcutis and periosteum are infiltrated with lidocaine.
- The needle is inserted into the bone with a rotating motion to a depth of 2 to 3 cm (less in foals).
- Marrow (0.5 mL) is aspirated into a 12-mL syringe containing one or two drops of EDTA.
- Smears can be stained with Wright's stain or any other Romanowsky's-type stain (see *Equine Medicine and Surgery, V*).

EVALUATING ERYTHROCYTES

Normal Values

Laboratory measurements of red cell mass (PCV, red cell count, hemoglobin concentration) are extremely variable in horses.

- A major contributing factor is the unique nature of the equine spleen, which holds up to one third of the red cell mass.
  - The spleen can sequester large numbers of red cells after tranquilization.
  - Splenic contraction associated with excitement or strenuous exercise can result in a substantial increase (up to 50%) in circulating red cell numbers.
- Red cell indices vary among light-horse breeds ("hot blooded") and draft and pony breeds ("cold blooded").
- The level and type of training also affect red cell values. Thoroughbreds in race training have values at the upper limits of normal.

Reference ranges for adult horses
Following are erythrocyte values for "hot-blooded" breeds:

- PCV (%): 32 to 53 (mean, 41 ± 4.5)
- RBC (× 10^6/µL): 6.8 to 12.9 (mean, 9.0 ± 1.2)
- hemoglobin (Hb) (g/dL): 11.0 to 19.0 (mean, 14.4 ± 1.7)
- mean corpuscular volume (MCV) (fl): 37.0 to 58.5 (mean, 45.5 ± 4.3)
- mean corpuscular hemoglobin (MCH) (pg): 12.3 to 19.7 (mean, 15.9 ± 1.5)
- mean corpuscular hemoglobin concentration (MCHC) (%): 31.0 to 38.6 (mean, 35.2 ± 1.4)

Erythrocyte values for "cold-blooded" breeds are as follows:

- PCV (%): 24 to 44 (mean, 35)
- RBC (× 10^6/µL): 5.5 to 9.5 (mean, 7.5)
- Hb (g/dL): 8.0 to 14.0 (mean, 11.5)

Foals and young horses
Measurements of red cell mass generally are higher at birth, decline rapidly within 12 to 24 hours, and then decline more gradually over the following 2 weeks. Thereafter, red cell values gradually increase to normal adult levels by 1 to 2 years of age. Table 19-9 in *Equine Medicine and Surgery V* lists erythrocyte values for foals 1 day, 2 to 7 days, 8 to 14 days, 21 to 30 days, 1 to 3 months, and 8 to 18 months of age.

Morphologic Changes

Rouleaux formation
Rouleaux formation (stacking of erythrocytes like coins) may be confused with autoagglutination in wet mounts. Rouleaux can be distinguished from autoagglutination by diluting the specimen with saline (one drop of blood with one drop of normal saline) before examination. Rouleaux disperse, whereas autoagglutinated erythrocytes remain clumped.

Howell-Jolly bodies
Howell-Jolly bodies (nuclear remnants that appear as small, round, basophilic red cell inclusions) are normal in a small percentage of horses. They may be slightly increased in anemic conditions.

Heinz bodies
Heinz bodies are clumps of denatured hemoglobin that form within erythrocytes exposed to oxidants such as phenothiazine, onions, and red maple leaves. They are readily

demonstrated by mixing an equal volume of blood with 0.5% new methylene blue and allowing the mixture to stand for 15 minutes before making a smear. Heinz bodies are small, round, blue-staining inclusions with erythrocytes.

Parasitic inclusions

Babesia caballi and *Babesia equi* appear as tear-shaped organisms within erythrocytes, using routine staining techniques. *B. caballi* are seen as paired pyriform bodies 2.5 to 4 μm in size. *B. equi* appear as four inclusions <2 μm in size, frequently in the form of a Maltese cross.

Anemia

Evaluation

Anemia most commonly is secondary to systemic disease or organ dysfunction. Thus critical evaluation of the entire patient and complete hematologic evaluation are indicated. Morphologic examination of the blood smear may give additional information regarding the pathogenesis of anemia.

* Refractile membrane inclusions (Heinz bodies) are associated with oxidative hemolysis.
* Spherocytosis suggests membrane damage that often is immune mediated.
* Evidence of red cell fragmentation suggests thrombotic disorders.

Sequential evaluation of the erythron may suggest whether blood loss is ongoing or whether the marrow is responding to the anemia. Examination of the bone marrow often is necessary to adequately characterize the anemia as regenerative or nonregenerative (see below).

Increased red cell destruction

This is a common cause of anemia in horses. Intravascular hemolysis and increased removal of red cells by the mononuclear phagocytic system generally are both involved. These disorders commonly are called hemolytic anemias. Causes include:

* immune-mediated mechanisms (e.g., equine infectious anemia [EIA], neonatal isoerythrolysis, autoimmune hemolytic anemia, transfusion reactions)
* certain bacterial infections (e.g., *Clostridium perfringens*)

* plant or chemical toxicity (e.g., red maple leaves, onions, phenothiazine)
* hyposmolarity
* blood parasites (e.g., *Babesia, Ehrlichia equi*)

Icterus is common, particularly with intravascular hemolysis; hemoglobinuria is a feature of severe intravascular hemolysis. Erythroid hyperplasia, reflecting increased red cell production, is found on bone marrow examination.

Depressed red cell production

This is the most common mechanism for development of anemia in horses. The anemia generally is more gradual and less severe than that caused by blood loss or hemolysis. Diminished red cell production may occur as a result of toxin-induced bone marrow suppression, but more typically it is secondary to a number of diseases (anemia of chronic disease). This nonregenerative, mild to moderate anemia may occur with chronic inflammatory of infectious processes such as pleuritis and abdominal abscessation, as well as with some forms of neoplasia. The anemia resolves after effective treatment of the underlying disorder.

Indicators of regeneration

Horses rarely release reticulocytes or polychromatophilic erythrocytes into the circulation in response to anemia; thus laboratory detection of regeneration is difficult. Techniques for evaluating red cells include:

* bone marrow examination (see *Equine Medicine and Surgery, V*)
* assessment of MCV
  · Increased MCV is more likely in horses with hemolytic anemias.
  · MCV may appear increased in animals with agglutinated erythrocytes, whether from laboratory artifact, immune-mediated hemolytic anemia, or high-dosage heparin therapy.
* red cell distribution width (coefficient of variation in red cell volume)
* erythrogram (histogram showing the volume spread of the red cell population in the sample)

Polycythemia

Polycythemia, or erythrocytosis, may represent an absolute increase in red cell mass, but more commonly it indicates hemoconcentration (e.g., dehydration) or splenic contraction. Absolute polycythemia can occur with myeloproliferative disease (polycythemia vera) or in conditions in which chronic hypoxia or abnormal erythropoietin production results in excessive red cell production. Sustained tissue hypoxia may be due to chronic pulmonary or cardiovascular disease, high-altitude exposure, or defective oxygen transport (e.g., methemoglobinemia).

EVALUATING LEUKOCYTES
Total White Blood Cell Count
The leukocyte, or WBC, count is routinely assessed as part of the complete blood count. In emergency situations the WBC count can be estimated from a stained blood smear.

* Using the 40 or 45× high-dry or 50× oil-immersion objective, the average number of WBCs per field of view is determined by examining 10 fields.
* A crude estimate of the WBC count/µL is calculated by multiplying the average number of WBCs/field by 1500 (40× objective) or 2000 (50× objective).

Differential Count
Following are the leukocyte reference intervals for adult horses used at the University of Georgia Veterinary Medical Teaching Hospital:

* total leukocyte count: 6000 to 12,000/µL
* neutrophils (segmented): 3000 to 6000/µL (30% to 75%)
* band neutrophils: 0 to 100/µL (0% to 1%)
* lymphocytes: 1500 to 5000/µL (25% to 60%)
* monocytes: 0 to 600/µL (0% to 8%)
* eosinophils: 0 to 800/µL (0% to 10%)
* basophils: 0 to 300/µL (0% to 3%)

Using absolute cell counts for leukogram interpretation results in fewer errors than relying on relative percentages alone.

Young foals
Total WBC counts in full-term foals average 7800 to 9500/µL.

* Neutrophil counts average 7940/µL at birth and decline to a mean of 4780/µL at 4 months.
* Band neutrophils, when present, are <150/µL.
* Lymphocyte counts gradually increase from a mean of 1340/µL at birth to 4730/µL at 3 months.
* Eosinophils, which are absent at birth, increase to a mean of 353/µL at 4 months. Basophil counts average <58/µL.
* Monocyte numbers in healthy animals apparently do not change with age.

Premature foals have total WBC counts of 4900 to 6800/µL, and lymphocytes generally outnumber neutrophils. The neutrophil:lymphocyte (N/L) ratio has prognostic value; nonsurviving premature foals have N/L ratios <1.3:1, while surviving premature foals have N/L ratios that increase from 1.1:1 at birth to 3.2:1 by 18 hours of age. In contrast, full-term healthy foals have N/L ratios >2.5:1.

Neutrophil Morphology
Band neutrophils
The presence of band (immature) neutrophils in peripheral blood is termed a *left shift*.

* If the neutrophil count is within the reference interval or is increased, >300 bands/µL indicates a clinically significant left shift.
* If neutropenia exists, a significant left shift is present if bands comprise >10% of the neutrophil population
* A "degenerative" or severe left shift exists when the number of immature neutrophils approaches, equals, or exceeds the number of segmented neutrophils.

Toxic changes
Toxic changes in neutrophil cytoplasm include basophilia, vacuolation, Döhle bodies (0.5- to 2.0-µm angular blue-gray particles in the periphery), and toxic granulation (small pinkish-purple granules). These changes usually denote severe, localized bacterial infection or septicemia. They also may be seen with sterile inflammation and phenylbutazone toxicity. Toxic granulation also has been seen in horses with hepatic lipidosis.

Ehrlichiosis

Ehrlichia equi infection may be diagnosed by finding characteristic morulae within neutrophils on Romanowsky-stained blood smears. These morulae have a mulberry-like appearance and stain with a grayish cast. They may be found in 20% to 50% of circulating neutrophils, and affected neutrophils may contain >1 morula. In leukopenic horses, buffy coat examination may be used to concentrate the leukocytes and facilitate the search for rickettsial inclusions.

Neutrophil Response Patterns

Neutrophilia

Neutrophilia is defined as the presence of >6000 neutrophils/µL of blood. There are four major causes:

- physiologic changes (excitement, fear, or brief but strenuous exercise)
  - Total WBC counts may reach 26,000/µL, and neutrophilia may exceed 14,000/µL.
  - Lymphocytosis often is present, but eosinophil and monocyte counts are unchanged or only slightly elevated.
  - Cell counts return to baseline within 30 minutes.
- corticosteroids (endogenous release or administration of corticosteroids or adrenocorticotropic hormone [ACTH])
  - Leukocytosis and neutrophilia occur, usually within 1 to 2 hours of administration.
  - Peak neutrophil counts range from 9000 to 15,400/µL.
  - Other characteristic changes include lymphopenia and eosinopenia.
  - Severe stress or acute disease must be present before endogenous corticosteroid release is sufficient to cause alterations in the leukogram.
- tissue inflammation and/or infection
  - The hallmark of inflammation is neutrophilia with a left shift.
  - The magnitude of the neutrophilia is greater with abscess formation or localized infection than with generalized inflammatory disorders.
  - The severity of the disease process is reflected in the intensity of the left shift and the degree of toxic change within neutrophils.
- hemorrhagic or hemolytic anemias (less common than the other three causes)
  - For example, the hemolytic anemia seen with red maple leaf toxicity may be accompanied by neutrophil counts reaching 35,000/µL with a left shift.

Persistence of neutrophilic leukocytosis with minimal left shift in the presence of clinical illness denotes a chronic suppurative disease. Associated changes typically include mild anemia (anemia of chronic disease) and hyperfibrinogenemia.

Neutropenia

Neutropenia is defined as <3000 neutrophils/µL of blood. It is a serious clinical problem because it may result in overwhelming bacterial infection. There are several possible causes.

- Neutropenia frequently is associated with bacterial infections involving the body cavities, respiratory tract, and gastrointestinal (GI) tract and with generalized septicemia.
  - It often is characterized by a left shift that may be degenerative and by toxic changes.
  - Causes include endotoxemia and intestinal disorders, such as blister beetle toxicosis, cecal perforation, monocytic ehrlichiosis, phenylbutazone toxicity, and salmonellosis.
- About 40% of foals with neonatal septicemia have leukopenia. Of these, 68% have neutrophil counts <4000/µL and 89% exhibit a left shift of at least 200 bands/µL.
  - Persistent neutropenia with a left shift and toxic changes over a 3- to 4-day period is a poor prognostic sign.
  - Persistent leukocytosis in conjunction with hyperfibrinogenemia denotes a chronic, persistent infection associated with arthritis, osteomyelitis, or pneumonia.
- Less commonly, neutropenia may occur with bone marrow necrosis or myelophthisis (obliteration of the marrow space).
  - Bone marrow aspiration and core biopsies are necessary to diagnose these disorders.

- Though neutropenia may occur alone, pancytopenia usually is present.
- Most instances of myelophthisis with secondary neutropenia can be attributed to neoplastic diseases, especially lymphosarcoma and leukemia.

Lymphocyte Morphology

Altered lymphocyte morphology may be apparent in neoplasia and plant toxicity.

- Lymphosarcoma and lymphocytic leukemia may cause increased numbers of small, well-differentiated lymphocytes or large, immature lymphocytes on a stained blood smear.
- Ingestion of *Swainsona* spp. causes appearance of vacuolated lymphocytes in the blood within 10 days, although neurologic signs are the predominant clinical manifestation.
  - Similar neurologic and hematologic changes may be seen with locoweed toxicity.

Lymphocyte Response Patterns

Lymphocytosis

Lymphocytosis is the presence of ≥5000 lymphocytes/μL of blood. In most instances, lymphocytosis can be attributed to physiologic states, chronic antigenic stimulation (e.g., chronic bacterial infection, vaccination), or lymphoid neoplasia.

- Physiologic lymphocytosis is transient and seen more often in young, high-strung horses.
- During excited states, lymphocyte counts may be >14,000/μL.
- Lymphoid neoplasia is a rare cause of lymphocytosis in horses.
  - Lymphocytosis may be observed in horses having lymphosarcoma with a leukemic blood picture and in lymphocytic leukemia.
  - Total WBC counts are highly variable but may reach 368,800/μL, with a differential count of 100% lymphocytes.

Lymphopenia

Lymphopenia is the presence of <1500 lymphocytes/μL of blood. It is a common finding with corticosteroid administration, acute infection, and combined immunodeficiency (see p. 508). With exogenous administration of corticosteroids or ACTH, changes in the leukogram appear within 2 hours; lymphocyte numbers return to baseline within 12 to 24 hours.

Monocytosis

Monocytosis is the presence of ≥600 monocytes/μL of blood. Monocytosis may be apparent with both acute and chronic diseases and usually accompanies neutrophilia. Causes include disorders associated with suppuration, necrosis, malignancy, hemolysis, hemorrhage, and pyogranulomatous inflammation.

Eosinophilia

Eosinophilia is the presence of >800 eosinophils/μL of blood. Possible causes include:

- parasitism
  - Eosinophilia is more likely with nematodes that migrate through tissues.
- allergic diseases
- inflammatory lesions of the skin, GI tract, lungs, or genitourinary tract
- hypereosinophilic syndromes, eosinophilic myeloproliferative diseases, and eosinophilic leukemias

Basophilia

Basophilia is the presence of >300 basophils/μL of blood. It is a rare finding and is most often seen with intestinal disturbances. Maximum cell counts seldom exceed 1700/μL.

EVALUATING PLATELETS

Normal platelet counts are in the range of 100,000 to 400,000/μL.

- Platelet numbers can be estimated from the blood smear.
  - The average number of platelets in a 100× oil-immersion field is multiplied by 15,000 or 20,000 to give an estimate of the number of platelets/μL of blood.
- Platelets exposed to EDTA may clump, the aggregates being concentrated in the feathered edge of the smear, artifactually decreasing platelet numbers in the remainder of the smear.
  - This spurious thrombocytopenia can be identified by collecting

an additional blood sample, using sodium citrate as the anticoagulant.

SEROLOGIC EXAMINATION

Diseases that can be diagnosed on serologic findings include equine infectious anemia, ehrlichiosis (infection with either *Ehrlichia risticii* or *E. equi*), and piroplasmosis (babesiosis). Although a single convalescent serum sample may document exposure to a given pathogen, paired (acute and convalescent) serum samples provide more definitive information.

EVALUATING THE IMMUNE SYSTEM

Humoral System

Total serum immunoglobin concentration

The total serum immunoglobulin (Ig) concentration can be determined from a routine blood chemistry panel by subtracting the albumin concentration from the total protein concentration. Total protein in normal adult horses usually is in the range of 5.2 to 7.9 g/dL. The normal range for albumin is 2.6 to 3.7 g/dL and for globulins, 2.6 to 4.2 g/dL.

Protein electrophoresis

Serum protein electrophoresis more accurately quantitates albumin and globulin concentrations and allows evaluation of the globulin classes.

- α-Globulins are acute phase proteins.
  - The normal range for serum α-globulins is 0.37 to 2.0 g/dL.
  - The plasma concentration rises in inflammatory states that accompany infection, neoplasia, immune-mediated disease, and parasitism.
- β-Globulins comprise acute phase proteins (including fibrinogen), complement, clotting factors, transferrin, and some immunoglobulins (IgM and IgG[T]).
  - The normal range for serum β-globulins is 0.69 to 2.47 g/dL.
  - Fibrinogen rises in response to the same types of conditions that increase α-globulins.
  - The transferrin concentration, measured as iron-binding ca-

pacity, sometimes is useful in evaluating anemic animals.
- γ-Globulins are the immunoglobulins.
  - The normal range of serum γ-globulins is 0.55 to 1.9 g/dL.
  - Hypogammaglobulinemia may occur with failure of passive transfer or hereditary immunodeficiency or during states causing nonspecific protein loss.
  - Increased concentrations of multiple immunoglobulin isotypes (polyclonal gammopathy) are displayed as a broad peak in the β and globulin region.
  - Polyclonal gammopathy is associated with chronic infectious or inflammatory diseases, immune-mediated diseases, chronic liver failure, and some lymphoid neoplasms.
  - Monoclonal gammopathies are the result of malignancy of a single plasma cell clone.

Quantitation of Ig classes and subclasses is discussed in *Equine Medicine and Surgery V.*

Evaluating passive transfer in neonates

A crude estimate of immunoglobulin concentration in neonates can be obtained by quantitation of total protein via refractometry. Values <5 g/dL indicate failure of passive transfer of maternal antibodies. More accurate tests include the following:

- The zinc sulfate turbidity test involves 0.1 mL of patient serum added to 6 mL of zinc sulfate solution (205 mg zinc sulfate/L distilled water).
  - Turbidity occurs at IgG concentrations of 400 to 500 mg/dL serum.
  - Hemolysis may falsely overestimate the serum IgG concentration.
- In the glutaraldehyde coagulation test, 50 μL of 10% glutaraldehyde is added to 0.5 mL of serum.
  - A positive reaction (gel formation) in <10 minutes is equated with a serum IgG >800 mg/dL, and a positive reaction in 60 minutes indicates >400 mg/dL.
  - Hemolysis may falsely overestimate the serum IgG concentration.
- The SRID test is the most accurate, sensitive, and quantitative test

available, but results are not available for 24 hours.

* The latex agglutination test kit and membrane-filter enzyme-linked immunosorbent assay (ELISA) kit are rapid and accurate field tests.

Failure of passive transfer is discussed in Chapter 6, Neonatal Evaluation and Management.

Cellular Defenses

Tests of lymphocyte, monocyte, and neutrophil function are described in *Equine Medicine and Surgery V*.

Autoimmune Disease

Following are the tests most commonly used in diagnosing autoimmune diseases in horses:

* Coombs' test determines whether the patient's red blood cells are coated with immunoglobulin, complement, or immune complexes.
  * The most common indication is for diagnosis of immune-mediated hemolytic anemia.
  * Because the endpoint is agglutination, autoagglutinated blood should not be tested.
  * The test may be falsely negative after severe, acute hemolysis or corticosteroid therapy.
* Platelet factor 3 test is used to detect antiplatelet antibodies.
  * Plasma from the patient is incubated with normal platelets; any antiplatelet antibody in the sample causes lysis of the platelets and accelerated clotting of the plasma.
  * Results are highly variable, and false negatives are common.
* Antinuclear antibody test uses indirect immunofluorescence to detect these antibodies.
* Rheumatoid factor test detects immunoglobulin directed against IgG.
  * Tests for rheumatoid factor are difficult to perform, and results can be variable.

EVALUATING THE HEMOSTATIC SYSTEM

Sample Collection

The minimum laboratory database needed to evaluate hemostasis in horses includes a platelet count and measurement of plasma fibrinogen, prothrombin time (PT), activated partial thromboplastin time (aPTT), and serum fibrin/fibrinogen degradation products (FDPs).

Proper collection and preparation of blood samples is paramount to obtaining accurate results.

* Blood must be collected by careful, accurate venipuncture to prevent contamination by tissue fluids that activate coagulation.
* Vacutainers containing trisodium citrate (1 part to 9 parts blood) are recommended for most tests (except FDPs).
  * Discarding the first tube of blood ensures that the sample does not contain tissue fluids.
  * Evacuated tubes should be allowed to fill until the vacuum has been expended because the ratio of anticoagulant to blood is critical in coagulation studies.
* For measurement of serum FDPs, blood must be collected into tubes containing thrombin and aminocaproic acid.
* Samples should be placed on ice and delivered to the laboratory within 1 hour of collection.
  * If the sample must be stored, plasma should be collected immediately by centrifugation, harvested with a plastic pipette, frozen, and assayed within a few days.
  * Blood for platelet counts cannot be stored and should be assayed within 2 hours of collection.

Reference Ranges

If the laboratory does not have normal reference values for horses, plasma from at least 2 healthy horses, preferably of similar age and sex, should be assayed for comparison. Following is a general guideline for normal hemostatic indices in adult horses:

* platelet count: 100,000 to 400,000/μL
* fibrinogen: 200 to 500 mg/dL
* PT: 9.5 to 13.5 seconds
* aPTT: 39 to 64 seconds
* FDPs: <10 μg/mL

Values for thrombin time, soluble fibrin monomer, factor V, factor VIII, antithrombin III, protein C, plasminogen, and α_2-antiplasmin are given in Table 19-3 of *Equine Medicine and Surgery V*.

Diseases Affecting Multiple Sites

(pages 2007-2020)
Debra D. Morris, Michelle H. Barton, Corrie Brown, and Debra C. Sellon

BONE MARROW APLASIA (APLASTIC ANEMIA)

Aplastic anemia represents failure of stem cells to undergo differentiation. The net result is marrow hypoplasia and peripheral pancytopenia of variable severity. Aplastic anemia is very uncommon; rare cases have been associated with phenylbutazone use. Myelophthisic anemia results when neoplastic or inflammatory tissue destroys the stem cell microenvironment. It has been described in horses with granulocytic leukemia and other myeloproliferative disorders.

Clinical signs
The onset of disease often is insidious, with vague complaints of poor performance, weight loss, and intermittent fever.

* Hemorrhagic diathesis (from thrombocytopenia) may be an early indicator.
  * Signs can include epistaxis, gingival bleeding, mucosal petechiae, hematomas, or prolonged hemorrhage after injections, trauma, or surgical procedures.
  * Thrombocytopenia also may cause mild edema.
* Pallor invariably is present, with tachycardia, a systolic heart murmur, and exercise intolerance, depending on the severity of anemia and rapidity with which it progresses.
* Neutropenia increases susceptibility to infection, especially bacterial invasion of the GI and respiratory tracts.

Laboratory findings
Hematologic evaluation reveals severe anemia, thrombocytopenia, and leukopenia (neutropenia and monocytopenia). The total lymphocyte count is variable, but lymphopenia is common. Occasionally the circulating lymphocytes are highly reactive, raising the question of neoplasia or a preleukemic syndrome. Plasma proteins may be low, normal, or reflect chronic antigenic stimulation. Blood chemistry values and clotting times are normal.

Diagnosis
Neutropenia without a left shift and thrombocytopenia are the earlier and most consistent manifestations of marrow aplasia, but diagnosis requires histologic examination of a bone marrow aspirate from the rib or ilial wing. The key feature is fatty marrow with essentially empty stroma. Nucleated red cells usually are the most numerous cell type.

Treatment
Treatment involves removal of suspected causative agents and supportive care until spontaneous remission occurs.

* The effectiveness of immunosuppressive (e.g., corticosteroids) or myelostimulatory drugs (e.g., androgens) is largely unproven in horses.
  * Most studies fail to show a benefit of high-dose corticosteroid therapy, and the increased risk of opportunistic infections makes their use potentially dangerous in these cases.
* Broad-spectrum antimicrobial therapy should be initiated after appropriate samples (e.g., blood cultures) have been taken for culture and sensitivity testing.
* Blood transfusions rarely are necessary and should be reserved for cases with life-threatening anemia (PCV <10%).

NEOPLASIA

Lymphosarcoma
* Lymphosarcoma is the most common type of neoplasia that affects the equine hemolymphatic system. Four anatomic forms (mediastinal, alimentary, cutaneous, multicentric) are reported, although there is considerable overlap. Lymphosarcoma occurs at any age, but it is most common in young adult horses.

Clinical signs

Clinical manifestations of lymphosarcoma are highly variable.

- Most affected horses have chronic weight loss, lethargy, anorexia, and subcutaneous edema, often with a history of fever.
- Peripheral lymphadenopathy of one or several nodes is common but is absent in a significant number of cases.
- Other presenting signs represent specific organ system involvement (e.g., colic, diarrhea, dyspnea, cough, dysphagia, chemosis, ataxia, jugular distention, lameness).
  - Signs usually are progressive over several weeks, but occasionally the onset is sudden.

Laboratory findings

Laboratory findings are variable, depending on the location and extent of tumor involvement.

- Many horses have indications of chronic inflammatory disease, such as neutrophilic leukocytosis, hyperglobulinemia, hyperfibrinogenemia, and nonresponsive anemia.
  - Lymphocytic leukocytosis is unusual, though reactive or abnormal lymphocytes in the peripheral blood are found in 30% to 50% of cases.
- Total plasma protein may be low, high, or normal. Frequently there is a reduction in the albumin:globulin ratio, particularly when there is GI involvement.

Other findings can include monoclonal gammopathy (causing hyperviscosity and hemorrhagic diathesis), immune-mediated hemolytic anemia (with clinical icterus), immune-mediated thrombocytopenia, and hypercalcemia (from pseudohyperparathyroidism).

Diagnosis

Diagnosis is made by finding neoplastic lymphocytes in affected tissues. Lymph nodes are most commonly involved, followed by the liver, spleen, kidney, and GI tract. Without enlarged lymph nodes or other masses that are accessible for biopsy, antemortem diagnosis can be difficult. Neoplastic cells occasionally are observed in blood, bone marrow aspirates, or thoracic or peritoneal effusions. Thoracic radiography and abdominal ultrasonography may be useful to identify and characterize masses in these cavities.

Treatment

Transient improvement has followed use of cytotoxic agents, immunostimulants, antiviral medication, and corticosteroids, but the prognosis is grave. Most horses die or must be euthanized for humane reasons within 6 months of the onset of signs.

PLASMA CELL MYELOMA

Plasma cell myeloma (multiple myeloma) is exceedingly rare in horses.

- It is characterized by proliferation of neoplastic plasma cells in the bone marrow and sometimes in the spleen, liver, lymph nodes, and kidneys.
- In addition to anemia (PCV 16% to 31%), laboratory findings often include hypercalcemia, leukopenia, thrombocytopenia, azotemia, and hyperproteinemia (monoclonal gammopathy).
- Multiple myeloma is diagnosed by identifying at least two of the following abnormalities:
  - plasmacytosis (>20% plasma cells) in the bone marrow
  - some indication of invasiveness (e.g., plasma cell infiltration of soft tissue lesions, radiographic evidence of osteolysis)
  - monoclonal gammopathy
  - light-chain (Bence-Jones) proteinuria
- Survival times range from 1 month to 2 years.

MYELOPROLIFERATIVE DISORDERS

Myeloproliferative syndromes described in horses include granulocytic, myelomonocytic, and monocytic leukemias and eosinophilic myeloproliferative disorder.

- Signs result from severe destruction of normal marrow architecture and inadequate production of erythrocytes, platelets, and normal leukocytes.
- Depression, weight loss, edema, mucosal petechiation, and signs of anemia predominate.

- Fever, peripheral lymphadenopathy, hemorrhagic diathesis,
  and oral ulcers are found in
  some horses.
- Most affected horses are anemic
  and thrombocytopenic. The WBC
  count may be elevated, normal, or
  decreased, but abnormal leukocytes
  invariably are found in the peripheral blood.
- Bone marrow aspirates are domi-
  nated by abnormal leukocytes.
- There is no effective treatment.

TRYPANOSOMIASIS

There are three trypanosomal diseases that affect horses; all are exotic
to the United States. Dourine is
spread venereally and is characterized initially by skin lesions and later
by central nervous system (CNS) impairment. Surra is a chronic wasting
disease transmitted by biting flies.
Nagana is a chronic disease characterized by anemia and weakness and
is transmitted by tsetse flies. These
diseases are discussed further in
Equine Medicine and Surgery V.

EQUINE INFECTIOUS ANEMIA

EIA is a viral disease of horses and
other equidae. It is transmitted primarily via biting insects (especially
horseflies) and potentially via blood-
contaminated instruments and equipment. Transmission also may occur
transplacentally or via colostrum. The
virus causes persistent infection in
horses. Although clinical disease may
not be evident, infected horses remain infected—and infective—for the
remainder of their life.
Clinical findings
Classically, clinical signs of EIA are
described as acute, chronic, or inapparent. However, in reality, differentiating these stages of infection can be
difficult.
- Within 7 to 28 days after infection,
  horses become viremic and febrile;
  rectal temperature may vary from
  38.5° C to 40.5° C (101.3° F to
  104.9° F).
  - Horses usually are lethargic and
    anorexic or inappetent during
    this period.

- Most acutely infected horses are
  at least transiently thrombocytopenic, and some may become
  anemic.
- Many horses never show clinical
  signs that are recognized by
  owners.
- Most horses recover from the initial episode within 1 to 7 days.
  Some never exhibit any additional
  signs, but others experience recurrent episodes of viremia and fever.
- Some horses progress to exhibit
  classic signs of chronic EIA or
  "swamp fever," which include
  fever, weight loss, dependent
  edema, lethargy, and depression.
  - Petechial hemorrhages and epis-
    taxis may develop.
  - These horses are anemic, throm-
    bocytopenic, hypoalbuminemic,
    and hyperglobulinemic; occasion-
    ally, serum liver enzyme activities
    (GGT and SDH) are increased.
  - These horses usually die.

*The majority of seropositive horses show
no overt signs of disease,* although most
have subtle laboratory abnormalities
such as mild anemia, intermittent
mild thrombocytopenia, increased
number of circulating B lymphocytes,
slight decrease in serum albumin,
and/or increase in serum globulins.
Diagnosis
EIA should be considered in all horses
with recurrent fever, thrombocytopenia, anemia, venstral edema,
and/or weight loss. Heinz body formation, autoagglutination, and impaired
bone marrow responsiveness may be
found during febrile episodes. There
are two serologic tests for diagnosis of
EIA: the agar gel immunodiffusion
(AGID) or Coggins' test and a compet-
itive ELISA (C-ELISA). In questionable cases, Western immunoblot and
PCR have been used to confirm infection. In the United States, testing for
EIA is performed only at state-
approved diagnostic laboratories.
Control
Isolation of infected horses and avoidance of mechanical transmission of
blood are important precautions to prevent the spread of EIA. Specific control
measures vary with the state (see *Equine
Medicine and Surgery, V*). Most states require that all horses must have a nega-

tive EIA test within 6 to 12 months of entering that state. Many states also require a negative EIA test for any change of ownership. The fate of an EIA seropositive horse is determined by the laws of the state in which that horse resides. Most states offer options of lifelong quarantine, euthanasia, or donation to a research facility.

Diseases Affecting Erythrocytes

(pages 2020-2025)
Ellen L. Zeimer and John C. Bloom

DISEASES WITH PHYSICAL CAUSES
Osmolar Hemolysis
Administration of hyposmolar intravenous (IV) fluids (e.g., water without electrolytes) can result in hemolytic anemia with hemoglobinemia and hemoglobinuria. The syndrome frequently is fatal. Treatment may be attempted with blood transfusion and fluid therapy.

INFLAMMATORY, INFECTIOUS, AND IMMUNE DISEASES
Neonatal Isoerythrolysis
Neonatal isoerythrolysis develops when there are blood group incompatibilities between the mare and the foal, particularly when the foal has the Aa or Qa red cell antigens and the mare does not.

* The mare becomes sensitized to the foal's alloantigens, and alloantibodies are concentrated in colostrum.
* Affected foals may die within the first 24 hours of life or develop tachypnea, depression, icterus, and progressive anemia 24 to 96 hours after colostrum ingestion.
* Hemoglobinuria and bilirubinuria may be detected on urinalysis, though hemoglobinuria may be transient.
* Treatment includes supportive care and blood transfusion if anemia is severe (PCV <12%).
  * Cross-matching of blood before transfusion is recommended but

may be difficult because of circulating alloantibodies.
* Thoroughly washed erythrocytes from the mare may be used for transfusion.

Autoimmune Hemolytic Anemia
Autoimmune hemolytic anemia is uncommon in adult horses.

* It may be a primary idiopathic condition or secondary to infection, drug administration, or neoplasia.
* Diagnosis is by antiglobulin testing (Coombs' test).
  * Negative antiglobulin tests may occur when low amounts of Ig are present, so do not necessarily rule out autoimmune hemolytic anemia.
* The condition often is corticosteroid responsive.
  * Initial treatment with dexamethasone (0.1 to 0.2 mg/kg/day IV or intramuscularly [IM], divided q12h) or prednisolone (2 to 3 mg/kg/day IM, divided q12h) is recommended.
  * Once a clinical response is noted (e.g., elevation in PCV), the dosage is gradually reduced to the lowest possible maintenance dosage.
* Blood transfusion may be required with severe anemia (PCV <12%) but should be avoided, since severe transfusion reactions, DIC, and renal failure may result.
* Underlying disease states should be treated and any preexisting drug therapy discontinued.

Transfusion Reactions
Massive or low-grade hemolysis may occur after transfusion, depending on the hemolytic potency of the immunoglobulin. Delayed hemolytic reactions may occur with low or undetectable immunoglobulin concentrations, resulting in partial or complete elimination of donor red cells within several days after transfusion. Cross-matching before transfusion is discussed in Chapter 4, Principles of Therapy.

Clostridiosis
Autoimmune hemolytic anemia has been reported as a complication of *Clostridium perfringens* infection.

Piroplasmosis (Babesiosis)

Piroplasmosis is caused by the protozoal parasites *Babesia caballi* and *Babesia equi*.

* It occurs worldwide, primarily in tropical and subtropical areas.
  * Equine piroplasmosis is enzootic in southern Florida, Puerto Rico, the Caribbean and U.S. Virgin Islands, Mexico, and Central and South America.
* Tick-borne transmission is of primary importance.
* Horses in enzootic areas may be inapparent carriers but can develop signs after stress.
* Signs include depression, anorexia, fever, pale or icteric mucous membranes, petechial or ecchymotic hemorrhages, edema, hemoglobinemia, hemoglobinuria, and death.
* During febrile episodes the parasite may be seen within erythrocytes (see p. 496).
* Serologic tests are available for diagnosis, the most reliable of which is complement fixation.

Treatment

Treatment recommendations vary with the circumstances and *Babesia* spp.

* If reexposure is possible, one dose of imidocarb dipropionate (2.2 mg/kg IM) may be given to suppress parasitemia and induce clinical remission.
* If the patient is to be maintained in a nonenzootic area, imidocarb should be given at 2 mg/kg/day IM for 2 days to eliminate *B. caballi* infections.
* *B. equi* is more resistant, and recommended therapy consists of imidocarb at 4 mg/kg IM every 72 hours for 4 treatments.
  * It may not be possible to completely clear the *B. equi* carrier state.

TOXIC DISEASES

Red Maple Leaf Toxicity

Red maple leaf toxicity has a seasonal occurrence, with most cases occurring in summer or early fall after ingestion of wilted leaves from the red maple tree *Acer rubrum*.

Sustained oxidative damage to erythrocytes results in Heinz-body formation and hemolytic anemia; methemoglobinemia also may occur.

Signs include anorexia, depression, fever, pale icteric and/or brown mucous membranes, and pigmenturia (methemoglobinuria and/or hemoglobinuria).

Treatment is largely supportive.

* Ascorbic acid (vitamin C) at 30 to 50 mg/kg IV q12h, added to IV fluids, may improve survival rates.
* Blood transfusion may be required because the anemia often is severe and progressive.
* Fluid and electrolyte therapy is indicated to prevent hemoglobin nephrosis.

Onion Poisoning

Ingestion of wild or cultivated onions (*Allium* spp.) can cause Heinz-body anemia. Signs include weakness, icterus, and hemoglobinuria. A marked onion odor may be apparent on the breath of affected horses. Mortality is high. Treatment involves removing horses from onion-contaminated pastures and providing stall rest with a balanced ration. Blood transfusion may be required with severe anemia.

Phenothiazine Toxicity

Phenothiazine-containing anthelmintics can cause hemolytic anemia, especially in debilitated horses on a poor plane of nutrition and in horses with renal or GI disease. Signs usually develop 24 to 72 hours after phenothiazine administration and include anorexia, depression, pale or icteric mucous membranes, colic, and hemoglobinuria. Treatment is supportive, including fluid and electrolyte therapy and, with severe anemia, blood transfusion.

MULTIFACTORIAL DISEASES

Iron-Deficiency Anemia

Iron-deficiency anemia is uncommon in horses.

* When present, it is virtually diagnostic of chronic hemorrhage.
* Iron deficiency is particularly common with gastric squamous cell carcinoma.

- Decreased marrow iron stores and serum iron concentration and increased total iron-binding capacity generally precede anemia and may be used to document the disorder.
  - Microcytic and hypochromic red cell changes usually are inapparent in horses.
- Oral administration of iron-containing supplements is recommended for treatment.
  - Fatal anaphylactic reactions have been reported with use of parenteral preparations.

Diseases Affecting Leukocytes *(pages 2025-2034)*
Kenneth S. Latimer

INFLAMMATORY, INFECTIOUS, AND IMMUNE DISEASES
Ehrlichiosis
Ehrlichia equi infections are most frequently documented in northern California but also have been reported in Florida, Colorado, Illinois, and New Jersey.

- Mortality is low and signs vary according to the age of the horse. Horses >3 years old are most severely affected.
- Signs may include fever, anorexia, depression, limb edema, ataxia, and mucosal petechiation.
- Hematologic findings frequently include leukopenia, thrombocytopenia, mild anemia, and cytoplasmic inclusions (morulae; see p. 498) within granulocytes. Diagnosis generally is based on the presence of *E. equi* morulae within granulocytes; serologic titers may be determined by indirect fluorescent antibody testing.
- Treatment comprises oxytetracycline at 7 mg/kg IV q24h or 20 mg/kg by mouth (PO) q12h for 7 days.

NEOPLASIA
Leukemia
Leukemia is neoplastic proliferation of hematopoietic cells.

- Acute leukemia implies a relatively short clinical presentation, variable numbers of immature (poorly differentiated or undifferentiated) cells in the blood and bone marrow, and short life expectancy.
- Chronic leukemia suggests a prolonged clinical course, an increased number of relatively mature (well-differentiated) cells on blood and bone marrow smears, and a longer life expectancy.
  - However, chronic leukemia may terminate acutely in a "blast crisis," characterized by many immature cells in the blood and bone marrow.
- Myeloproliferative disorders include neoplastic proliferation of granulocytes, monocytes, erythrocytes, megakaryocytes, and mast cells.
  - These disorders are exceedingly rare in horses.
  - Myelomonocytic leukemia (proliferation of the stem cells that generate neutrophils and monocytes) is the most common type of myeloproliferative disorder in horses.
- Lymphoproliferative disorders are limited to neoplastic proliferation of lymphocytes and plasma cells.
  - Confirmed cases of lymphocytic leukemia are rare; most cases with a leukemic blood picture are associated with lymphosarcoma.

Clinical findings
Clinical signs of leukemia in horses are variable and vague.

- Signs include depression, inappetence, weight loss, weakness, ventral edema, respiratory distress, fever, peripheral lymphadenopathy, colic, pallor of mucous membranes, and evidence of bleeding.
  - Signs in some horses may be related to specific tissue or organ dysfunction secondary to neoplastic infiltration.
- Horses with myelomonocytic leukemia usually are young (2 to 5 years of age).
- Laboratory abnormalities may include anemia (PCV 9% to 30%), thrombocytopenia (<5000 to 78,000/µL), and a variable leukocyte count (1900 to 184,000/µL).
  - Blast cells may be prominent on blood and bone marrow smears.

• The suggestion of leukemia on CBC may be confirmed by bone marrow biopsy.

Treatment and prognosis

Leukemia warrants a poor prognosis because chemotherapy is prohibitively expensive and too few cases are recorded to suggest an effective chemotherapy protocol.

Diseases of the Immune System *(pages 2034-2040)*

Lance E. Perryman

CONGENITAL AND FAMILIAL DISEASES

Combined Immunodeficiency

Combined immunodeficiency (CID) is an autosomal recessive condition primarily found in Arabian foals. As a result of the absence of T and B lymphocytes, these foals are unable to generate antigen-specific immune responses. However, affected foals have an intact complement system and produce normal numbers of neutrophils and macrophages with phagocytic activity.

Clinical findings

Foals with CID appear normal at birth, grow well, and remain free of infections for 3 to 8 weeks if passive transfer of maternal immunoglobulin is adequate.

• However, waning of maternal antibodies leaves the foal susceptible to various infections.

• Initially these foals respond well to antimicrobial therapy, but inevitably they succumb to infections for which effective antimicrobials are not available.

  • Major problems are caused by equine adenovirus, *Pneumocystis carinii*, and other opportunists, including *Cryptosporidium* spp.

• Signs most often are referable to the respiratory system, although a few foals show primary signs of enteritis or hepatitis.

• Without immune system reconstitution, the foal invariably dies, usually before 5 months of age.

• Necropsy findings include lymphoid hypoplasia in lymph nodes, spleen, and thymus, and lesions referable to secondary infection in various organ systems.

  • Lymph nodes are small unless they are edematous.

  • The spleen is small and lacks grossly evident splenic corpuscles.

  • The thymic remnant merely consists of a thin band of adipose tissue.

Diagnosis

Three criteria are required to establish a definitive diagnosis of CID:

• absence of IgM

  • Demonstration of IgM in a presuckling serum sample excludes a diagnosis of CID.

  • Maternal (colostral) IgM usually is undetectable by 18 days of age but may persist for 30 days, so suspect foals with detectable IgM should be retested if younger than 30 days.

• lymphopenia (<1000/µL)

  • Normal newborn foals often are lymphopenic, but the lymphocyte count should increase to >1000/µL by 24 to 48 hours of age.

  • Foals with CID have persistent lymphopenia.

• lymphoid hypoplasia, confirmed histologically after necropsy

  • Formalin-fixed spleen is the preferred sample.

  • The thymic remnant also should be submitted (in formalin). It is useful but not essential to submit lymph nodes.

No single criterion is adequate to establish the diagnosis. Fulfillment of any two criteria allows the foal to be identified as a CID suspect, but *all three criteria must be satisfied for the diagnosis to be definitive.*

Clinical management

Affected foals invariably die unless their immune system is reconstituted by transplant of histocompatible lymphoid stem cells (see *Equine Medicine and Surgery, V*). It is now possible to test Arabian horses to determine which are clear of, or heterozygous for, the CID trait. Testing is commercially available.

Agammaglobulinemia

This uncommon immunodeficiency disorder has been diagnosed in a few

Quarter Horse, Standardbred, and Thoroughbred males.

- Affected horses lack mature B lymphocytes and cannot synthesize immunoglobulins, although they produce normal numbers of functional T lymphocytes.
- Clinical signs are observed as early as 2 months of age.
  - Pneumonia, arthritis, and enteritis are typical findings; dermatitis and laminitis are seen in some cases.
- A tentative diagnosis is suggested in male horses with normal lymphocyte counts, absence of serum IgM and IgA, low and declining serum concentrations of IgG and IgG(T), and normal T lymphocyte responses to phytolectin stimulation (see *Equine Medicine and Surgery, V*).
- Clinical management consists of IV administration of suitably matched plasma and symptomatic treatment with appropriate antibiotics.

Selective IgM Deficiency

This disorder affects both males and females, usually of Arabian and Quarter Horse breeds. It is characterized by serum IgM concentrations >2 standard deviations *below* mean levels of age-matched control horses. All other immune system values are within normal limits.

Three clinical manifestations have been observed:

- horses >2 years of age at the time of initial diagnosis, with no history of recurrent infections as foals or yearlings but development of respiratory signs as adults
  - About 50% of these horses have or eventually develop lymphosarcoma.
- foals with a history of infections that usually respond to antimicrobial therapy but recur when treatment is stopped
  - Growth is inhibited and athletic potential is decreased.
  - These foals survive for 1 to 2 years before death from infections or euthanasia.
- young foals with severe pneumonia, enteritis, or arthritis, resulting in death before 1 year of age (the most common syndrome)

Diagnosis requires quantitation of serum immunoglobulin classes (see *Equine Medicine and Surgery, V*). Management is long-term, frustrating, and usually unrewarding.

Diseases Affecting Plasma Proteins

(pages 2040-2045)
Susan Clark Eades

DIAGNOSTIC AND THERAPEUTIC CONSIDERATIONS

Hypoproteinemia

Causes of hypoproteinemia involve decreased production or increased loss of plasma proteins.

- Decreased production occurs with immunodeficiency states and liver disease, although hypoproteinemia is not common in horses with even severe liver disease.
- Loss of plasma proteins usually is due to blood loss, acute severe peritonitis, GI disease, or renal disease.

Signs of severe hypoproteinemia may include dependent edema, diarrhea, and dyspnea (pulmonary edema, identified by hearing crackles on auscultation). When total protein concentration decreases below 4 g/dL, it may be necessary to administer plasma from a compatible donor (see Chapter 4, Principles of Therapy).

Hyperproteinemia

Hyperproteinemia generally is caused by either dehydration or increased globulin production.

- Chronic inflammation resulting from bacterial or chronic viral infections, parasitism, neoplasia, or immune-mediated disorders increases production of all globulin fractions.
  - *Polyclonal* gammopathy is more common with chronic infections.
  - Increased globulin concentrations during chronic disease may decrease albumin synthesis, causing hypoalbuminemia.
- Any inflammatory disease can increase production of complement, fibrinogen, and immunoglobulins that migrate in the β-globulin region, so the β-globulinemia seen with intestinal parasitism is a nonspecific finding.

◆ *Monoclonal* gammopathy may occur in horses with plasma cell myeloma or lymphosarcoma.

MULTIFACTORIAL DISEASES
Protein-Losing Enteropathy

Protein-losing enteropathy is most commonly associated with granulomatous enteritis, GI neoplasia (lymphosarcoma, squamous cell carcinoma), intestinal parasitism (especially cyathostomes), eosinophilic gastroenteritis, and nonsteroidal antiinflammatory drug (NSAID) toxicity. Other causes include acute enterocolitis and congestive heart failure. Hypoalbuminemia with decreased, increased, or normal plasma globulin concentrations characterizes the plasma protein changes. Diagnosis and management are discussed in Chapter 10, Alimentary System.

Diseases Affecting the Hemostatic System

(pages 2045-2056)

Ian B. Johnstone, Debra D. Morris, and Michelle H. Barton

CONGENITAL AND FAMILIAL DISEASES
Hemophilia A

Hemophilia A is a rare inherited blood disorder that has been reported in Thoroughbreds, Standardbreds, and a Quarter Horse–crossed foal.

◆ The basic defect is an abnormality in factor VIII, which affects blood clotting through the intrinsic coagulation pathway.
◆ The PTT is prolonged, usually to at least twice the control time; frequently, the activated clotting time also is prolonged.
  • Platelet counts, PT, and thrombin clotting time usually are normal.
◆ Definitive diagnosis requires measurement of factor VIII activity (see *Equine Medicine and Surgery, V*).
◆ There is no effective long-term therapy, and the prognosis is grave; most affected horses die or are euthanized by 6 months of age.

• Bleeding episodes may be controlled in the short term by transfusions of fresh blood or fresh or fresh-frozen plasma.

Von Willebrand's Disease

Von Willebrand's disease is a rare inherited bleeding disorder resulting from a deficiency of von Willebrand factor (vWF).

◆ Deficiency impedes platelet adhesion at sites of vascular injury, thus delaying the formation of a primary hemostatic plug and prolonging the bleeding time.
◆ The disease in horses presents as a mild hemorrhagic diathesis, with increased surface bleeding after surgery or trauma, or recurrent epistaxis.
  • Unlike hemophilia A, von Willebrand's disease may not be recognized early in life, and both sexes are equally at risk.
◆ The skin/mucosal bleeding time generally is prolonged.
  • PTT may be prolonged if there also is a reduction in factor VIII.
◆ The platelet count, prothrombin time, and thrombin clotting time, usually are normal.
◆ Definitive diagnosis relies on assessments of vWF activity (see *Equine Medicine and Surgery V*).
◆ Management is targeted at minimizing injury and avoiding the use of drugs known to suppress equine platelet function (e.g., NSAIDs, sulfonamides).
  • Transfusions of fresh blood or fresh or fresh-frozen plasma may be of value in the control of bleeding episodes.
◆ Affected animals should not be used for breeding.

INFLAMMATORY, INFECTIOUS, AND IMMUNE DISEASES
Immune-Mediated Thrombocytopenia

Thrombocytopenia (platelet count $<90,000/\mu L$) results from one or a combination of three basic mechanisms: decreased or ineffective platelet production; sequestration, usually in the spleen; or shortened platelet survival time. Decreased platelet production may occur secondary to marrow replacement (myelophthisis), aplastic anemia, or congenital disorders.

Shortened platelet life span is the most common cause of thrombocytopenia in horses and usually occurs by immune-mediated mechanisms.

◆ Immune-mediated thrombocytopenia often is primary (idiopathic).

◆ Causes of secondary immune-mediated thrombocytopenia include the following:
  • bacterial infections
  • viral disease (e.g., EIA)
  • other systemic immunologic disorders (e.g., autoimmune hemolytic anemia, neonatal isoerythrolysis)
  • neoplasia (e.g., lymphosarcoma)
  • certain drugs (thiazides, digoxin, gold salts, aspirin, phenylbutazone, heparin, quinidine, rifampin, penicillin, sulfas, tetracycline, and erythromycin)

Clinical signs

Thrombocytopenia leads to hemorrhagic diathesis, which is characterized by multiple sites of small vessel bleeding.

◆ Petechial hemorrhages generally are found on the oral, nasal, and/or vaginal mucosae, as well as the nictitans and sclera.
  • Epistaxis, melena, hyphema, and/or microscopic hematuria also may occur.

◆ Prolonged bleeding from injections or wounds and the propensity to form hematomas after minor trauma are common, especially when the platelet count is <40,000/µL.
  • Spontaneous hemorrhage is unusual unless the platelet count is <10,000/µL.

◆ Horses with idiopathic immune-mediated thrombocytopenia usually are bright and afebrile and may not manifest overt signs of hemorrhage despite severe thrombocytopenia.

◆ Horses with thrombocytopenia secondary to sepsis or neoplasia are particularly susceptible to bleeding.

Laboratory findings

Abnormalities include severe thrombocytopenia (<40,000µL), prolonged bleeding time, and abnormal clot retraction.

◆ PT, aPTT, and plasma fibrinogen are normal.
  • Serum FDPs may be mildly increased (10 to 40 µg/mL).

◆ Feces and urine frequently are positive for occult blood.

◆ Anemia and mild hypoproteinemia occur if there has been significant ongoing blood loss.

◆ In most cases, megakaryocytic hyperplasia is evident on examination of bone marrow.

Diagnosis

Diagnosis is based on small vessel hemorrhagic diathesis and severe thrombocytopenia in a horse with normal coagulation times and no other evidence of DIC (see p. 501). Response to treatment supports the diagnosis.

Treatment and prognosis

Wherever possible, therapy should be directed against the underlying cause.

◆ Use of any implicated medication should be stopped immediately.
  • Drug-induced thrombocytopenia usually responds within 4 to 14 days of drug withdrawal.

◆ Persistent life-threatening hemorrhage or signs of CNS hemorrhage should be treated with a transfusion of fresh whole blood or platelet-rich plasma (see *Equine Medicine and Surgery, V*).

◆ Most horses improve when treated with corticosteroids.
  • Dexamethasone at 0.05 to 0.2 mg/kg IV or IM, given each morning, usually results in an elevated platelet count within 4 to 7 days; the full effect may not be seen for up to 3 weeks.
  • Once the platelet count is >100,000/µL, the dosage can be reduced by 0.01 mg/kg/day while closely monitoring the platelet count for relapse.
  • Treatment usually can be discontinued after 10 to 21 days, provided the platelet count has been normal for at least 5 days.

◆ Horses refractory to corticosteroids may be successfully treated with a single dose of vincristine at 0.01 to 0.025 mg/kg IV, added to ongoing corticosteroid therapy.

In most horses with immune-mediated thrombocytopenia the prognosis is good.

Vasculitis

Vasculitis is a general term that refers to blood vessel inflammation. Some infectious agents (e.g., equine arteritis virus), chemicals, and endotoxins may directly damage blood vessel walls. More commonly, infections or drugs cause vasculitis by immunologic mechanisms. Most vasculitic syndromes in horses have characteristics of hypersensitivity (allergic) vasculitis, distinguished by predominant involvement of small vessels in the skin.

Clinical signs

Clinical manifestations may include:

◆ demarcated signs of dermal and/or subcutaneous edema that often progress to skin infarction, necrosis, and exudation

◆ mucosal hyperemia, hemorrhages (petechial and ecchymotic), and/or ulceration

◆ numerous adverse sequelae, including localized infections (e.g., cellulitis, pneumonia), thrombophlebitis, and laminitis

Vasculitic syndromes with predominant cutaneous involvement include purpura hemorrhagica, equine viral arteritis, equine infectious anemia, and ehrlichiosis. These conditions are discussed in other sections or chapters.

Laboratory findings

Laboratory findings are determined by the underlying disease, length of illness, multiplicity of organ involvement, and secondary complications. Chronic inflammation is attended by neutrophilia, mild anemia, hyperglobulinemia, and hyperfibrinogenemia. The platelet count usually is normal.

Diagnosis

Definitive diagnosis relies on demonstration of characteristic histopathologic lesions. Full-thickness punch biopsies of the skin, preserved in 10% formalin, are the appropriate samples. One or more biopsies should be preserved in Michel's transport medium and submitted for immunofluorescence studies.

TOXIC DISEASES

Vitamin K Antagonist Toxicity

Warfarin and its congeners are odorless and tasteless chemicals commonly used as rodenticides.

◆ The major effect of these vitamin K antagonists is hemorrhagic diathesis.

◆ Signs range from epistaxis and subcutaneous hematomas (particularly over pressure points) to lameness and muscle soreness associated with joint or muscle bleeding.

  • Persistent bleeding from or swelling at injection sites is common.

  • Sudden death occasionally occurs as a result of massive internal bleeding.

◆ Diagnosis is based on a history of possible exposure and a laboratory profile consistent with multiple clotting factor deficiencies.

  • Prolongation of PT tends to occur first, followed by an increase in PTT.

  • Values for thrombin clotting time, fibrinogen, platelet numbers, and FDPs are normal.

◆ Treatment with vitamin K_1 at 0.5 mg/kg subcutaneously (SC) q6-8h is recommended.

  • PT and PTT should be checked daily.

  • The effects of warfarin may be reversible in 2 to3 days, but the effects of its congeners are much more persistent, requiring weeks of therapy.

  • *Vitamin K_3 must not be used because it is highly nephrotoxic in horses.*

◆ When severe anemia or life-threatening bleeding is evident, blood or plasma transfusions to replace red cells and/or clotting proteins may be necessary.

Sweet Clover Poisoning

Sweet clover poisoning is caused by ingestion of spoiled sweet clover hay or silage.

◆ Coumarin is a normal (and innocuous) constituent of sweet clover (*Melilotus* spp.), but it is converted to dicoumarol by fungi and/or molds in spoiled sweet clover hay.

◆ The action of dicoumarol is similar to that of warfarin, so signs of sweet clover poisoning are similar to those described above for vitamin K antagonist toxicity.

◆ Diagnosis is based on clotting abnormalities (prolonged PT and PTT but normal thrombin clotting time) and a history of exposure to sweet clover.

- A favorable response to vitamin K₁ therapy or detection of high dicoumarol levels in feed samples also is useful.
- Treatment consists of removing the likely source of dicoumarol and treating with vitamin K₁.
  - In cases of severe anemia and/or profuse bleeding, supportive therapy with fresh whole blood or plasma may be indicated.

MULTIFACTORIAL DISEASES
Disseminated Intravascular Coagulation

DIC is a syndrome characterized by widespread fibrin generation and deposition within the microcirculation and resultant ischemic tissue and organ damage. Paradoxically, a systemic hemorrhagic tendency caused by depletion of platelets and clotting factors and hyperactivity of the fibrinolytic mechanism usually dominates the clinical picture. DIC almost invariably is a complication of a primary pathologic process, such as:

- endotoxemia or septicemia
- intestinal accidents
- intravascular hemolysis (hemolytic anemia)
- immune-mediated or drug-induced thrombocytopenia
- retained dead fetus and/or placenta
- malignancy
- hepatitis or pancreatitis
- various infectious processes (e.g., equine viral arteritis, rickettsial diseases)

Clinical findings
Findings vary with the phase of DIC and subsequent complications.

- Initially, signs are indicative of widespread microcirculatory occlusion and ischemic injury.
  - This thrombotic phase may be reflected by an increased tendency for IV catheters to occlude, peripheral vascular thrombosis to occur, and laminitis to develop.
  - In addition, there may be evidence of renal impairment (increased blood creatinine and/or urea) or muscle damage (increased serum creatine kinase [CK] and aspartate aminotransferase [AST]).

- The most common clinical picture is spontaneous bleeding from multiple sites (in acute DIC) or an increased bleeding tendency (in the more chronic forms).
  - Bleeding ranges from superficial petechiation and ecchymosis to mucosal bleeding (epistaxis, melena, hematuria) to hematoma formation and hemarthrosis.
  - Often the first sign noticed is prolonged bleeding from venipuncture sites.
- Nonspecific signs, such as fever, hypotension, acidosis, hypoxia, or proteinuria, may be evident.
- In addition, signs of the primary disease or pathologic process usually are evident.

Laboratory findings
No single laboratory abnormality is diagnostic for DIC.

- In acute DIC, PT and PTT usually are prolonged, the platelet count is reduced, and serum FDPs are elevated.
  - The thrombin clotting time (TCT) usually is prolonged.
- In subacute and chronic forms, the PT, PTT, and TCT may be normal or even decreased.
- Plasma fibrinogen may be decreased in advanced cases, but earlier in the syndrome it usually is normal or even elevated.
- Thrombocytosis frequently is associated with malignancy, so a normal platelet count does not necessarily rule out DIC in these cases.

Diagnosis
DIC often is a clinical diagnosis based on bleeding in a specific clinical setting and supported by indirect evidence of intravascular thrombin generation. The most practical screening profile consists of a platelet count, and measurement of PT, PTT, FDPs, and, if available, TCT.

Treatment
Use of thrombin inhibitors, particularly heparin, has been advocated, although heparin use remains controversial.
The recommended dosage of heparin varies widely.

- One suggested schedule begins with an initial dose of 150 U/kg SC, followed by 125 U/kg q12h for 3 days, then a further reduction to 100 U/kg q12h.

- It is advisable to give plasma concurrently to ensure adequate levels of ATIII.

The inciting cause(s) must be removed, if possible, and adequate organ perfusion maintained. To these ends, antimicrobial drugs, IV fluid therapy, and surgical intervention may be beneficial.

Liver Disease

Though hemostatic abnormalities can be detected in many individuals with liver disease, the frequency of overt bleeding in animals with liver disease is relatively low. Detectable hemorrhage as a result of liver disease usually indicates severe hepatic insult. In such cases, other changes indicative of liver dysfunction would be anticipated. Liver disease is discussed in Chapter 10, Alimentary System.

Diseases of the Spleen

(pages 2058-2062)

Catherine J. Savage

INFLAMMATORY, INFECTIOUS, AND IMMUNE DISEASES

Splenic Abscessation

Abscesses in the spleen may result in weight loss, inappetence, fever, and abdominal pain.

- Leukocytosis with or without a left shift, monocytosis, hyperfibrinogenemia, and hyperglobulinemia are common.
- Abnormalities on abdominal fluid analysis often include increased protein and cell counts (>80% of which are neutrophils) and toxic changes with intracellular and even free bacteria.
- The peritoneal fluid should be cultured.
  - The three most common isolates are *Streptococcus equi* var. *equi*,

S. equi var. *zooepidemicus,* and *Corynebacterium pseudotuberculosis* (in the Western United States).

- It may be possible to palpate the abscess per rectum, although splenic ultrasonography (and ideally laparoscopy) may be necessary to reveal the mass.
- Therapy consists of long-term (e.g., 6 to 24 weeks) antimicrobial therapy.

MULTIFACTORIAL DISEASES

Splenic Rupture or Puncture

Hemoabdomen with or without fatal hemorrhage can result from splenic trauma.

- Abdominocentesis is a useful tool in cases of splenic rupture.
  - If the peritoneal fluid PCV is >10%, the bleeding is significant, if and the PCV is >20%, the bleeding may be fatal.
- Although bleeding may be successfully arrested in some horses with ruptured spleens, the source of bleeding often cannot be identified.
- The horse should be stabilized by IV administration of isotonic fluids or a blood transfusion from a cross-matched horse.
  - Another source of whole blood can be the injured horse's abdomen (autotransfusion).

Neoplasia

Splenic lymphosarcoma has been reported in horses. Melanomas and hemangiosarcomas involving the spleen also have been documented. Anemia may be present in horses with splenic neoplasia.

Splenomegaly

Splenomegaly may result from neoplasia, equine infectious anemia, salmonellosis, and anthrax. Rarely, primary splenomegaly may occur with splenic cirrhosis, cardiac failure, or active sequestration of erythrocytes.

Index

Tables are indicated by t.